ORTHOPAEDIC SURGERY ESSENTIALS

ADULT RECONSTRUCTION

ORTHOPAEDIC SURGERY ESSENTIALS

ORTHOPAEDIC SURGERY ESSENTIALS

Foot and Ankle
David B. Thordarson, MD
Paul Tornetta III, MD
Thomas A. Einhorn, MD

Hand and Wrist
James R. Doyle, MD
Paul Tornetta III, MD
Thomas A. Einhorn, MD

Oncology and Basic Science
Timothy A. Damron, MD
Carol D. Morris, MD

Sports Medicine
Anthony A. Schepsis, MD
Brian Busconi, MD
Paul Tornetta III, MD
Thomas A. Einhorn, MD

Pediatrics
Kathryn E. Cramer, MD
Susan A. Scherl, MD
Paul Tornetta III, MD
Thomas A. Einhorn, MD

Spine
Christopher M. Bono, MD
Steven R. Garfin, MD
Paul Tornetta III, MD
Thomas A. Einhorn, MD

Trauma
Charles Court-Brown, MD
Margaret M. McQueen, MD
Paul Tornetta III, MD
Thomas A. Einhorn, MD

ORTHOPAEDIC SURGERY ESSENTIALS

ADULT RECONSTRUCTION

Series Editors

PAUL TORNETTA III, MD
Professor and Vice Chairman
Department of Orthopaedic Surgery
Boston University School of Medicine;
Director of Orthopaedic Trauma
Boston University Medical Center
Boston, Massachusetts

THOMAS A. EINHORN, MD
Professor and Chairman
Department of Orthopaedic Surgery
Boston University School of Medicine
Boston, Massachusetts

Editors

DANIEL J. BERRY, MD
Professor and Chairman
Department of Orthopedic Surgery
Mayo Clinic
Rochester, Minnesota

SCOTT P. STEINMANN, MD
Associate Professor of Orthopedics
Department of Orthopaedics
Mayo Clinic College of Medicine;
Mayo Medical School
Rochester, Minnesota

Wolters Kluwer | Lippincott Williams & Wilkins
Health
Philadelphia • Baltimore • New York • London
Buenos Aires • Hong Kong • Sydney • Tokyo

Acquisitions Editor: Robert Hurley
Managing Editor: Michelle LaPlante
Senior Project Manager: Rosanne Hallowell
Senior Manufacturing Manager: Benjamin Rivera
Marketing Manager: Sharon Zinner
Creative Director: Doug Smock
Illustrator: Wendy Beth Jackelow, MFA, CMI
Production Services: Aptara, Inc.
Printer: Quebecor World-Bogotà

530 Walnut Street
Philadelphia, PA 19106
LWW.com

Printed in Colombia

Library of Congress Cataloging-in-Publication Data.

Adult reconstruction / editors, Daniel J. Berry, Scott P. Steinmann.
p. ; cm.—(Orthopaedic surgery essentials)
Includes bibliographical references and index.
ISBN-13: 978-0-7817-9638-5
ISBN-10: 0-7817-9638-5
1. Orthopedic surgery. I. Berry, Daniel J. II. Steinmann, S. (Scott) III. Series.
[DNLM: 1. Joint Diseases–surgery. 2. Arthroplasty—methods. 3. Reconstructive Surgical Procedures—methods. WE 312 A2435 2007]
RD731.A38 2007
617.4'7–dc22

2007013075

To purchase additional copies of this book, call our customer service department at (800) 639-3030 or fax orders to (301) 824-7390. International customers should call (301) 714-2324. Lippincott Williams & Wilkins customer service representatives are available from 8:30 am to 6:00 pm, EST, Monday through Friday, for telephone access. Visit Lippincott Williams & Wilkins on the Internet: http://www.lww.com.

10 9 8 7 6 5 4 3 2 1

To my students, residents, fellows, colleagues, and teachers, all of whom have enriched my life and taught me the science and art of orthopedic surgery.

—Daniel J. Berry

To my mother, Alice, for guiding me with wisdom, support, and love and my brother, Bruce, for being my best friend and providing understanding and constant support.

—Scott P. Steinmann

CONTENTS

SECTION III: SHOULDER RECONSTRUCTION

SECTION IV: ELBOW RECONSTRUCTION

CONTRIBUTORS

Julie E. Adams, MD
Resident in Orthopaedic Surgery
Mayo Clinic
Rochester, Minnesota

Arash Aminian, MD
Northwestern University
Chicago, Illinois

George S. Athwal, MD
Assistant Professor
University of Western Ontario
Hand and Upper Limb Centre
St. Joseph's Health Care
London, Ontario
Canada

Christopher P. Beauchamp, MD
Associate Professor
Mayo Clinic College of Medicine;
Chair
Department of Orthopaedics
Mayo Clinic
Scottsdale, Arizona

Paul E. Beaulé, MD
Associate Professor
Head, Adult Reconstruction Service
Division of Orthopaedic Surgery
University of Ottawa
Ottawa Hospital
Ottawa, Ontario
Canada

John-Erik Bell, MD
Center for Shoulder, Elbow and Sports Medicine
Columbia Presbyterian Medical Center
New York Orthopaedic Hospital
New York, New York

Keith R. Berend, MD
Clinical Assistant Professor
Department of Orthopaedics
The Ohio State University
Columbus, Ohio;
Orthopaedic Surgeon
New Albany Surgical Hospital
New Albany, Ohio

Daniel J. Berry, MD
Professor and Chairman
Department of Orthopedic Surgery
Mayo Clinic
Rochester, Minnesota

Hari P. Bezwada, MD
PENN Orthopaedics
Pennsylvania Hospital
Philadelphia, Pennsylvania

Theodore A. Blaine, MD
Center for Shoulder, Elbow, and Sports Medicine
Columbia Presbyterian Medical Center
New York Orthopaedic Hospital
New York, New York

Robert E. Booth, Jr., MD
PENN Orthopaedics
Pennsylvania Hospital
Philadelphia, Pennsylvania

Kevin J. Bozic, MD, MBA
Department of Orthopaedic Surgery
University of California, San Francisco
San Francisco, California

Patrick Chin, MD
Clinical Instructor
Division of Athletic Injuries/Arthroscopy and Upper Extremity Reconstruction
Department of Orthopaedics
British Columbia, Vancouver
Canada

Henry D. Clarke, MD
Mayo Clinic Scottsdale
Scottsdale, Arizona

John C. Clohisy, MD
Barnes-Jewish Hospital at Washington
University School of Medicine
Department of Orthopaedic Surgery
St. Louis, Missouri

Brian J. Cole, MD, MBA
Associate Professor
Departments of Orthopaedics and Anatomy and Cell Biology
Section Head, Cartilage Restoration Center at Rush
Rush University Medical Center
Chicago, Illinois

Gilbert Csuja, MD
National Naval Medical Center
Bethesda, Maryland

Don D'Alessandro, MD
Chief of Sports Medicine
OrthoCarolina
Charlotte, North Carolina

Diane L. Dahm, MD
Assistant Professor
Department of Orthopaedic Surgery
Mayo Clinic College of Medicine
Rochester, Minnesota

Craig J. Della Valle, MD
Assistant Professor
Department of Orthopaedic Surgery
Rush University Medical Center
Chicago, Illinois

Paul Di Cesare, MD
Professor of Orthopaedic Surgery and Cell Biology
Director, Musculoskeletal Research Center
Chief, Adult Reconstructive Service
NYU–Hospital for Joint Diseases
New York, New York

Scott Duncan, MD, MPH
Assistant Professor of Orthopaedic Surgery
Mayo Medical School;
Consultant, Mayo Clinic Scottsdale
Scottsdale, Arizona

Xavier Duralde, MD
Assistant Clinical Professor
Department of Orthopaedics
Emory University
Peachtree Orthopaedic Clinic
Atlanta, Georgia

Sara L. Edwards, MD
Center for Shoulder, Elbow, and Sports Medicine
Columbia Presbyterian Medical Center
New York Orthopaedic Hospital
New York, New York

Bassem Elhassan, MD
Fellow
Harvard Shoulder Fellowship
Boston, Massachusetts

Robert J. Esther, MD, MSc
Fellow in Orthopedic Oncology
Mayo Clinic
Rochester, Minnesota

Kenneth J. Faber, MD
Associate Professor of Surgery
Hand and Upper Limb Centre
University of Western Ontario
London, Ontario
Canada

Thomas Fehring, MD
Co-director
Ortho Carolina Hip and Knee Center
Charlotte, North Carolina

Larry D. Field, MD
Co-Director, Upper Extremity Service
Mississippi Sports Medicine and Orthopaedic Center
Clinical Instructor, Department of Orthopaedic Surgery
University of Mississippi School of Medicine
Jackson, Mississippi

Wolfgang Fitz, MD
Associate Orthopaedic Surgeon
Brigham and Women's and Falkner Hospitals
New England Baptist Hospital
Instructor of Orthopaedic Surgery
Harvard Medical School
Brigham and Women's Orthopaedic and Arthritis Center
Chestnut Hill, Massachusetts

Kyle R. Flik, MD
Sports Medicine
Northeast Orthopaedics, LLP
Albany, New York

David R. J. Gill, MD
Consultant Orthopaedic Surgeon
Royal Perth Hospital
Perth, Western Australia;
Clinical Lecturer
Faculty of Medicine and Dentistry
University of Western Australia
Perth, Western Australia

Dan Ginat, MD
Clinical Research Assistant
Musculoskeletal Research Center
NYU–Hospital for Joint Diseases
New York, New York

Michele T. Glasgow, MD
Orthopaedic Surgeon
Midwest Orthopaedic Institute
Sycamore, Illinois
Orthopaedic Surgeon
Department of Surgery
Kishwaukee Hospital
Dekalb, Illinois

Andreas H. Gomoll, MD
Fellow in Orthopaedic Sports Medicine
Department of Orthopaedic Surgery
Rush University Medical Center
Chicago, Illinois

Eric M. Gordon, MD
Center for Shoulder, Elbow, and Sports Medicine
Columbia University Medical Center
New York, New York

Andrew Green, MD
Department of Orthopaedic Surgery
Brown University School of Medicine
Providence, Rhode Island

Carlos A. Guanche, MD
Southern California Orthopedic Institute
Van Nuys, California

George Haidukewych, MD
Florida Orthopedic Institute
Tampa, Florida

Michael Hartman, MD
Orthopedic Resident
Mayo Clinic
Rochester, Minnesota

Jason R. Hull, MD
Assistant Professor of Orthopaedic Surgery
Virginia Commonwealth University School of Medicine;
Medical College of Virginia Hospitals/Virginia Commonwealth University Health System
Richmond, Virginia

David Jacofsky, MD
Chairman
The CORE Institute
The Center for Orthopedic Research and Education
Sun City West, Arizona

Srinath Kamineni, MD
Professor of Bioengineering
Brunel University;
Consultant Surgeon
Cromwell Upper Limb Unit;
Consultant Surgeon
London, United Kingdom
Clementine Churchill Hospital
Middlesex, United Kingdom

Edward W. Kelly, MD
Minnesota Orthopaedic Specialists
Minneapolis, Minnesota

Kang-Il Kim, MD, PhD
Rothman Institute of Orthopedics
Thomas Jefferson University
Philadelphia, Pennsylvania

Hervey L. Kimball, MD
New England Baptist Hospital
Department of Orthopaedics and Hand Surgery
Boston, Massachusetts

Jeffrey C. King, MD
Clinical Assistant Professor
College of Human Medicine
Michigan State University;
Healthcare Midwest
Division of Hand and Elbow Surgery
Kalamazoo, Michigan

Jason Koh, MD
Associate Professor
Northwestern University
Chicago, Illinois

Michael A. Kuhn, MD
New England Baptist Hospital
Department of Orthopaedics and Sports Medicine
Boston, Massachusetts

Mauricio Largacha, MD
Shoulder and Elbow Surgery
Clinica del Country Bogota
Colombia

Cyrus Lashgari, MD
Orthopaedics and Sports Medicine Center
Anne Arundel Medical Center
Annapolis, Maryland

Mark Lazarus, MD
Thomas Jefferson University Medical College
Philadelphia, Pennsylvania

William N. Levine, MD
Vice Chairman, Education
Associate Professor, Orthopaedic Surgery
Columbia University
New York, New York

Jay R. Lieberman, MD
Chair
Department of Orthopedic Surgery
University of CT, Hartford, CT
Los Angeles, California

Jess H. Lonner, MD
Director of Knee Replacement Surgery
Booth Bartolozzi Balderston Orthopaedics;
Pennsylvania Hospital
Philadelphia, Pennsylvania

Steven J. MacDonald, MD
London Health Sciences Centre
University Hospital
London, Ontario
Canada

Pierre Mansat, MD, PhD
Associate Professor
Department of Orthopaedic Surgery
University Hospital of Toulouse-Purpan
Toulouse, France

Guido Marra, MD
Chief of Shoulder Elbow Surgery
Loyola Medical Center
Maywood, Illinois

J. Bohannon Mason, MD
OrthoCarolina Hip and Knee Center
Charlotte, North Carolina

Simon C. Mears, MD, PhD
Assistant Professor
Department of Orthopaedic Surgery
Johns Hopkins Bayview Medical Center
Baltimore, Maryland

Vip Nanavati, MD
Assistant Professor
Department of Orthopaedic Surgery
SUNY Upstate Medical University
Syracuse, New York

Douglas D. R. Naudie, MD
Assistant Professor
Division of Orthopaedic Surgery
University of Western Ontario;
London Health Sciences Center
University Campus
London, Ontario
Canada

Gregory P. Nicholson, MD
Assistant Professor
Department of Orthopaedic Surgery
Rush University Medical Center
Chicago, Illinois

Andrew R. Noble, MD
Fellow of Adult Reconstruction
Department of Orthopaedic Surgery
Brigham and Women's Hospital
Boston, Massachusetts

Mark W. Pagnano, MD
Associate Professor of Orthopedic Surgery
Mayo College of Medicine
Mayo Clinic
Rochester, Minnesota

Rick F. Papandrea, MD
Orthopaedic Associates of Wisconsin
Clinical Instructor of Orthopaedic Surgery
Medical College of Wisconsin
Waukesha, Wisconsin

Javad Parvizi, MD
Rothman Institute of Orthopedics
Jefferson University
Philadelphia, Pennsylvania

Frank A. Petrigliano, MD
Department of Orthopaedic Surgery
David Geffen School of Medicine
University of California Los Angeles
Los Angeles, California

Roger G. Pollock, MD
Assistant Professor of Clinical Orthopaedic Surgery
Columbia University Medical Center
New York, New York

Vaishnav Rajgopal, MD
Senior Resident
Division of Orthopaedic Surgery
University of Western Ontario
London Health Sciences Center
London, Ontario
Canada

J. Randall Ramsey, MD
Upper Extremity Service
Mississippi Sports Medicine and Orthopaedic Center
Jackson, Mississippi

Kevin J. Renfree, MD
Consultant, Department of Orthopaedic Surgery
Assistant Professor
Mayo Medical School
Mayo Clinic
Scottsdale, Arizona

Robert S. Rice, MD
Resident in Orthopedic Surgery
Mayo College of Medicine
Mayo Clinic
Rochester, Minnesota

Glen Ross, MD
New England Baptist Hospital
Department of Orthopaedics and Sports Medicine
Boston, Massachusetts

Joaquin Sanchez-Sotelo, MD, PhD
Adult Reconstruction
Department of Orthopedic Surgery
Mayo Clinic Rochester;
Assistant Professor
Mayo Graduate Medical School
Rochester, Minnesota

Sathappan S. Sathappan, MD
Adult Reconstruction Fellow
NYU–Hospital for Joint Diseases Department of Orthopaedic Surgery
New York, New York

Felix H. Savoie, III, MD
Co-Director, Upper Extremity Service
Mississippi Sports Medicine and Orthopaedic Center
Clinical Associate Professor, Department of Orthopaedic Surgery
University of Mississippi School of Medicine
Jackson, Mississippi

Perry L. Schoenecker, MD
Department of Orthopaedic Surgery
Barnes-Jewish Hospital at Washington University School of Medicine;
St. Louis Shriner's Hospital for Children
St. Louis Children's Hospital
St. Louis, Missouri

Jonathan B. Shook, MD
Loyola University Medical Center
Department of Orthopaedic Surgery and Rehabilitation
Maywood, Illinois

M. Wade Shrader, MD
Chief
Deer Valley Campus
The CORE Institute
The Center for Orthopaedic Research and Education
Sun City West, Arizona

Michael Skutek, MD
Hannover Medical School
Hannover, Germany

Adam M. Smith, MD
Kentucky Sports Medicine Clinic
Lexington, Kentucky

Mark J. Spangehl, MD
Assistant Professor of Orthopaedics
Department of Orthopaedics
Mayo Clinic College of Medicine
Mayo Clinic Scottsdale, Mayo Foundation
Scottsdale, Arizona

John W. Sperling, MD
Associate Professor of Orthopaedic Surgery
Department of Orthopedic Surgery
Mayo Clinic
Rochester, Minnesota

Andrew I. Spitzer, MD
Associate Director
Joint Replacement Institute at Cedars Sinai Medical Center
Kerlan-Jobe Orthopaedic Clinic
Los Angeles, California

Bryan D. Springer, MD
Charlotte Hip and Knee Center
OrthoCarolina
Charlotte, North Carolina

Scott P. Steinmann, MD
Associate Professor of Orthopaedics
Department of Orthopaedics
Mayo Clinic College of Medicine
Mayo Medical School
Rochester, Minnesota

Justin Strickland, MD
Department of Orthopaedic Surgery
Mayo Clinic
Rochester, Minnesota

Robert T. Trousdale, MD
Consultant
Department of Orthopaedic Surgery
Mayo Clinic
Professor
Department of Orthopaedic Surgery
Mayo Clinic College of Medicine
Rochester, Minnesota

Melissa A. Yadao, MD
Sports Medicine Fellow
Mississippi Sports Medicine and Orthopaedic Center
Jackson, Mississippi

Jeffrey S. Zarin, MD
Fellow in Adult Reconstruction
Department of Orthopaedic Surgery
Brigham and Women's Hospital
Harvard Medical School
Boston, Massachusetts

PREFACE

Adult reconstructive surgery of the hip, knee, shoulder, and elbow encompasses much of the core of orthopedic practice. The field is large and the pace of change has been rapid. The goal of *Adult Reconstruction* is to provide the practicing orthopedic surgeon, fellow, or resident with a concise volume that provides a framework for understanding how to evaluate, diagnose, and treat common problems encountered in these four joints. The chapters explain not only which treatments are preferred but also summarize the latest information about controversies in management and treatment.

Chapter topics have been chosen to cover subjects that are most pertinent and germane to orthopedic surgeons in training and in practice. Each chapter is written to provide the reader with a solid understanding of both fundamentals and a consensus perspective on the latest topics of interest. Chapter authors have been selected for their known expertise in the subject field. The book is not intended to be a comprehensive text that covers every aspect of every subject; more comprehensive but less concise references are available for that purpose. Those who read the book from cover to cover should come away with a foundation of essential knowledge of these subjects and an appreciation of the current areas of controversy. For those who use the text on an as-needed basis to refresh memory or provide deeper understanding of a topic, the information is presented in a concise and organized manner to facilitate this form of learning.

We hope this book becomes a well-worn companion for those learning the practice of orthopedic surgery and those practicing the art and science of orthopedic surgery.

Daniel J. Berry, MD
Scott P. Steinmann, MD

ACKNOWLEDGMENTS

We would like to thank and acknowledge Acquisitions Editor, Mr. Robert Hurley, and Senior Project Editor, Ms. Michelle LaPlante, both of Lippincott Williams & Wilkins, for the vision to create this book and for the great effort put into making this book well-organized, well-illustrated, and user-friendly. We are indebted to the many contributors who spent a tremendous amount of their valuable time—and provided their great expertise—writing each chapter. The excellent authors are the foundation of this book. We also would like to thank our assistants, Ms. Norma Mundt, Ms. Julie Schuster, and Ms. Karen Fasbender, for their many efforts during the process of creating this book.

ORTHOPAEDIC SURGERY ESSENTIALS

ADULT RECONSTRUCTION

PHYSICAL EVALUATION OF THE HIP

BRYAN D. SPRINGER

A wide array of tests and diagnostic tools are available to the surgeon to aid in the diagnosis of hip disease. Thorough history and physical examination, however, remain the most important tools that a physician possesses when evaluating a painful hip joint. Diagnostic tests and procedures should be used *in addition to and not as a substitute for* a careful history and complete physical examination.

HISTORY

Obtaining a thorough and complete history from the patient with suspected hip disease is the first and one of the most critical steps in being able to properly diagnose pathology. This can often lead to a preliminary diagnosis and will allow for a more directed physical examination. A patient with hip pathology most frequently complains of pain. True hip pathology usually presents with pain located in the groin, anterior thigh, deep buttock, and occasionally knee. Every patient who presents with knee pain or medial thigh pain should have a thorough hip evaluation to rule out hip pathology as a source of referred pain to the knee. Important questions regarding the characteristics of pain include location, severity, frequency, and radicular features. It is also important to note circumstances that aggravate or relieve the pain. Arthritic pain generally is aggravated by activity and relieved by rest. Pain that occurs at night or during rest is less common in degenerative arthritis and may indicate the presence of an inflammatory process or infection. Referred pain from the lumbosacral region is common. This type of pain is often located in the gluteal or posterior iliac crest region and may present with radicular signs and symptoms. Several other conditions may refer pain to the hip (Table 1-1). Nonarthritic hip conditions should also be evaluated (Table 1-2).

Other important details that should be obtained include the following:

- Previous history of hip pathology (Perthes disease, slipped capital epiphysis, hip dysplasia, sepsis) including surgery or other treatment
- History of trauma
- Medication history including use of pain medications (e.g., narcotics) or corticosteroids.
- Limitations of activities of daily living (walking, going up and down stairs, sitting)
- Limitation of functional activities (getting into or out of car, getting shoes and socks on, foot hygiene)
- Limitation of occupational and recreational activities

PHYSICAL EXAMINATION

The evaluation should begin immediately with the first encounter. Noting how the patient rises from a chair, walks to the exam room, and assumes certain postures can provide valuable information in a non-exam-specific setting. Every patient should be disrobed and appropriately gowned to allow for a thorough inspection of the hip and surrounding areas.

Evaluation of Gait

The phases of the gait cycle include the *stance phase* (60%): heel strike, midstance, toe-off; and the *swing phase* (40%): initial, midswing, and terminal swing. Several types of abnormal gait patterns can be indicative of hip pathology and are listed in Table 1-3. Patients who experience pain with weight bearing on the affected limb (antalgic or avoidance gait) will try to minimize the time on this limb during the stance phase of gait, resulting in a limp. Abductor muscle weakness will result in the pelvis tilting away from the affected limb when that limb is in the stance phase of gait (Fig. 1-1). To compensate, patients may lean over their affected hip to shift the center of gravity, resulting in a so-called Duchenne gait. Patients with a true leg length discrepancy may circumduct the long leg during the swing phase of gait to allow for the limb to clear the floor.

Leg Length Determination

Leg lengths should be measured in all patients, but particularly those planning to undergo arthroplasty. Several different methods can be used.

TABLE 1-1 CONDITIONS THAT MAY REFER PAIN TO THE HIP

- Lumbosacral pathology
- Intra-abdominal pathology
- Hernia
- Ovarian cyst
- Vascular ischemia
- Chronic prostatitis
- Tumor (primary and metastatic)

TABLE 1-2 NONARTHRITIC HIP CONDITIONS

- Trochanteric bursitis
- Ischiogluteal bursitis
- Iliopsoas bursitis
- Osteitis pubis
- Transient osteoporosis
- Snapping hip syndrome

TABLE 1-3 ABNORMAL GAIT PATTERNS

- Antalgic or avoidance gait: Pain with weight bearing on the affected limb
- Trendelenburg or Duchenne gait: Abductor muscle weakness
- Circumduction: Leg length discrepancy
- Steppage: Peroneal nerve weakness resulting in foot drop

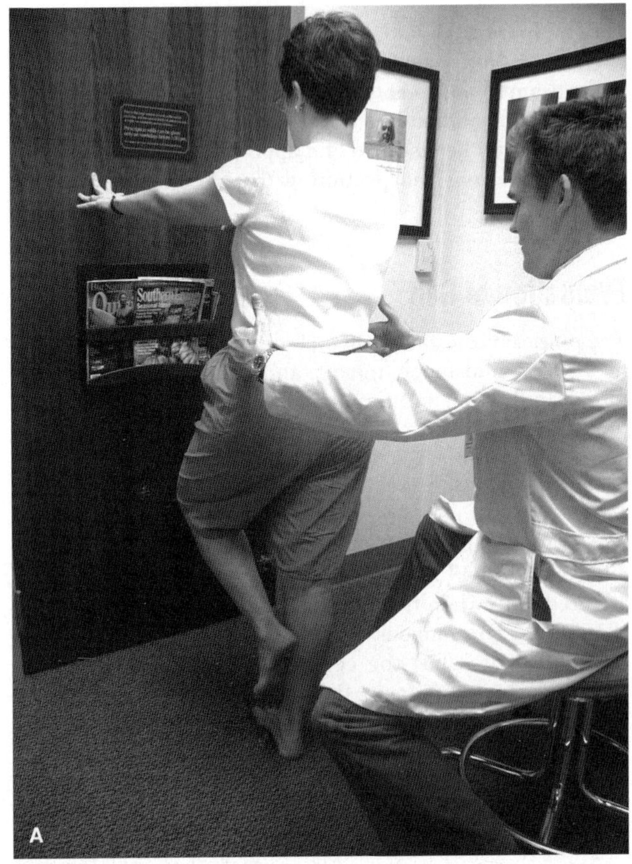
A

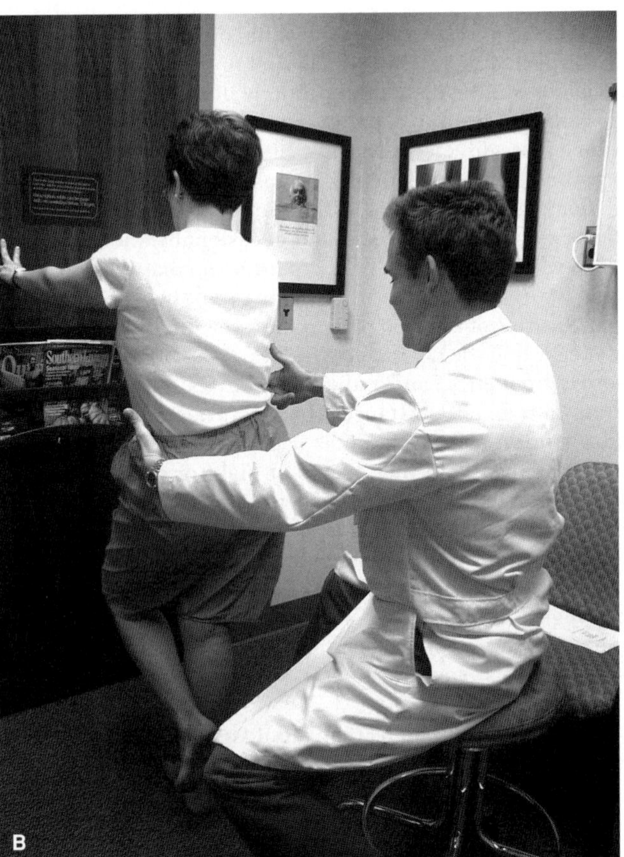
B

Figure 1-1 The examiner places his hands on the patient's pelvis. The patient is then asked to stand on the affected limb. If the abductors are functioning properly, the pelvis will remain level. With a weak or deficient abductor mechanism, the pelvis will tilt away from the affected limb.

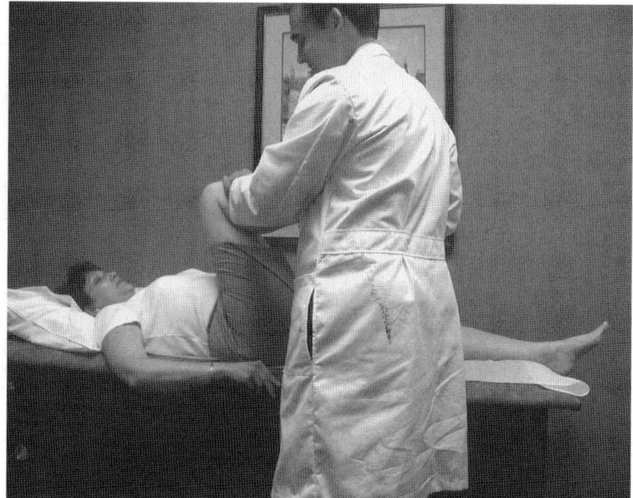

Figure 1-2 Hip flexion: Average ROM is 0 to 125 degrees.

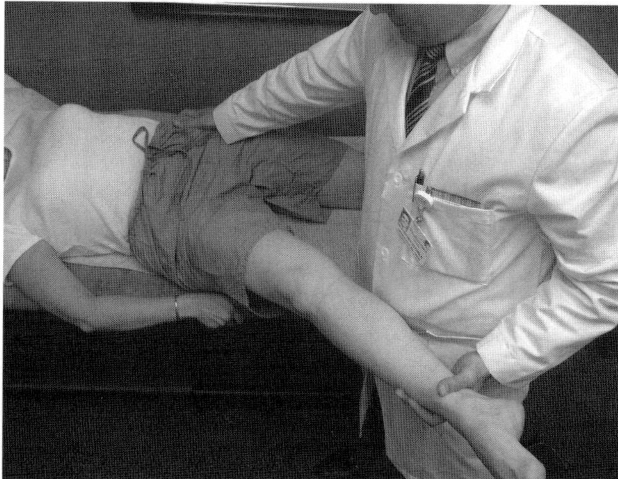

Figure 1-4 Abduction: Average ROM is 0 to 40 degrees. Note that examiner's hand stabilizes pelvis to prevent pelvic tilt.

- With the patient standing flat on ground, the examiner sits behind the patient and places his or her hands on the pelvic brim. Any asymmetry in pelvic height is noted. Measured blocks can be placed under the short limb until the pelvis becomes level. The height of the block used to level the pelvis can give an estimation of the leg length discrepancy. *The measurement will be affected by a fixed pelvic obliquity.*
- *Apparent leg length*: With the patient supine on the exam table, measure each leg from the umbilicus to a fixed point on the medial malleolus. *This measurement will also be affected by a fixed pelvic obliquity.*
- *True leg length*: With the patient supine on the exam table, measure each leg from the anterior superior iliac spine (ASIS) to a fixed point on the medial malleolus. *This measurement will not be affected by a fixed pelvic obliquity.*

Inspection and Palpation

The overlying skin should be inspected and palpated to look for outward signs of trauma (swelling, ecchymosis) and infection (warmth, erythema). All previous scars should be evaluated and noted. Other sources of cutaneous pain about the hip such as lesions associated with herpes zoster should be evaluated. Palpation of soft tissue and bony landmarks around the hip is important to rule out nonarticular causes of pain such as bursitis. Important bony landmarks that may be palpated include the following:

Lumbar spine and sacrum
Greater trochanter
Anterior superior iliac spine (ASIS)
Posterior superior iliac spine (PSIS)
Ischial tuberosity

Range of Motion

Range of motion about the hip joint should be noted and compared with the unaffected side. Patients with osteoarthritis will have limited range of motion, and the extremes of motion may cause pain and discomfort that is similar to their symptoms. In general, patients with osteoarthritis tend to lose hip flexion and internal rotation first (Figs. 1-2 through 1-7).

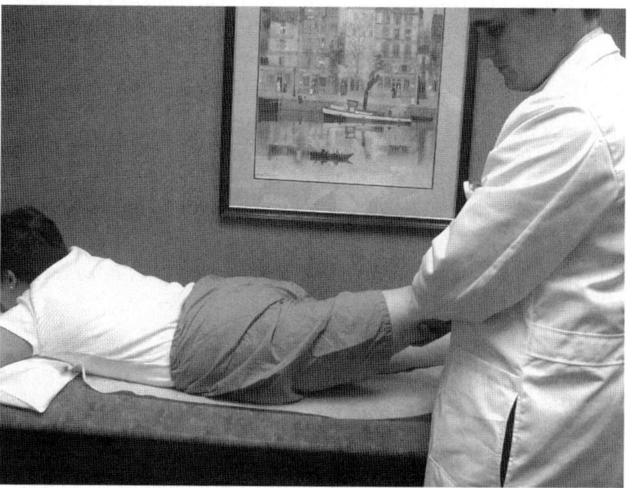

Figure 1-3 Hip extension: Average ROM is 0 to 25 degrees.

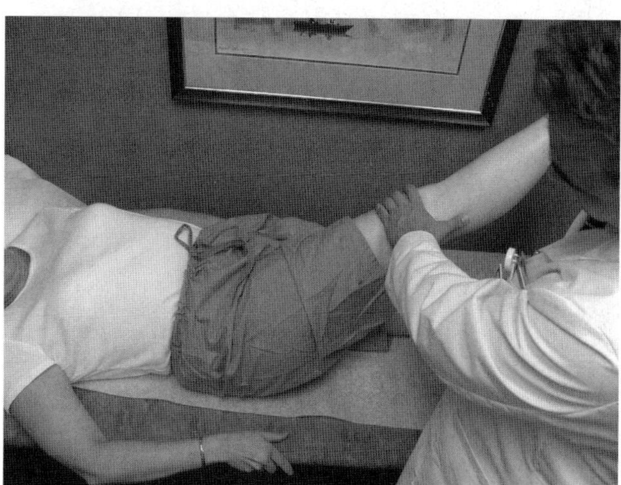

Figure 1-5 Hip adduction: Normal ROM is 0 to 30 degrees.

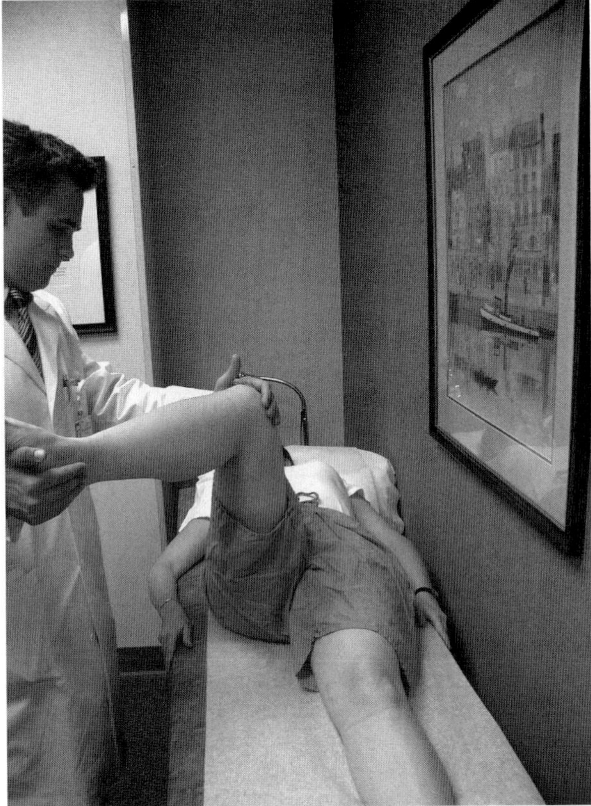

Figure 1-6 Internal rotation of the hip: Normal ROM is 0 to 30 degrees.

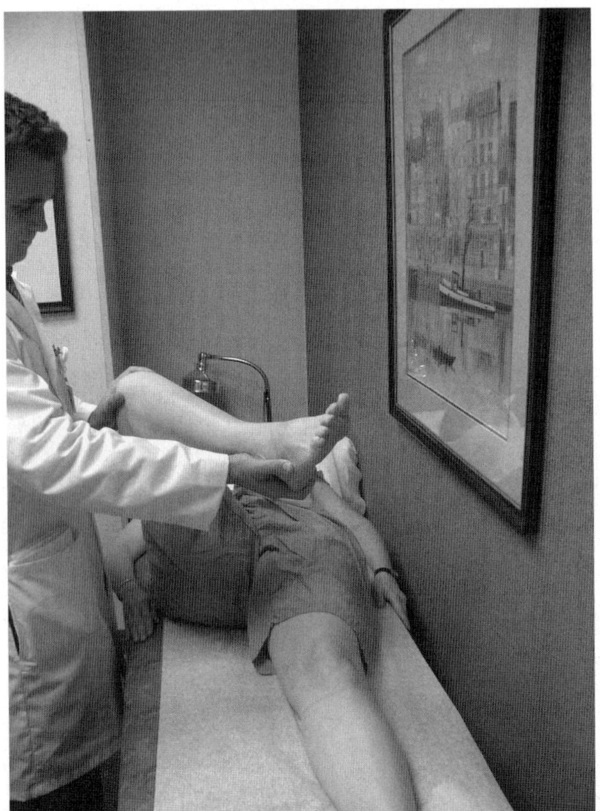

Figure 1-7 External rotation of the hip: Normal ROM is 0 to 60 degrees.

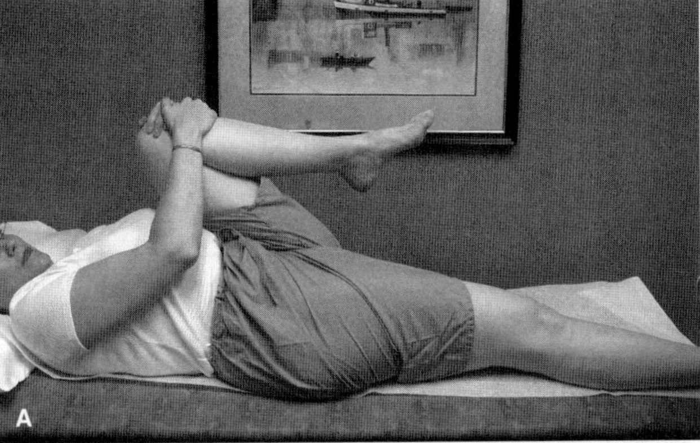

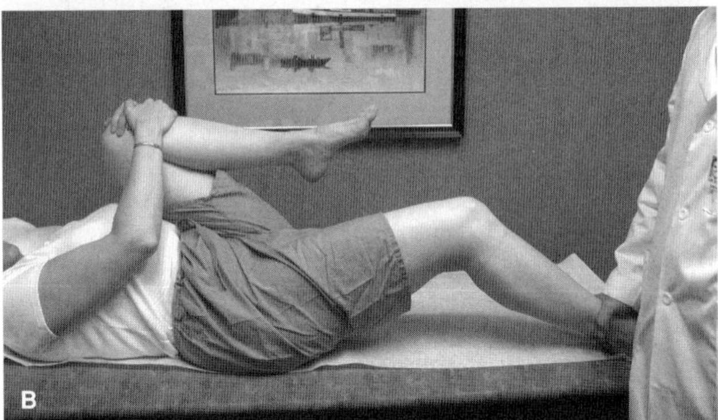

Figure 1-8 **A.** Normal test. **B.** Hip flexion contracture.

Hip-Specific Tests

Thomas Test. The patient is supine on the exam table (Fig. 1-8). Both knees are brought to the chest and held with the arms (this removes any lumbar lordosis). The leg to be tested is then released and allowed to come back to the table while the opposite leg remains held to the chest. A patient with a hip flexion contracture will be unable to fully extend the hip back to the exam table. Estimate the contracture by measuring the angle created by the patient's leg and the exam table.

Ely Test. With the patient in the prone position (Fig. 1-9), the affected leg is flexed at the knee. A patient with a rectus femoris contracture will spontaneously flex at the hip.

Ober Test. With the patient in the lateral decubitus position and the affected leg facing up (Fig. 1-10), the leg is slowly abducted with the knee flexed. From this position, the leg is released. A patient with a tight iliotibial band will remain in the abducted position whereas for those with a normal iliotibial band, the leg will fall into an adducted position.

Patrick Test or FABER Test. With the patient in the supine position (Fig. 1-11), the affected leg is *f*lexed, *ab*ducted, and *e*xternally *r*otated so the foot is placed against the contralateral knee. Pressure can then be applied by placing one hand on the opposite pelvis and pressing down the affected limb. Posterior pain indicates sacroiliac

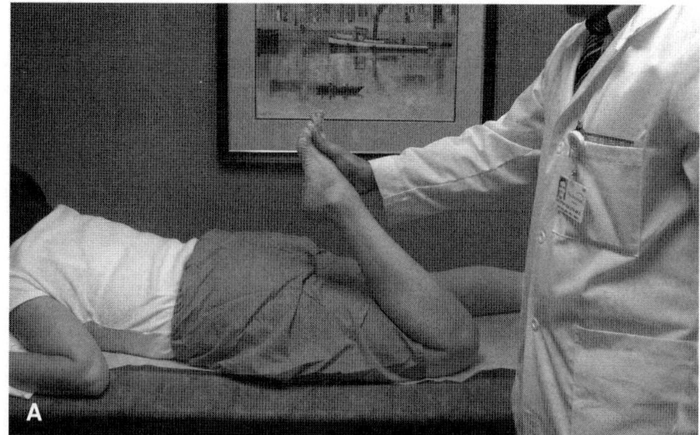

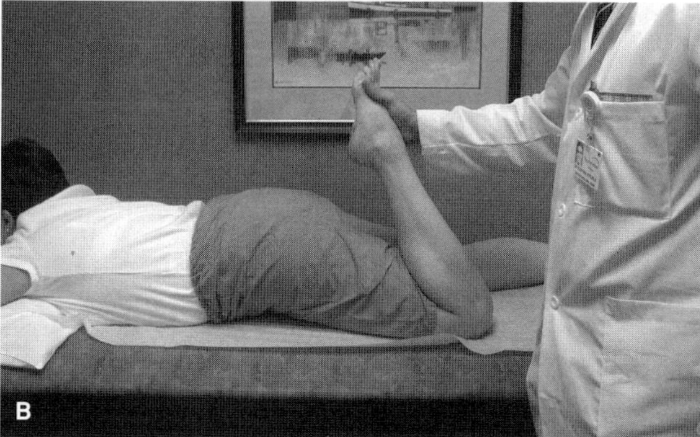

Figure 1-9 **A.** Normal test. **B.** Rectus femoris contracture.

joint pathology, whereas anterior groin pain is indicative of hip pathology.

The Stinchfield Maneuver. With the patient in the supine position (Fig. 1-12), the hip is flexed approximately 30 degrees with the knee fully extended. The patient is then asked to resist the examiner's downward force by maintaining the hip in the flexed position. A positive test reproduces pain across the hip joint.

Neurovascular Examination

Every patient should undergo a directed neuromuscular and vascular examination. Palpation and documentation of pulses in both extremities is mandatory. This may include palpation of the femoral, popliteal, and posterior tibialis and dorsalis pedis pulses.

Neuromuscular examination of the hip should include muscle testing and assessment of sensation. Hip muscles can be grouped into flexors, extensors, and medial and lateral rotators. Table 1-4 lists the muscles, innervation, and nerve root derivation of the hip muscles. The strength of pertinent muscle groups should be graded and documented. Strength can be graded on a standard scale of 0 to 5:

5/5: normal strength against resistance
4/5: normal strength against gravity with some resistance
3/5: strength against gravity with no resistance
2/5: movement with gravity eliminated
1/5: muscle contractility
0/5: no muscle contractility

Sensation is tested by assessment of superficial touch over dermatomes of the hip and lower extremities (Fig. 1-13). If any abnormalities are noted, a more thorough examination to include assessment of pain, temperature, and vibration may be conducted. Reflexes including the patellar (L2-4) and Achilles (S1) may be evaluated and compared with the contralateral side.

Evaluation of the Painful Total Hip Arthroplasty

When evaluating a patient with a painful total hip arthroplasty, several questions are important in evaluating the cause. Symptoms prior to surgery, dates of surgery, pain-free period after surgery and onset of new symptoms must be evaluated. Patients who never had any pain relief after surgery should be evaluated for other causes of referred pain to the hip (Tables 1-1 and 1-2). All preoperative and immediate postoperative radiographs should be obtained and evaluated. Patients with no or only a limited

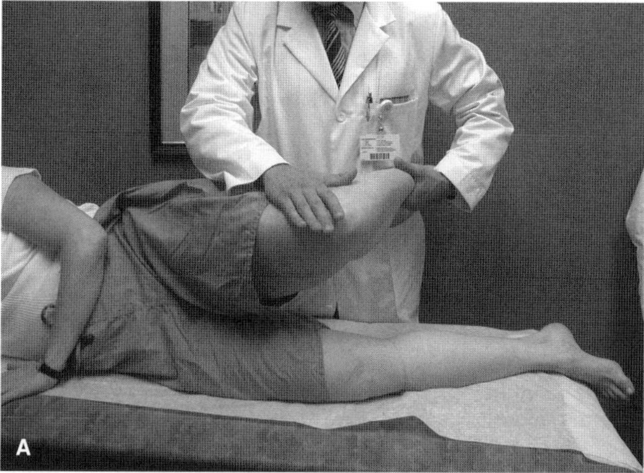

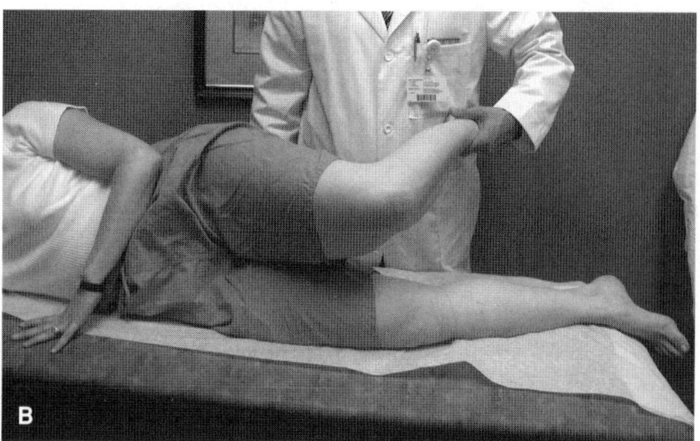

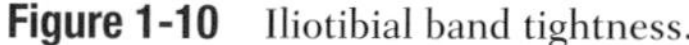

Figure 1-10 Iliotibial band tightness.

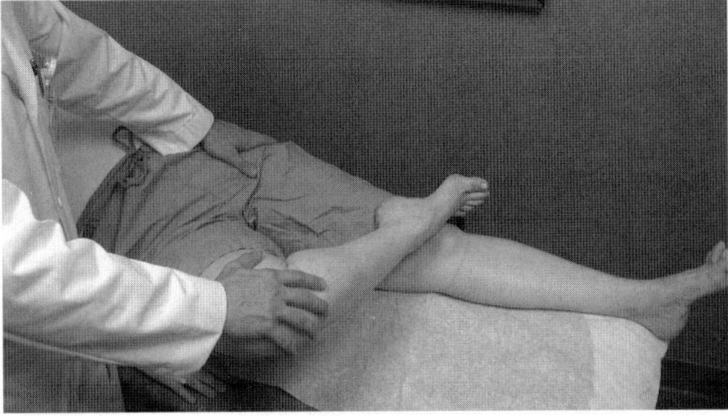

Figure 1-11 Sacral and hip joint pathology.

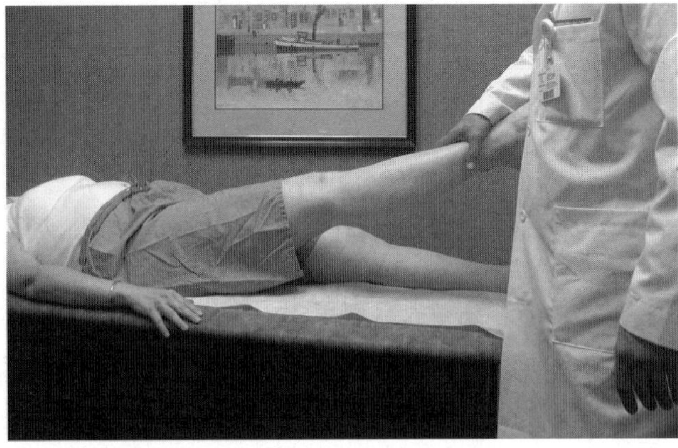

Figure 1-12 Loading hip joint in supine position.

TABLE 1-4 ACTIONS AND INNERVATIONS OF THE MUSCLES OF THE HIP

Action	Muscles	Nerve Innervation
Hip flexion	1. Psoas	L1-3
	2. Iliacus	Femoral
	3. Rectus femoris	Femoral
	4. Sartorius	Femoral
	5. Pectineus	Femoral
	6. Adductor longus	Obturator
	7. Adductor brevis	Obturator
	8. Gracilis	Obturator
Hip extensors	1. Biceps femoris	Sciatic
	2. Semimembranosus	Sciatic
	3. Semitendinosus	Sciatic
	4. Gluteus maximus	Inferior gluteal
	5. Gluteus medius (posterior)	Superior gluteal
	6. Adductor magnus	Sciatic
Hip abduction	1. Tensor fascia lata	Superior gluteal
	2. Gluteus minimus	Superior gluteal
	3. Gluteus medius	Superior gluteal
	4. Gluteus maximus	Inferior gluteal
	5. Sartorius	Femoral
Hip adduction	1. Adductor longus	Obturator
	2. Adductor brevis	Obturator
	3. Adductor magnus	Obturator
	4. Gracilis	Obturator
	5. Pectineus	Femoral
Medial (internal) rotation of hip	1. Adductor longus	Obturator
	2. Adductor brevis	Obturator
	3. Adductor magnus	Obturator
	4. Gluteus minimus (anterior)	Superior gluteal
	5. Gluteus medius (anterior)	Superior gluteal
	6. Tensor fascia lata	Superior gluteal
	7. Pectineus	Femoral
Lateral (external) rotation of hip	1. Gluteus maximus	Inferior gluteal
	2. Obturator internus	Nerve to obturator internus
	3. Obturator externus	Obturator
	4. Quadratus femoris	Nerve to quadratus femoris
	5. Piriformis	L5, S1-2
	6. Gemellus superior	Nerve to obturator internus
	7. Gemellus inferior	Nerve to quadratus femoris
	8. Sartorius	Femoral
	9. Gluteus medius	Superior gluteal nerve

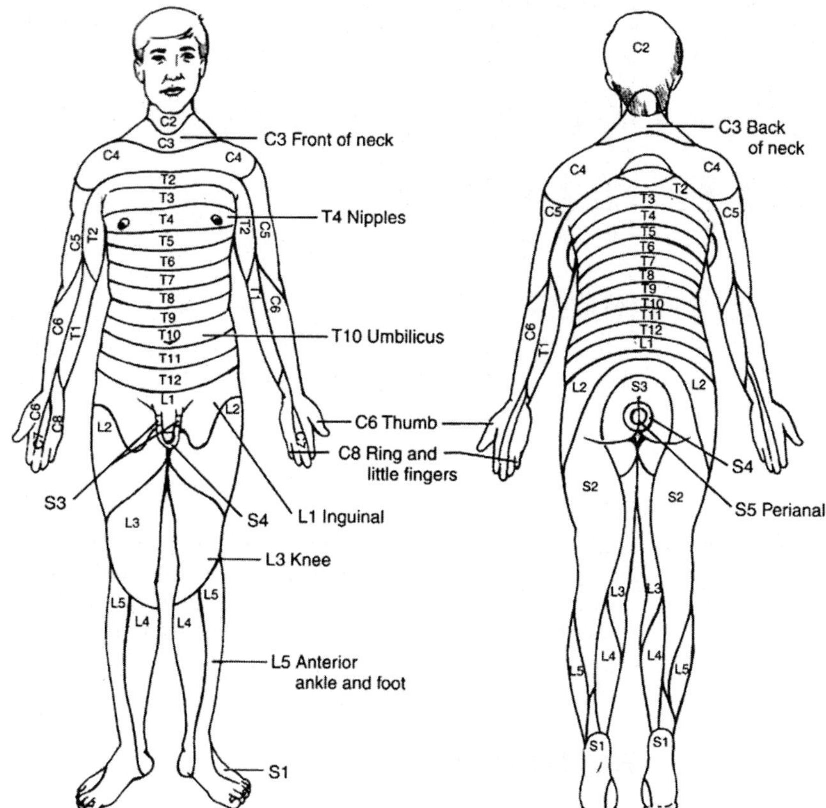

Figure 1-13 Dermatomes of the upper and lower extremity.

period of pain relief who continue to have discomfort that is not relieved by rest sould be evaluated for infection.

Patients with mechanical symptoms (i.e., loosening of the femoral or acetabular component) have generally had a pain-free period, then developed pain that has become progressive in frequency, duration, and intensity over time. Patients generally do not have pain at rest. They will often demonstrate a triphasic pain pattern, characterized by pain with initial weight bearing that subsides as they continue to walk (and the prosthesis finds a stable position) and then returns as the patient continues to bear weight.

On physical examination, patients with a painful total hip arthroplasty may demonstrate an antalgic gait or weakness of surrounding muscles. They also may demonstrate instability or apprehension at the extremes of motion.

SUGGESTED READINGS

Garvin KL, McKillip TM. History and physical examination. In: Callaghan JJ, Rosenberg AG, Rubash HE. *The Adult Hip*. Philadelphia: Lippincott–Raven Publishers; 1998:315–332.

Hoppenfeld S. *Orthopaedic Neurology: A Diagnostic Guide to Neurologic Levels*. Norwalk: Appleton and Lange; 1977.

Hoppenfeld S. *Physical Examination of the Spine and Extremities*. New York: Appleton-Century-Crofts; 1976.

Magee DJ. *Orthopaedic Physical Assessment*. 4th ed. Philadelphia: WB Saunders; 2002.

Thompson JC. *Netter's Concise Atlas of Orthopaedic Anatomy*. Icon Learning Systems, Teterboro, NJ; 2002.

IMAGING OF THE HIP

BRYAN D. SPRINGER

Over the past several decades there have been significant technologic advances in the field of radiology including computed tomography, magnetic resonance imaging, and nuclear medicine. Plain radiography, however, remains the initial diagnostic imagining study of choice and should serve as the first step in the radiographic evaluation of the hip.

The goal of any imaging study is to confirm or provide a diagnosis of a disorder. For any imaging modality to be useful, it must be performed and interpreted accurately. This chapter outlines the screening radiography of the hip along with special views and additional modalities that may be useful in evaluating a patient with suspected hip pathology.

PLAIN RADIOGRAPHY (X-RAY VIEW)

Every patient with suspected hip pathology should undergo a screening radiographic examination. For evaluation of the pelvis and hips, this should include anterior-posterior pelvis (AP pelvis) and cross-table or frog-leg lateral views. The findings on screening radiography allow for identification of initial pathology and enable the physician to make a more directed radiographic evaluation with special views or other imaging modalities.

AP Pelvis

The AP pelvis radiograph (Fig. 2-1) is performed with the patient supine on the x-ray table. The legs are internally rotated 15 degrees to compensate for normal femoral anteversion. The beam should be directed centrally to view the entire pelvis. This view allows for imaging of the iliac bones, sacrum, pubis, ischium, femoral heads, and acetabulum and the proximal aspect of the femur including the greater and lesser trochanter.

Cross-Table Lateral

The cross-table lateral or groin lateral view (Fig. 2-2) is obtained with the patient supine on the examination table and the opposite hip flexed and abducted. The x-ray cassette is placed on the outside of the affected hip, and the beam is angled from the opposite side toward the patient's groin. This view provides a lateral image of the femoral head allowing for assessment of anteversion angle of the femoral neck, which can range from 25 to 30 degrees. It also allows for visualization of the ischial tuberosity and the anterior and posterior margins of the acetabulum.

Frog-Leg Lateral

The frog-leg lateral view (Fig. 2-3) is performed with the patient supine on the x-ray table with the knees flexed and the thigh maximally abducted. The beam is directed either vertically or with 10 to 15 degrees of cephalad tilt. This projection demonstrates the lateral aspect of the femoral head and both trochanters.

Special Views

Ancillary views for the pelvis and hips can often provide essential additional information to screening radiography.

Pelvis

The inlet and outlet views of the pelvis are used in addition to the AP pelvis for evaluation of the bony pelvis. The inlet view (Fig. 2-4) projects the rings of the pelvis and allows for evaluation of rotational alignment of the pelvis. The outlet view (Fig. 2-5) projects parallel to the pelvic rim and perpendicular to the sacrum and allows for evaluation of vertical translation or malalignment.

Acetabulum

Judet oblique views of the pelvis and acetabulum are obtained by rotating the patient 45 degrees from the supine position with the beam directed anteroposteriorly. They allow for visualization of the columns and walls of the acetabulum and are used in evaluation and classification of acetabular fractures as well as in the evaluation of bone loss and osteolysis in patients with a failed acetabular component. The two views are as follows:

Anterior oblique. The anterior oblique or "obturator oblique" view (Fig. 2-6) demonstrates the anterior column and the posterior wall of the acetabulum.

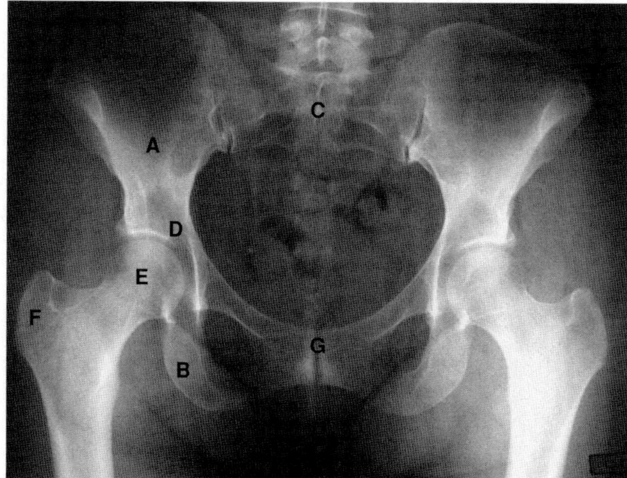

Figure 2-1 Anterior-posterior (AP) view of the pelvis. *A*, ilium; *B*, ischium; *C*, sacrum; *D*, acetabulum; *E*, femoral head; *F*, greater trochanter; *G*, pubic symphysis.

Posterior oblique. The posterior oblique or "iliac oblique" view (Fig. 2-7) demonstrates the posterior column and the anterior wall of the acetabulum.

Radiographic Landmarks of the Pelvis and Femur

Pelvis

Radiographic landmarks of the pelvis (Fig. 2-8) are as follows:

A. Iliopectineal line: denotes anterior column
B. Ilioischial line: denotes posterior column
C. Teardrop: inferior margin of the medial acetabular border.
D. Anterior acetabular rim
E. Posterior acetabular rim

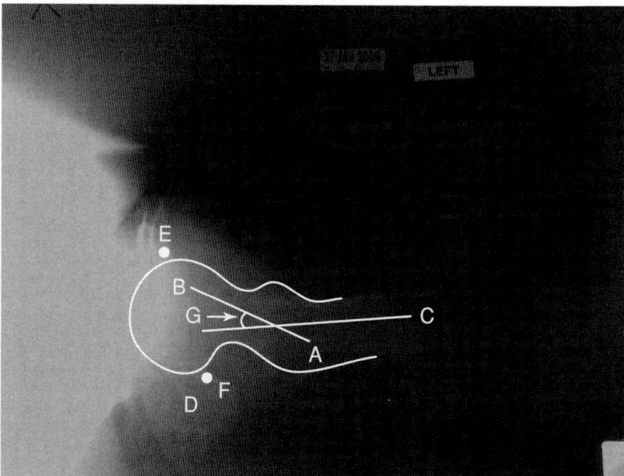

Figure 2-2 Cross-table lateral view of the pelvis and femur. *A*, greater trochanter; *B*, femoral head; *C*, femoral shaft; *D*, ischium; *E*, anterior margin of acetabulum; *F*, posterior margin of acetabulum; *G*, angle of femoral anteversion.

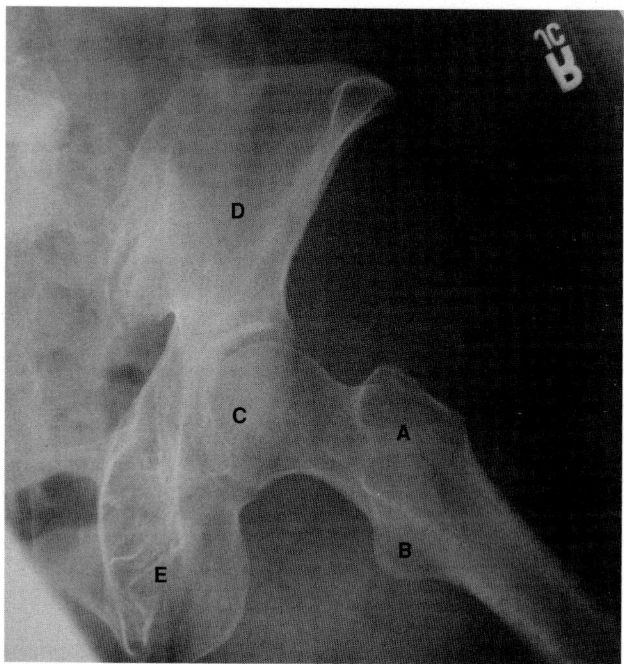

Figure 2-3 Frog-leg lateral view of the pelvis and femur. *A*, greater trochanter; *B*, lesser trochanter; *C*, femoral head; *D*, ilium; *E*, ischium.

Femur

Radiographic landmarks of the femur (Fig. 2-9) are as follows:

A. Greater trochanter
B. Lesser trochanter
C. Calcar femoris: intramedullary lamellar (compact) bone along medial femoral neck through the lesser trochanter
D. Primary compressive trabecular bands
E. Primary tensile trabecular bands

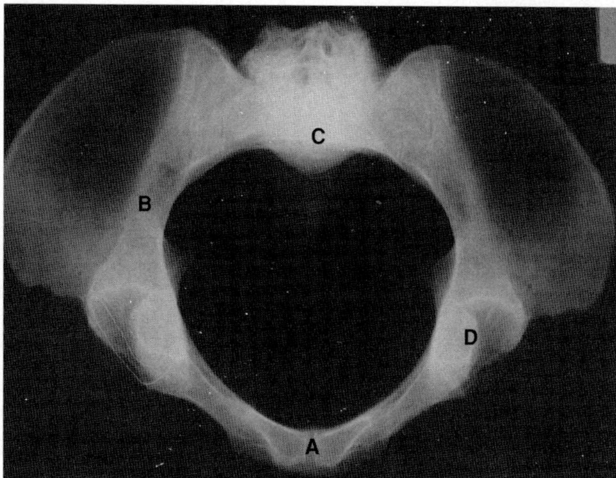

Figure 2-4 The inlet view of the pelvis. *A*, pubic symphysis; *B*, ilium; *C*, sacral promontory; *D*, acetabulum.

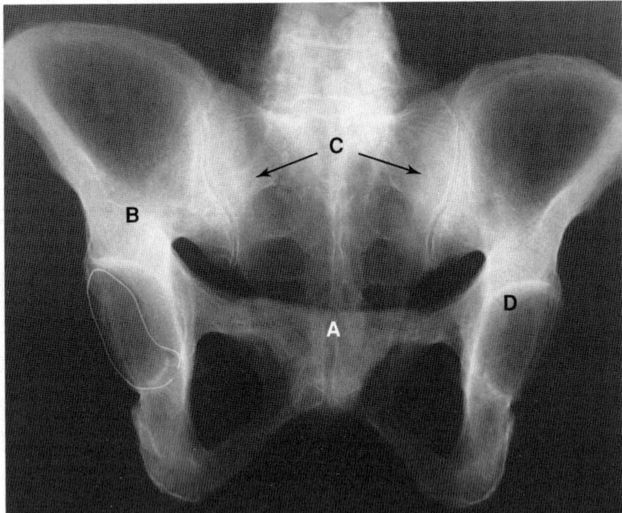

Figure 2-5 The outlet view of the pelvis. *A*, pubic symphysis; *B*, ilium; *C*, sacrum/sacroiliac (SI) joints; *D*, acetabulum.

Radiographic Measurement of the Hip

Radiographic measurement of the hip (Fig. 2-10) involves examination of the following:

Femoral offset: Horizontal distance from the center of the femoral head to the center of the femoral shaft.

Femoral neck shaft angle: Angle measured between the central line of the femoral neck and shaft. Normal 125 degrees with a range of 120 to 140 degrees.

Shenton line: Observed as a confluent arch between the inferior border of the superior pubic ramus and the medial border of the femoral neck. Helpful in evaluating the relationship of the femoral head to the acetabulum. A break in the Shenton line indicates migration of the femoral head.

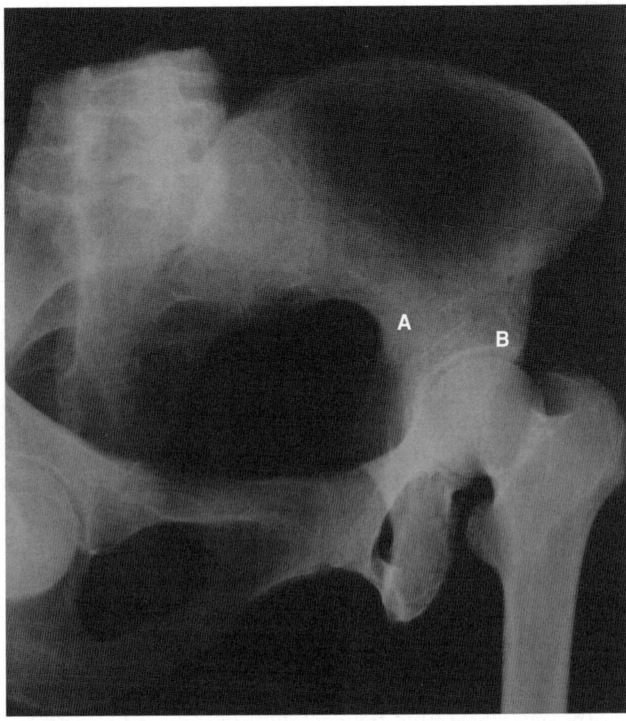

Figure 2-7 The posterior oblique or iliac oblique Judet view of the pelvis. *A*, posterior column of pelvis; *B*, anterior wall of acetabulum.

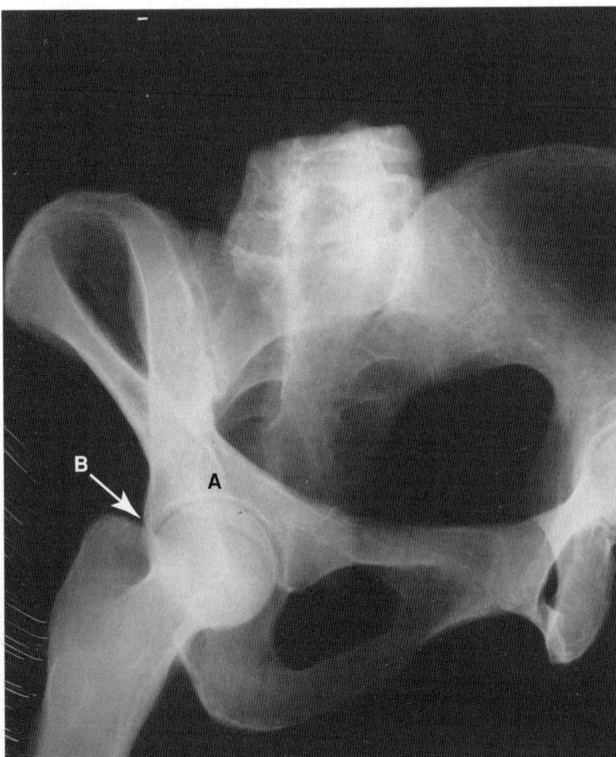

Figure 2-6 The anterior oblique or obturator oblique Judet view of the pelvis. *A*, anterior column of pelvis; *B*, posterior wall of acetabulum.

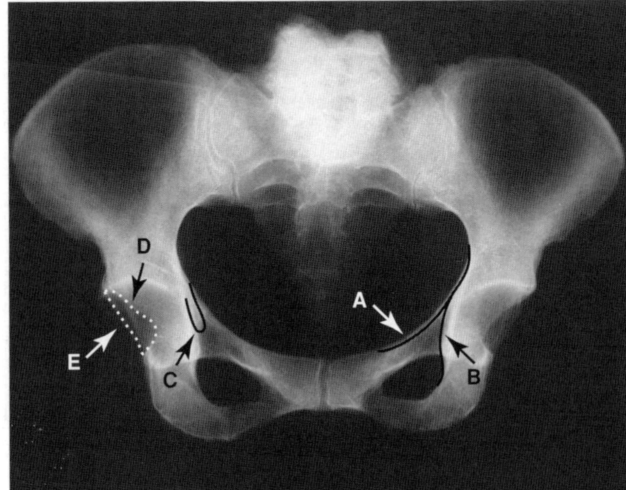

Figure 2-8 Radiographic landmarks of the pelvis. *A*, iliopectineal line; *B*, ilioischial line; *C*, acetabular teardrop; *D*, anterior acetabular rim; *E*, posterior acetabular rim.

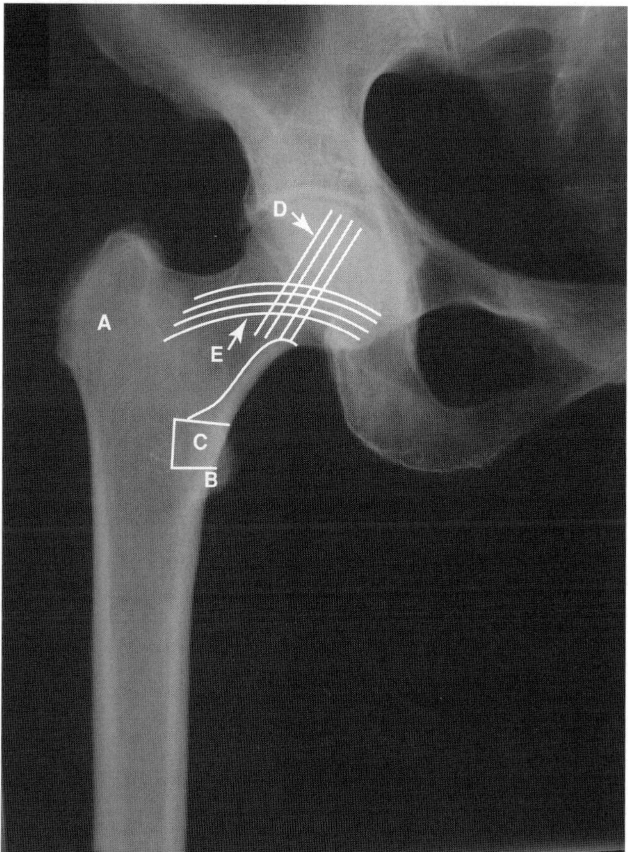

Figure 2-9 Radiographic landmarks of the femur. *A*, greater trochanter; *B*, lesser trochanter; *C*, calcar femoris; *D*, primary compressive trabecular bands; *E*, primary tensile trabecular bands.

Center edge angle of Wiberg: A line is drawn from the center of the femoral head to the edge of the acetabulum. A second line is drawn vertically to the center of the femoral head to form the incident angle.

Kohler Line: A line is drawn from the medial border of ischium to the medial border of ilium. Penetration medial to this line indicates protrusion.

Radiographic Characteristics of Osteoarthritis of the Hip

The hip and knee are the most common sites of osteoarthritis (Fig. 2-11). Symptoms may vary from stiffness to pain to difficulty walking. The severity of symptoms may not always correlate with radiographic severity. The classic radiographic features of osteoarthritis include the following:

- Joint space narrowing as a result of articular cartilage loss
- Subchondral sclerosis or eburnation of bone
- Osteophyte (bone spur) formation as a result of an attempted reparative process in areas subject to stress. Osteophytes often develop at the periphery or margin of the joint.
- Formation of bone cyst from intrusion of synovial fluid into the bone.
- Migration of the femoral head relative to the acetabulum.

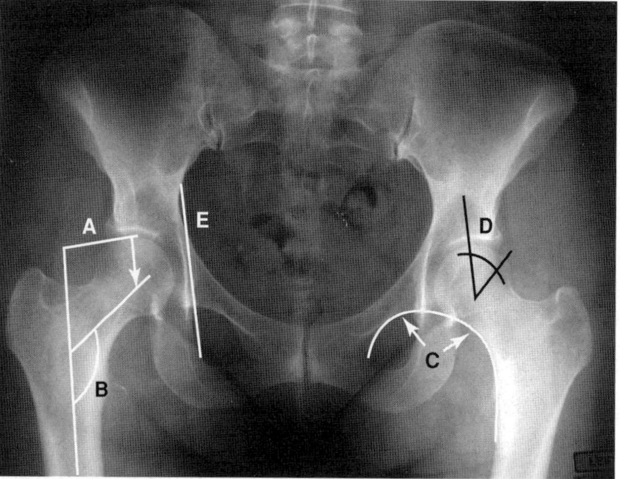

Figure 2-10 Radiographic landmarks of the femur. *A*, femoral offset; *B*, femoral neck shaft angle; *C*, Shenton line; *D*, center edge angle of Wiberg; E, Köhler line.

Imaging of the Prosthetic Hip

Evaluation of a patient with a prosthetic hip requires a thorough and complete radiographic assessment. Adequate radiographs should show the entire prosthesis and any surrounding cement. In most cases, plain radiographs will provide adequate information for the diagnosis, and ancillary

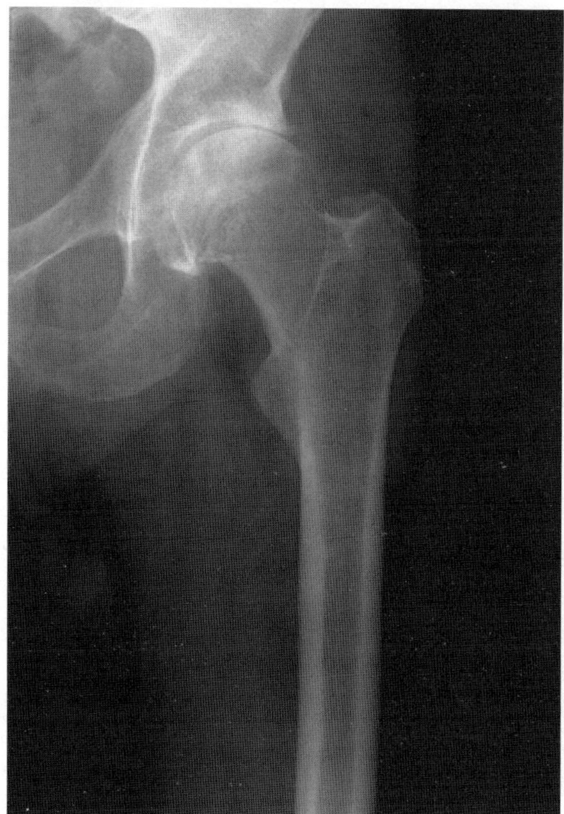

Figure 2-11 Radiographic characteristics of osteoarthritis of the hip.

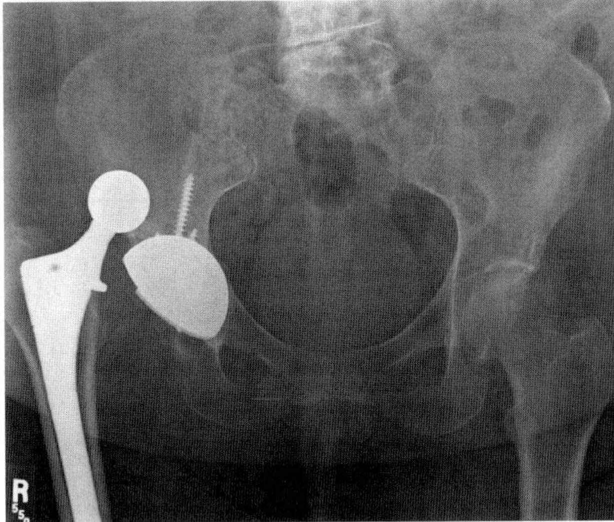

Figure 2-12 Anteroposterior pelvis radiograph demonstrating a dislocated total hip arthroplasty.

imaging (CT scan, bone scan) is needed only in selected circumstances.

Some common complications of arthroplasty often identified on plain radiographs include the following:

- Component malposition or dislocation
- Aseptic loosening of cemented or uncemented prostheses
- Osteolysis or bone reabsorption secondary to wear debris of prosthetic materials
- Infection
- Periprosthetic fracture

Component dislocation may occur at any time after surgery (Fig. 2-12). A common cause of early dislocation is component malposition. AP radiograph should demonstrate approximately 45 degrees of abduction (Fig. 2-13). Assessment of acetabular anteversion can be obtained from a true lateral radiograph. Appropriate acetabular component anteversion is 10 to 30 degrees. Occasionally CT scan to directly demonstrate femoral and acetabular component position may be required.

Aseptic loosening (Fig. 2-14) of either the femoral or acetabular components is a common cause of failure of the prosthetic hip. Radiographic changes can be subtle and

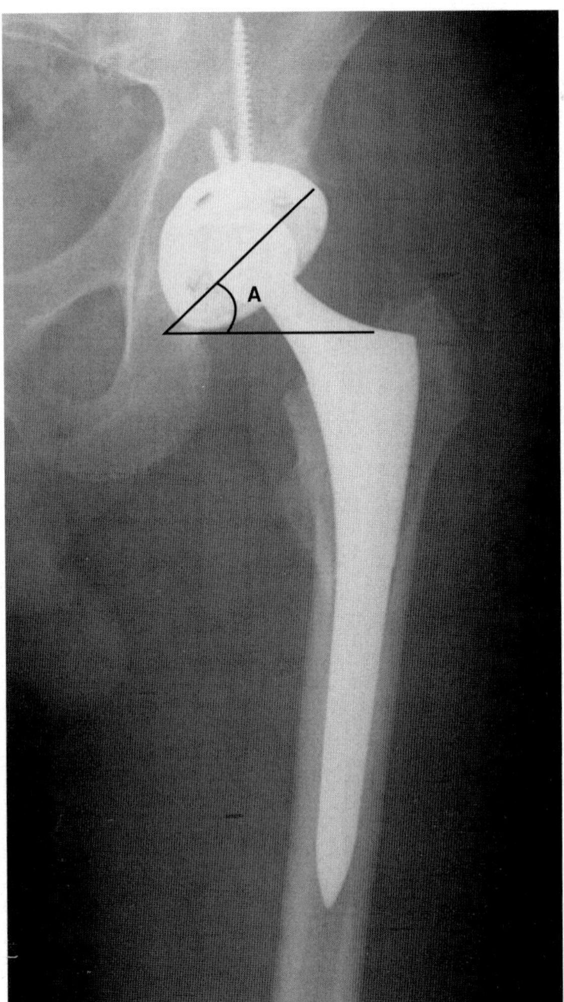

Figure 2-13 Anteroposterior pelvis radiograph demonstrating appropriate acetabular abduction. A, abduction angle of acetabular component.

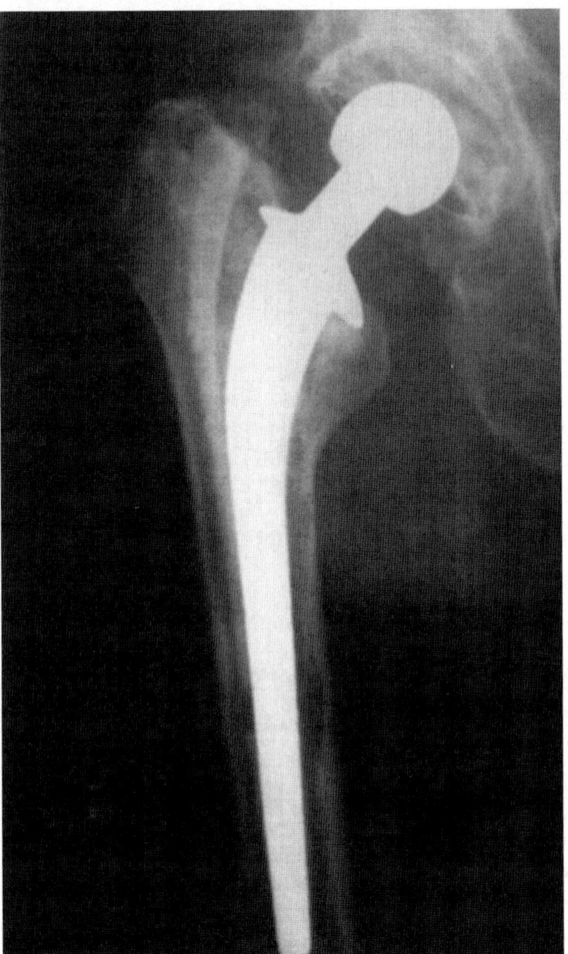

Figure 2-14 Anteroposterior radiograph of the femur demonstrates aseptic loosening of the femoral component.

TABLE 2-1 RADIOGRAPHIC CRITERIA OF ASEPTIC LOOSENING

Femoral components
Migration or subsidence of the prosthesis within the cement or bone
Migration/subsidence of the cement mantle within bone
Fracture/fragmentation of the cement mantle
Fracture of the femoral prosthesis
Complete radiolucent line at the bone/cement interface surrounding the prosthesis
Presence of radiolucent lines adjacent to the porous surface of the prosthesis
Shedding of metallic particles from the implant.

Acetabular components
Component migration
Fracture/fragmentation of cement mantle
Presence of complete radiolucent line between the bone and cement interface surrounding the component

often require the evaluation of serial radiographs taken over a period of time. Different mechanisms and patterns of failure exist for loosening of cemented and uncemented prosthesis. Table 2-1 lists the common radiographic findings of aseptic loosening of a total hip arthroplasty.

Infection (Fig. 2-15) continues to be one of the most devastating complications for the patient and surgeon following prosthetic hip replacement. Infection may be seen as an acute process or may be chronic. Radiographic findings in the acute setting are often absent and in the chronic setting may be subtle. The chronically infected prosthetic joint may present with periprosthetic bone resorption, frank bony destruction, and mechanical failure of the prosthesis.

Periprosthetic fractures (Fig. 2-16) are often the result of a fall or trauma resulting in a fracture of the bone around the prosthesis. The pattern is often described as being around the implant, at the tip of the implant, or distal to the implant. The prosthesis may continue to be well fixed despite the fracture or be loose as a result of the fracture of the surrounding supportive bone.

Ancillary Imaging

The cause of hip pain can be occult. Additional information not available on plain radiographs oftentimes is required to properly diagnose and treat certain disorders. In these situations, ancillary imaging techniques may be helpful. The most commonly used techniques include computed tomography, magnetic resonance imaging, and bone scintigraphy.

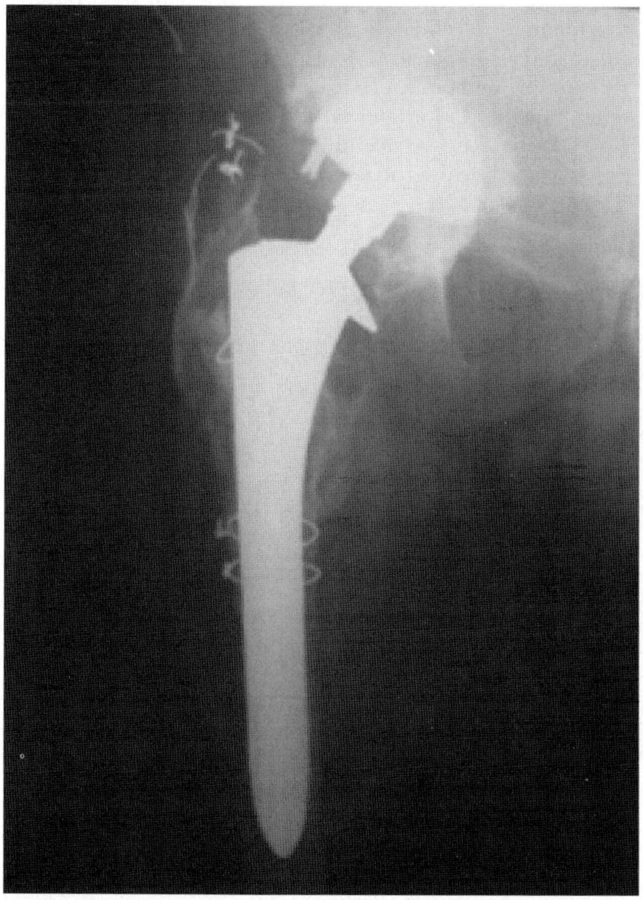

Figure 2-15 Anteroposterior radiograph of the femur demonstrates periprosthetic bone resorption secondary to infection.

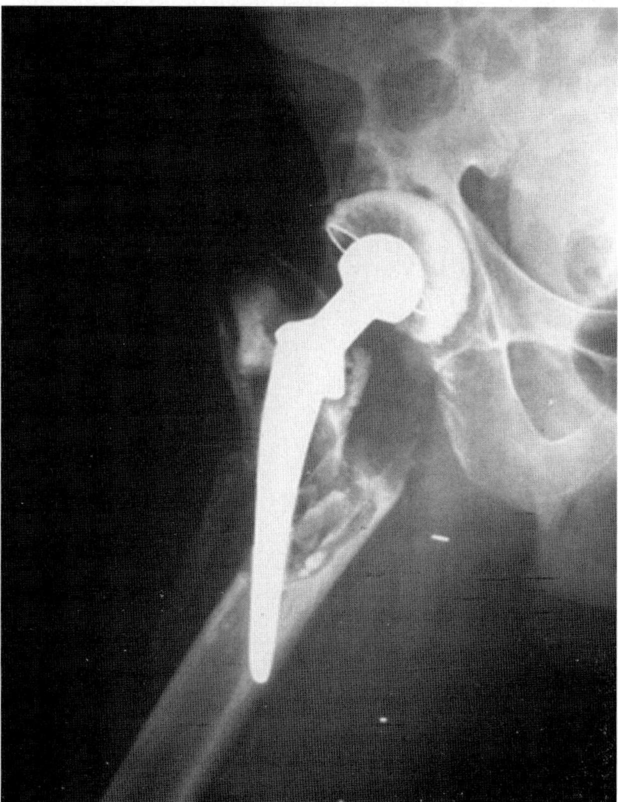

Figure 2-16 Periprosthetic fracture around the stem of a total hip arthroplasty.

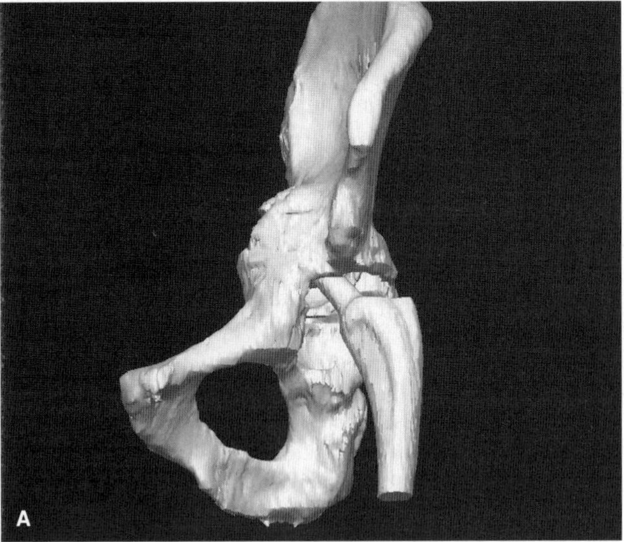

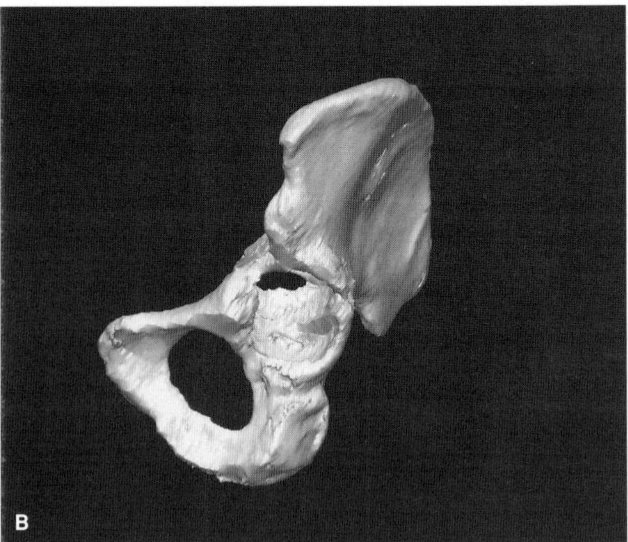

Figure 2-17 Computer tomography 3D reconstruction of the pelvis with components in place (A) and with prosthesis subtracted (B) demonstrating severe protrusion defect of acetabular bone but intact anterior and posterior columns.

COMPUTED TOMOGRAPHY

Computed tomography is most commonly used to evaluate primary disorders of the hip, assess pelvic bone quality, and aid in the postoperative evaluation of prosthetic component positioning. The latest generation of CT scanners use multiple detectors that allow for improved resolution. Reconstruction algorithms allow the generation of reformatted and three-dimensional images (Fig. 2-17A, B). These techniques are particularly useful in regions with complex anatomy such as the pelvis.

For patients who present for complex revision of a failed acetabular component, CT scans can aid in determining the adequacy of remaining bone stock in patients with protrusio defects or pelvic discontinuity. In addition, CT allows for localization of intrapelvic cement and retained hardware in relationship to intrapelvic vasculature (Fig. 2-18A, B). A CT scan may also be useful for assessing component position in the clinical setting of recurrent prosthetic instability.

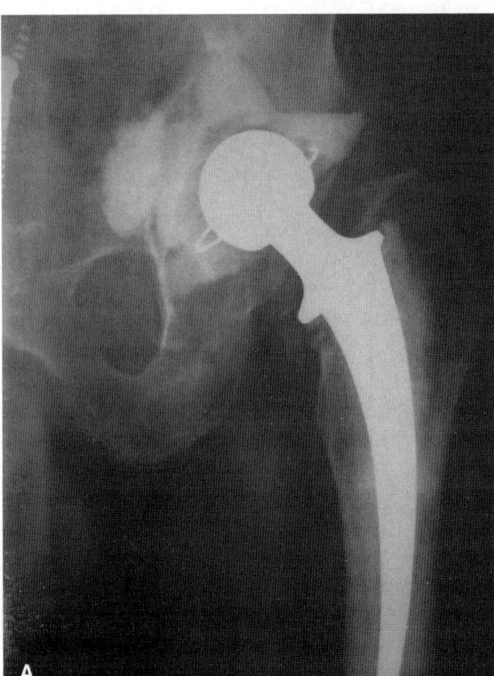

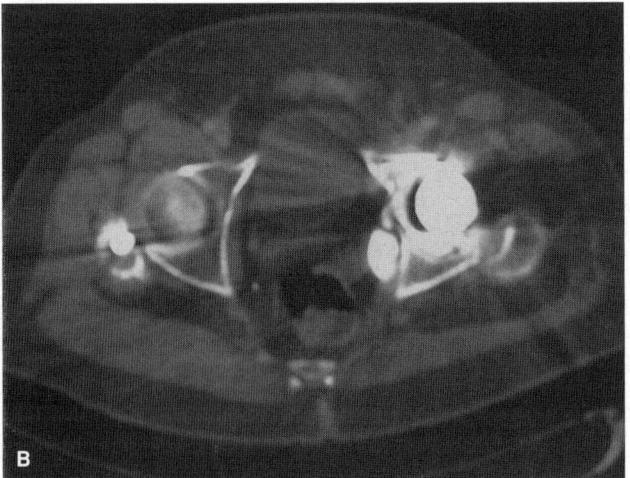

Figure 2-18 Preoperative radiograph of a 68-year-old man with an infected left total hip arthroplasty (A) with retained intrapelvic cement confirmed on CT scan (B) that required removal during surgery.

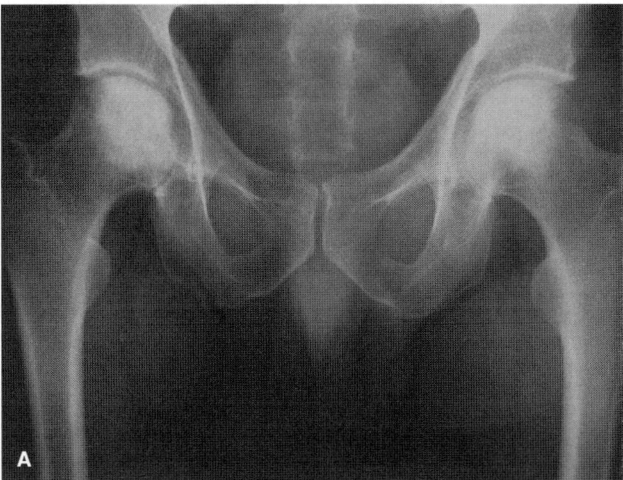

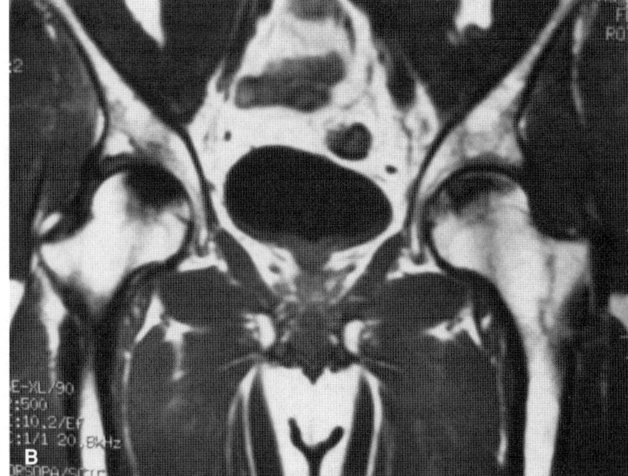

Figure 2-19 Radiographs (A) and T1-weighted magnetic resonance imaging (B) of a 50-year-old man with bilateral avascular necrosis of the hips.

The evaluation of acetabular or femoral component anteversion in relationship to fixed bony landmarks may provide useful information prior to revision surgery.

MAGNETIC RESONANCE IMAGING

Magnetic resonance imaging (MRI) has gained wide acceptance in the evaluation of the painful total hip. Pathologic conditions in which MRI may be useful include: avascular necrosis, labral pathology, occult fractures, infection, and tumors. Multiplanar capability combined with superior soft tissue resolution allows for accurate visualization of bone and soft tissue structures surrounding the hip joint.

MRI is the diagnostic modality of choice for early detection and evaluation of osteonecrosis (ON). MRI has proven to be the most sensitive and specific test for the diagnosis of ON. It is useful in the detection of early disease, asymptomatic disease, and bilateral disease present in approximately 80% of patients. The characteristic MRI appearance is a focal, segmental signal abnormality in the subchondral bone of the femoral head (Fig. 2-19A, B). In contrast, transient osteoporosis of the femur, a clinical and diagnostic entity often confused with avascular necrosis, has signal abnormality involving the head and neck diffusely without discrete signal abnormality.

The addition of paramagnetic intravenous contrast agents such as gadolinium to MRI increases the signal in vascular structures around the hip. In the setting of avascular necrosis, this may help to distinguish between areas of reparative and necrotic tissue. Intravenous (IV) contrast may also help in identifying focal fluid collections. After contrast administration, rim enhancement of a nonvascularized abscess can be differentiated from diffusely enhancing inflammatory tissue. MRI arthrography, consisting of the direct installation of gadolinium into the hip joint, has proven valuable in the diagnosis of labral and chondral pathology of the hip (Fig. 2-20).

Magnetic Resonance Imaging and Prosthetic Evaluation

Previously, large artifacts and noise prevented useful magnetic resonance imaging of the total hip prosthesis. Recently, new imaging protocols have allowed for less artifact and more accurate depiction of soft tissue and bone around the prosthesis. One area where this technology may prove particularly useful is in the early detection and assessment of periprosthetic osteolysis. Preliminary data suggests that metal suppression MRI techniques may be more sensitive and specific than plain radiographs in determining the presence and volume of periprosthetic osteolysis.

NUCLEAR IMAGING

Nuclear imaging studies (bone scintigraphy) remain useful tools for detecting areas for abnormal metabolic activity in

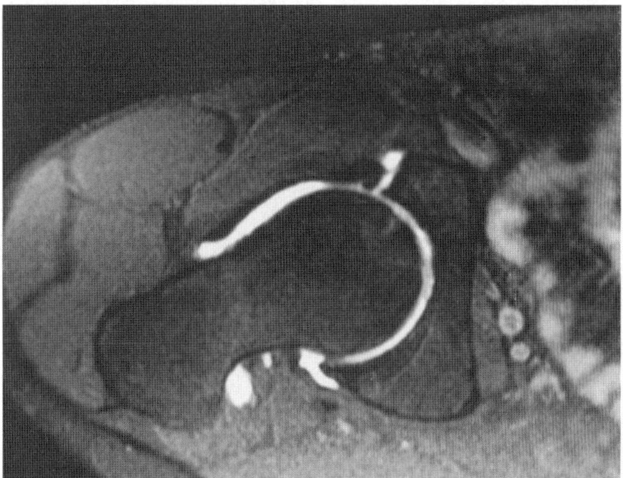

Figure 2-20 MRI arthrography of the hip demonstrating anterior labral tear.

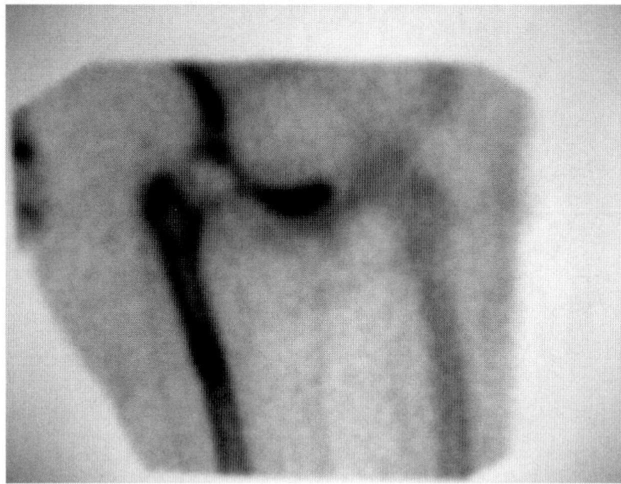

Figure 2-21 Tech 99 bone scan demonstrating symmetric uptake of tracer around the femoral component of a right total hip arthroplasty consistent with loosening of the prosthesis.

bone. The bone scan is typically performed in three phases after administration of technetium 99:

Vascular phase: images performed at 2 to 5 seconds indicate areas of increased or decreased blood flow

Blood pool phase: images to determine areas of hyperemia (osteomyelitis)

Delayed phase: images to determine areas of increased or decreased tracer uptake

Bone scintigraphy may be useful in evaluating the suspected loose or infected total hip prosthesis when other clinical modalities (laboratory values, x-ray views) are equivocal. Although this technique has high sensitivity, it also has poor specificity. Increased tracer uptake can be seen surrounding a normal hip prosthesis for ≤24 months after surgery. A loose hip prosthesis will commonly show abnormal tracer uptake at the trochanters, tip of the prosthesis, and acetabulum (Fig. 2-21).

Although infection at the site of prosthesis will generally show diffuse uptake, bone scintigraphy is not specific enough to differentiate infection from loosening. The addition of indium-111–labeled leukocyte scan that accumulates in regions of infection by chemotaxis has been shown to improve both the sensitivity and specificity of identifying periprosthetic infection, especially when combined with technetium-99 bone scan. Because indium-111 may also accumulate at the site of bone marrow distribution, the addition of a sulphur colloid bone marrow scan may also aid in improving the sensitivity and specificity. If abnormal uptake of white blood cells on an indium scan is not matched by congruent uptake on a bone marrow scan, the findings more likely correlate with infection.

SUGGESTED READINGS

Garvin KL, McKillip TM. History and physical examination. In Callaghan JJ, Rosenberg AG, Rubash HE. *The Adult Hip*. Philadelphia: Lippincott-Raven Publishers; 1998:315–332.

Greenspan A. *Orthopaedic Imaging: A Practical Approach*. Philadelphia: Lippincott Williams and Wilkins; 2004.

3 OSTEOARTHRITIS AND INFLAMMATORY ARTHRITIS OF THE HIP

MARK J. SPANGEHL

Osteoarthritis and inflammatory arthritis are the most frequently encountered diseases in orthopaedics. They are the leading causes of joint disease in the hip, resulting in joint destruction, and often in the need for hip replacement. Symptomatic osteoarthritis of the hip is prevalent in 3% to 5% of the adult white population. Radiographic evidence of osteoarthritis is more common (9% to 10%), indicating that roughly half of the patients with some radiographic evidence of osteoarthritis are asymptomatic.

Degenerative joint disease (DJD) is a historic term, still often used, that implies degenerative changes owing to various causes. The term DJD can be confusing because it is often used synonymously for osteoarthritis, but can be applied to any condition that results in degenerative changes of the joint. A more correct use of terminology would be to avoid the use of DJD and use the correct underlying diagnosis instead.

Degenerative conditions of the hip can be broadly grouped into noninflammatory and inflammatory arthritis. Osteoarthritis is by far the most common condition of the noninflammatory group. Osteoarthritis results from a primary failure of the cartilage, whereas with inflammatory arthritis, the cartilage failure is secondary to the inflammatory response. Table 3-1 outlines the more common arthritides that can affect the hip joint.

PATHOGENESIS

Etiology

The development of osteoarthritis (OA) results from a multitude of conditions, with the end result being failure of the weight-bearing cartilage. Because of its various potential causes, OA can be thought of as a syndrome rather than a single entity. In the past, it was felt that most patients who developed osteoarthritis had primary OA without any identifiable cause, arising as a result of a yet unidentified weakness of the cartilage. Now, it is more evident that most patients with OA likely have an underlying mechanical cause that results in damage and subsequent degeneration of cartilage. However, still there are patients in whom no cause can be clearly identified, and these may represent a biologic condition that results in cartilage failure. These patients represent primary osteoarthritis, which can be considered a diagnosis of exclusion.

In recent years there has been a much clearer understanding of various mechanical problems, which may be termed prearthritic conditions, whose natural histories show progression to osteoarthritis. These conditions include mild hip dysplasia as well as femoroacetabular impingement (FAI). FAI has become recognized as a mechanical abnormality of the hip in which the anterior femoral neck impinges on the acetabulum, leading to shear damage of the articular cartilage. Two types of impingement have been described: cam type and pincer type. Originally felt to possibly represent an asymptomatic or subclinical slipped epiphysis, the cam type of impingement has been shown to be a developmental abnormality. During development the femoral head epiphysis and trochanteric apophysis share one physis, which separates into two distinct growth plates around 4 years of age. A delayed separation or abnormal, eccentric closure results in an abnormal morphology typically affecting the anterolateral femoral neck. The effect is a decreased head/neck offset, reducing the head/neck ratio in this region and resulting in impingement of the anterior femoral neck with the anterior rim of the acetabulum (Fig. 3-1). The pincer type of impingement is more a result of an acetabular abnormality. Approximately 16% of dysplastic acetabula are retroverted. This retroversion results in a relatively prominent anterior rim, also causing impingement in flexion. Additionally, a deep acetabulum (coxa profunda) may result in a prominent acetabular rim, causing impingement. Both cam and pincer types of impingement may coexist.

TABLE 3-1 ARTHRITIDES AFFECTING THE HIP

- Noninflammatory arthritis
  - Osteoarthritis
    - Primary (idiopathic)
    - Secondary
      - Dysplasia
      - Femoroacetabular impingement
        - Cam type
        - Pincer type
      - Slipped capital femoral epiphysis
      - Legg-Perthes
      - Traumatic
  - Osteonecrosis of the femoral head
  - Neuropathic
  - Multiple epiphyseal dysplasia
- Paget disease
- Pigmented villonodular synovitis
- Chondrocalcinosis
- Hemophilic arthropathy

- Inflammatory
  - Rheumatoid arthritis
  - Systemic lupus erythematosus
  - Spondyloarthropathies
    - Psoriatic arthritis
    - Ankylosing spondylitis
    - Reactive arthritis (Reiter syndrome)
    - Enteric spondyloarthropathy

Table 3-1 summarizes various types of inflammatory arthritides. Rheumatoid arthritis is the most common form of inflammatory arthritis. It has a prevalence of 0.3% to 1.5% in North America and is approximately 2.5 times more common in women. The cause is thought to be an autoimmune cell-mediated response. Further pathogenesis is discussed later. The inciting event that begins the inflammatory response has yet to be identified, but is likely an extrinsic factor (e.g., infectious, environmental) in a genetically susceptible host. A genetic predisposition (HLA-B27) has also been shown in seronegative (defined as rheumatoid factor–negative) arthropathies; however, an infectious cause has been more closely linked to certain types. Reactive and enteric spondyloarthropathies have been associated with various gastrointestinal and genitourinary infections.

Epidemiology

Although mechanical abnormalities may be the etiologic factor responsible for most osteoarthritis, there are epidemiologic factors as well. These epidemiologic factors may result in a predisposition of the joint to osteoarthritis as a result of altered mechanics or other yet to be defined biologic factors. Family and twin studies have shown an increased prevalence of osteoarthritis within families. Familial studies have documented an increased incidence in first degree relatives, with 8% to 13% requiring hip replacement or having symptoms of coxarthrosis. Twin studies further underscore the hereditary component of osteoarthritis. Monozygotic female twins older than 50 years of age have been shown to have an approximately 60% heritability or genetic factor for the development of hip osteoarthritis. Additional risk factors for the development of osteoarthritis include increased age (older), race (whites [3% to 5% prevalence] greater than in Asians), as well as gender. In those younger than 50 years of age, men have a higher risk of developing hip osteoarthritis; in those older than 50 years of age, women have a greater incidence of the disease.

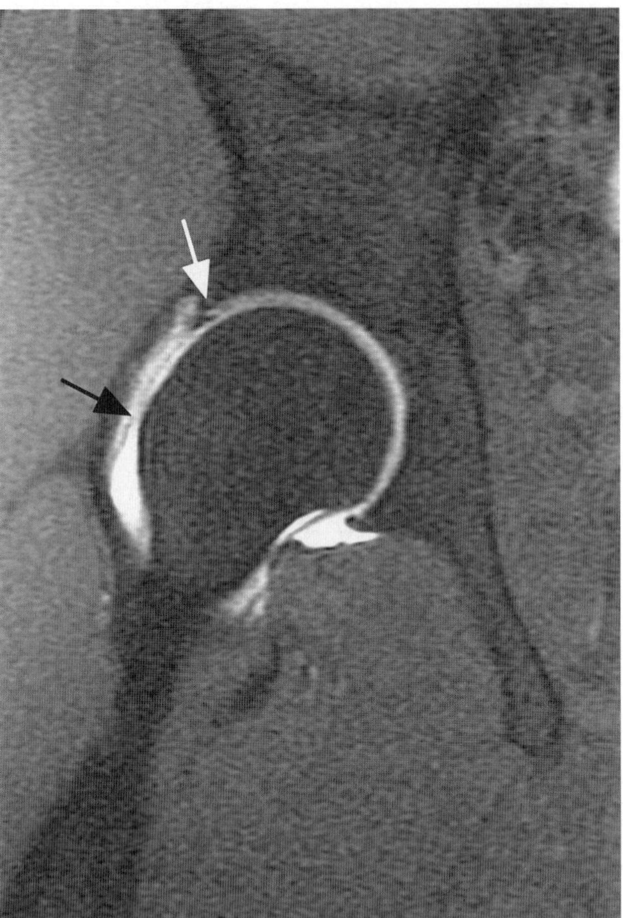

Figure 3-1 Coronal oblique view of patient with cam type femoroacetabular impingement. Note the prominence of bone anteriorly (*black arrow*) resulting in poor head–neck offset and reduced head/neck ratio. Note also anterior labral tear (*white arrow*).

Although there is clear evidence that obesity is associated with osteoarthritis of the knee, the literature linking obesity to hip disease is less well defined. Nevertheless, a growing body of evidence now more strongly supports the relationship of obesity to hip osteoarthritis. This relationship seems to be important even at a younger age; increased body mass index (BMI) earlier in life (age 18) is a stronger predictor for the development of osteoarthritis than increases in BMI later in life and is associated with increased risk for requiring hip replacement. Increased BMI is also associated with changes in gait patterns. When comparing gait patterns of nonobese and obese persons, changes in gait symmetry, stride width, and hip abduction angles were noted,

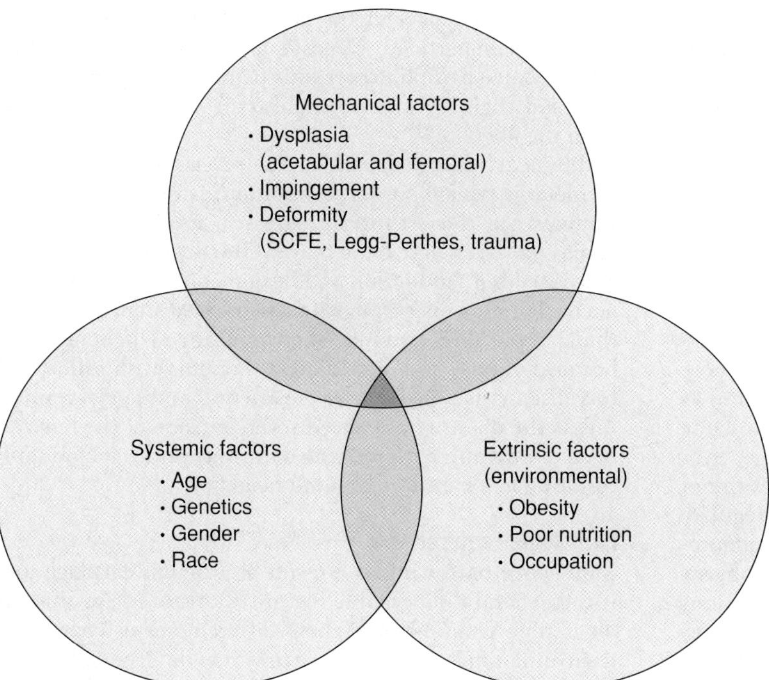

Figure 3-2 Etiologic factors associated with the development of osteoarthritis.

suggesting that a mechanical effect in obese patients could also result in the development of OA. Yet other studies suggest that patients who are obese suffer more hip complaints at the same radiographic stage than nonobese patients, therefore making them more likely to seek hip replacement at an earlier stage than nonobese patients. Possibly therefore, the incidence of radiographic OA is similar in obese and nonobese populations; however, obese populations are more symptomatic and seek treatment sooner for a given stage of osteoarthritis. In summary, studies have shown that obesity is a risk factor in the development of hip osteoarthritis. This association is stronger for women, in whom increased BMI early in life has been shown to be associated with an increased incidence of OA.

Similarly, occupational factors show less association with osteoarthritis of the hip than that of the knee. However, some population studies do suggest that occupation may have some influence on the development of hip osteoarthritis such as the higher prevalence of hip osteoarthritis in European farmers. Other studies have suggested that high-demand recreational activities (professional soccer, track and field, racket sports) may also contribute to hip arthritis. Figure 3-2 outlines various factors that contribute to the development of osteoarthritis.

Rheumatoid arthritis affects women more than men (2.5 times more common in women). A genetic predisposition is supported by studies that show familial clustering and a higher prevalence in monozygotic twins versus dizygotic twins, with monozygotes having a 3.5 greater chance of developing the disease. Further genetic predisposition is supported by the higher prevalence in Native American populations (5% to 6%). Seronegative arthropathies have a genetic predisposition that is dependent on the prevalence of HLA-B27 in a given population. Generally, the greater the prevalence of HLA-B27 in a given population, the higher the prevalence of spondyloarthropathies. HLA-B27 is common in certain Native American populations (up to 50% positive), relatively common in Europeans (7% to 20%), less prevalent in Asians and North American whites (7%), and uncommon in African Americans (1% to 2%). Spondyloarthropathies occur in approximately 5% to 14% of HLA-B27–positive individuals. Seronegative spondyloarthropathies can also occur, less commonly, in individuals who are HLA-B27–negative.

Pathophysiology

Osteoarthritis is a condition that begins as a result of overload of the cartilage. In rare situations there is a true genetic basis to joint destruction in which a generalized joint destruction occurs as a result of a mutation that codes for type II collagen. Much more commonly, the cartilage may be predisposed to damage because of various mechanical conditions in the joint that result in a gradual destruction of the cartilage. There is a failure of the chondrocytes to maintain or repair damaged cartilage. Although chondrocytes are metabolically more active in osteoarthritis, it is postulated that the increased response is inadequate against the increased degradation of products synthesized by the chondrocytes. Characteristic changes occur within the cartilage structure, including changes in water content (increased) and changes in proteoglycan concentrations (overall decrease with shorter chains and increased chondroitin/keratin sulfate ratio). Another characteristic change is collagen destruction: Interleukin 1 (IL-1) from various cells (chondrocytes, synovial cells, neutrophils) regulates the production of catabolic enzymes, e.g., metalloproteinases that degrade the core protein of proteoglycans and collagenase resulting in collagen destruction. IL-1 also influences the cartilage matrix by causing a decreased synthesis of types II and IX collagen and an increase in types I and III collagen.

In inflammatory arthritides, the cartilage degeneration is secondary to the inflammatory response, which begins in the synovium. In early rheumatoid arthritis (RA), a microvascular synovial injury appears to occur, resulting in edema and synovial cell proliferation. Lymphocytes and macrophages infiltrate the synovium early on, forming organized lymphoid tissue. Plasma cells are found in more advanced disease. With synovial hyperplasia, the pannus of synovium that extends to the edge of cartilage and bone begins to invade and destroy the bone and cartilage. Synovial macrophages produce cytokines (interleukin 1, tumor necrosis factor [TNF]-α and -β), which in turn regulate the production of various degradative enzymes (metalloproteinases, collagenase, stromelysin) by synovial fibroblasts and chondrocytes, resulting in cartilage destruction. Bony erosions result from multinucleated giant cells, which may originate from the pannus, which is rich in macrophages. Rheumatoid synovial T cells have been shown to produce osteoclast differentiation factor, which may be responsible for the transformation of synovial macrophages into multinucleated giant cells and the subsequent erosion of bone.

DIAGNOSIS

Physical Examination and History

Clinical Features

Pain is the usual presenting feature of hip arthritis, regardless of the cause. Occasionally, there are symptoms that may differentiate osteoarthritis from inflammatory arthritis; however, both may present with similar symptoms of hip pathology.

Symptoms, at least initially, tend to be mostly mechanical with activity-related pain or pain with certain motions resulting from mechanical irritation or impingement. As the disease progresses and becomes more severe, symptoms may also become more constant and may include pain at rest.

Inflammatory arthritis most commonly has multijoint involvement, either polyarticular or oligoarticular. It is rarely monoarticular involving the hip. Although patients with inflammatory disease may have hip symptoms that are mechanical in nature, these patients tend to have a higher occurrence of constant hip pain or rest pain because of chronic synovitis and hip joint effusion.

Symptoms are typically localized to the groin and proximal anterior thigh (roughly 80% to 90% of patients). Pain often radiates down the anterior thigh toward the knee. Buttock and lateral thigh symptoms also occur in many patients, but these symptoms in isolation are less common. The lateral proximal thigh pain is usually felt more deeply and often more proximally (over the abductor muscles), than symptoms of trochanteric bursitis, which are typically over the posterolateral aspect of the greater trochanter and somewhat more superficial. Occasionally patients present with isolated knee pain; however, this pain tends to be more diffuse and slightly more proximal than pain that originates from the knee.

Physical findings depend on the severity of disease. Loss of motion, typically internal rotation, is one of the initial findings. As the arthritis progresses, motion usually becomes more restricted and may eventually result in a nearly ankylosed hip. Adduction and flexion contractures typically occur. Patients may limp, with a decreased stance phase on the affected side, and may show a positive Duchenne sign because of pain and/or weakness. Patients with inflammatory disease usually have less restriction in range of motion unless the disease has caused severe erosion of the femoral head or a significant protrusio deformity of the acetabulum resulting in a captured femoral head.

Radiologic Features

Joint space narrowing as a result of articular cartilage loss is the general radiographic feature of arthritis. Specific radiographic characteristics help differentiate osteoarthritis from inflammatory arthritis. However, differentiation between these two conditions occasionally can be difficult, and both may be present radiographically.

The radiographic features of osteoarthritis of the hip are joint space narrowing, subchondral sclerosis, degenerative subchondral cysts, and peripheral osteophytes. Occasionally the joint space may still be well maintained, but the appearance is somewhat irregular and other features such as peripheral osteophytes or evidence of prearthritic conditions such as femoroacetabular impingement may be present. Initially, the joint space narrowing is often asymmetrical with either a superomedial or superolateral wear pattern. Eventually the entire joint space may disappear. Radiographic features are more hypertrophic than those seen with inflammatory arthritis (Fig. 3-3).

Inflammatory arthritis tends to show more diffuse symmetrical joint space narrowing with fewer hypertrophic changes. Peripheral osteophytes, although often visible, are usually small. Cystic changes are more evident than with osteoarthritis. Diffuse osteopenia is characteristic of inflammatory changes. The wear pattern is often symmetrical at onset, but may eventually lead to a more medial wear pattern with a protrusio deformity of the acetabulum and superomedial migration of the femoral head (Fig. 3-4).

Radiographic Grading of Osteoarthritis

Various grading systems of osteoarthritis have been described. It must be remembered that approximately 40% to 50% of patients with radiographic changes of osteoarthritis are asymptomatic. Joint space narrowing has been shown to correlate most strongly with clinical symptoms. A number of grading systems are presented in Table 3-2.

Diagnostic Workup Algorithm

The most important investigation for patients presenting with hip pain is to obtain good quality, properly exposed and oriented radiographs with the appropriate views. In a properly oriented anteroposterior pelvis radiograph, the

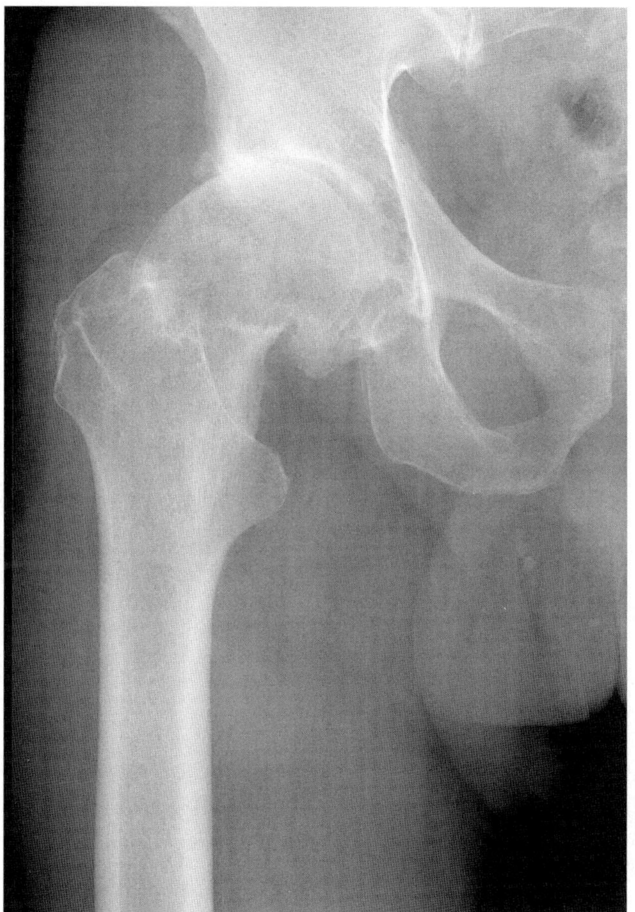

Figure 3-3 Radiographic example of patient with osteoarthritis. Note the superolateral joint space narrowing, bony sclerosis, and large osteophytes. The changes are much more hypertrophic than that seen in inflammatory arthritis.

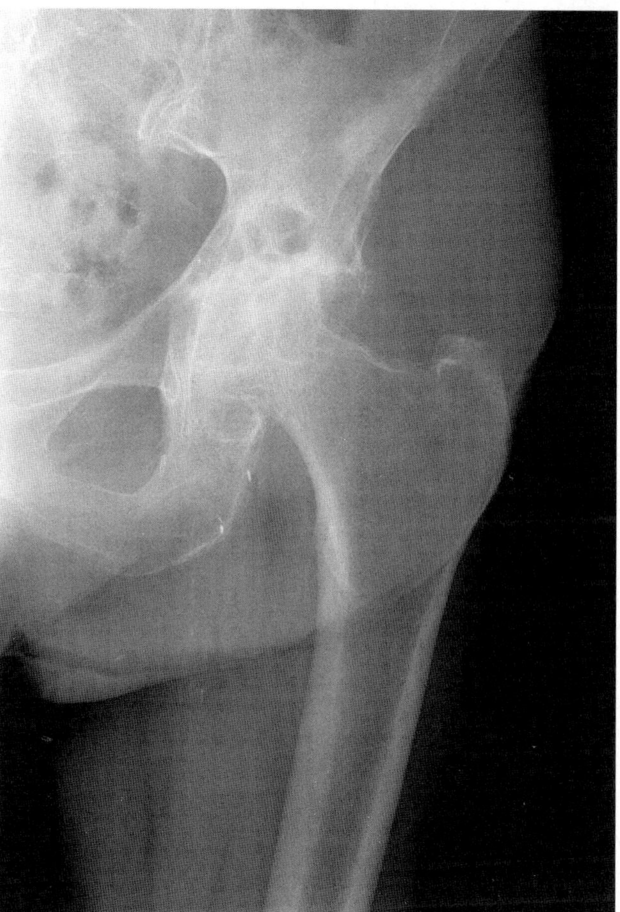

Figure 3-4 Radiographic example of patient with rheumatoid arthritis. Note the symmetrical joint space narrowing with an early protrusio deformity, and cystic changes. Large osteophytes are not present.

TABLE 3-2 RADIOGRAPHIC GRADING OF OSTEOARTHRITIS OF THE HIP

Grade	Tönnis[a]	Kellgren and Lawrence[b]		Croft[c]
0	No signs	None	No features	No changes
1	Slight narrowing of joint space, slight lipping at joint margin, slight sclerosis of femoral head or acetabulum	Doubtful	Minute osteophytes, doubtful significance	Osteophytosis only
2	Small cysts, increased narrowing of joint space, moderate loss of femoral head sphericity	Minimal	Definite osteophytes, unimpaired joint space	Joint space narrowing only
3	Large cysts, severe narrowing or obliteration of joint space, severe deformity of femoral head, avascular necrosis	Moderate	Moderate diminution of joint space	Two of: osteophytosis, joint space narrowing, subchondral sclerosis, and cyst formation
4		Severe	Joint space greatly impaired with subchondral sclerosis	Same as grade 3 but requires three features
5				Same as grade 4, plus deformity of the femoral head

[a]Busse J, Gasteiger W, Tönnis D. Eine neue Methode zur röntgenologischen Beurteilung eines Hüftgelenkes—Der Hüftwert. *Arch Orthop and Trauma Surg*. 1972;72:1–9.
[b]Kellgren JH, Lawrence JS. Radiological assessment of osteoarthrosis. *Ann Rheum Dis*. 1957;16:494–502.
[c]Croft P, Cooper C, Wickham C, Coggan D. Defining osteoarthritis of the hip for epidemiologic studies. *Am J Epidemiol*. 1990;132:514–522.

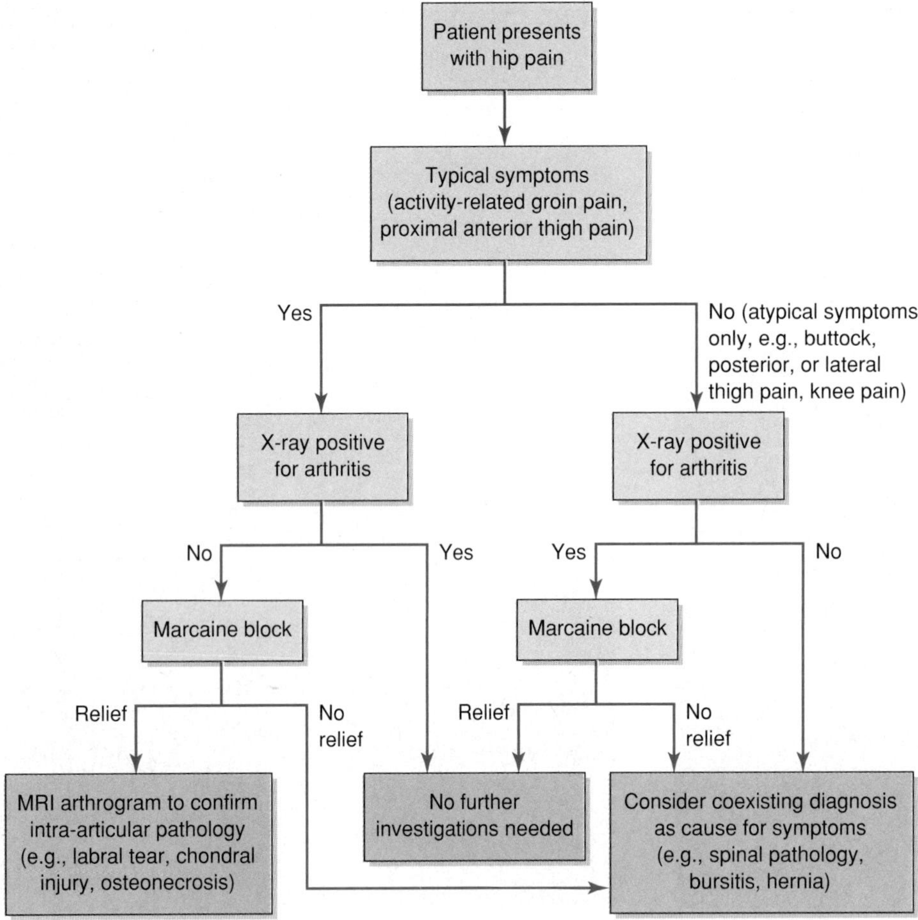

Figure 3-5 Diagnostic algorithm for patients presenting with hip pain.

obturator foramina appear symmetrical and the coccyx projects approximately 1 cm above the pubic symphysis. A true lateral radiograph also should be obtained with attention focused on the contour of the anterior femoral head/neck junction and also the anterior acetabulum. Together with a thorough history, the large majority of conditions can be diagnosed with the use of plain radiographs.

Many patients who present with hip pain will have radiographic features of arthritis. If the clinical presentation correlates with the radiographs, then no further investigations are necessary. Patients who present with radiographic changes of arthritis but whose symptoms are atypical (isolated buttock, lateral hip or knee pain) may be further evaluated with an intra-articular local anesthetic injection placed under fluoroscopic guidance. If the symptoms are temporarily relieved by the injection, then hip pathology is highly likely. Patients who present with symptoms of hip pathology but whose radiographs appear normal, despite close scrutiny for conditions such as mild dysplasia, femoroacetabular impingement, or retroverted acetabulum, may require further investigation, usually with an MRI scan. If intra-articular pathology such as a labral tear is suspected, then a gadolinium arthrogram MRI is most valuable. Figure 3-5 outlines a diagnostic algorithm for patients presenting with hip pain.

TREATMENT

The most common surgical procedure for hip arthritis is total hip replacement. However, various other procedures are indicated for certain conditions. A more detailed discussion of specific management will be presented in subsequent chapters. For an overview, see Table 3-3.

Surgical Indications

Persistent hip pain, despite nonoperative management, is the usual indication for surgery. Occasionally patients complain more of restricted function and less of pain, but it is generally the pain that results in the restricted function and is the reason why patients seek hip replacement surgery. Prior to surgery, patients should receive an appropriate coarse of nonoperative management. For osteoarthritis, this includes activity modification, weight control if feasible, the use of walking aids, and medications (nonnarcotic analgesics and nonsteroidal anti-inflammatory medications). Presently, the routine use of corticosteroid or hyaluronate hip injections cannot be recommended. Patients with inflammatory arthritis are generally under the care of a rheumatologist or internist for nonoperative

TABLE 3-3 SURGICAL OPTIONS FOR PATIENTS WITH OSTEOARTHRITIS OR PREARTHRITIC CONDITIONS

Procedure	Condition
Labral debridement	- Labral tear in isolation (likely a very rare situation—tears are usually associated with other boney conditions)
Anterior acetabular rim resection	- Acetabular torsion/version abnormality (pincer type FAI, coxa profunda, retroverted acetabulum)
Anterolateral femoral neck resection	- Poor femoral head/neck offset (cam type FAI)
Proximal femoral osteotomy	- Proximal femoral deformity (e.g., trauma, slipped epiphysis, Legg-Perthes)
Periacetabular osteotomy (PAO)	- Classic dysplasia (correct anterolateral deficiency)
	- Retroverted acetabulum (reverse PAO for posterior deficiency)
Total hip replacement	- Moderate and advanced arthritis

FAI, femoral acetabular impingement; PAO, periacetabular osteotomy.

management. However, when considering surgery, certain considerations must be addressed; these are discussed below.

When total hip replacement is being considered, there is rarely a disadvantage in delaying surgery as long as the patient is able to maintain function. However, for conditions that may be considered prearthritic (e.g., femoroacetabular impingement, dysplasia without arthritic changes) there may be some merit in recommending joint-sparing surgery when symptoms initially begin or are relatively mild, rather than have the patient undergo a protracted coarse of nonoperative treatment. Symptoms should still be significant enough to justify the risks of surgery, but a long extensive coarse of nonoperative management may be counterproductive because further cartilage damage may occur during this time period. The goal of nonarthroplasty joint-preservation surgery is to relieve symptoms and if possible, also to alter the natural history and prevent or delay the onset of arthritic changes; hence there may be an optimum window of time in which such surgery is most successful. Unfortunately, definitive data on altering of the natural history by joint-preservation surgery is still lacking.

Surgical Considerations

Prior to surgery, patients with both noninflammatory and inflammatory arthritis should be counseled as to the risks, possible complications, and usual recovery related to the procedure. Patients should be medically stable, and any chronic medical conditions should be assessed preoperatively and optimized prior to surgery. This includes maintaining proper nutrition and also eliminating potential sources of infection by specifically asking about their dental history or any urinary problems. A careful skin evaluation is also necessary.

Patients with inflammatory arthritis have unique concerns that require consideration before surgery. These concerns include polyarticular disease, medication used for management of inflammatory disease, as well as unique reconstructive challenges because of bone deformity or loss. Patients with inflammatory arthritis, particularly rheumatoid disease, generally have polyarticular involvement. Prior to surgery, C-spine lateral flexion and extension views are necessary to exclude C1-C2 instability. Additionally, in most circumstances, lower extremity surgery should be planned prior to upper extremity surgery and hip replacement prior to knee replacement when both are needed. It is more difficult for the patient to regain knee motion if there is significant hip disease. Patients with inflammatory disease are often on immunosuppressive agents (corticosteroids, disease-modifying antirheumatic drugs—e.g., methotrexate, TNF-α antagonists). The use of these before surgery should be reduced if possible or temporarily discontinued. This is particularly true for TNF-α antagonists, which are potent immune suppressors; continued use during the perioperative period may increase the risk of infection. Last, patients with rheumatoid arthritis often have osteopenic bone, which is at increased risk of intraoperative fracture. These patients may also have acetabular bone loss related to a protrusio deformity, which may require bone grafting or the use of special implants (e.g., deep profile cup or in severe cases an acetabular reconstruction cage). As in all reconstructive cases, appropriate surgical planning is necessary to anticipate and have available any special implants, instruments, or bone graft that may be required.

SUGGESTED READINGS

Felson DT. Obesity and vocational and avocational overload of the joint as risk factors for osteoarthritis. *J Rheumatol*. 2004;31 (suppl 70):2–5.

Ganz R, Parvizi J, Beck M, et al. Femoroacetabular impingement. A cause for osteoarthritis of the hip. *Clin Orthop*. 2003;417:112–120.

Gelber AC. Obesity and hip osteoarthritis: the weight of the evidence is increasing. *Am J Med.* 2003;114:158–159.

Giori NJ, Trousdale RT. Acetabular retroversion is associated with osteoarthritis of the hip. *Clin Orthop.* 2003;417:263–269.

Harris WH, Bourne RB, Oh I. Intra-articular acetabular labrum: a possible etiological factor in certain cases of osteoarthritis of the hip. *J Bone Joint Surg.* 1979;61A:510–514.

Karlson EW, Mandl LA, Aweh GN, et al. Total hip replacement due to osteoarthritis: the importance of age, obesity and other modifiable risk factors. *Am J Med.* 2003;114:93–98.

Klippel JH, ed. *Primer on the Rheumatic Diseases.* 12th ed. The Arthritis Foundation, Altanta, Georgia; 2001.

Li PLS, Ganz R. Morphologic features of congenital acetabular dysplasia. One in six is retroverted. *Clin Orthop.* 2003;416:245–253.

MacGregor AJ, Antoniades L, Matson M, et al. The genetic contribution to radiographic hip osteoarthritis in women. *Arthritis Rheum.* 2000;43:2410–2416.

Radin EL. Who gets osteoarthritis and why? *J Rheumatol.* 2004;31(suppl 70):10–15.

Reynolds D, Lucas J, Klaue K. Retroversion of the acetabulum: a cause of hip pain. *J Bone Joint Surg.* 1999;81B:281–288.

Siebenrock KA, Wahab KHA, Werlen S, et al. Abnormal extension of the femoral head epiphysis as a cause of cam impingement. *Clin Orthop.* 2004;418:54–60.

OSTEONECROSIS OF THE FEMORAL HEAD

4

FRANK A. PETRIGLIANO
JAY R. LIEBERMAN

Osteonecrosis (ON) of the femoral head is a progressive disease that if left untreated often results in subchondral fracture, collapse of the femoral head, and debilitating arthrosis. The precise pathophysiology of ON remains unclear; however, it appears to be the final common pathway of either traumatic or atraumatic factors that compromise the tenuous circulation of the femoral head. The disease typically affects young patients, thereby significantly impacting both work and leisure activity. Accordingly, early diagnosis and treatment are crucial to limit the progression of ON and the subsequent need for total hip arthroplasty. In many cases, however, diagnosis is made in later stages of the disease, when femoral head–preserving treatments are no longer effective. This chapter discusses the natural history of ON, the current diagnostic and treatment options for both early and late stages of the disease, and the limitations of these existing therapies.

PATHOGENESIS

Epidemiology

Osteonecrosis is observed in 10% to 25% of hip dislocations, with increased risk associated with prolonged duration of dislocation.[1,2] The incidence of traumatic ON of the femoral head following nondisplaced femoral neck fractures is approximately 10%, whereas the incidence following displaced fractures ranges from 15% to 50% and generally correlates with the degree of displacement, time until reduction, and accuracy of reduction.[3,4] The true incidence of atraumatic ON is unknown; however, some studies in Western populations show that about 10% of all total hip arthroplasties are performed for ON, leading to estimates that there are at least 20,000 to 30,000 new cases per year in the United States.[5] The disease affects men four times more frequently than women and generally presents in the third to fifth decades of life. Atraumatic ON is bilateral in 30% to 70% of patients at the initial time of presentation; however, the stage of disease typically presents asymmetrically.[6]

Etiology

A number of traumatic and atraumatic factors are associated with the development of ON of the femoral head. Mechanical interruption of the blood supply to the femoral head has been identified as the causative factor of ON following femoral neck fracture or hip dislocation.[7] Conversely, the precise genesis of atraumatic ON is unclear, but it has been associated with numerous risk factors and underlying clinical conditions (Table 4-1). It is hypothesized that these etiologic factors either result in a compromise of the blood supply of the subchondral region of the femoral head or have direct toxic effect on cells, resulting in cellular necrosis and impaired remodeling potential of the subchondral bone with eventual collapse of the compromised region.

Corticosteroid and alcohol use, thrombophilias, gout, hyperlipidemia, renal osteodystrophy, sickle cell anemia, caisson disease, and other systemic disorders have all been associated with ON of the femoral head. Of these recognized risk factors, corticosteroid use and alcohol abuse are the most commonly implicated, representing 90% of new cases of ON.[8] High-dose oral steroid regimens have a stronger association with ON as compared with low-dose therapy.[7,9] However, in a study of liver transplant patients receiving immunosuppressive corticosteroids, no association was noted between steroid dose and the development of ON.[10] It appears that transplant patients who develop ON demonstrate an idiosyncratic response to the drug secondary to an underlying hypercoagulability or hypofibrinolysis. With some diseases such as liver and renal failure, it is difficult to separate the effects of corticosteroids on bone from those of the underlying disease. Defining the quantity of alcohol intake that increases the risk of ON has been problematic. One prospective study suggested that patients who consume over 400 mL of alcohol per week were 9.8 times likely to develop ON versus nondrinkers.[11] Additionally, an increasing number of reports document a relationship between human immunodeficiency virus (HIV) infection and ON of the hip.[12] The causal relationship is difficult to establish because many of these patients have numerous concomitant risk factors; however, there is some evidence implicating antiviral therapy as a causative agent.[13]

TABLE 4-1 RISK FACTORS ASSOCIATED WITH OSTEONECROSIS OF THE FEMORAL HEAD

Traumatic
Displaced hip fractures
Hip dislocation
Iatrogenic injury secondary to anterograde medullary nailing

Atraumatic
High-dose corticosteroid use
Alcohol abuse
Smoking
Thrombophilias
Renal osteodystrophy
Solid organ transplantation
Hemoglobinopathies
Human immunodeficiency virus infection
Gaucher disease
Hyperlipidemia
Pancreatitis
Radiation therapy
Chemotherapy
Liver disease
Gout
Systemic lupus erythematosus
Caisson disease

Although each of the etiologic possibilities must be considered, it is important to recognize that the vast majority of patients with the aforementioned risk factors do not develop ON, and in other patients, no risk factor is identified, underscoring the multifactorial genesis of this disease.

Pathophysiology

The exact mechanisms underlying the pathophysiology of atraumatic ON of the femoral head are not clearly defined; however, several theories have implicated both intravascular and extravascular factors that may contribute to this pathologic process. Each of these phenomena shares the final outcome of ischemia, cellular necrosis, and failure of remodeling of the subchondral bone. Osteocyte death has been attributed to alterations in blood flow that may be the result of local or systemic factors. Following fracture or dislocation, disruption of the lateral retinacular arteries may compromise the primary blood supply of the femoral head. This precarious arterial blood supply may also be altered by intravascular microemboli that are generated by systemic diseases including the thrombophilias, sickle cell disease, fat emboli resulting from hyperlipidemia, or air embolization secondary to dysbaric phenomena.[7,8,12] Local hyperlipidemia and intravascular lipid deposits have also been noted in patients with corticosteroid and alcohol use, suggesting a causal role for these agents.

The local osseous architecture of the femoral head may predispose the region to extravascular compression and local ischemia. The cancellous bone within the subchondral region of the femoral head is enclosed within rigid cortical bone. This system is particularly susceptible to increases in pressure, and the venous outflow can be exquisitely sensitive to compression. Disorders in fat metabolism, generated by corticosteroid or alcohol use, may cause both adipocytes and osteocytes to hypertrophy, resulting in local microvascular compression.[7,8,12] In Gaucher disease, macrophages enlarge as they accumulate sphingolipids, resulting in a similar compressive phenomenon. The direct cytotoxic effects of alcohol and corticosteroids have also been implicated in osteocyte necrosis and may inhibit osteogenic differentiation of mesenchymal stromal cells.[14,15]

DIAGNOSIS

Physical Examination and History

Clinical Features

A prompt diagnosis of ON allows for earlier treatment, which may result in a more favorable outcome. A thorough history focused on determining associated risk factors should be undertaken. Patients may not have any specific complaints during the early stages of the disease; however, with progression, patients will complain of deep groin pain with ambulation or pain referred to the knee. The onset of pain may be insidious or acute in nature and is typically described as throbbing; night pain and morning stiffness are not uncommon. The findings on physical examination are variable. Some patients have a complete, pain-free, range of motion of the hip and walk without a limp. Others have a limp and discomfort with active and passive range of motion. Collapse of the femoral head is associated with painful internal rotation and a limited range of motion. Individuals with chronic symptoms may have a flexion contracture. It is of utmost importance that the contralateral hip be examined, as bilateral disease is common. Because some patients may develop ON without the existence of any risk factors, an index of suspicion must be developed for young patients with persistent groin pain that is unresponsive to rest and activity modification.

Radiographic Features

Plain Radiographs. The primary diagnostic workup should include plain anteroposterior and frog-leg lateral radiographs to determine the status of the femoral head. The early stages of the disease may not be visible on plain radiographs, but over time, a predictable pattern of radiographic change becomes evident. This sequence begins with radiolucencies and sclerosis in the femoral head, resulting from bone resorption and new bone formation. Progressive microfractures may result in a pathognomonic crescent sign, most readily visible on frog-leg lateral views (Fig. 4-1A). This represents precollapse of the weakened necrotic subchondral bone. The necrotic angle (measured referencing the center of the femoral head) can be calculated from plain films to stage the size of the necrotic region. This value is the sum of the angle of the necrotic segment as measured on both the anteroposterior and lateral radiographs. Patients with a necrotic angle >200 degrees

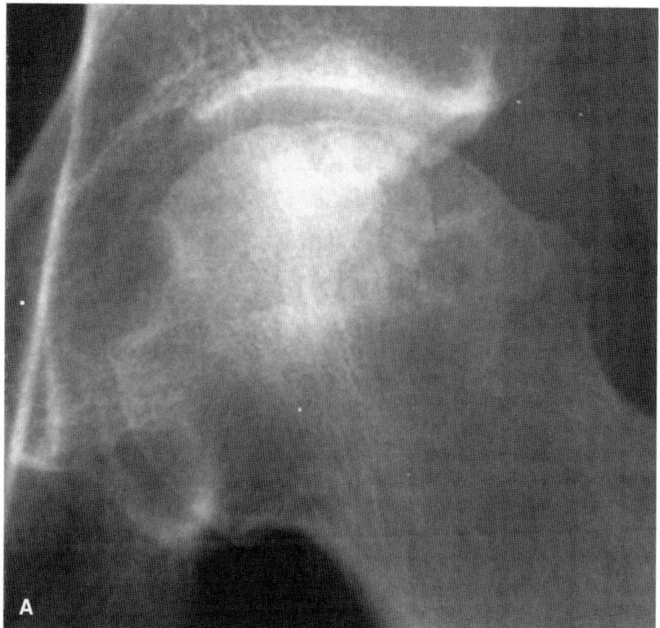

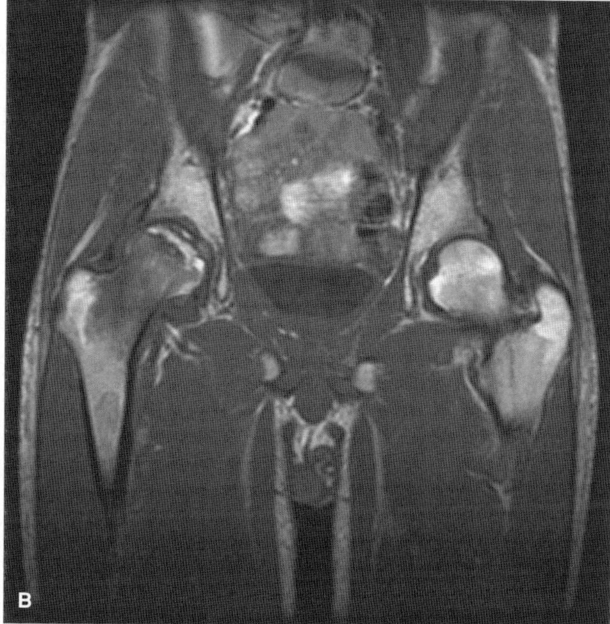

Figure 4-1 Plain radiograph of the hip demonstrating adjacent sclerosis and lucency along with subchondral collapse or crescent sign (**A**). T1-weighted MRI illustrating low signal at the normal-ischemic bone interface (**B**).

have less favorable results following certain femoral-head sparing procedures.[16] The end stage of the disease manifests as a complete collapse of the femoral head and subsequent arthritic changes noted on both the femoral head and acetabulum.

Magnetic Resonance Imaging. Magnetic resonance imaging (MRI) has become the standard in diagnosing ON and should be obtained in all suspected cases in which the plain radiographs are normal. In such cases, examination of both hips should be performed because more than half of all cases are bilateral. The changes noted on T1-weighted images typically include subchondral signal changes located in the anterior superior quadrant of the femoral head with a single-density line demarcating the normal-ischemic bone interface (Fig. 4-1B). The T2-weighted images may demonstrate a high-signal line inside a low-signal region (double-line sign). As lesion size has been associated with prognosis and response to therapy, MRI can be used to determine lesion size or volume.[17]

Radiographic Staging

The most widely recognized radiographic staging system was proposed by Arlet and Ficat in the 1960s and has undergone subsequent modification (Table 4-2).[18] This classification relies solely on plain radiographs, which are often unrevealing early in the disease. Steinberg et al. have proposed a radiographic classification that incorporates plain x-ray, bone scan, and MRI findings to create a comprehensive and specific description that may be more effective in characterizing the progression of the disease (Table 4-2).[19] Moreover, this system considers volumetric assessment of femoral head involvement that may have predictive value in the outcomes of specific interventions.

Diagnostic Workup Algorithm

For young patients presenting with hip pain, a thorough history focused on delineating risk factors for the development of ON should be obtained. However, other causes of hip pain should be considered. An examination of the spine should be performed to rule out lumbar pathology. In cases where infection is suspected, hip aspiration may prove useful. Plain anteroposterior and frog-leg lateral radiographs of both hips should be obtained to evaluate for sclerosis or collapse of the femoral head in ON, but these studies may also reveal other painful conditions including hip dysplasia or neoplasm. When plain radiographs are normal, or sclerosis of the femoral head is noted, MRI examination of the affected and the contralateral hip should be undertaken. In pregnant females or males in the fifth decade of life, it is important to consider transient osteoporosis of the hip (TOH), which, if diagnosed, is self-limited. Unlike the localized changes found in ON, TOH demonstrates diffuse osteopenia on plain radiographs, and the MRI often has a global decrease in T1-weighted signal throughout the femoral head and neck metaphysis (Fig. 4-2) and a global increase in the T2-weighted signal in the same regions. Treatment includes protected weight bearing until the condition resolves, which may take up to 6 months.[9] Figure 4-3 presents a diagnostic workup algorithm.

TREATMENT

Patient age, activity level, and general constitution must be considered in conjunction with radiographic and clinical

TABLE 4-2 RADIOGRAPHIC CLASSIFICATIONS OF OSTEONECROSIS OF THE FEMORAL HEAD

Ficat and Arlet
Stage I
Normal
Stage II
Sclerotic or cystic lesions
Stage III
Subchondral collapse
Stage IV
Osteoarthritis with articular collapse

University of Pennsylvania
Stage 0
Normal or nondiagnostic radiograph, bone scan, and MRI
Stage I
Normal radiograph; abnormal bone scan and/or MRI
A: Mild (<15% of head affected)
B: Moderate (15% to 30% of head affected)
C: Severe (>30% of head affected)
Stage II
Lucent and sclerotic changes in the femoral head
A: Mild (<15% of head affected)
B: Moderate (15% to 30% of head affected)
C: Severe (>30% of head affected)
Stage III
Subchondral collapse (crescent sign) without flattening
A: Mild (<15% of head affected)
B: Moderate (15% to 30% of head affected)
C: Severe (>30% of head affected)
Stage IV
Flattening of the femoral head
A: Mild (<15% of head affected)
B: Moderate (15% to 30% of head affected)
C: Severe (>30% of head affected)
Stage V
Joint narrowing and/or acetabular changes
A: Mild
B: Moderate
C: Severe
Stage VI
Advanced degenerative changes

(Modified from Ficat P, Arlet J. Functional investigation of bone under normal conditions. In: Ficat P, Arlet J, Hungerford DS, eds. *Ischemia and Necroses of Bone*. Baltimore: Williams & Wilkins; 1961; and Steinberg ME, Hayken GD, Steinberg DR. A quantitative system for staging avascular necrosis. *J Bone Joint Surg Br*. 1995;77[1]:34–41.)

findings to formulate a treatment plan. Young, healthy patients without significant acetabular disease will generally be better served by procedures that attempt to preserve the femoral head. Conversely, arthroplasty may be an excellent option for patients with collapse of the femoral head or acetabular involvement. It is important to recognize that the indications for existing treatment regimens remain controversial and are often dictated by the surgeon's clinical expertise and familiarity with available surgical options.

Nonoperative Management

The role of nonoperative modalities in the treatment of ON of the femoral head remains limited. The prescription of protected weight-bearing regimens in forestalling the progression of disease has proven ineffective in most cases.[6,20] This approach may be reserved for those patients who are incapable of tolerating a surgical intervention or are of limited life expectancy. Other nonoperative modalities including electrical stimulation and hyperbaric oxygen have been evaluated in the treatment of ON. These modalities have demonstrated varying success in preventing collapse of the femoral head.[21,22] More recently, the results of extracorporeal shock-wave therapy were compared with those of core decompression and bone grafting. The authors concluded that extracorporeal shock-wave treatment appeared to be more effective than core decompression and nonvascularized fibular grafting in patients with early-stage ON of the femoral head.[23] The role of pharmacologic therapies in the treatment of ON has not been well defined and requires further investigation. Antihyperlipidemic, antihypertensive, and anticoagulant medications all have been proposed as candidate treatment agents. Most recently, the bisphosphonate alendronate has been shown to be effective in delaying the progression of femoral head collapse in a cohort of patients with early-stage disease.[24] Again, long-term evaluation is mandated to determine if this agent truly prevents, rather than merely retards, collapse of the femoral head.

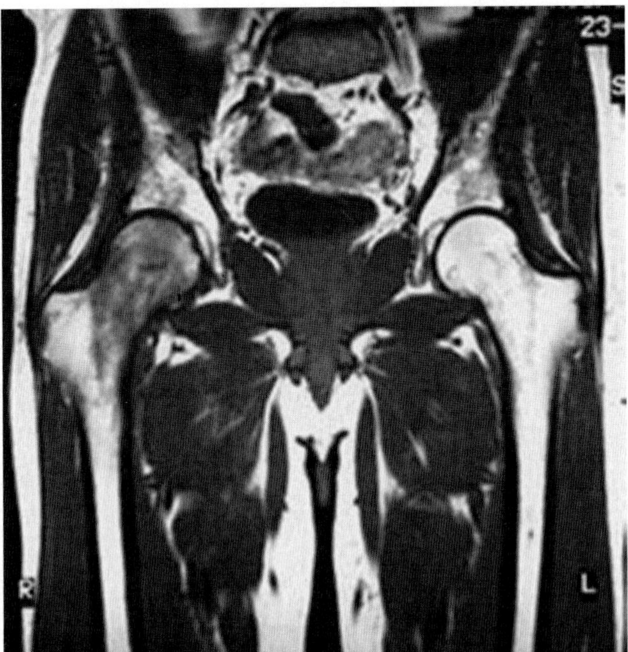

Figure 4-2 T1-weighted MRI with low-intensity signal representing bone marrow edema in the femoral head, neck, and metaphysis consistent with transient osteoporosis of the hip. The left hip appears normal.

Operative Management

Many femoral head–sparing procedures have been used in attempts to prevent collapse, arthrosis, and the subsequent need for arthroplasty. Currently, core decompression is the most commonly used and most comprehensively studied treatment for early-stage ON of the femoral head. Originally described by Ficat and Arlet as a diagnostic intervention,

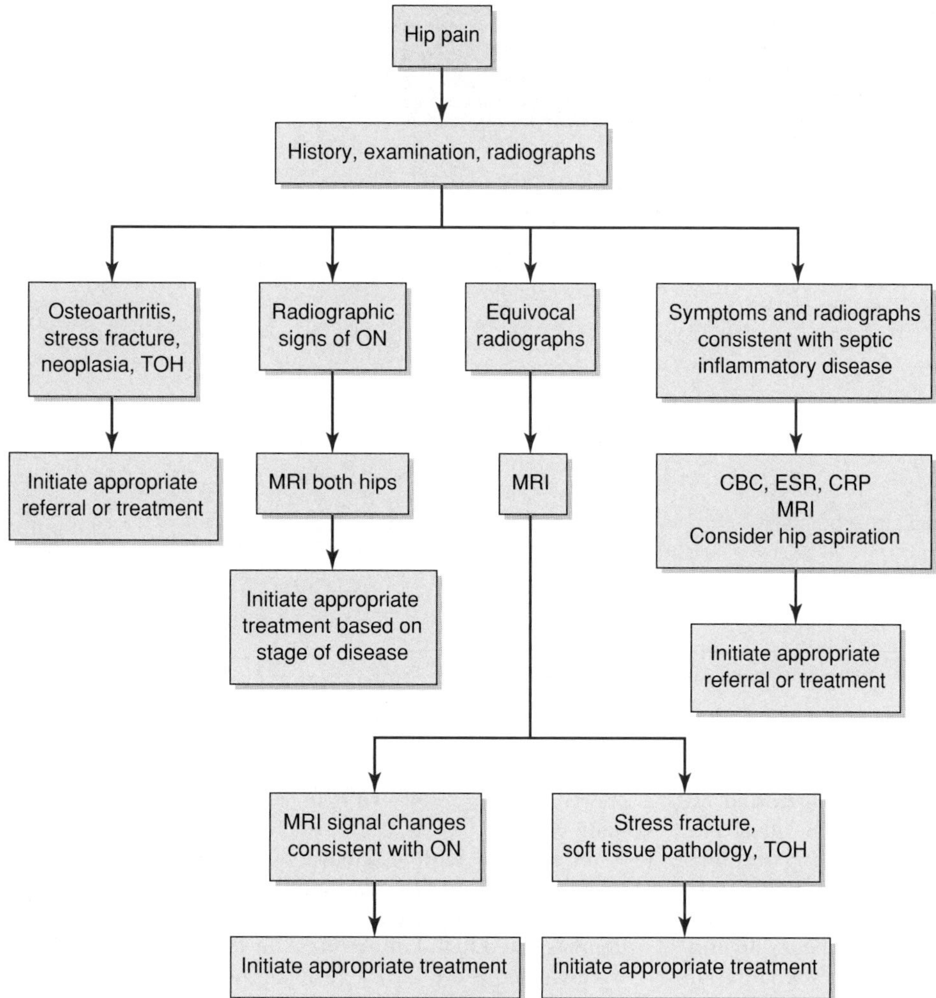

Figure 4-3 Diagnostic algorithm for osteonecrosis of the hip. CBC, complete blood count; ESR, erythrocyte sedimentation rate; CRP, C-reactive protein; MRI, magnetic resonance imaging; ON, osteonecrosis; TOH, transient osteoporosis of the hip.

core decompression was found to alleviate pain, presumably by reducing femoral head pressure and restoring physiologic blood flow.[7] Eventually core decompression was adopted as a treatment modality. The procedure involves creating a decompression tract from the lateral cortex of the femur to the area of necrosis, the diameter of which can range from 9 to 12 mm depending on the diameter of the femoral neck. A biopsy is usually obtained at the time of surgery, and protected weight bearing is advised for a minimum of 6 weeks following the procedure. Although the success rates following the procedure are variable, for small and medium-sized precollapse lesions, the results of core decompression are generally 80% to 90% successful.[25] However, the results are poor in the presence of a crescent sign or definitive collapse of the femoral head.[26,27]

More recently, vascularized fibular bone grafting has been advocated for treating early-stage disease. Vascularized fibular grafts have the potential advantage of providing structural support, osteoconductive factors, osteoinductive factors, and a vascular supply to the necrotic region. However, this procedure requires a longer operation and is associated with donor site morbidity, ankle instability, peroneal nerve palsy, heterotopic ossification, and subtrochanteric fracture.[28–30] Patients may not bear weight for a minimum of 6 weeks following the procedure and may be only partially weight bearing for an additional 3 to 5 months. The relative benefit of vascularized fibular graft versus nonvascularized graft or core decompression has yet to be conclusively proven. However, reported results are satisfactory in hips that do not have significant head depression.[28–30]

Bone grafting of the femoral head with demineralized bone matrix is an appealing option because it may enhance healing without significantly altering the anatomy of the femoral neck if arthroplasty is necessary. Biologic adjuvants including growth factors (such as VEGF, BMP) and autologous bone marrow cells may also play a role in treating osteonecrotic lesions and have prompted a great deal of clinical interest. Lieberman et al. demonstrated that allograft bone grafts in combination with BMP prevented radiographic progression of ON in 14 of 17 hips at an average follow-up of 53 months.[31] Randomized trials evaluating the efficacy of these agents in preventing femoral head collapse are necessary.

Intertrochanteric osteotomy is an effective treatment option for carefully selected patients with ON of the femoral head. The goal of osteotomy in these patients is to reposition the necrotic segment away from the weight-bearing

TABLE 4-3 TREATMENT ALGORITHM ACCORDING TO THE UNIVERSITY OF PENNSYLVANIA SYSTEM OF CLASSIFICATION AND STAGING (RADIOGRAPHIC STAGE, SYMPTOMS, AND PROCEDURE)

I and II
Asymptomatic
Observation, pharmacologic treatment, possible core decompression ± bone grafting

IA, IB, IC, IIA, IIB, and IIC
Symptomatic
Core decompression ± bone grafting, vascularized graft

IC, IIC, IIIA, IIIB, IIIC, and IVA
Symptomatic
Bone grafting (vascularized or nonvascularized), osteotomy, limited femoral head resurfacing, total hip arthroplasty

IVB and IVC
Symptomatic
Limited femoral head resurfacing, total hip arthroplasty

V and VI
Symptomatic
Total hip arthroplasty

(Adapted from Lieberman JR, et al. Osteonecrosis of the hip: management in the 21st century. *J Bone Joint Surg Am*. 2002;84-A:834–853.)

surface and bring normal articular cartilage supported by healthy bone into the weight-bearing area. The ideal patient for this procedure is a young adult possessing a mobile hip with a small isolated lesion who does not require corticosteroids or abuse alcohol.[20,32] The type of osteotomy will be contingent on the size and location of the lesion and may include intertrochanteric, rotational transtrochanteric, valgus flexion, or varus intertrochanteric osteotomies. Outcomes following osteotomies are better in small or medium-size lesions of early stage whereas these procedures are less predictable following femoral head collapse.[20] These technically demanding procedures should be performed only by experienced surgeons, and subsequent conversion to a total hip arthroplasty may be difficult.

Collapse of the femoral head and the development of arthrosis are indications for reconstructive procedures. Failure rates for total hip arthroplasties (THA) and hemiarthroplasties in this cohort are higher than failure rates for other diagnoses, which is most likely attributable to the relative youth of the patients and the lack of other factors limiting physical activity.[33] Accordingly, temporizing procedures have evolved to address this difficult-to-treat group of patients. Joint resurfacing, or surface arthroplasty, has been proposed as a means of providing pain relief to patients who are deemed too young for conventional arthroplasty. Hemiresurfacing uses a cemented hemispheric femoral head prosthesis that is matched to the patient's native acetabulum. This mode of resurfacing may be considered for patients with little or no acetabular disease. In the presence of significant articular cartilage degeneration, a total resurfacing procedure (which incorporates a prosthetic acetabular component in addition to the femoral resurfacing) may be considered. Although these resurfacing procedures have demonstrated clinical promise, the current short- and long-term results for resurfacing procedures remain variable.[33–35]

In patients with extensive femoral head involvement and end-stage arthrosis, total hip replacement is indicated. Although early studies evaluating THA in patients demonstrated high failure rates, newer surgical techniques have yielded more favorable results.[36,37] With the advent of highly cross-linked polyethylene, metal-on-metal, and ceramic-on-ceramic weight-bearing surfaces, patients with ON may have more favorable success rates with total hip arthroplasty, obviating the need for multiple surgeries. A treatment algorithm based on radiographic stage and clinical symptom proposed by Lieberman et al. is outlined in Table 4-3.[9]

REFERENCES

1. Brav EA. Traumatic dislocation of the hip. Army experience and results over a twelve year period. *J Bone Joint Surg Am*. 1962;44:1115–1134.
2. Upadhyay SS, Moulton A. The long-term results of traumatic posterior dislocation of the hip. *J Bone Joint Surg Br*. 1981;63B(4):548–551.
3. Barnes R, Brown JT, Garden RS, et al. Subcapital fractures of the femur. A prospective review. *J Bone Joint Surg Br*. 1976;58(1):2–24.
4. Garden RS. Malreduction and avascular necrosis in subcapital fractures of the femur. *J Bone Joint Surg Br*. 1971;53(2):183–197.
5. Hungerford DS, Jones LC. Asymptomatic osteonecrosis: should it be treated? *Clin Orthop Relat Res*. 2004(429):124–130.
6. Bradway JK, Morrey BF. The natural history of the silent hip in bilateral atraumatic osteonecrosis. *J Arthroplasty*. 1993;8(4):383–387.
7. Lavernia CJ, Sierra RJ, Grieco FR. Osteonecrosis of the femoral head. *J Am Acad Orthop Surg*. 1999;7(4):250–261.

8. Mont MA, Hungerford DS. Non-traumatic avascular necrosis of the femoral head. *J Bone Joint Surg Am*. 1995;77(3):459–474.
9. Lieberman JR, Berry DJ, Mont MA, et al. Osteonecrosis of the hip: management in the 21st century. *Instr Course Lect*. 2003;52:337–355.
10. Lieberman JR, Scaduto AA, Wellmeyer E. Symptomatic osteonecrosis of the hip after orthotopic liver transplantation. *J Arthroplasty*. 2000;15:767–771.
11. Matsuo K, Hirohata T, Sugioka Y, et al. Influence of alcohol intake, cigarette smoking, and occupational status on idiopathic osteonecrosis of the femoral head. *Clin Orthop Relat Res*. 1988;234:115–123.
12. Jones LC, Hungerford DS. Osteonecrosis: etiology, diagnosis, and treatment. *Curr Opin Rheumatol*. 2004;16(4):443–449.
13. Siddiqui SA, Smith AM, Mashoof AA, et al. Osteonecrosis of the femoral head in patients infected with HIV: a report of 4 cases and literature review. *Am J Orthop*. 2004;33:618–622.
14. Hernigou P, Beaujean F, Lambotte JC. Decrease in the mesenchymal stem-cell pool in the proximal femur in corticosteroid-induced osteonecrosis. *J Bone Joint Surg Br*. 1999;81(2):349–355.
15. Suh KT, Kim SW, Roh HK, et al. Decreased osteogenic differentiation of mesenchymal stem cells in alcohol-induced osteonecrosis. *Clin Orthop Relat Res*. 2005;431:220–225.
16. Beaule PE, Amstutz HC. Management of Ficat stage III and IV osteonecrosis of the hip. *J Am Acad Orthop Surg*. 2004;12(2):96–105.
17. Cherian SF, Laorr A, Saleh KJ, et al. Quantifying the extent of femoral head involvement in osteonecrosis. *J Bone Joint Surg Am*. 2003;85-A(2):309–315.
18. Ficat P, Arlet J. Functional investigation of bone under normal conditions. In: Ficat P, Arlet J, Hungerford DS, eds. *Ischemia and Necrosis of Bone*. Baltimore: Williams & Wilkins; 1961.
19. Steinberg ME, Hayken GD, Steinberg DR. A quantitative system for staging avascular necrosis. *J Bone Joint Surg Br*. 1995;77(1):34–41.
20. Khanuja HS, Mont MA, Etienne G, et al. Treatment algorithm for osteonecrosis of the hip. *Tech Orthop*. 2001;16(1):80–89.
21. Aaron RK. Treatment of osteonecrosis of the femoral head with electrical stimulation. *Instr Course Lect*. 1994;43:495–458.
22. Reis ND, Schwartz O, Militianu D, et al. Hyperbaric oxygen therapy as a treatment for stage-I avascular necrosis of the femoral head. *J Bone Joint Surg Br*. 2003;85(3):371–375.
23. Wang CJ, Wang FS, Huang CC, et al. Treatment for osteonecrosis of the femoral head: comparison of extracorporeal shock waves with core decompression and bone-grafting. *J Bone Joint Surg Am*. 2005;87:2380–2387.
24. Lai KA, Shen WJ, Yang CY, et al. The use of alendronate to prevent early collapse of the femoral head in patients with nontraumatic osteonecrosis. A randomized clinical study. *J Bone Joint Surg Am*. 2005;87:2155–2159.
25. Lieberman JR. Core decompression for osteonecrosis of the hip. *Clin Orthop Relat Res*. 2004;418:29–33.
26. Smith SW, Fehring TK, Griffin WL, et al. Core decompression of the osteonecrotic femoral head. *J Bone Joint Surg Am*. 1995;77:674–680.
27. Fairbank AC, Bahtia D, Jinnah RH, et al. Long-term results of core decompression for ischaemic necrosis of the femoral head. *J Bone Joint Surg Br*. 1995;77(1):42–49.
28. Kim SY, Kim YG, Kim PT, et al. Vascularized compared with nonvascularized fibular grafts for large osteonecrotic lesions of the femoral head. *J Bone Joint Surg Am*. 2005;87:2012–2018.
29. Marciniak D, Furey C, Shaffer JW. Osteonecrosis of the femoral head. A study of 101 hips treated with vascularized fibular grafting. *J Bone Joint Surg* Am. 2005;87:742–747.
30. Zhang C, Zeng B, Xu Z, et al. Treatment of femoral head necrosis with free vascularized fibula grafting: a preliminary report. *Microsurgery*. 2005;25(4):305–309.
31. Lieberman JR, Conduah A, Urist MR. Treatment of osteonecrosis of the femoral head with core decompression and human bone morphogenetic protein. *Clin Orthop Relat Res*. 2004;429:139–145.
32. Shannon BD, Trousdale RT. Femoral osteotomies for avascular necrosis of the femoral head. *Clin Orthop Relat Res*. 2004;418:34–40.
33. Schmalzried TP. Total resurfacing for osteonecrosis of the hip. *Clin Orthop Relat Res*. 2004;429:151–156.
34. Adili A, Trousdale RT. Femoral head resurfacing for the treatment of osteonecrosis in the young patient. *Clin Orthop Relat Res*. 2003;417:93–101.
35. Grecula MJ. Resurfacing arthroplasty in osteonecrosis of the hip. *Orthop Clin North Am*. 2005;36(2):231–242.
36. Kim YH, Oh SH, Kim JS, et al. Contemporary total hip arthroplasty with and without cement in patients with osteonecrosis of the femoral head. *J Bone Joint Surg Am*. 2003;85-A(4):675–681.
37. Nich C, Sariali el-H, Hannouche D, et al. Long-term results of alumina-on-alumina hip arthroplasty for osteonecrosis. *Clin Orthop Relat Res*. 2003;417:102–111.

SUGGESTED READINGS

Kim YH, Oh SH, Kim JS, et al. Contemporary total hip arthroplasty with and without cement in patients with osteonecrosis of the femoral head. *J Bone Joint Surg Am*. 2003;85-A:675–681.

Kim SY, Kim TG, Kim PT, et al. Vascularized compared with nonvascularized fibular grafts for large osteonecrotic lesions of the femoral head. *J Bone Joint Surg Am*. 2005;87:2012–2018.

Lavernia, CJ, Sierra RJ, Grieco FR. Osteonecrosis of the femoral head. *J Am Acad Orthop Surg*. 1999;7(4):250–261.

Lieberman JR. Core decompression for osteonecrosis of the hip. *Clin Orthop Relat Res*. 2004;418:29–33.

Lieberman JR, Berry DJ, Mont MA, et al. Osteonecrosis of the hip: Management in the 21st century. *J Bone Joint Surg Am*. 2002;84-A:834–853.

Mont MA, Hungerford DS. Non-traumatic avascular necrosis of the femoral head. *J Bone Joint Surg Am*. 1995;77:459–474.

Shannon BD, Trousdale RT. Femoral osteotomies for avascular necrosis of the femoral head. *Clin Orthop Relat Res*. 2004;418:34–40.

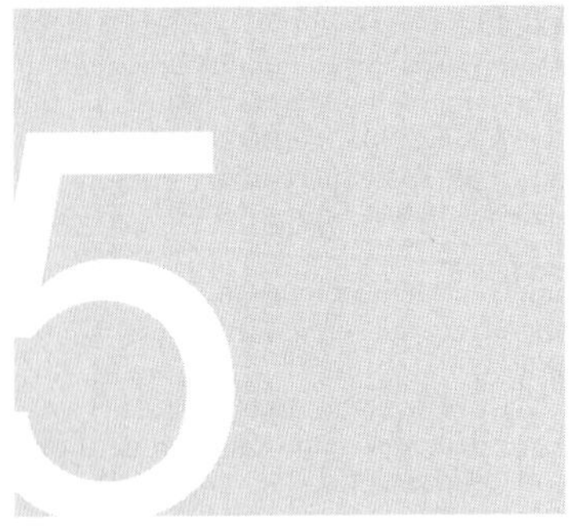

DEVELOPMENTAL DYSPLASIA

MICHAEL SKUTEK
STEVEN J. MACDONALD

Developmental dysplasia of the hip (DDH) is one of the most common neonatal orthopaedic problems, and it has variable morphologic patterns. The term refers to an abnormal relationship between the femoral head and the acetabulum and includes the fetal, neonatal, and infantile periods. It results in anatomic abnormalities leading to increased contact pressure in the joint and, eventually, coxarthrosis. Abnormal mechanical forces on the head of the femur may contribute to DDH; however, the primary cause is still unknown. The pathomorphologic appearance commonly includes an increased femoral neck/shaft angle, increased anteversion of the proximal femur and a shallow acetabulum. In untreated or unsuccessfully treated cases, pain and disability commonly necessitate reconstructive surgery or hip replacement at some time during adult life. However, many patients with hip dysplasia become symptomatic before the development of severe degenerative changes because of abnormal hip biomechanics, hip instability, impingement, or associated labral pathology. Several nonarthroplasty treatment options are available. The primary deformity is most commonly acetabular; therefore, for many patients; a reconstructive osteotomy that restores more nearly normal pelvic anatomy is often considered. Total hip arthroplasty for the treatment of DDH can be complex with technical challenges on both the acetabular and femoral sides.

PATHOGENESIS

Etiology

There are many theories as to the primary cause and pathogenesis of DDH. During embryonic development the hip joint, both femoral head and acetabulum, develop from the same primitive mesenchymal cells, and after 11 weeks the hip joint is fully formed. At birth the femoral head is deeply seated in the acetabulum and is difficult to dislocate. In a dysplastic hip, however, the femoral head can easily be subluxated or dislocated. Several theories regarding the cause of congenital dysplasia have been proposed, including mechanical factors, hormone-induced joint laxity, primary acetabular dysplasia, and genetic inheritance. Breech delivery, with the mechanical forces of abnormal flexion of the hips, can be seen as a cause of dislocation of the femoral head. It has been observed that in boys, DDH often occurs in association with concomitant deformities and oligohydramnios, whereas in girls it has been attributed to hormone-induced laxity of the hip capsule.

Although most dislocations occur during the first 2 weeks after birth, occasionally a dislocation will occur up to 1 year of age in patients documented to be normal previously. This is particularly true among infants with either a positive family history of DDH, breech presentation, or a persistent hip click on clinical examination. Hence, it is important to screen for DDH even after the newborn period.

Epidemiology

The prevalence of DDH varies considerably depending on genetic factors, habits, and cultural practices of different populations. The historical incidence was between 0.5 and 1.5 cases per 1,000 live births. By current clinical testing almost 10 to 20 newborns per 1,000 are considered to have abnormal hips and therefore normally receive some type of treatment. DDH is approximately five to eight times more common in girls than in boys with the ratio of reported prevalences ranging from 2.4:1 to 9.2:1. Breech deliveries make up approximately 3% to 4% of all deliveries, and the incidence of congenital dysplasia of the hip is increased in this patient population. A family history of DDH of the hip increases the likelihood of this condition to approximately 10%. The risk of a genetic influence was noted by Ortolani, who reported a 70% incidence of a positive family history in children with congenital dysplasia of the hip. Infants treated in a neonatal intensive care unit are also at higher risk. The incidence of DDH is as high as 50 per 1,000 births in Lapps and North American Indians; however, it is almost nonexistent among Chinese and those of African descent. In general, it is more common in white children than in black children. An increased incidence of congenital dysplasia of the hip has been reported in cultures that place infants in swaddling clothes with the hip in constant extension.

Pathophysiology

There is evidence that the presence of a spherical femoral head, concentrically reduced in the acetabulum, is a very important stimulus for the normal growth of the triradiate cartilage and the three ossification centers of the acetabular portion of the pubis, ilium, and ischium to form a concave acetabulum. The altered growth and bony deformities characteristically include increased neck/shaft and anteversion angles in the proximal femur. The femoral head is usually small, the neck may be short, the greater trochanter is displaced posteriorly, and the femoral canal is narrow. On the pelvic side, the true acetabulum is typically shallow, lateralized, anteverted, and deficient anteriorly and superiorly. Occasionally the whole hemipelvis is underdeveloped. Retrotorsion problems of the acetabulum and/or femur are also seen rarely and may lead to anterior impingement. In combination, these abnormalities lead to a decreased contact area between the femoral head and acetabulum and to lateralization of the center of hip rotation, which increases the body-weight lever arm.

The natural history of untreated DDH is variable; however, the longer DDH goes undetected, the greater is the developmental impairment of both the femoral head and the acetabulum. In adults, the natural history of untreated complete dislocation depends on the presence or absence of a well-developed false acetabulum as well as bilaterality. Back pain eventually occurs in patients with bilateral dislocations. This is thought to be secondary to associated hyperlordosis of the lumbar spine. In unilateral hip dislocations, secondary problems of limb-length inequality, deformity of the hip, ipsilateral knee pain, scoliosis, and gait disturbances are common.

Classification

The degree of hip joint pathology varies from capsular laxity to severe acetabular, femoral head, and femoral neck dysplasia. The anatomical definition of dysplasia refers to inadequate development of the acetabulum, the femoral head, or both. Anatomical classification is performed using the system of Severin (Table 5-1). It has been shown that this classification, a simultaneous evaluation of acetabular dysplasia, femoral head deformity and subluxation, correlates well with long-term radiographic, clinical, and functional outcome.

TABLE 5-1 SEVERIN CLASSIFICATION FOR RADIOGRAPHIC RESULTS

Class	Radiographic Appearance
I	Spherical femoral head
II	Moderate deformity of femoral head, neck, or acetabulum
III	Dysplastic hip, no subluxation
IV	Subluxation
V	Articulation with secondary false acetabulum
VI	Complete redislocation

TABLE 5-2 CLASSIFICATION OF HIP DYSPLASIA BY HARTOFILAKIDIS

Type	Description
I: Dysplasia	Femoral head, despite some degrees of subluxation, is still contained within the original acetabulum.
II: Low dislocation	Femoral head articulates with a false acetabulum that partially covers the true acetabulum.
III: High dislocation	Femoral head has migrated superiorly and posteriorly.

The classification of Crowe is a method to categorize the degree of dysplasia, i.e., the grade of subluxation. It is calculated using an anteroposterior radiograph by measuring the vertical distance between the interteardrop line and the junction between the femoral head and the medial edge of the neck. The amount of subluxation is the ratio between this distance and the vertical diameter of the undeformed head. When the femoral head is deformed, the predicted vertical diameter of the femoral head has been found to be 20% of the height of the pelvis as measured from the highest point on the iliac crest to the inferior margin of the ischial tuberosity. It is graded as grade I (<50% subluxation), grade II (50% to 75% subluxation), grade III (75% to 100% subluxation), or grade IV (>100% subluxation). An alternate classification by Hartofilakidis (Table 5-2) has also been suggested.[1]

DIAGNOSIS

Physical Examination and History

Patients with DDH should be followed carefully and regularly to detect early signs of coxarthrosis following the increased contact pressure in the joint secondary to the anatomic abnormalities. Growth disturbance of the proximal femur, which may be associated with femoral head avascular necrosis, may be a problem after treatment of DDH. History should be taken, and differential diagnosis that includes inflammatory disease, neuromuscular disease, traumatic epiphyseal slip, congenital coxa vara, and abnormal joint laxity should be considered. Incomplete femoral head coverage can also be observed in various conditions other than DDH (cerebral palsy, pelvic tilt). The natural history of dysplasia should be discussed with the patients and radiographs evaluated periodically to monitor the joint for development of arthritis.

The physical examination of the skeletally mature will have distinct features from that of the child. A careful documentation of the leg length and evaluation of impingement signs should be performed. A thorough examination is essential in eliciting signs that confirm clinical suspicions. Clinical examination begins with inspection of the lower extremity and includes assessment of gait, limb lengths, muscle power, range of motion, and special tests.

On initial inspection of the leg, any muscle wasting should be noted. Quadriceps atrophy can be indicative of severe or chronic hip problems. The position that the leg spontaneously takes should be carefully observed. This is true not only for abduction and adduction but also for rotation, as for example a leg maintained in internal rotation can be associated with femoroacetabular impingement. Range of hip motion is commonly normal in early hip dysplasia and will begin to decrease as the degree of secondary coxarthrosis increases. A fixed adduction contracture or very limited abduction that reproduces hip pain and may produce a palpable clunk is a sign of hinge abduction present in residual Perthes disease deformity. Macnicol[2] has described the "gear stick" sign, which will help differentiate trochanteric overgrowth from other sources of decreased hip abduction. With this test hip abduction is full in flexion but is limited in extension by impingement of the greater trochanter on the ilium or posterior wall of the acetabulum.

The external rotators of the hip are examined with the patient prone, the knee flexed, and the hip undergoing rotation. The piriformis and the posterior border of the gluteus medius may be tender on direct palpation, and occasionally this tenderness may extend to the lateral border of the sacrum. In patients with coxa vara with decreased femoral anteversion, tight external rotators as well as hamstrings may be demonstrated. Tight external rotators can also be seen in patients with acetabular retroversion because they maintain their leg in external rotation to minimize anterior impingement and can subsequently develop contractures.

Hip pain exacerbated by hip extension alone, or by external rotation in full extension, is seen in femoroacetabular impingement of various causes. If there is already a lack of full extension, the extension maneuver may force the hip into internal rotation to avoid posteroinferior contact between the acetabulum and the femoral head. If there is an osteophyte present on the posterior aspect of the femoral head, then full extension may become possible only with hip abduction.

Special Tests

The impingement test is used to delineate the acetabular rim syndrome. The hip is internally rotated as it is flexed 90 degrees and adducted 15 degrees (Fig. 5-1). This combination of movement brings the proximal and anterior part of the femoral neck into contact with the anterior rim of the acetabulum, which is the usual location for labral disease. This will elicit sharp pain from a mobile os acetabuli or a torn, degenerative, or ossified anterior acetabular labrum. An uncommon cause for a positive impingement test is acetabular retroversion or decreased femoral neck anteversion, as both of these anatomic variants result in early acetabular-femoral neck impingement with internal rotation.

The apprehension test is used to demonstrate anterior instability. The patient lies supine and the hip is adducted and externally rotated, producing discomfort and a sense of instability as the femoral head experiences deficient anterior acetabular coverage (Fig. 5-2). In a very thin patient this external rotation in extension can produce a mass in the inguinal region referred to as a "lump sign," which represents the femoral head pushing against the anterior hip capsule.

Abductor fatigue is tested by having the patient examined in the lateral position with the affected hip up and a bicycle pedaling maneuver performed as the lateral and posterior margins of the trochanter are palpated. Provocation of this maneuver can be performed by increasing the load on the pedaling foot, which may exacerbate the pain (Fig. 5-3). Tenderness is most commonly palpable along the posterior border of the gluteus medius. Under direct palpation, often a crepitation may be felt over the trochanteric bursa, which the patient may have previously described as a sensation of "sand in the joint."

A true hip click or clunk has been described by some authors as a sign of labral disease. Our experience, however, has demonstrated that in dysplastic hips with deficient anterior coverage, or in other causes of anterior femoral head prominence such as increased femoral neck anteversion, if the extremity is actively flexed and externally rotated and then brought back slowly toward extension and neutral rotation, at between 40 degrees and 50 degrees of external rotation, the iliopsoas tendon snaps over the uncovered femoral head. With the same maneuver in neutral or internal rotation, this click is eliminated.

Clinical Features

Activity-related groin pain is a common sign in patients with DDH. It is often reported with hyperextension and external rotation of the hip and thought to be secondary to subluxation of the femoral head. Locking, giving way symptoms, and catching may indicate associated labral or chondral pathology. Patients with subluxated hips usually have symptom onset at a younger age than those with complete dislocations. Invariably, radiographic subluxation leads to degenerative joint disease. The rate of deterioration is related directly to the severity of the subluxation and the age of the patient. Patients with the most severe subluxations usually develop symptoms during the second decade of life. Those with moderate subluxation often present at 30 to 40 years of age, and those with minimal subluxations experience symptoms usually in their 40s or 50s. Patients with complete dislocations and high-riding hips often will not develop problems until the fifth or sixth decades of life. It is rare to see radiographic changes of degenerative joint disease such as joint space narrowing, osteophyte formation, or subchondral cysts at symptom onset. The only radiographic signs may be subchondral sclerosis in the weight-bearing area. After clinical symptoms and radiographic signs of degenerative joint disease appear, progression is rapid.

Diagnostic Workup Algorithm

The diagnostic workup consists of the history and clinical examination already described and the radiographic imaging as described below. DDH-related problems such as back pain, secondary problems of limb-length inequality,

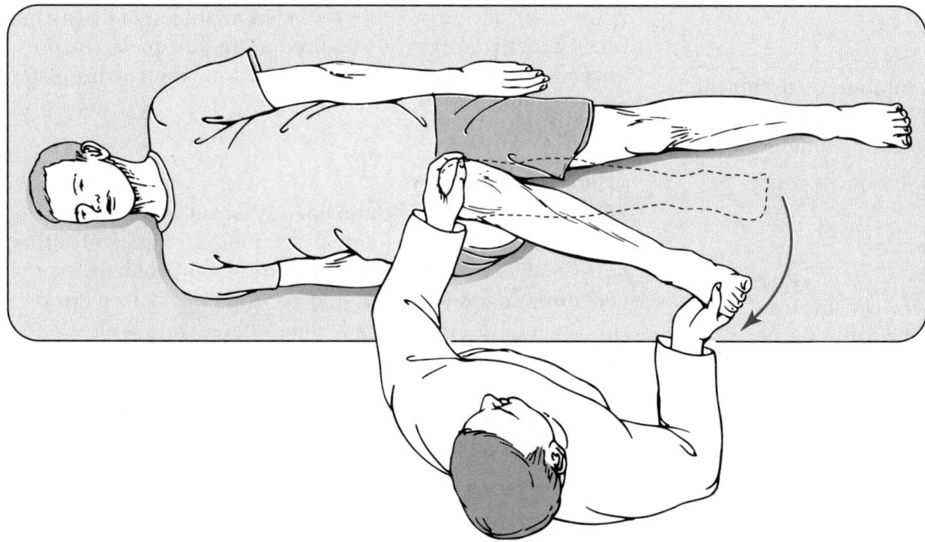

Figure 5-1 Impingement test.

deformity of the hip, ipsilateral knee pain, scoliosis, and gait disturbances need to be considered.

Radiologic Features

Selection of appropriate imaging techniques in patients with DDH depends on age and differs for diagnostic versus management situations. Plain radiographs, including an anteroposterior view of the pelvis and lateral view of the hip, are the first steps in imaging evaluation.

Patients with severe degenerative changes in which an arthroplasty is indicated will not routinely require additional imaging. However, occasionally with complex cases a three-dimensional CT scan with reconstructions may give additional information. Further imaging is required in patients in whom joint salvage procedures are being considered. A false profile image, which is a standing lateral hip image, will give valuable information on anterior femoral head coverage and aids in preoperative planning. Abduction and adduction views should also be obtained to assess joint congruency and containment. Labral pathology is best evaluated with MR/MR arthrogram. It is normally indicated in the rare patient presenting with labral pathology with minimal dysplasia in whom arthroscopy alone may be given consideration. MRI can also be helpful in the evaluation of loose bodies, chondral defects, and synovial disease.

The anteroposterior radiograph should be evaluated by the assessment of the Shenton line, the Tonnis angle, the center edge (CE) angle, and the extrusion index. The Shenton line is drawn between the medial border of the neck of the femur and the superior border of the obturator foramen. In the normal hip this line is an even, continuous arc, whereas in a dislocated hip with proximal displacement of the femoral head, it is broken and interrupted.

A standard anteroposterior pelvic radiograph may not demonstrate the full degree of hip dysplasia that is clearly present on a false profile view. The false profile image should be evaluated with regard to the ventral center edge angle.

The Severin anatomical classification is a simultaneous evaluation of acetabular dysplasia, femoral head deformity, and subluxation (Table 5-1). It has been shown to correlate well with long-term radiographic, clinical, and functional outcomes. Degenerative changes are classified according to Tonnis on a scale from absent (grade 0) to severe (grade III).

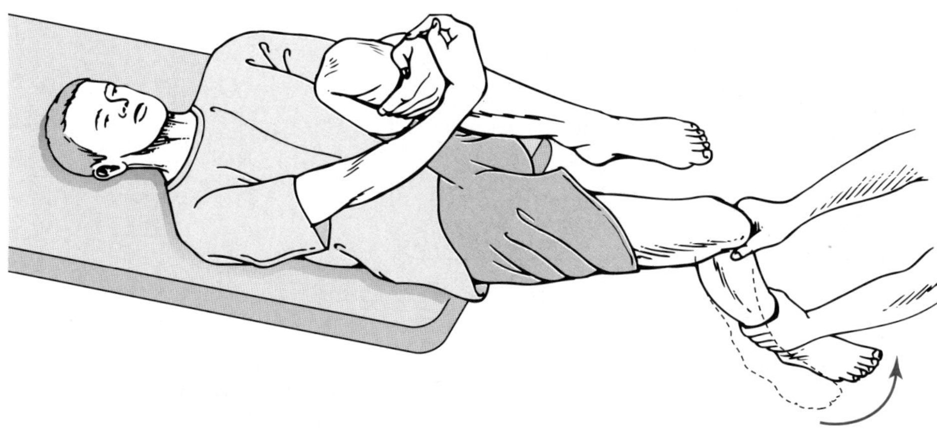

Figure 5-2 Apprehension test.

TREATMENT

There is great variability in the presentation of dysplastic patients with regard to age, severity of radiographic changes, symptoms, and patient expectations. Treatment alternatives vary with each of these factors.

Nonoperative Options

Nonsteroidal anti-inflammatory agents can be used, and high-impact activities should be avoided. Although controversy does exist, most would agree that the surgical alternatives should be reserved for symptomatic patients with severe limitation of their daily activities.

Surgical Options

The nonarthroplasty surgical procedures include arthroscopic surgery, pelvic osteotomy, femoral osteotomy, arthrodesis, and resection arthroplasty. The main goal of these procedures is to decrease pain. Arthroscopy can be beneficial when symptoms seem to be related only to labral tears or lose bodies in the absence of severe structural abnormalities about the hip. Fusion and resection arthroplasty are rarely, if ever, indicated given current treatment alternatives. The operative treatment of residual dysplasia of the hip after skeletal maturity is based on the assumption that the dysplasia, if left untreated, will lead to secondary osteoarthritis of the hip.

Many surgical procedures on the pelvis have been described for late salvage in cases of persistent acetabular maldevelopment and instability (Table 5-3). The common goals of such interventions are the provision of improved acetabular coverage, enhanced femoral head–acetabular congruence and containment, and improved joint biomechanics. Some osteotomies are also expected to slow down progression of degenerative changes by better distributing forces applied through the hip joint, and they may provide better distribution of bone stock that might facilitate further reconstructive surgery if required in the future. In the presence of severe degenerative changes, total joint arthroplasty gives the most predictable outcomes.

Arthroscopic Surgery

Hip arthroscopy may be considered for selected, mildly dysplastic hips with mechanical symptoms related to either loose bodies or labral tears. Retrotorsion problems of the acetabulum and femur should be ruled out before offering this procedure. Arthroscopic debridement and lavage in the presence of degenerative changes is a less predictive procedure. Arthroscopy alone has limited applications in the dysplastic hip because the underlying bony deformities cannot be addressed.

Osteotomy

Procedures to reorient the articulating surfaces of the hip joint are attractive in the patient with hip dysplasia. Increased joint congruity after reorientation of the osteotomized fragment allows load transmission through a broader area, which can reduce articular surface pressure. In general, osteotomies should be offered to young patients who have symptomatic hip dysplasia without excessive proximal migration of the center of rotation, reasonably well-preserved range of motion, and no more than mild degenerative changes on the articular surface (Fig. 5-4, Table 5-3). The Salter single innominate osteotomy is beneficial in children, but often is insufficient in adults because it allows limited correction (approximately 10-degree change in Tonnis angle) owing to the decreased flexibility of the symphysis pubis. It also lateralizes the hip joint, which is undesirable in dysplastic hips. So-called salvage procedures such as the Chiari iliac osteotomy and shelf procedures still may be indicated in some severely dysplastic hips that cannot be rendered congruent by a reconstructive osteotomy because of the discrepancy in sizes and shapes between the femoral head and the acetabulum.

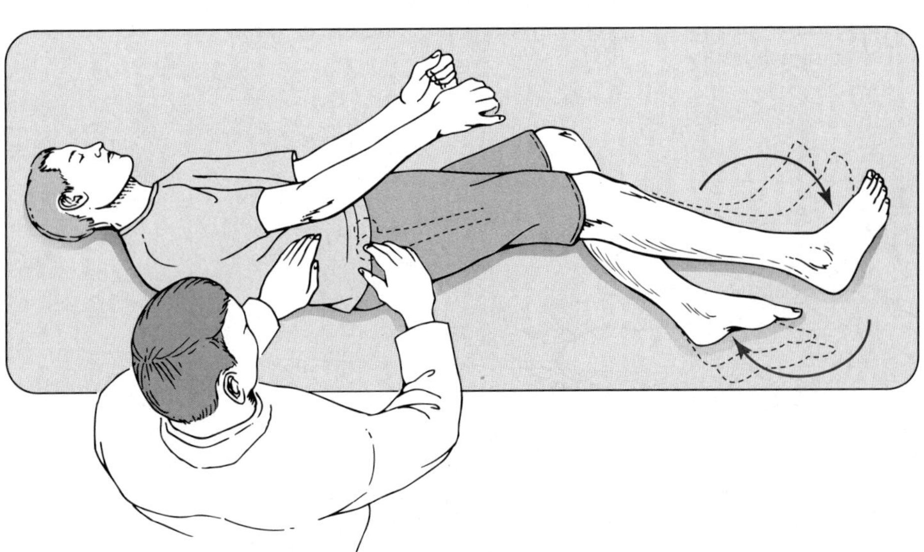

Figure 5-3 Abductor fatigue test (bicycle test).

TABLE 5-3 OSTEOTOMIES FOR DEVELOPMENTAL DYSPLASIA OF THE HIP (DDH) IN ADULTS

Osteotomy	Advantages/Disadvantages
Bernese-Ganz periacetabular	Allows large corrections of the osteotomized acetabular fragment in all directions. Posterior column of the hemipelvis remains intact; minimal internal fixation required. Age: 12–40 years
Salter single innominate osteotomy	Beneficial in children but often insufficient in adults because it allows limited correction owing to stiffness of the symphysis pubis.
Double/triple osteotomy	Improvement in coverage is often limited by the size of the fragments and ligamentous and muscular attachments to the sacrum. All triple osteotomies can lead to marked deformity of the pelvis if significant amount of correction is obtained.
Spherical osteotomies	Provide good lateral coverage. Often limited amount of anterior coverage and limited ability to medialize the hip joint. Concerns regarding osteonecrosis of osteotomized fragment.
Chiari osteotomy	Reconstructive pelvic osteotomies place a greater area of the acetabular surface in contact with the femoral head and have supplanted the so-called salvage osteotomies such as Chiari and shelf. Consideration might be given in severely dysplastic hips with significant discrepancy between the sizes and shapes of the femoral head and acetabulum, where hips cannot be rendered congruent by a reconstructive osteotomy.
Shelf procedure	Creates a buttress intended to increase joint stability but does not change the relationship of the femoral head and the true acetabulum.
Femoral osteotomy	Indicated when femur is the primary site of deformity or when a pelvic osteotomy does not provide enough correction

Bernese-Ganz Osteotomy

This osteotomy is currently the acetabular procedure preferred by many reconstructive surgeons. The procedure is indicated in patients with a closed triradiate cartilage. It requires only one incision and is performed with a series of straight, relatively reproducible extra-articular cuts.[3] It allows large corrections of the osteotomized acetabular fragment in all directions. The osteotomy includes a partial osteotomy of the ischium, a complete osteotomy of the superior pubic ramus, an incomplete osteotomy of the ilium, and a final cut connecting the ileal cut to the ischial cut. The posterior column of the hemipelvis remains intact, allowing early ambulation. The periacetabular fragment is mobilized once the osteotomies are completed.

Correction is considered satisfactory when the acetabular sourcil is horizontal, the femoral head is congruous, appropriate version has been obtained, the femoral head is medialized to within 5 to 15 mm of the ilioischial line, and the Shenton line is near normal. The joint may be opened and evaluated for labral lesions.

The periacetabular osteotomy has proven to be an effective technique for surgical correction of a severely dysplastic acetabulum in adolescents and young adults (Fig. 5-5). The early clinical results have been reported in several series, including a series by Clohisy et al.[4] in which results were reported as very good at an average of 4.2 years postoperatively. If a total hip arthroplasty is necessary at a later stage, this can be done safely in patients with a previous periacetabular osteotomy and should provide excellent results.[5] The Bernese periacetabular osteotomy can also be used successfully to treat neurogenic acetabular dysplasian skeletally mature patients.[6]

Chiari Osteotomy

The Chiari osteotomy is a capsular interposition arthroplasty and should be considered only in those instances in which other reconstructions are impossible: when the femoral head cannot be centered adequately in the acetabulum or in painfully subluxated hips with early signs of osteoarthritis. This procedure deepens the deficient acetabulum by medial displacement of the distal pelvic fragment and improves superolateral femoral coverage. The Chiari procedure is an operation that places the femoral head beneath a surface of joint capsule and cancellous bone with the capacity for regeneration and corrects the lateral pathologic displacement of the femur. The biomechanical effect of medial weight-bearing transfer is to unload the femoral head and reduce the demands on the abductor musculature. The angle of osteotomy is 10 to 20 degrees relative to the plane of the upper acetabular margin, and the lower segment is displaced medially by approximately half its width. The superior fragment of the osteotomy then becomes a shelf, and the capsule is interposed between it and the femoral head.

Shelf Operations

Shelf procedures are useful for subluxations and dislocations that have been reduced and in which no other osteotomy will establish a congruous joint with apposition of the articular cartilage of the acetabulum to the femoral head. In a classic shelf operation, the acetabular roof is extended laterally, posteriorly, or anteriorly, either by a graft or by turning the acetabular roof and part of the lateral cortex of the ilium distally over the femoral head.

Femoral Osteotomy

An intertrochanteric osteotomy is indicated when the femur is the primary site of deformity or when a pelvic osteotomy alone does not provide sufficient correction. Several requirements must be fulfilled before proposing an isolated femoral osteotomy. First, the osteotomy must be able to provide satisfactory correction of the deformity. Second, the preoperative range of motion

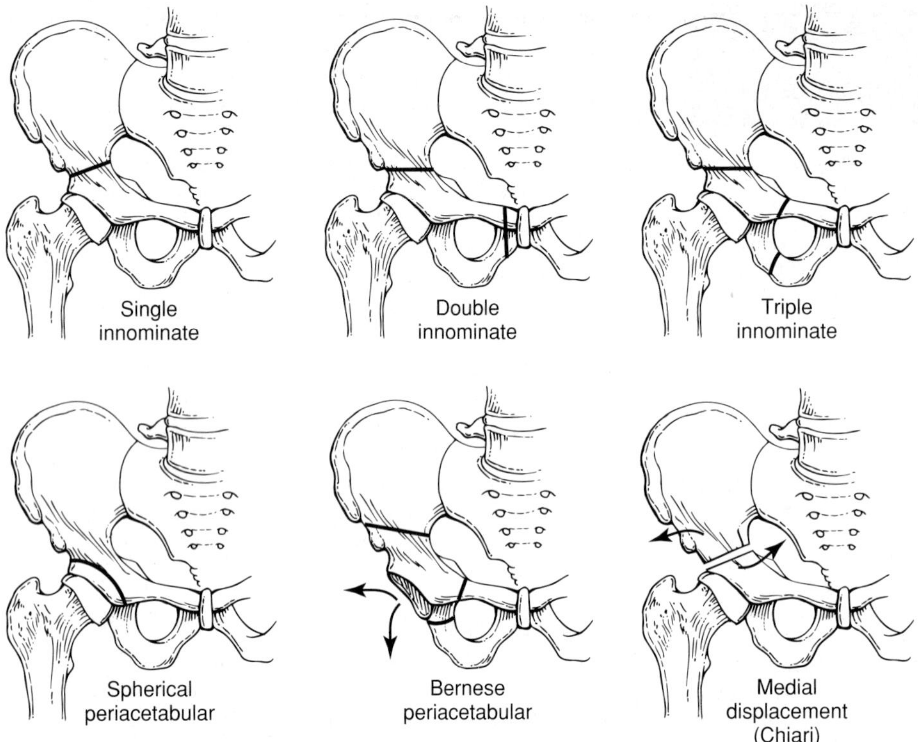

Figure 5-4 Osteotomy options.

should be sufficient to allow a functional arc of hip motion after correction. Third, the joint should be congruent in the proposed position of correction. Most patients with hip dysplasia who are candidates for isolated femoral osteotomy have coxa valga with mild acetabular deformity.

Arthroplasty

Total Hip Replacement. In patients with symptomatic end-stage coxarthritis secondary to hip dysplasia, total hip arthroplasty (THA) is the procedure of choice. As described elsewhere in the text, there are specific challenges on both the acetabular and femoral sides of the reconstruction. Based on the severity of subluxation, a number of different options are available for acetabular/femoral reconstruction (Table 5-4).

Surgical Technique. The goal of acetabular reconstruction is to place the acetabular component in the true acetabulum. There may be bone stock deficiency superiorly depending on the degree of dysplasia and additionally the true acetabulum may have increased, or rarely decreased,

TABLE 5-4 TOTAL HIP ARTHROPLASTY RECONSTRUCTION OPTIONS BASED ON SEVERITY OF HIP DYSPLASIA (CROWE CLASSIFICATION)

Crowe Classification	Acetabulum	Femur	Approach
I	Uncemented, true acetabular region, slight medialization	Cemented or uncemented stem based on patient age, bone quality, and bone geometry	Anterolateral or posterolateral
II, III	Uncemented at or near true acetabular region, if necessary autograft or high hip center or medialization	Cemented or uncemented stem based on patient age and bone geometry	Anterolateral, posterolateral, or subtrochanteric approach
IV	Small uncemented, true acetabular region	Greater trochanteric osteotomy with sequential proximal shortening and cemented DDH stem, or shortening subtrochanteric osteotomy and uncemented stem	Transtrochanteric or posterior approach with shortening subtrochanteric osteotomy

DDH, developmental dysplasia of the hip.

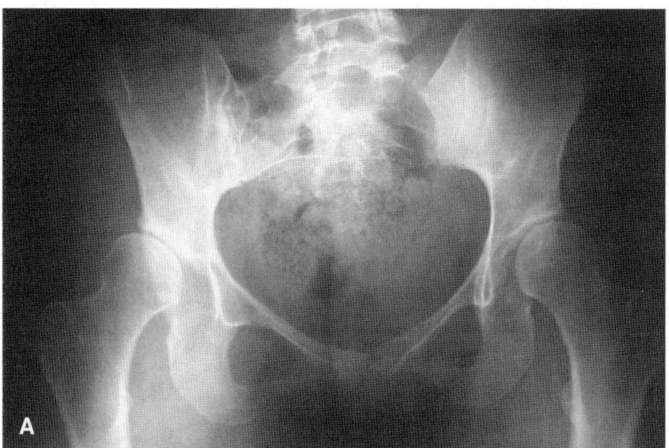

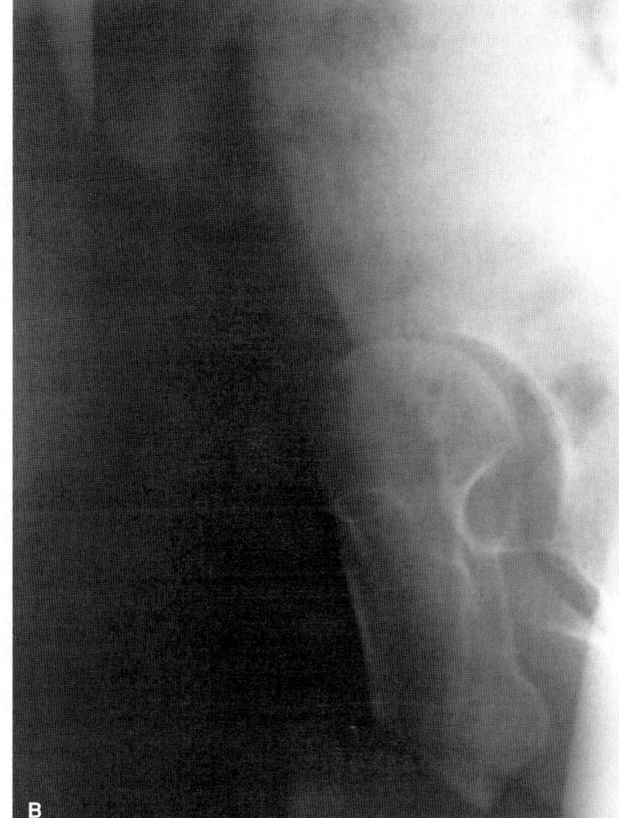

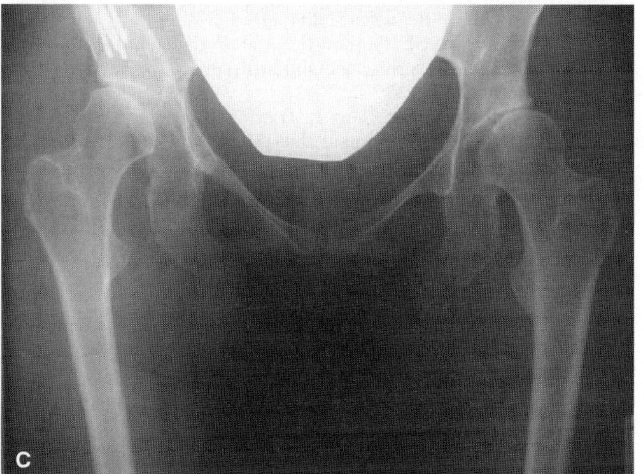

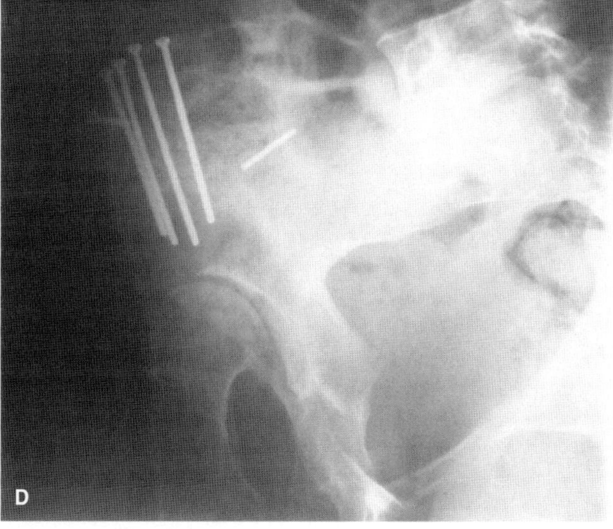

Figure 5-5 Preoperative anteroposterior and false views demonstrating acetabular dysplasia. Postoperative images 6 years following corrective Bernese pelvic osteotomy with preservation of joint space.

version, which has to be assessed at the time of component placement. Occasionally the patient's femoral head may be used as an autograft if the component is excessively uncovered (>25%) superolaterally. Cementless acetabulum components with screw fixation are preferred. When choosing the optimal location of acetabular component placement, the advantages of a normal anatomic location must be balanced with the need to provide sufficient acetabular implant coverage. Whenever possible, the acetabular reconstruction should seek normalization of the hip center. Extra-small acetabular implant sizes often are required. Small femoral head sizes to preserve adequate polyethylene thickness may be needed. Because most of these patients are younger, an alternate bearing such as highly cross-linked polyethylene, ceramic on polyethylene, ceramic on ceramic, or metal on metal may be considered.

The femoral anatomy may demonstrate excessive femoral neck anteversion, a valgus neck/shaft angle, metaphyseal-diaphyseal mismatch (with a very narrow medullary canal) and prominent greater trochanter in cases of high dislocation. A shortening femoral osteotomy may have to be performed to minimize injury to the sciatic nerve owing to leg lengthening. Often a modular cementless femoral component is ideally suited to address the host bone abnormalities.

THA has proven to be a reliable procedure, even in patients younger than 30 years of age, especially when other alternatives such as arthrodesis or resection arthroplasty are considered. Pain relief in patients with hip dysplasia after total hip arthroplasty parallels the excellent results of total hip arthroplasty in the general population. Long-term survivorship remains a challenge in this often younger patient population; however, with the advent of alternate bearings with improved wear characteristics this may improve in the future.

CONCLUSION

Developmental dysplasia in the adult presents as a varied and complex clinical scenario to the adult reconstruction surgeon. A thorough knowledge of the natural history, the physical and radiographic evaluation, and the various treatment alternatives is required to manage these challenging cases.

REFERENCES

1. Hartofilakidis G, Stamos K, Karachalios T, et al. Congenital hip disease in adults. Classification of acetabular deficiencies and operative treatment with acetabuloplasty combined with total hip arthroplasty. *J Bone Joint Surg Am*. 1997;78:683–692.
2. Macnicol MF, Makris D. Distal transfer of the greater trochanter. *J Bone Joint Surg Br*. 1991;73:838–841.
3. Ganz R, Klaue K, Vinh TS, et al.A new periacetabular osteotomy for the treatment of hip dysplasias: technique and preliminary results. 1988. *Clin Orthop Relat Res*. 2004;418:3–8.
4. Clohisy JC, Barrett SE, Gordon JE, et al. Periacetabular osteotomy for the treatment of severe acetabular dysplasia. *J Bone Joint Surg Am*. 2005;87(2):254–259.
5. Parvizi J, Burmeister H, Ganz R. Previous Bernese periacetabular osteotomy does not compromise the results of total hip arthroplasty. *Clin Orthop Relat Res*. 2004;423:118–122.
6. MacDonald SJ, Hersche O, Ganz R. Periacetabular osteotomy in the treatment of neurogenic acetabular dysplasia. *J Bone Joint Surg Br*. 1999;81:975–978.

POSTTRAUMATIC CONDITIONS

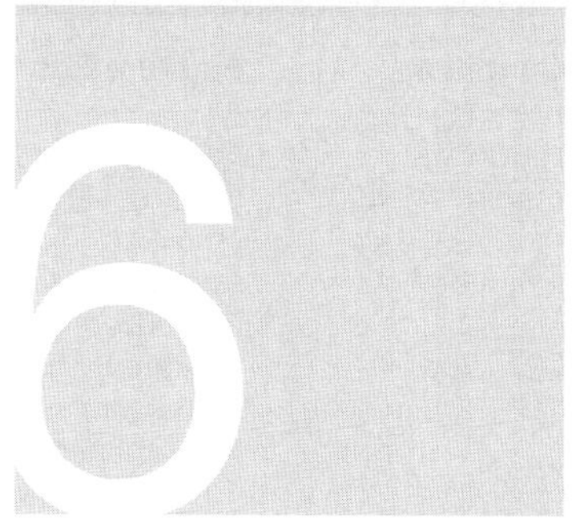

SIMON C. MEARS

Trauma to the hip can lead to long-term dysfunction from posttraumatic arthritis, osteonecrosis, malunion, and nonunion. End-stage arthritis may develop quickly after the injury or it may develop years later. In many patients, treatment involves removal of the current hardware and conversion to total hip arthroplasty. Osteoporosis, bone loss, and heterotopic bone formation complicate total hip arthroplasty. Hip salvage via other procedures such as refixation of the fracture, valgus osteotomy, or femoral head reshaping may be considered for patients with a viable femoral head.

PATHOGENESIS

Etiology

All hip fractures may lead to posttraumatic conditions (Table 6-1). Hip dislocations may damage the blood supply to the femoral head, leading to late osteonecrosis, a risk increased in direct proportion to the length of time the hip remains dislocated. Cartilage damage from the initial injury predisposes patients to later arthritis. Surgical treatment of acetabular fractures may lead to iatrogenic arthritis from intra-articular hardware or malreduction. Elderly patients are at risk for osteoporotic fracture patterns that are difficult to reduce and stabilize effectively.

Femoral neck fractures can lead to osteonecrosis of the femoral head, malunion, nonunion, and severe arthritis. In the older patient, these conditions are treated with hip replacement, whereas in the younger patient hip salvage may be possible. Hip salvage may be achieved by revision fixation, bone grafting, or femoral head reshaping. Intertrochanteric fractures typically are treated with a hip screw and side plate or an intramedullary hip screw. In the young patient, nonunion can occur, and revision internal fixation with bone grafting may be indicated. In the elderly patient, a nonunion or malunion is best treated with arthroplasty.

Epidemiology

Posttraumatic arthritis of the hip can result from trauma to the acetabulum or proximal femur. Acetabular fractures are thought to occur at a rate of 3 per 100,000 population per year. The rate of posttraumatic arthritis for all acetabular fractures is 20% to 30%. Posterior wall fractures represent about 25% of all fractures and are at high risk for late arthritis. The elderly patient and those with more comminuted fractures have worse results from initial reduction and fixation than younger patients with simple fracture patterns. Almost 10% of fractures have severe initial damage to the femoral head or acetabulum, which is best treated with acute arthroplasty.

Of the approximately 250,000 hip fractures that occur each year in the United States, approximately 40% involve the femoral neck. Femoral neck fractures are especially common in the elderly patient. Of those treated with open reduction and internal fixation, 15% develop osteonecrosis, 30% develop nonunion, and 20% to 35% require revision surgery. Intertrochanteric fractures also are common in the osteoporotic individual, and rates in elderly women are estimated at 63 per 100,000 population. Failure of fixation is related to fracture stability and the amount of comminution. In one study, 43% of fractures were classified as unstable and up to 50% of unstable intertrochanteric fractures may develop nonunion after internal fixation.

Pathophysiology

Damage to the cartilage of the femoral head and/or acetabulum resulting from an acetabular fracture or a hip dislocation can lead to arthritic changes in the hip. Cartilage damage occurs to the area of the joint next to the fracture and is termed marginal impaction. Impacted cartilage must be elevated and supported with bone graft during fixation. Postfracture damage to the femoral head also can occur secondary to nonconcentric reduction or intra-articular bodies while the patient awaits surgical fixation. Damage to 40% or more of the weight-bearing articular cartilage, the femoral head, or acetabular surface is an indication for acute total hip replacement.

Osteonecrosis of the femoral head occurs by disruption of the blood supply to the femoral head. Disruption can occur by traumatic dislocation of the femoral head, by traumatic injury from hip fracture displacement, from elevated

TABLE 6-1 CONDITIONS AFTER HIP TRAUMA

Condition	Fracture Site
Hardware pain	Femoral neck (cannulated screws) Intertrochanteric fractures (sliding hip screws)
Infection	Acetabular, femoral neck, and intertrochanteric fractures
Malunion	Acetabular fractures (leading to joint step-off) Femoral neck (leading to femoroacetabular impingement) Intertrochanteric fractures (leading to leg-length discrepancy, abductor weakness)
Nonunion	Acetabular fractures (pelvic dissociation) Femoral neck and intertrochanteric fractures
Osteonecrosis	Acetabular, femoral neck, and intertrochanteric fractures
Posttraumatic arthritis	Acetabular, femoral neck, and intertrochanteric fractures

intracapsular pressure, or by surgical injury to the blood supply. The lateral epiphyseal artery (the end branch of the medial circumflex artery), which supplies the femoral head, enters the femoral head through the obturator externus muscle on the posterior aspect of the femoral neck. The risk of femoral head osteonecrosis is directly proportional to both the length of time that a hip is dislocated and the amount of displacement of a femoral neck fracture. Increased pressure in the hip joint by bleeding from an intracapsular femoral neck fracture tamponades the blood supply to the femoral head and also may contribute to the development of osteonecrosis.

The acetabulum is supplied by multiple arteries, including the superior and inferior gluteal, medial femoral circumflex, obturator, fourth lumbar, and iliolumbar arteries. Disruption of the entire blood supply requires stripping of the soft tissues from the inner and outer tables of the acetabulum. Avoidance of excessive stripping during extensile approaches is critical when stabilizing complex acetabular fractures.

Malunion can lead to several posttraumatic conditions, including posttraumatic arthritis, femoroacetabular impingement, and limb-length discrepancy. Malreduction of an acetabular fracture causes joint incongruity. Residual fracture step-off increases contact pressure in the hip and leads to cartilage wear, arthritis, and poor clinical outcomes. Malunion of a femoral neck or intertrochanteric fracture leads to shortening of the hip with resultant limb-length discrepancy and Trendelenburg gait. Shortening can occur when a fracture is treated with parallel screw or sliding hip screw fixation. Malunion of a femoral neck fracture results in an abnormal head/neck angle, with retroversion and varus deformity of the femoral neck. The abnormal neck/shaft angle causes the anterior aspect of the neck to impinge on the acetabulum and is termed femoroacetabular impingement. Impingement damages the superior anterior

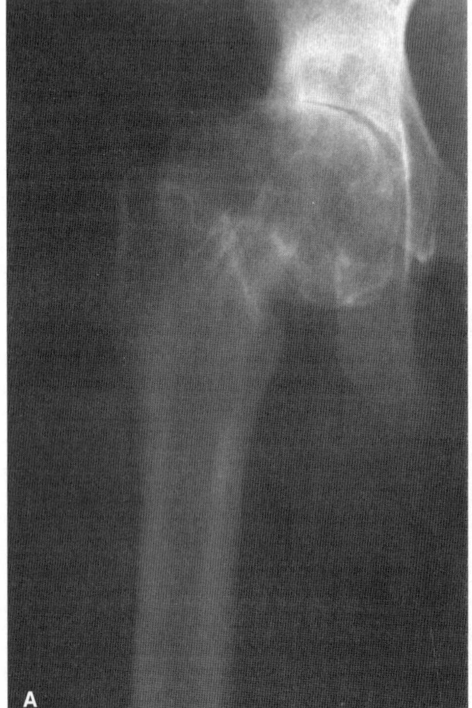

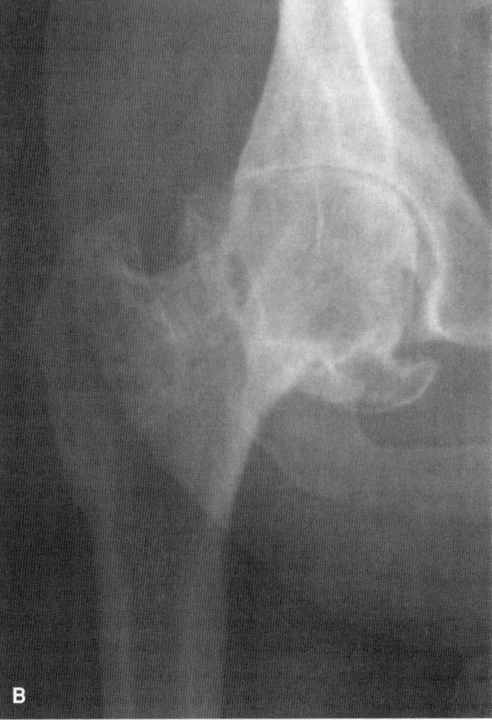

Figure 6-1 Patient with malunion of the femoral neck after pinning of a slipped capital femoral epiphysis. **A:** Anteroposterior radiograph showing the development of severe arthritis from femoroacetabular impingement. **B:** An oblique view gives a "true" view of the femoral neck and osteophytes and is helpful for preoperative templating.

acetabular labrum and leads to osteophyte formation and arthritis through a cam mechanism (Fig. 6-1).

Femoral neck and intertrochanteric fracture nonunions are more common after unstable fractures. Factors related to the nonunion include the stability and comminution of the initial fracture and the quality of the reduction and fixation of the fracture. Technical problems of initial fixation such as malreduction and incorrect hardware selection or placement can lead to nonunion. The role of bone mineral density is controversial.

Classification

There are no classification systems specific to posttraumatic conditions of the hip. Osteoarthritis is graded radiographically by an evaluation of the minimal joint space or by the system of Kellgren and Lawrence. Osteonecrosis is graded according to the modified system of Ficat by its appearance on scans and plain radiographs ranging from grade 1 (a lesion seen only on magnetic resonance imaging) to grade 4 (severe degenerative joint disease on radiographs). Nonunions are graded as atrophic or hypertrophic. Individual fracture patterns can be classified using the Arbeitsgemeinschaft fur Osteosyntheses/Orthopaedic Trauma Association (AO/OTA) classification system, which numerically lists fractures by site and pattern. Acetabular fractures are classified using the system of Letournel and Judet into elementary and associated fracture patterns. Femoral neck fractures are classified as stable or unstable based on the amount of fracture displacement. Intertrochanteric fractures are classified as stable or unstable depending on the number of fracture fragments, the presence of an intact medial or lateral buttress, and the direction of the fracture. Many fracture classification systems lack interobserver and intraobserver reliability.

DIAGNOSIS

Physical Examination and History

Clinical Features

It is important for the clinician to understand the specifics about the energy (high or low) that caused the fracture, patient age, comorbidities, and a determination of the presence of osteoporosis. Any patient who fractured a bone after the age of 50 years is at high risk for osteoporosis and should be considered for assessment with bone densitometry. Other evaluations should include the patient's gait to determine if a limp is present, measurement of limb lengths for discrepancy, measurement of hip motion, and examination of the patient and signs of infection. Patients should be questioned carefully about severity and pattern of pain, the level of hip dysfunction, and infection issues, including previous wound healing problems.

Imaging Studies

If possible, existing radiographs should be reviewed to evaluate the initial injury and to assess serial changes in the hip over time. Up-to-date anteroposterior and lateral views of the hip and an anteroposterior view of the pelvis are required. If substantial rotational contracture of the hip exists, oblique views can be helpful (Fig. 6-1). In the case of an acetabular fracture, Judet views of the pelvis can help assess the columns and walls of the acetabulum. A computed tomography scan is used to assess for nonunion of the acetabulum or hip, bone defects of the acetabulum, and heterotopic ossification. In particular, a transverse nonunion of the acetabulum, termed a pelvic discontinuity, requires refixation of the pelvis and must be evaluated on the Judet views and computed tomography scan.

Diagnostic Workup Algorithm

A diagnostic workup algorithm is shown in Figure 6-2.

TREATMENT

Nonoperative

For patients with posttraumatic hip arthritis, nonoperative modalities should be the first line of treatment. Interventions include activity modification, weight reduction if the patient is obese, ambulatory assistance devices (walker, wheelchair, or motorized scooter, especially if the patient is elderly and infirm), pain medications (such as acetaminophen, nonsteroidal anti-inflammatory medications, and narcotic agents), and shoe lifts for limb-length discrepancy. Patients with healing fractures require careful radiographic follow-up until fracture union. In the event of a malunion or nonunion, the younger patient may be at risk for early posttraumatic arthritis and the older patient may be at risk for substantial bone loss from screw cutout. In either case, earlier surgery may lead to a better outcome.

Surgical

Preoperative Considerations

All patients who have had previous surgery to the hip should be assessed for infection. Infection may have caused the failure of previous treatment, and if present, it will affect the management of the patient. Erythrocyte sedimentation rate and C-reactive protein serve as screening tools. Any patient with elevation of these values should undergo hip aspiration under fluoroscopy. White blood cell–tagged bone scans also may be used to evaluate for infection. In all cases, intraoperative frozen sections should be sent to assess for infection, and intraoperative cultures should be taken.

Surgery on the previously traumatized hip is not routine, and the treatment plan should be made well in advance of the surgical date. Templating should be performed on the preoperative radiographs ahead of time to help determine what implant systems will be required. Operative reports from previous surgeries facilitate ordering the correct tools for hardware removal. A broken-screw removal set and a high-speed metal cutting burr should be available in case screw heads are stripped.

Elderly patients with failed fracture repair are frail and usually have been in poor health since their initial injury. Contractures or bed sores may have developed from lack of activity. The patient should be evaluated for systemic problems, may require preoperative evaluation by a cardiologist, and may need an intensive care unit bed postoperatively. It is

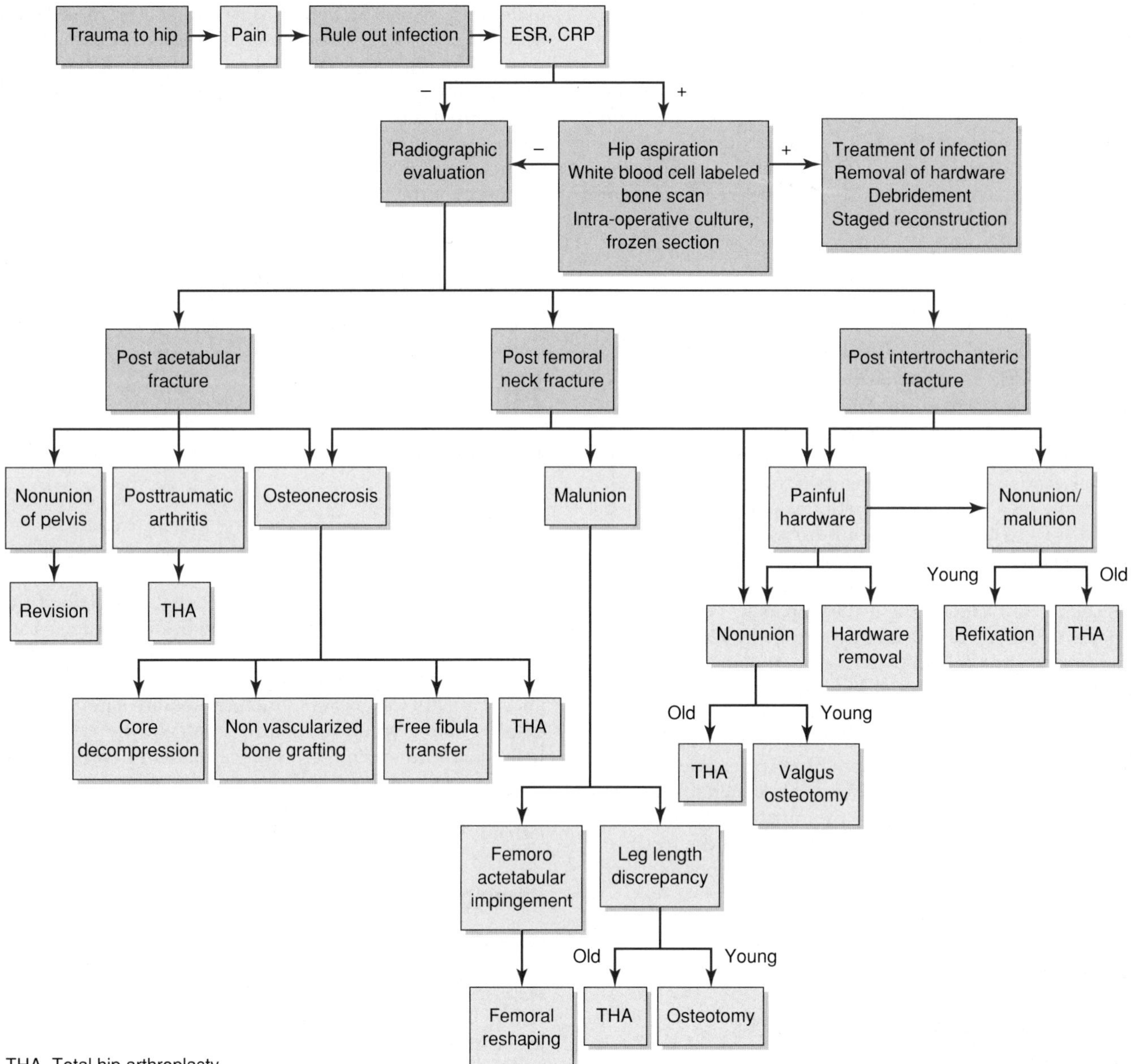

Figure 6-2 Diagnostic workup algorithm.

helpful to plan for a geriatrician or hospitalist to follow the patient in the postoperative period because postoperative medical complications such as delirium are common. The patient and family should be prepared for a lengthy recovery and the possibility of complications, including death.

Goals/Approaches

Joint arthrosis may be the end result of osteonecrosis of the femoral head, malunion, or cartilage damage. Because total hip replacement has been so successful, it is now the most commonly used treatment option. Alternate options include hip resection or fusion, but both lead to substantial leg-length discrepancy and hip dysfunction and are not well accepted by patients.

Acetabular Fracture. Hip arthroplasty after acetabular fracture is difficult, and an uncemented acetabular component with additional screw fixation should be used. Existing hardware from the previous fixation, including posterior wall plates or column screws, should be removed only if they impede reaming or cup insertion. The sciatic nerve is at great risk when a posterior column plate is removed, and care must be taken with retractor placement. Bone defects must be expected, depending on the initial fracture pattern: The most common defects occur posteriorly after posterior wall fractures or anteriorly and medially after osteoporotic acetabular fractures. Bone graft from the arthritic femoral head should be used first, and then cancellous allograft chips as needed. Each patient should be examined intraoperatively for pelvic dissociation; if present, the posterior column must be stabilized with a contoured reconstruction plate. The defect then is packed with bone graft, and an uncemented cup is inserted with multiple screws. For very large defects, an acetabular autograft (protected by a cage) may be required.

Femoral Neck Fracture. Femoral neck fracture complications, such as arthritis, nonunion, or malunion, generally are treated with hip arthroplasty. Arthroplasty requires removal of the existing screws, but a standard femoral stem usually can be inserted. Pain after hip fracture repair may occur directly over hardware such as a sliding hip screw or cannulated screw or it may be secondary to screws having backed out substantially. However, before considering hardware removal, fracture nonunion should be excluded by computed tomography scan.

Young patients with a viable concentric femoral head should be considered for hip salvage surgery. For the young patient with femoral neck nonunion, an intertrochanteric valgus producing osteotomy converts shear forces into compression forces, allowing for fracture healing (Fig. 6-3). The osteotomy is performed on a fracture table with fluoroscopy, and a 95-degree blade plate is used for fixation.

Femoral neck malunion may result in femoroacetabular impingement. A femoral reshaping procedure can remove impinging osteophytes to prevent additional arthritic

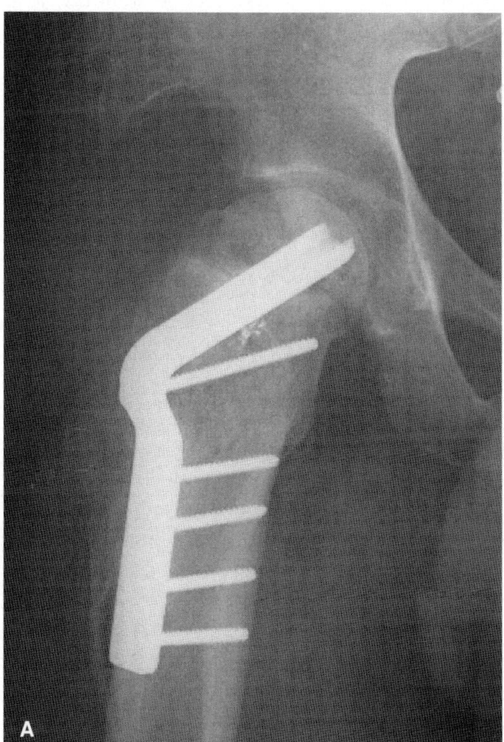

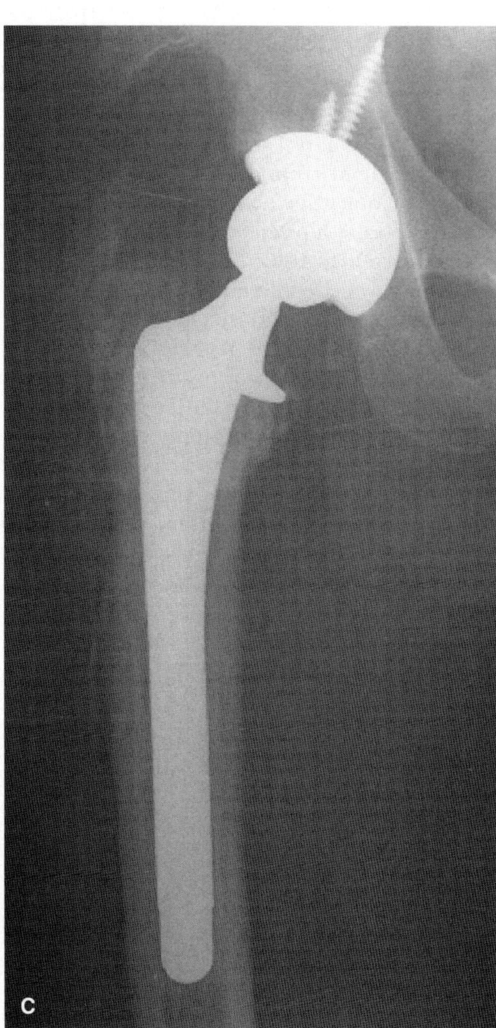

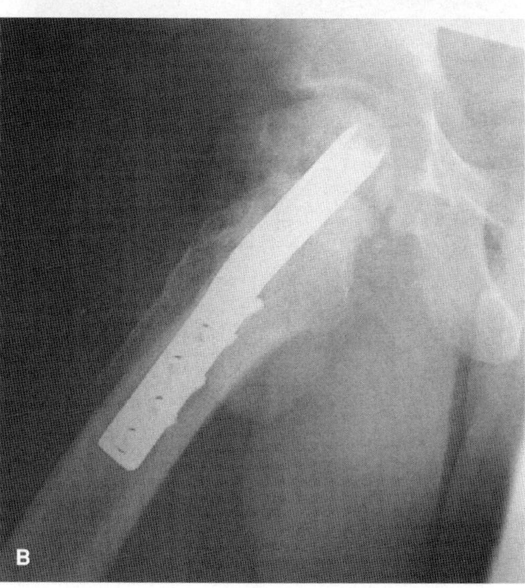

Figure 6-3 Young patient with femoral neck nonunion treated with valgus osteotomy and blade plate fixation. **A:** Anteroposterior view of the hip showing the blade plate. **B:** Lateral view of the hip reveals that the femoral head has collapsed from osteonecrosis. **C:** Anteroposterior view of the hip showing the uncemented total hip arthroplasty after blade plate removal.

TABLE 6-2 TIPS FOR TOTAL HIP REPLACEMENT AFTER FAILED TREATMENT FOR INTERTROCHANTERIC FRACTURE

Template preoperatively.
Prepare patient for complications and extended recovery time.
Bypass implant screw holes with long-stem prosthesis.
Restore length with calcar buildup.
Consider large head size for increased stability.
Be prepared for trochanteric reattachment.

changes. A trochanteric slide osteotomy approach to the hip avoids damage to the femoral head's blood supply. A burr is used to remove the impinging osteophytes.

Intertrochanteric Hip Fracture. In the elderly patient, intertrochanteric nonunion and malunions should be treated with prosthetic replacement. Hemiarthroplasty may be used in the elderly patient with intact acetabular cartilage. Some technical difficulties of total hip replacement should be recognized and are summarized in Table 6-2. The previous scar from internal fixation may be too far anterior, requiring a second incision. Care must be taken during exposure because a hip contracture is usually present, making exposure difficult. Fracture of the femur or ankle may occur by overzealous retraction. The greater trochanter usually is widened and partially healed with callus and heterotopic ossification. A modified direct lateral or posterior approach can be used per surgeon preference. In some cases, the trochanteric fragment has not healed to the femur, and a trochanteric slide approach can be used. The hip should be exposed and dislocated before hardware removal.

Often, the hip screw has cut out through the femoral head, producing cartilage damage and a bony defect in the acetabulum. In such a case, the remains of the femoral head should be used to graft the defect, and an uncemented cup should be inserted. A bony defect of the medial proximal femur often is present, leading to the need for a calcar-replacing femoral prosthesis. A cemented or uncemented prosthesis can be used, but the stem should extend past the final screw hole to avoid a stress riser (Fig. 6-4). Previous screw holes should be plugged to prevent cement extravasation. Careful trial reduction and intraoperative radiographs are recommended to help ascertain whether the appropriately sized calcar buildup has been used. If the calcar buildup is too small, the hip will remain short and instability may result. Because instability is a larger concern than wear in these elderly patients, a large femoral head should be used. During closure, care should be taken with the greater trochanter. If unstable fracture lines remain, the trochanter can be stabilized with a claw and cables or wires.

In the young patient with an intact femoral head and acetabulum, revision fixation with bone grafting is an option. A 95-degree fixed-angle blade-plate device can be inserted using the intact inferior portion of the femoral head for fixation.

Results and Outcome

Most reports of the results and outcomes of treatment of posttraumatic hip problems are case series. Little is known about outcome measures in these patient groups, and no studies in the literature are randomized or controlled. This lack of large, investigative studies may reflect the fact that the numbers of patients with these posttraumatic problems is small and that the spectrum of failure mechanisms is wide.

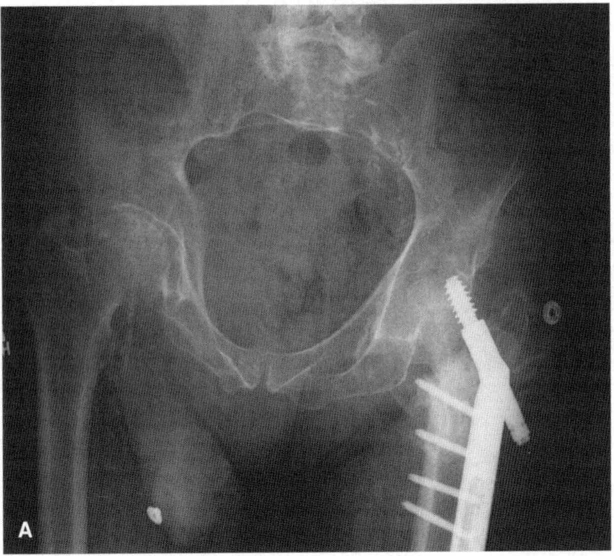

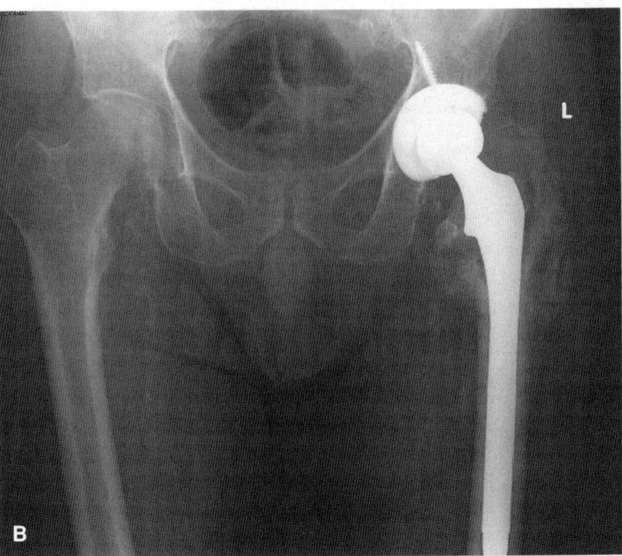

Figure 6-4 Elderly man with intertrochanteric fracture nonunion and sliding hip screw cutout. **A:** Anteroposterior view of the hip shows nonunion of the fracture and collapse. **B:** Anteroposterior view of the hip showing a long-stemmed uncemented prosthesis used to bypass screw holes with calcar buildup for leg-length restoration.

Conditions after Acetabular Fracture. Limited information is available about the acute treatment of acetabular fractures with total hip arthroplasty. In one case series, 80% of patients had good or excellent results at intermediate follow-up. Excessive medialization of the acetabular component occurred in 10% of patients, and the difficulty of acute arthroplasty was stressed. Several authors have reported the results of late total hip arthroplasty for acetabular fractures: With modern implants, 90% have good to excellent results at intermediate follow-up. The procedures were noted to be more difficult with more blood loss than with primary hip arthroplasty. Extended liners and additional bone grafts often were required. Some reports have shown increased evidence of component loosening that is thought to be related to the young age and activity of patients at the time of hip replacement.

Conditions after Femoral Neck Fracture. Excellent results have been reported for the treatment of femoral neck nonunion or osteonecrosis with total hip replacement. Results are slightly inferior to those of primary total hip arthroplasty, with higher rates of dislocation and trochanteric complications. Valgus-producing osteotomies have been reported as leading to healing of femoral neck nonunions in 80% of cases. However, patients often continue to have a limp from abductor weakness. Osteonecrosis may occur later after osteotomy, requiring subsequent hip replacement. The results of femoral reshaping procedures for femoroacetabular impingement from malunion of the femoral neck are preliminary: One case series of the use of a trochanteric flip osteotomy and femoral head reshaping showed excellent pain relief. Long-term follow-up is needed to determine whether arthrosis is prevented.

Conditions after Intertrochanteric Fracture. The results of treating failed intertrochanteric fractures with bone grafting and revision fixation are limited, but available reports show 80% to 95% healing rate after the use of a fixed-angle 95-degree blade-plate device in selected patients. Arthroplasty for failed intertrochanteric fractures has been reported to have 90% good to excellent results at intermediate follow-up. These cases were technically difficult, and long-stemmed and calcar-replacing implants commonly were used.

Postoperative Management

Total Hip Replacement. After hip replacement, intraoperative cultures should be followed for 5 days. Postoperative radiographs should be scrutinized carefully for iatrogenic fractures. Hip dislocation precautions relative to the specific operative approach should be followed. Weight-bearing restrictions depend on the stability of the components achieved intraoperatively. If at all possible, weight bearing should be allowed as tolerated because elderly patients often have difficulty following weight-bearing restrictions. Radiographs should be obtained and assessed during the postoperative year to document component stability and bone in-growth.

Osteotomy. After valgus osteotomy of the hip, weight bearing is restricted for 6 weeks after surgery and then may be advanced per the patient's tolerance. Radiographs must be assessed carefully to monitor healing of the femoral neck and osteotomy and to monitor for the development of osteonecrosis of the femoral head. If the fracture does not heal or if substantial osteonecrosis develops, the patient is best treated with hip replacement.

Femoral Reshaping. After femoral head reshaping, partial weight bearing may be started immediately. Active hip abduction exercises should be restricted, and hip flexion >90 degrees should be restricted for 6 weeks to allow for osteotomy healing. Strengthening, stretching, and full weight bearing begin thereafter. The hip should be followed radiographically for trochanteric healing, osteonecrosis, and arthritic changes.

SUGGESTED READINGS

Bachiller FG, Caballer AP, Portal LF. Avascular necrosis of the femoral head after femoral neck fracture. *Clin Orthop Relat Res.* 2002;399:87–109.

Bellabarba C, Berger RA, Bentley CD, et al. Cementless acetabular reconstruction after acetabular fracture. *J Bone Joint Surg.* 2001;83A:868–876.

Eijer H, Myers SR, Ganz R. Anterior femoroacetabular impingement after femoral neck fractures. *J Orthop Trauma.* 2001;15:475–481.

Haidukewych GJ, Berry DJ. Hip arthroplasty for salvage of failed treatment of intertrochanteric hip fractures. *J Bone Joint Surg.* 2003;85A:899–904.

Mabry TM, Prpa B, Haidukewych GJ, et al. Long-term results of total hip arthroplasty for femoral neck fracture nonunion. *J Bone Joint Surg.* 2004;86A:2263–2267.

Mathews V, Cabanela ME. Femoral neck nonunion treatment. *Clin Orthop Relat Res.* 2004;419:57–64.

Mears DC, Velyvis JH. Acute total hip arthroplasty for selected displaced acetabular fractures: two to twelve-year results. *J Bone Joint Surg.* 2002;84A:1–9.

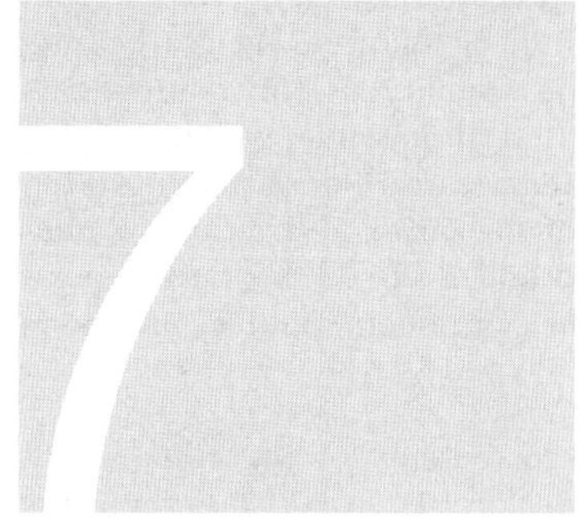

MISCELLANEOUS DISORDERS OF THE HIP JOINT

CHRISTOPHER P. BEAUCHAMP

The list of miscellaneous disorders that can affect the hip is lengthy. This section addresses some of the unique and more troublesome problems. Patients can present with symptoms of pain and functional loss or may simply present with a radiographic abnormality discovered incidentally (Table 7-1). Some of these problems are rare and can be difficult to treat. Some disorders have characteristic radiographic features that can be diagnostic (Table 7-1).

PIGMENTED VILLONODULAR SYNOVITIS OF THE HIP

Pigmented villonodular synovitis (PVNS) of the hip is an uncommon disorder characterized by an effusion, thickened hyperplastic synovium with joint erosions and cysts. It can present with an insidious onset, and the ultimate diagnosis can be difficult to make as it may mimic other inflammatory disorders. Patients who present with a nontraumatic monoarticular effusion should be suspected of having PVNS.

Etiology

The cause is unknown. It is debatable whether this disorder is the result of a true neoplastic process or whether it is merely a reactive monoarticular arthritis. The fact that it is monoarticular supports the concept that it is a neoplastic disease. Although rare, polyarticular disease can occur.

Epidemiology

PVNS occurs equally in males and females and is most common in the third to fifth decade of life. The incidence of this disorder is 1.5 per million; it most commonly affects the knee, hip, ankle, hand, and foot.

Pathology

The gross appearance is characteristic: the joint fluid is blood tinged and the synovium is thickened, nodular, and stained reddish brown with yellow nodules. Histologically, there is a mononuclear stromal cell infiltrate with multinucleated giant cells and foamy histiocytes and there are areas of macrophages containing hemosiderin.

Presentation

Patients usually present with an irritable hip, with pain and diminished range of motion. Symptoms can be insidious.

Radiographic Examination

Plain radiographs range from being normal to end-stage arthritis. The classic radiographic changes that are present include bone erosions in the head and neck of the femur and the acetabulum. The MRI typically shows an effusion with hypertrophic synovium with areas of low signal on T1 and bright areas on T2. Because of the hemosiderin present, there will be other small areas of low signal intensity of T1- *and* T2-weighted images.

Diagnosis

The diagnosis is most often made with MR imaging. The differential diagnosis may include infection or other inflammatory arthritis and an aspiration may be appropriate. Histologic changes from other inflammatory arthritis disorders can often mimic PVNS, particularly if there have been recurrent hemarthroses; thus this condition is often overdiagnosed on pathology reports.

Treatment

The preferred treatment for PVNS is open synovectomy. Attempts at radionucleotide synovectomy have been disappointing. The surgical recurrence rate is high, especially with the diffuse form; therefore, thorough synovectomy, curettage of the cystic lesions, and bone grafting of cavitary defects must be meticulously performed. To visualize the joint completely, the hip must be dislocated. Surgical dislocation of the hip is safe, and the risk of avascular necrosis is very low if the procedure is done correctly. I prefer a

TABLE 7-1 RADIOGRAPHIC DIAGNOSES ANY ORTHOPAEDIC SURGEON SHOULD BE ABLE TO MAKE

Geode
Paralabral degenerative cyst
Enchondroma
Synovial herniation pit
Bone island
Paget disease
Chondroblastoma
Osteoid osteoma
Pigmented villonodular synovitis
Chondromatosis

classic trochanteric slide osteotomy. Care is taken to avoid dissection of any of the posterior capsular structures. The anterior hip capsule is exposed, and an arthrotomy is made in line with the femoral neck. Flaps are then created at the base of the neck toward the lesser trochanter anteriorly and posteriorly along the superior aspect of the capsule just distal to the labrum. A Z-shaped capsular arthrotomy now permits an anterior dislocation of the hip. The ligamentum teres is avulsed or transected, and the dislocation is complete. Adequate visualization now permits a complete synovectomy.

For recurrent disease or aggressive extensive initial disease, moderate dose radiation therapy can be considered. Older patients or those with associated substantial degenerative arthritis are best managed with complete synovectomy and an arthroplasty. Fortunately, with more choices in implant materials, such as metal on metal or ceramic on ceramic bearing surfaces, younger patients can enjoy the reduced recurrence rate and better function that total joint arthroplasty can offer.

Long-Term Outcome

The risk of local recurrence is significant. Patients need to be followed radiographically with periodic MRI scans. A baseline scan is done 6 weeks postsynovectomy. Asymptomatic small local recurrences can be observed. Patient counseling is very important with this disease, because there is risk of progressive arthritis and subsequent need for a total hip arthroplasty. At times this can be a frustrating, progressive, difficult-to-control disease, and patients need to understand this at the beginning of treatment.

Case Presentation

The patient is a 22-year-old man who presents with a one month history of increasing hip pain with episodes of severe hip pain. His physical examination reveals a limp and a painful restricted range of motion. His plain x-ray films and CT scan (Fig. 7-1A–C) demonstrate subtle soft tissue swelling and multiple radiolucent lesions affecting the femoral head and acetabulum. His MRI shows hypointensity on T1 and increased intensity on T2 with low T1 and T2 areas consistent with hemosiderin deposits (Fig. 7-1D–F). He was treated with an open arthrotomy with surgical dislocation of the hip, complete synovectomy, and curettage and bone grafting of the head and acetabular lesions (Fig. 7-1G). Nine months later he underwent removal of the screws in the event a total hip was ever required in the future. Currently 4 years later he remains in remission and has maintained a normal joint space (Fig. 7-1H).

SYNOVIAL CHONDROMATOSIS

This disease of unknown cause is characterized by a metaplastic transformation of synovial tissue. The disease can affect any synovial tissue. The synovium becomes thickened with the formation of nodules of cartilage. The cartilage nodules can grow and become fixed nodules or break off and become loose bodies. Bathed in synovial fluid, they can grow and ossify. The loose fragments can range from tiny radiolucent pieces of cartilage to large bony masses centimeters in diameter.

Epidemiology

The typical age group for this disorder is in the third to fifth decade. Males outnumber females four to one.

Presentation

Patients present usually with an insidious onset of pain, limp, and restricted range of motion. Symptoms of a loose body with locking and giving way are common. Occasionally patients present with end-stage osteoarthritis. The disease is monoarticular affecting the knee, shoulder, elbow, and hip most commonly. Extra-articular disease can occur anywhere there is synovial tissue.

Radiographic Examination

Plain radiographs can range from normal to end-stage osteoarthritis with numerous ossified loose bodies. However, the many loose bodies may be cartilage and unossified, and therefore not visible on plain radiographs. In the early stages, differentiation between other causes of an irritable hip can be difficult.

Computed tomography and magnetic imaging can often be diagnostic. These can demonstrate synovial proliferation with the presence of nodular disease and numerous loose bodies. Once calcified and ossified, the loose bodies can be more readily seen. Occasionally a large synovial extension into the soft tissues can result in an impressive collection of loose bodies.

Treatment

The preferred treatment is removal of all loose bodies and a complete synovectomy. This can be accomplished arthroscopically in some cases, but an open synovectomy allows a more thorough debridement. Arthroscopy has the

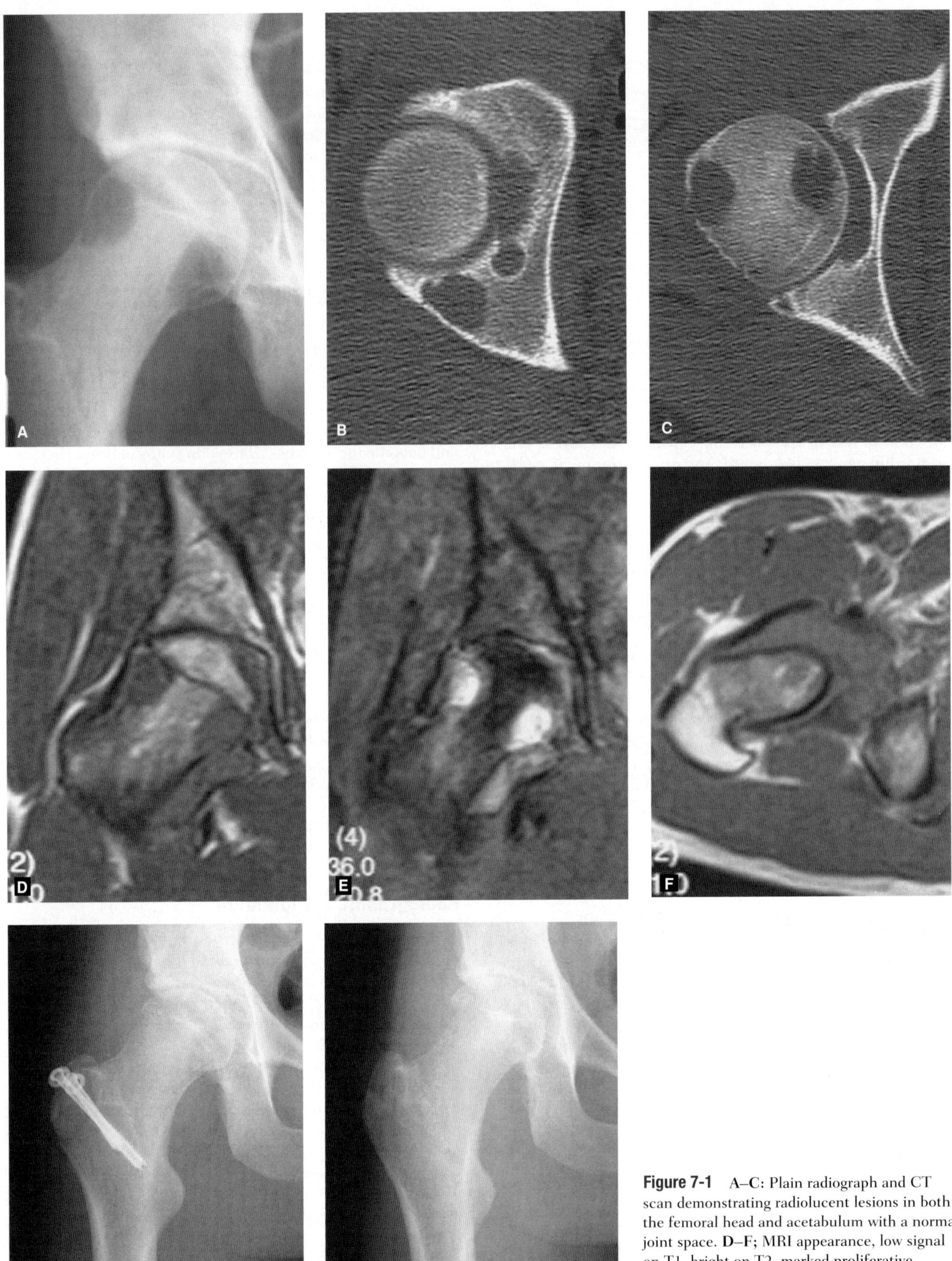

Figure 7-1 A–C: Plain radiograph and CT scan demonstrating radiolucent lesions in both the femoral head and acetabulum with a normal joint space. D–F; MRI appearance, low signal on T1, bright on T2, marked proliferative synovitis, and small areas of dark signal on both T1 and T2 from hemosiderin. G–H: Immediate postoperative and 4-year follow-up films showing cavitary lesions following curettage and grafting.

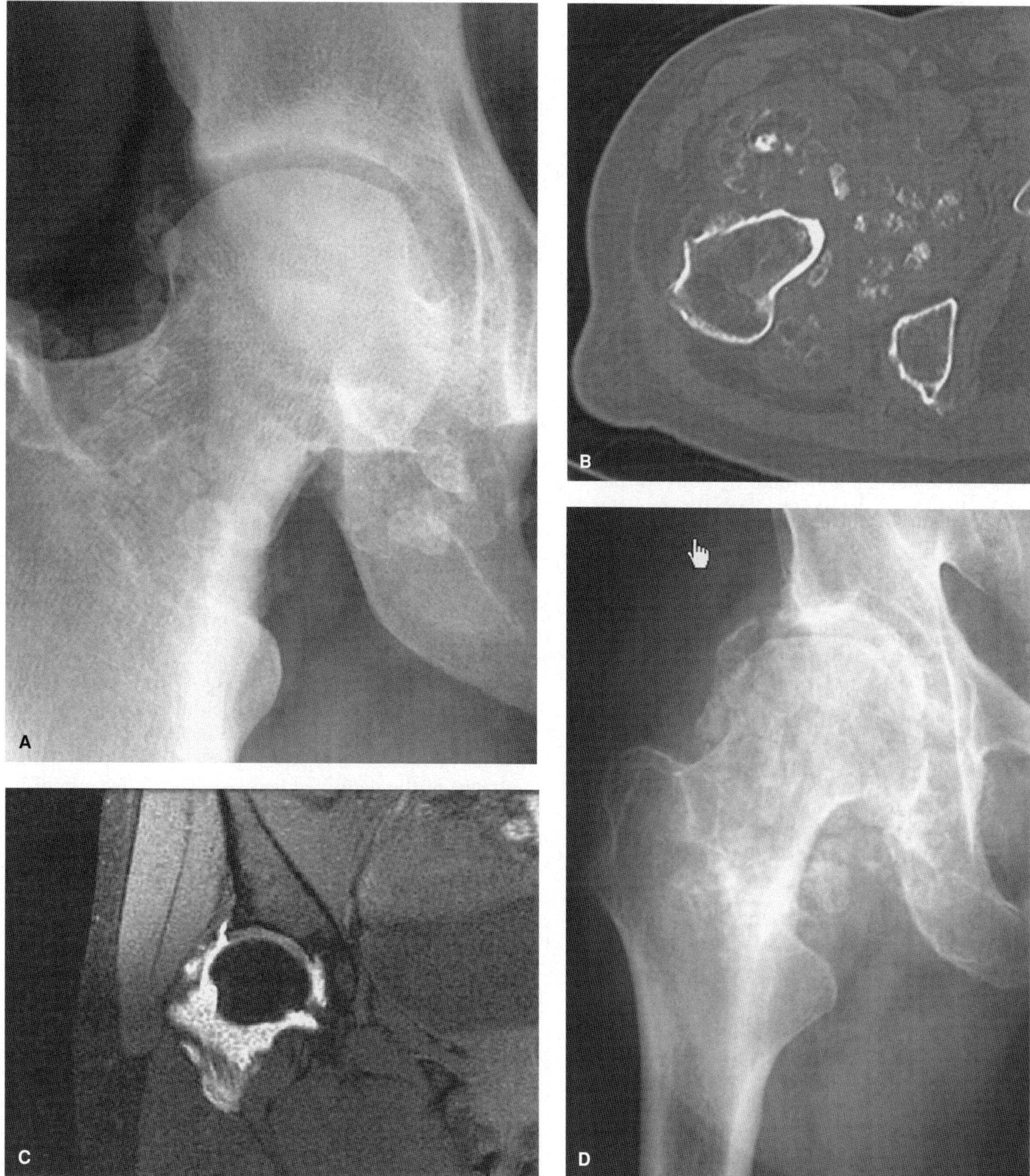

Figure 7-2 A: Plain radiograph demonstrating numerous ossified loose bodies. B: CT scan showing marked synovial proliferation and ossified loose bodies C: MRI T2-weighted image revealing numerous nonossified, noncalcified cartilaginous loose bodies. D: Progression of chondromatosis to advanced secondary degenerative arthritis 4 years later. (Photos A, B, and D courtesy of John Hunter, MD.)

advantage of lower morbidity with less subsequent scarring. Repeat arthroscopy also is more easily performed for recurrent disease. If an adequate debridement and synovectomy cannot be performed with a scope, an open synovectomy with dislocation of the hip as described above should be performed. This disease has a high chance of local recurrence.

Case Presentation

The patient is a 55-year-old man who presents with a 3-year history of increasing pain, a limp and diminished range of motion of his right hip. He has had numerous episodes of locking and giving way of his leg, but these events were short lived and are occurring less frequently now. His physical examination reveals a limp and a markedly reduced painful range of motion. His plain radiographs, CT, and MRI scan demonstrated minimal osteoarthritis with numerous ossified loose bodies (Fig. 7-2A–C). The radiographic features are diagnostic of synovial chondromatosis. Four years later the patient developed progressive osteoarthritis. (Fig. 7-2D). Treatment at this stage consisted of a total hip arthroplasty with synovectomy and removal of the loose bodies.

FIBROUS DYSPLASIA

Fibrous dysplasia is a benign developmental abnormality affecting bone. It can be solitary (monostotic) or multiple (polyostotic) and can have a wide variation in severity. It can sometimes be associated with other medical conditions. This developmental abnormality results in the failure of primitive bone remodeling. The immature bone is imbedded in dysplastic fibrous tissue and is poorly mineralized; it therefore contains the normal constituents of bone but in a very disorganized form, resulting in marked reduction in mechanical strength. The bone is therefore prone to slowly developing deformities and pathologic fractures.

Etiology

The cause of fibrous dysplasia is now believed to be a post-fertilization somatic cell line gene mutation. The severity of the disease is dependent on when and where the mutation occurs during embryogenesis.

Epidemiology

Males and females are equally affected. The disease may present at any age and is nonhereditary. The most common sites of involvement are the long bones, pelvis, ribs, and craniofacial bones.

Clinical Features

Patients present with fibrous dysplasia as an incidental finding, pain, deformity, or fracture. The pain can be owing to the mechanical insufficiency caused by the abnormal tissue or the lesion itself. The degree of deformity depends on the severity and location of the bone involved. The proximal femur is a common location, and the mechanical weakness can result in severe angular deformities with limb-length inequality. This is especially so in polyostotic fibrous dysplasia as it tends to progress in adult life. The classic deformity of the proximal femur is the so-called "shepherd's crook" deformity, a pronounced varus deformity with bowing of the femur and shortening of the limb.

Radiologic Features

Most lesions are noted incidentally. The plain radiograph is usually diagnostic, and the x-ray film characteristics are so distinctive that a diagnosis can be made with confidence. The lesion is usually well demarcated and consists of fairly homogenous fibro-osseous calcified material that has a ground-glass appearance. Occasionally the plain radiographs can be nonspecific owing to cystic degeneration, multiple fractures, or deformity. Patients with a nonspecific radiographic appearance require further investigation and sometimes a biopsy.

Computed Tomography

Computed tomography gives a detailed high-resolution view of the bone, and a diagnosis can often be made at this point. If the radiographic appearance is atypical, an MRI study and a biopsy may be needed.

Magnetic Resonance Imaging

The magnetic resonance image is usually a low-signal T1-weighted image and a T2 signal of higher intensity. The signal intensity is determined by the relative composition of fibrous tissue and mineralized immature bone. There may also be areas of cystic degeneration with a high T2 signal.

Treatment

The role of surgery is not to "remove the tumor" as it is not a neoplastic condition but rather to deal with the mechanical consequences of a relatively weak and deformed bone. Treatment of the deformed bone is difficult because of its poor mechanical strength, and eradication of the fibrous dysplasia usually is not possible.

Case Presentation

The patient is a 20-year-old woman with a history of increasing activity-related pain affecting the right groin and thigh. She has mild pain at rest and moderate pain at night. Her physical examination is essentially normal. Her CT scan shows a lesion in the femoral neck, largely radiolucent with a deficiency in the medial aspect of the cortex (Fig. 7-3A). There is a well-defined reactive rim with increased bone density. The radiographic differential is large, favors a benign process, and includes nonossifying fibroma, fibrous dysplasia, unicameral bone cyst, and eosinophilic granuloma, and so on. Owing to her symptoms, the location of the lesion, and the cortical defect, the patient underwent an open biopsy via a transtrochanteric window under fluoroscopic guidance. Frozen section was consistent with fibrous dysplasia. The lesion was then curetted, and a fibular strut graft was passed up through the neck along the medial cortex of the neck (Fig. 7-3B). A cortical fibular allograft strut was selected for the reconstruction to reduce the risk of dysplastic bone remodeling of the graft. Her follow-up radiograph 4 years later demonstrated a healed graft without replacement by fibrous dysplasia (Fig. 7-3C).

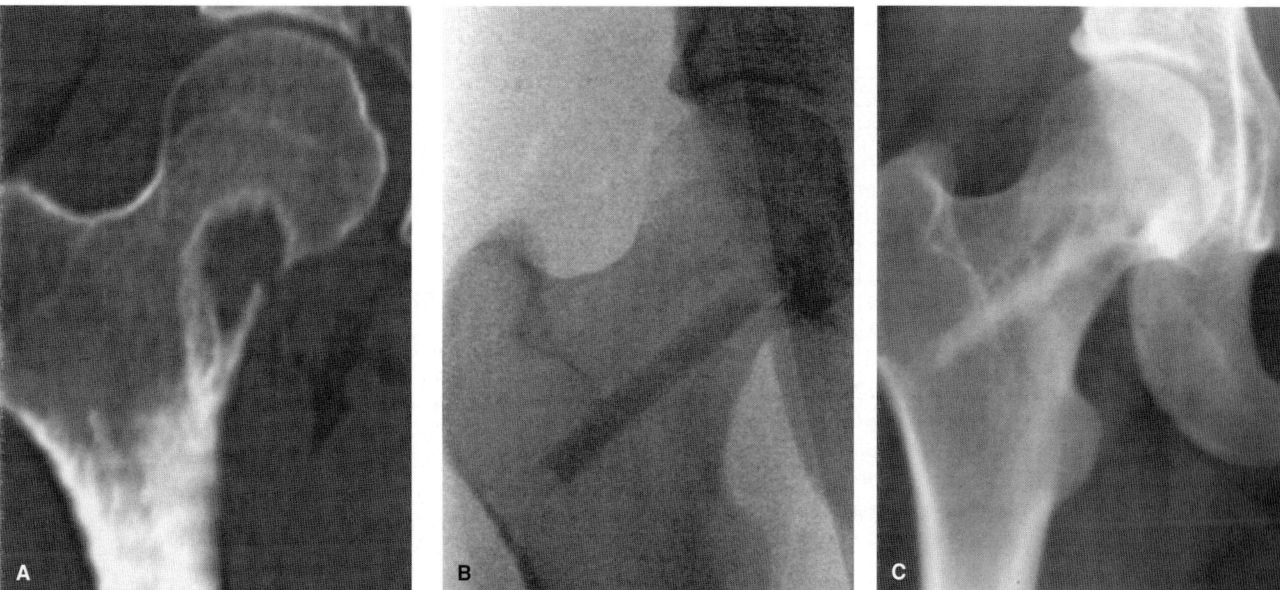

Figure 7-3 A: Coronal CT scan demonstrating relatively nonspecific lesion with a pronounced rim of reactive bone surrounding a radiolucent lesion with a defect in the femoral neck. **B:** Intraoperative image following biopsy and curettage of fibrous dysplasia with insertion of an allograft fibular strut. **C:** Four-year follow-up radiograph showing healing of the graft and no evidence of graft erosion by fibrous dysplasia.

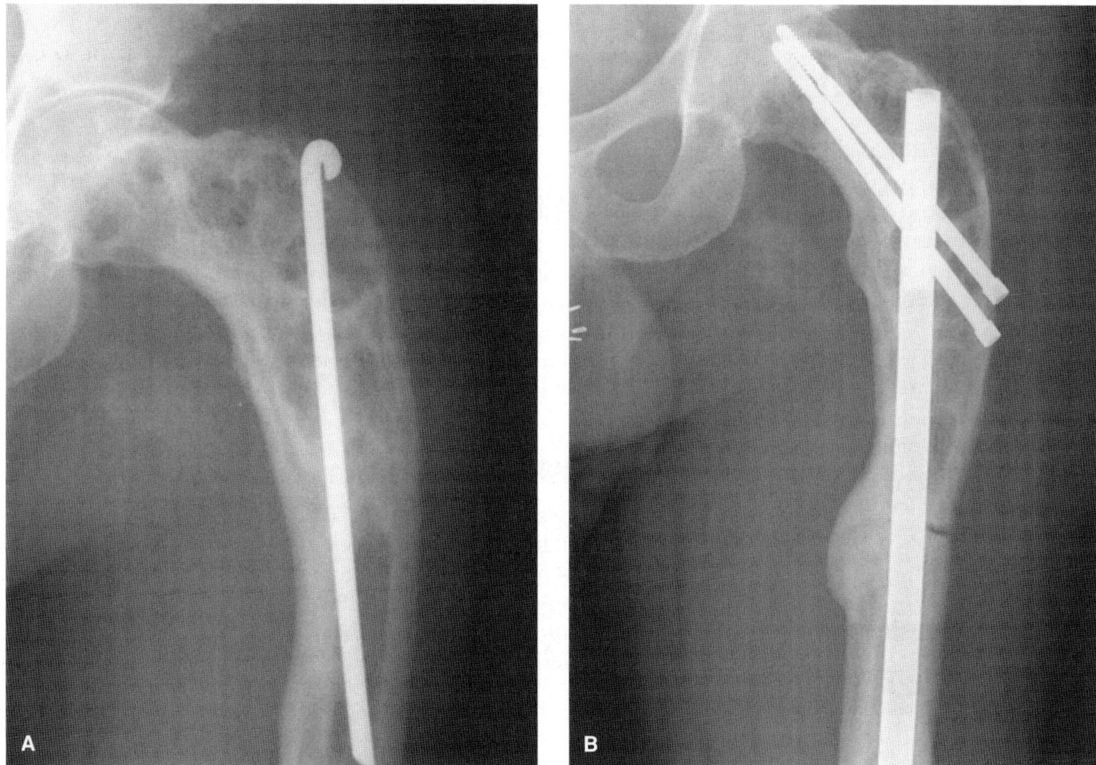

Figure 7-4 A: Plain radiograph of previously treated fibrous dysplasias. Some areas of radiolucency with a ground glass appearance. Previous Rush rod and surgical changes. Note the varus deformity. **B:** Follow-up radiograph 2 years following corrective osteotomy and reconstruction nail fixation.

Case Presentation

A 46-year-old man presents with a long history of episodes of his right hip and thigh pain. He has had episodes of severe pain sometimes requiring crutches. As a child he underwent a surgical procedure because of recurrent pain. His physical examination revealed a 1.5-cm. limb-length discrepancy with shortening in the femur. He had a nearly full range of motion of his hip with minimal pain at the extremes. His radiographs demonstrate mild osteoarthritis, a varus deformity of the femoral neck and proximal femur, evidence of previous surgery, and a mixed radiolucent/radiodense lesion. On close inspection, the bone has a ground-glass appearance (Fig. 7-4A.) His previous surgical records included a pathology report describing fibrous dysplasia. Given his symptoms and the varus deformity, a corrective osteotomy with intramedullary fixation was performed (Fig. 7-4B). The patient has since enjoyed a marked reduction in his symptoms.

METASTATIC DISEASE OF THE FEMORAL NECK

Metastatic malignant disease commonly affects the proximal femur and acetabulum. The role of the orthopaedic surgeon in the management of a patient with metastatic disease is to establish the diagnosis, identify those patients at risk for fracture, and reconstruct bone defects following fracture (Table 7-2).

The management of a pathologic fracture is very different compared with a traumatic fracture in normal bone. Every effort must be directed to the restoration of the patient's function and relief of pain as quickly as possible. Fixation choices should include those options that permit immediate full weight bearing, with the assumption that the fracture itself will never heal. The surgeon must recognize that further local progression of the metastatic lesion may occur.

Femoral neck metastatic disease is rarely treated with retention of the femoral head. Curettage, cementation, and screw fixation of femoral neck lesions is rarely performed. Reduction and fixation of femoral neck fractures should not be performed. These lesions are best managed with either a total hip arthroplasty or hemiarthroplasty. Consideration should be given to using a long cemented stem. This permits predictable immediate fixation, allows for postoperative radiation therapy, and extends the scope of the reconstruction to prophylactically strengthen the remaining femur. The management of an impending femoral neck fracture is the same as for a completed fracture. However, palliative radiotherapy may be offered first as some patients may have a very good response and thus avoid surgery.

TABLE 7-2 METASTATIC BONE DISEASE BASIC SURGICAL PRINCIPLES

Be certain of the diagnosis.
Define the extent of disease.
Assume the fracture will not heal.
Plan for an immediate return of full function.
Fix with a high chance of success.
Anticipate the mode of failure.

Case Presentation

The patient is a 56-year-old woman with known metastatic breast cancer. She has had increasing right hip pain for the past month. The pain was initially present only with weight bearing, but it is now present at rest and she is using crutches and a wheelchair. She has had radiation therapy to that area 4 weeks ago. Her physical exam demonstrated an otherwise healthy-appearing female, but her hip examination revealed a painful range of motion. Her plain radiographs and CT scan show widespread disease affecting the head, neck, and proximal femur. The patient has failed radiation therapy and is at risk of fracture. The intent of treatment is to fix the problem predictably, permit immediate return to function, and avoid future problems related to progression of the disease. Consequently, an arthroplasty was chosen. In this case, a total hip arthroplasty was performed; a hemiarthroplasty would work as well, but a total hip avoids the possibility of a painful hemiarthroplasty in a young patient. A long cemented stem was chosen to permit predictable immediate fixation, antibiotic delivery, and prophylactic stabilization of as much of the femur as possible (Fig. 7-5A–C).

OSTEOID OSTEOMA

Osteoid osteoma is a benign bone tumor with an often characteristic presentation. The lesion is typically ≤1 cm in diameter. It is characterized by a radiolucent nidus with surrounding reactive bone formation. The diagnosis is easy to make histologically.

Epidemiology

This lesion can occur at any age but is more common in children and young adults, with a male predilection of two to one; it can occur in any bone. The lesion produces prostaglandins, which mediate pain and produce new bone formation. Aspirin and other anti-inflammatories block the production of prostaglandin, hence controlling the symptoms.

Presentation

Patients classically present with a deep distressing throbbing pain, typically worse at night. The pain is particularly responsive to aspirin, something patients often stumble on by themselves. Patients may medicate themselves to the

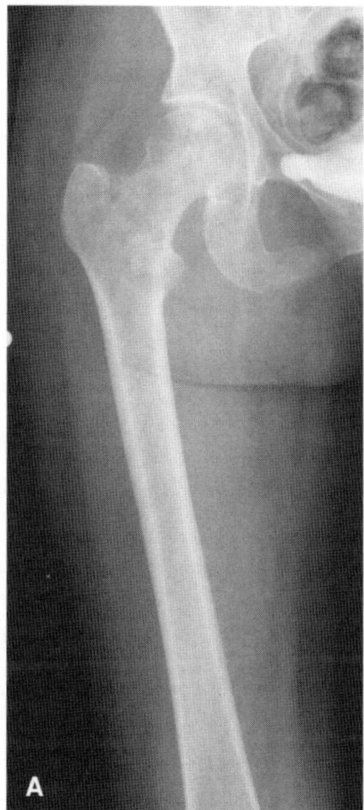

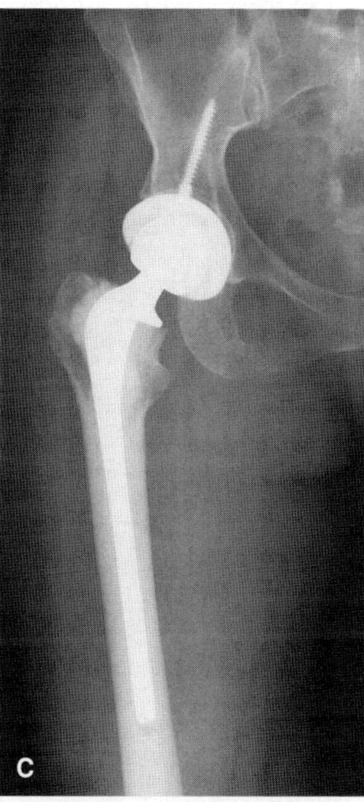

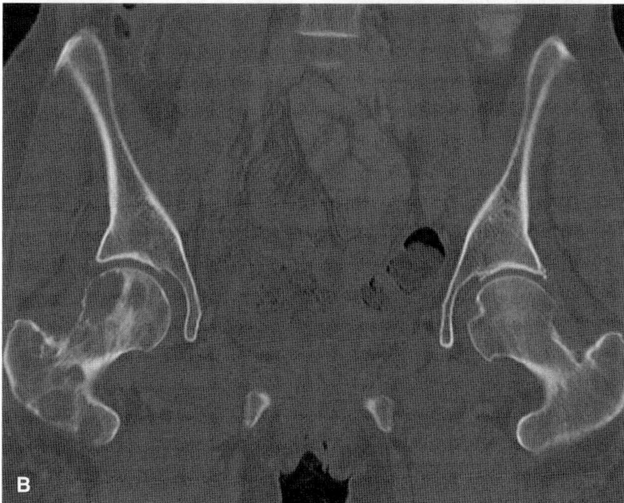

Figure 7-5 A: Multiple radiolucent destructive lesions affecting the femoral head and neck B: CT scan demonstrating diffuse disease from metastatic breast carcinoma C: Pose operative radiograph, long stemmed cemented total hip arthroplasty.

point of developing tinnitus. If the tumor is present in the neck or head of the femur, it can present with typical pain as well as an irritable hip.

Radiographic Evaluation

Plain radiographs are often diagnostic, with the lesion classically demonstrating a radiolucent nidus with a surrounding area of reactive bone produced by prostaglandin production. Technetium bone scanning typically shows a hot spot. A bone scan is helpful when the lesion is not readily apparent on plain radiographs. Computed tomography is often diagnostic and is helpful in locating the lesion in difficult anatomic locations. Dynamic enhanced (gadolinium angiography) magnetic resonance imaging is helpful in differentiating an osteoid osteoma from other similar-appearing lesions. The nidus of an osteoid osteoma will show a bright blush from the gadolinium.

Osteoid osteoma involving the hip joint can have a dramatic appearance on magnetic imaging with edema involving the bone and surrounding soft tissues. A prominent and florid synovial reaction can occur if the lesion is intra-articular, on the surface of the femoral neck, or near the synovium. This can mimic other synovial proliferative disorders both clinically and radiographically.

Treatment

The treatment of choice when medical management fails or is not acceptable is radiofrequency ablation. With the precise guidance of computed tomographic fluoroscopy under general anaesthesia, a radiofrequency needle is placed within the center of the nidus and heated to 90°C for 6 minutes. The morbidity is low, the failure rate is low, and typically the patient is painfree the next day. A biopsy is done at the time of needle insertion, but because of the small size of the needle used, representative tissue is seen only 40% of the time. More than 95% of patients can be expected to be cured with a single treatment. The risk of relapse is low. The patient may resume full unrestricted activity immediately following treatment.

Case Presentation

The patient is a 12-year-old boy with an 8-month history of intermittent hip pain. It has been increasing over the last 2 months and is particularly worse at night. The patient has been taking ibuprofen with moderate pain relief. Physical examination reveals a marked restriction in range of motion of the hip and muscular atrophy. MR imaging reveals a lesion on the neck of the femur with an effusion, synovitis, and surrounding edema (Fig. 7-6A). The image was initially suggestive of either infection or Ewing sarcoma. The clinical and radiographic features were more consistent with osteoid osteoma with a brisk inflammatory reactive response (Fig. 7-6B–D). The patient was treated with a CT-guided radiofrequency thermal ablation (Fig. 7-6E). The patient had an excellent response and remains symptomfree 2 years later.

CHONDROBLASTOMA

Chondroblastoma is a rare benign cartilaginous tumor that classically arises in the epiphysis and accounts for <1% of all primary bone tumors. Most tumors arise in patients with active epiphyses, and the most common location is the proximal humerus, followed by the knee and hip.

Presentation

Patients typically present with symptoms; it is rarely an incidental finding. Symptoms include pain, swelling, and a painful range of motion.

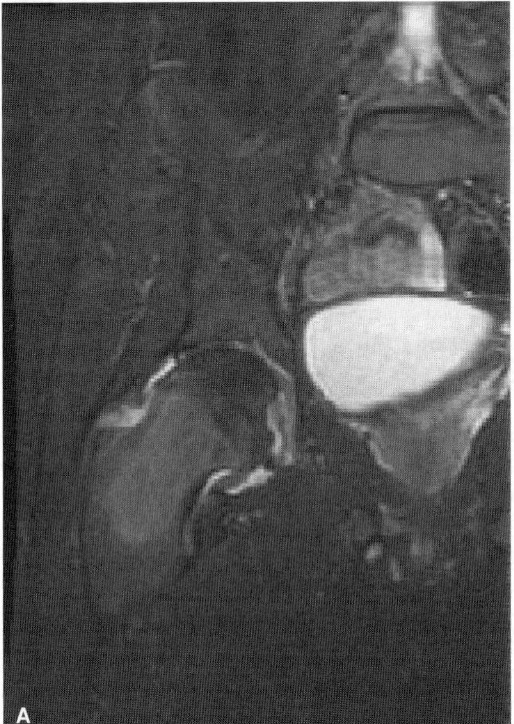

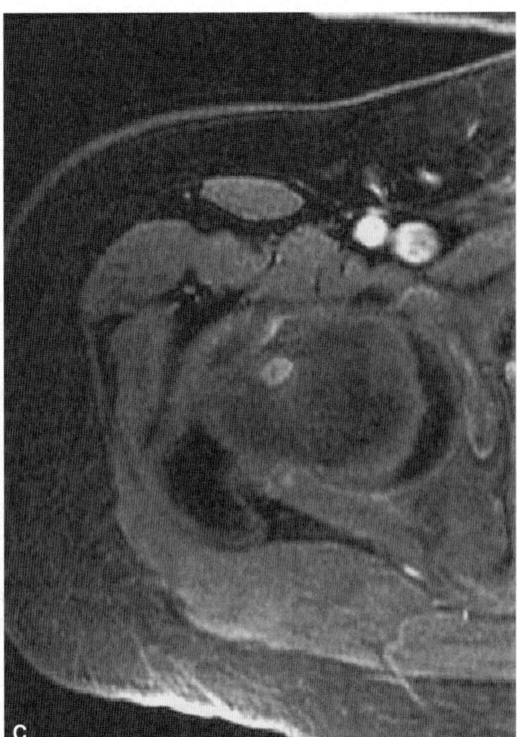

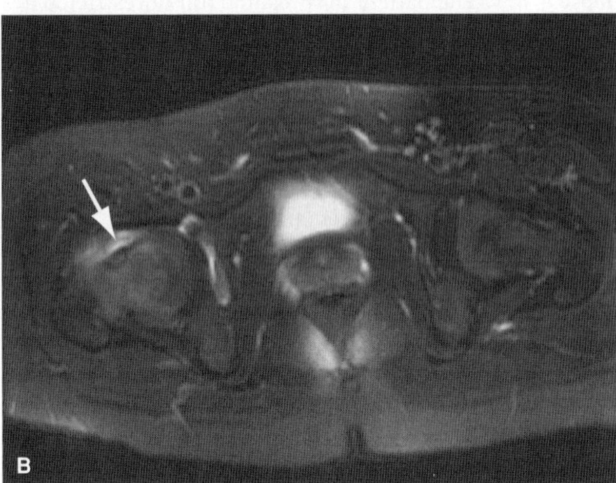

Figure 7-6 **A:** T2-weighted MR image demonstrating marrow signal changes in the proximal femur with a large effusion. **B:** Axial MR image demonstrating the nidus. **C:** Dynamic enhanced MRI showing characteristic blush from gadolinium.

Radiologic Evaluation

The lesion is typically radiolucent with a sharply defined reactive rim. The lesion may show subtle areas of calcification within it, and its location is usually indicative of the diagnosis. The lesion is hot on bone scan, and generalized uptake around the affected joint is not uncommon.

Computed tomography is helpful in demonstrating intralesional calcification and better defines the plain radiographic appearance. Magnetic resonance imaging demonstrates a homogenous hypointense appearance on T1-weighted imaging and variable to hyperintense signal on T2-weighted images. A secondary aneurysmal bone cyst component is not uncommon with chondroblastoma. This is evident by an area of high signal on T2 suggestive of blood and fluid levels on both MRI and CT scans. A large amount of reactive edema in the bone and synovitis in the joint is often seen as well and explains the symptoms of pain and joint irritability seen with often relatively small lesions. Giant cell tumor and clear cell chondrosarcoma are in the differential, but these tend to occur in older patients. Clear cell chondrosarcoma can have a similar MRI appearance to chondroblastoma but is usually in an older age group, is larger, and extends beyond the epiphysis.

Treatment

Chondroblastoma usually responds well to intralesional curettage and bone grafting. This disorder has a local

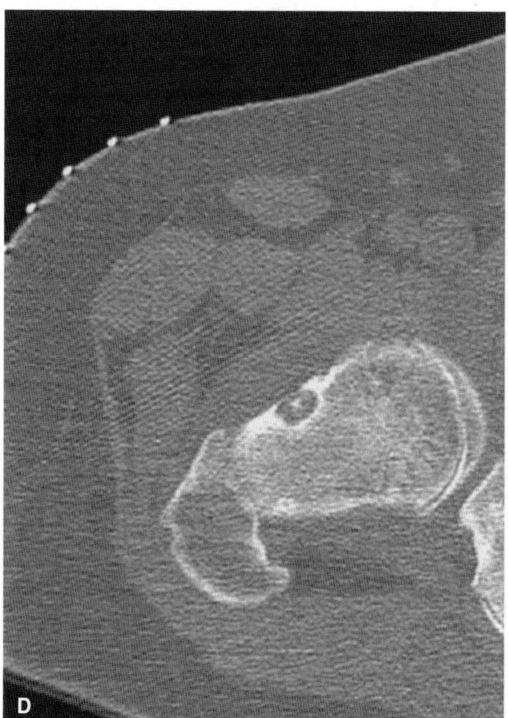

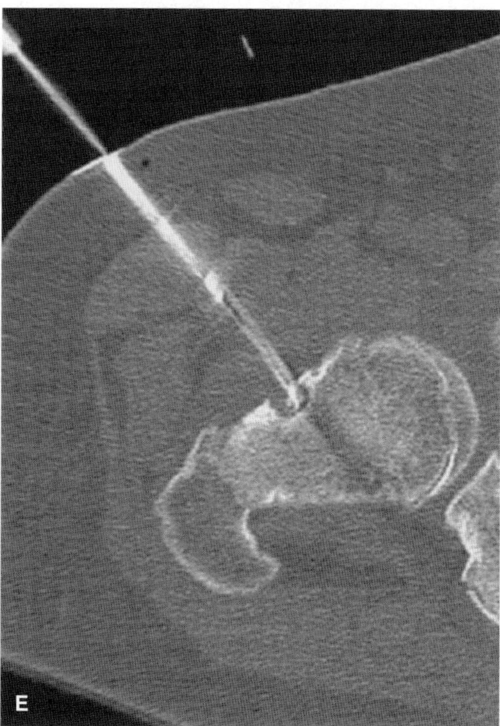

Figure 7-6 ***(Continued)*** D–E: CT images demonstrating the nidus and placement of the radiofrequency probe.

recurrence rate of 5% to 15%, largely depending on the thoroughness of resection. Chondroblastoma of the femoral head presents a challenge in all aspects of its management. In patients in whom the diagnosis is unlikely to be a clear cell chondrosarcoma, treatment can consist of open biopsy, frozen section, and immediate curettage and bone grafting. The surgical approach can include arthrotomy, surgical dislocation, and approaching the lesion from a window in the neck below the articular cartilage or a transtrochanteric tunnel through the neck of the femur. Open arthrotomy has a higher morbidity but would most likely allow for a more complete curettage. A transtrochanteric approach has a lower morbidity but a higher chance of local recurrence. The older patient with a radiolucent epiphyseal tumor is a more difficult problem. The differential diagnosis would include a clear cell chondrosarcoma. A biopsy has the potential to contaminate either the joint or the intertrochanteric region depending on the approach. If the index of suspicion is very high or if the femoral head is so involved and the joint is not contaminated, an excisional biopsy and total hip arthroplasty can be considered on very rare occasions.

Case Presentation

The patient is a 19-year-old female college student who presents with a 4-month history of left hip pain. Activity related, it is increasing in severity and is present at rest and at night. Physical examination reveals a limp and a generally diminished range of motion of her hip with severe pain at the extreme of motion. Plain radiographs demonstrate a radiolucent lesion arising solely in the epiphysis of the proximal femur (Fig. 7-7A). MRI demonstrates a well-defined lesion with a modest amount of edema (Fig. 7-7B,C). The clinical and radiographic features strongly favored a chondroblastoma. The patient was treated by an intralesional curettage and bone grafting. This was done via a transtrochanteric approach with fluoroscopic guidance. A core of bone was removed with a 16-mm trephine. The bone was reserved, and the curettage was guided by fluoroscopy with direct visualization using a laparoscope through the tunnel. Once completed, the core was reinserted into the defect and the lateral deficiency was grafted with morselized allograft. The postoperative MRI at 18 months shows the transtrochanteric approach and the resolution of the lesion with healing of the graft. (Fig. 7-7D–E).

SEPTIC ARTHRITIS WITH PRE-EXISTING JOINT DISEASE

Septic arthritis in adults occurs infrequently. Occasionally, severe joint destruction can occur, most often when the diagnosis is delayed. This problem usually is managed with a resection arthroplasty and a delayed total hip arthroplasty.

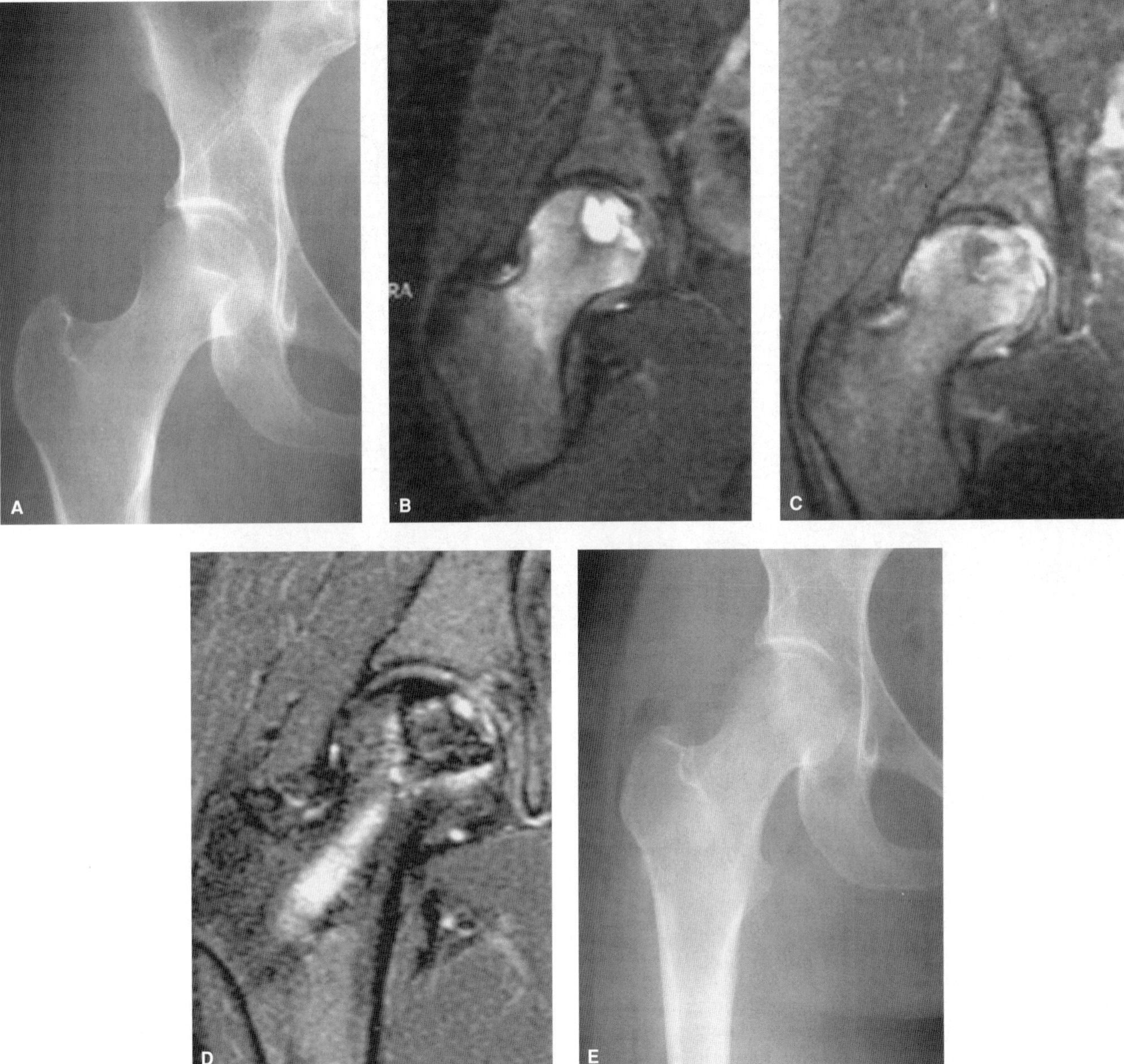

Figure 7-7 A: Plain radiograph showing a subtle radiolucent epiphyseal lesion. B–C: MR image demonstrating marrow edema involving the head and neck. D: Two-year postoperative MRI. The track made by the trephine to obtain access to the lesion is seen on this image. The bone graft is evident in the cavity. E: The corresponding plain radiograph showing the grafted lesion.

Epidemiology

Approximately 20,000 cases per year occur in the United States. The incidence is increased in immunocompromised and elderly patients with comorbidities. Forty-five percent of patients are older than 65 years of age. The morbidity and mortality rate is dependent on the organism.

Diagnosis

This disorder may present with a range of symptoms from subtle joint irritability to fulminant systemic sepsis. Typically, the presentation is monarticular and is usually acute in onset. Patients with pre-existing joint disease report a sudden increase in their joint symptoms.

Physical Examination

On examination, typically the hip is guarded in flexion and external rotation and any motion of the joint is extremely painful. With severely immunocompromised patients, the signs may be less obvious, and in patients with severe sepsis, the diagnosis of polyarticular sepsis may be difficult to make. Ninety percent of cases are monarticular.

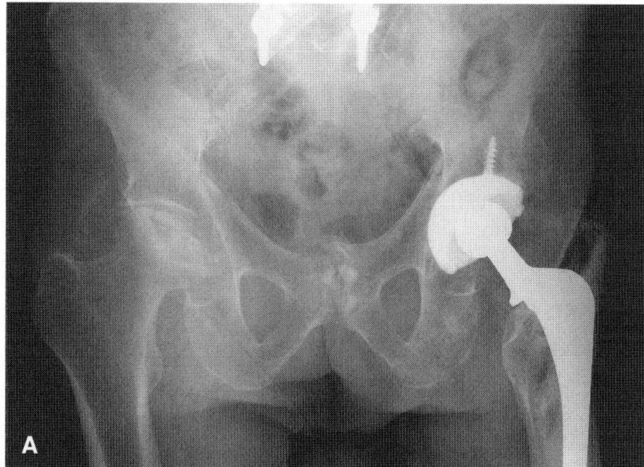

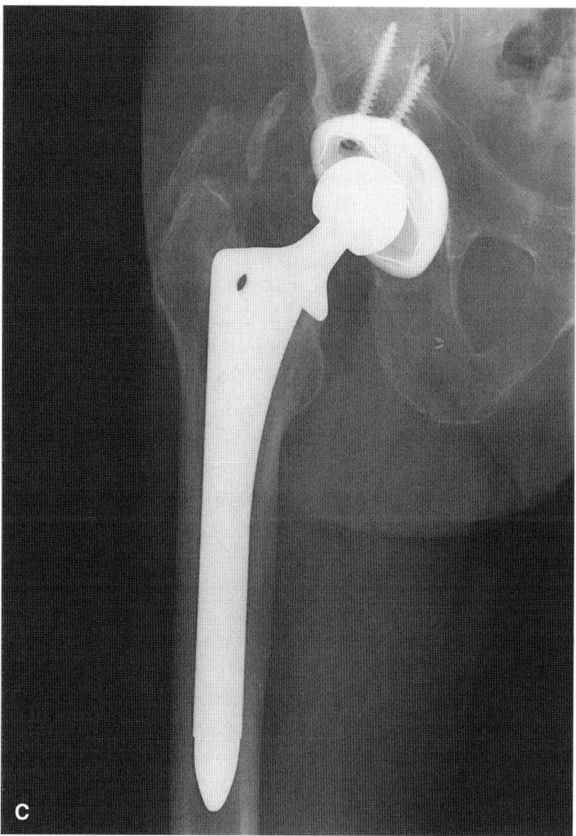

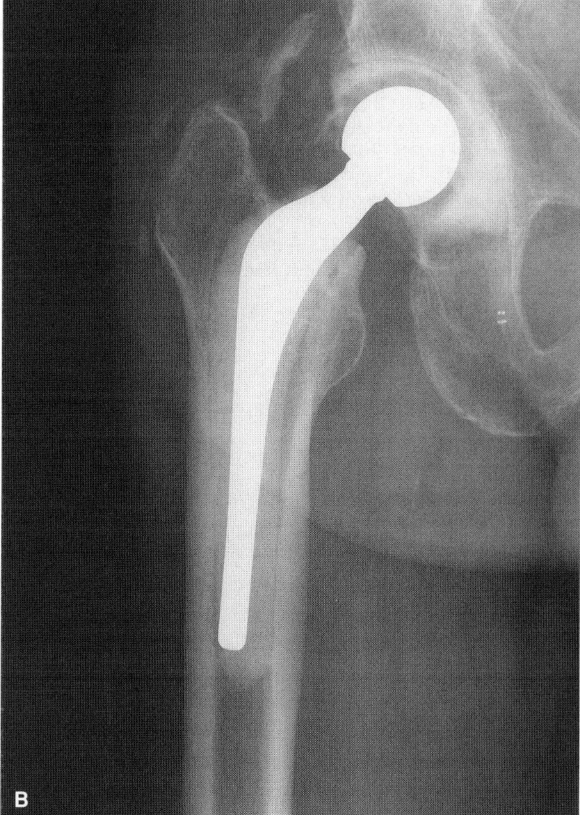

Figure 7-8 A: Plain radiograph showing advanced avascular necrosis and soft tissue swelling around the right hip joint. B: Interval antibiotic spacer prosthesis. The patient was allowed full weight bearing on this device. C: Subsequent definitive reconstruction with a cementless implant.

Diagnosis

The plain radiographs usually are normal. An MRI is very helpful in demonstrating an effusion with reactive edema. Patients with pre-existing hip pathology can present more of a challenge radiographically, as the underlying arthritic problem can be the source of pain.

Aspiration for culture, cell count, and joint fluid analysis is the test of choice. Treatment is based on the clinical findings and the preliminary joint fluid analysis. If the suspected diagnosis is sepsis, the treatment is arthrotomy, debridement, and antibiotic therapy.

Various approaches can be used, but I prefer an anterolateral approach, excision of the anterior capsule of the hip, and a synovectomy without dislocating the hip. In patients who have pre-existing end-stage hip disease or those patients with persistent infection with a destroyed hip joint, I resect the femoral head and insert a primary functional antibiotic-impregnated spacer total hip prosthesis. Various spacers are now available. I prefer to use a therapeutic dosage of antibiotics in the bone cement, typically 4.8 g of gentamicin and 2.0 g of vancomycin per 40-g package of cement. The patient receives 6 weeks of parenteral antibiotics followed by a definitive arthroplasty, usually a minimum of 8 weeks later. The second stage can be deferred indefinitely in patients who are elderly and frail and have other significant comorbidities.

Case Presentation

The patient is a 68-year-old man with a recent diagnosis of a low-grade gastrointestinal (GI) lymphoma and has been receiving chemotherapy. He has had right hip pain for the past 5 months. It began suddenly and has been getting worse. Over the past 3 days the pain has become severe, and he has been unable to get out of bed for the past 24 hours. On physical examination he appears unwell and his temperature was 39.5°C. His hip is extremely painful to any motion, and he has marked tenderness in his right groin. His hip was aspirated, revealing a white count of 65,000 cells with 80% nucleated polymorphonuclear cells. A Gram stain revealed Gram-positive cocci. His plain radiograph showed stage four avascular necroses (Fig. 7-8A). The patient was treated with surgical debridement and a two-stage total hip replacement, first using a functional antibiotic-impregnated spacer prosthesis (Fig. 7-8B). He was treated with 6 weeks of intravenous vancomycin and oral rifampin for methicillin-resistant staph aureus. He continued his chemotherapy, and initially it was planned to leave the temporary device in indefinitely. He did well with his lymphoma, was allowed to be as active as possible, and finally a year later his hip was replaced with a definitive prosthesis (Fig. 7-8C).

SUGGESTED READINGS

Chaarani MW. Percutaneous extra-articular excision of femoral neck osteoid osteoma: report of a new method. *J R Coll Surg Edinb.* 2002;47:705–708.

Ganz R, Gill TJ, Gautier E, et al. Surgical dislocation of the adult hip: a technique with full access to the femoral head and acetabulum without the risk of avascular necrosis. *J Bone Joint Surg Br.* 2001;83:1119–1124.

Goldman AB, DiCarlo EF. Pigmented villonodular synovitis. Diagnosis and differential diagnosis. *Radiol Clin North Am.* 1988;26:1327–1347.

Knoeller SM. Synovial osteochondromatosis of the hip joint. Etiology, diagnostic investigation and therapy. *Acta Orthop Belg.* 2001;67(3):201–210.

Krebs VE. The role of hip arthroscopy in the treatment of synovial disorders and loose bodies. *Clin Orthop Rel Res.* 2003;406:48–59.

Masri BA, Duncan CP, Beauchamp CP. Long-term elution of antibiotics from bone-cement: an in vivo study using the prosthesis of antibiotic-loaded acrylic cement (PROSTALAC) system. *J Arthroplasty.* 1998;13(3):331–338.

Parekh SG, Donthineni-Rao R, Ricchetti E, et al. Fibrous dysplasia. *J Am Acad Orthop Surg.* 2004;12(5):305–313.

Stricker SJ. Extraarticular endoscopic excision of femoral head chondroblastoma. *J Pediatr Orthop.* 1995;15:578–581.

Vastel L, Lambert P, De Pinieux G, et al. Surgical treatment of pigmented villonodular synovitis of the hip. *J Bone Joint Surg Am.* 2005;87:1019–1024.

Weber KL, Lewis VO, Randall RL, et al. An approach to the management of the patient with metastatic bone disease. *Instr Course Lect.* 2004;53:663–676.

HIP ARTHROSCOPY INTERVENTION IN EARLY HIP DISEASE

8

J. BOHANNON MASON

In the late 1970s and early 1980s, the acetabular labrum was implicated in the evolution of hip arthritis and was cited as a potential cause for hip pain with normal-appearing radiographs. On the heels of clinical success with knee and shoulder arthroscopy, hip arthroscopy emerged in the mid 1980s, predominantly as a treatment modality for removal of loose bodies and evaluation and resection of acetabular labral defects.

With the development of arthroscopic techniques and the recognition of the considerably wider spectrum of intra-articular hip pathology amenable to arthroscopic evaluation, the techniques of hip arthroscopy have continued to evolve. Most recently, with renewed interest in minimally invasive surgical techniques, hip arthroscopy is being explored as a potential adjunct to other surgical interventions designed to address a wider array of hip pathology.

ANATOMIC CONSIDERATIONS

The acetabulum represents the convergence and subsequent fusion of the three ossification centers of the pelvis: the pubis, ischium, and ilium. Normal hip anatomy includes a ball-and-socket configuration with deep intrinsic stability. The femoral head articulates at a neck shaft angle typically of 130 degrees and 10 degrees of anteversion. Developmental variances provide a wide spectrum of head coverage. This variability is compounded by the degree of anteversion of the acetabular opening and the flexural position of the pelvis relative to the lumbar spine. The motion of the hip is typically considered in three planes: sagittal, frontal, and transverse. The greatest degree of motion occurs in the sagittal plane.

The acetabular labrum is a triangular cartilaginous structure that rims the edge of the acetabulum. The labrum originates anteriorly at the transverse acetabular ligament. The anterior and superior aspects of the acetabular labrum are typically triangular. Posteriorly, the labrum is less pronounced and more rounded. A small sulcus is present between the labrum and the articular margin of the acetabular cartilage. This sulcus is typically more pronounced posteriorly. The hip capsule is composed of dense fibrous tissue and can anatomically be divided into three ligaments. These include the iliofemoral ligament or Y ligament of Bigelow, which extends from anterior superiorly on the ileum down to the anterior intertrochanteric ridge. The ischial femoral ligament is typically considered a capsular thickening, which wraps forward from the posterior acetabular rim to the piriformis fossa. The third component of the hip capsule is a pubofemoral ligament, which extends inferiorly from the pubis to the posterior inferior femoral neck. The patulence of the hip capsule is greatest inferiorly, and is constricted around the neck of the femur by circular oriented fibers of the hip capsule, forming the zona orbicularis.

The arthroscopic approach to the hip must transverse the subcutaneous tissues, abductor muscle mass, and the capsular structures. Because of the intimate configuration of the ball-and-socket joint, arthroscopic visualization of the articular surface generally requires distraction of the hip to allow access between the femoral head and the acetabulum. The thick muscular envelope and often thick subcutaneous layer require exacting techniques of portal placement to ensure optimal mobility of the instruments within the hip joint.

The acetabular labrum derives its blood supply from vessels originating from the acetabular bony rim. Nociceptors are present within the labral tissue. Consequently, damage to the acetabular labrum can result in pain, and tearing of the acetabular labrum away from the acetabular rim may devascularize the labral fragment. The dysvascular labral tear has limited potential for spontaneous healing.

The iliofemoral and ischiofemoral ligaments both are tighter in hip extension than in slight hip flexion.

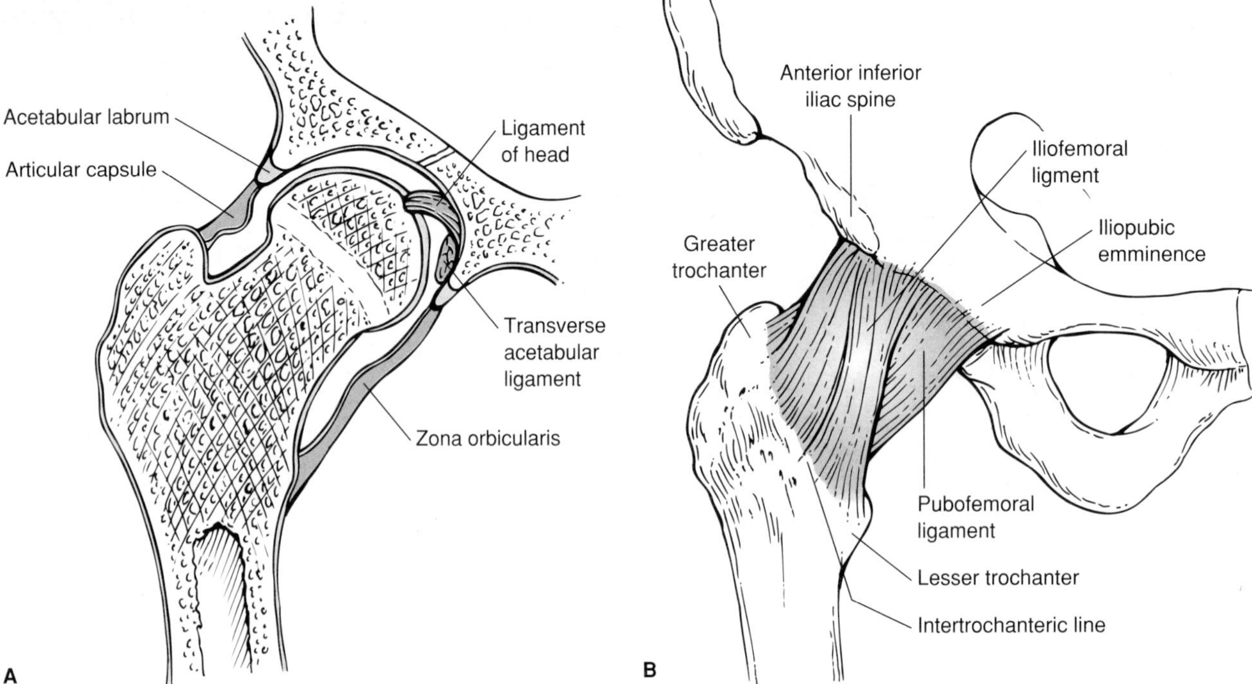

Figure 8-1 **A:** Midcoronal cross-sectional drawing of the right hip. **B:** Right hip pericapsular structures.

Consequently, hip distraction typically is best achieved with slight hip flexion. The ligamentum teres remains recessed within the acetabular fossa. In the neonate, blood supply to the femoral epiphysis occurs via the terminal branches of the medial femoral circumflex artery via the ligamentum teres. In the adult, the ligamentum teres exists primarily as a tendinous structure attached to the base of the acetabulum at the confluence of the transverse acetabular ligament and the fovea on the femoral head. In the adult, the artery of the ligamentum teres supplies only a vestige of blood supply to the femoral head (Fig. 8-1A, B).

SURGICAL INDICATIONS

Hip arthroscopy has benefited from an increased understanding of hip anatomy, improvements in distraction techniques, and instrumentation designed specifically to address hip pathology arthroscopically. Prior to hip arthroscopy, open exploration of the hip with dislocation of the hip was the only method to address many intra-articular problems including loose bodies, acetabular labral tears, bone spurs, and synovial pathology.

Proposed current indications for hip arthroscopy include diagnostic evaluation of the painful hip, excision of loose bodies, management of synovial chondromatosis, resection of labral tears and chondral flaps, diagnostic evaluation of osteonecrosis, treatment of torn ligamentum teres, partial synovectomy, foreign body removal, posttraumatic excision of osteochondral fragments, lavage in crystalline arthropathy or early sepsis as well as capsular shrinkage in conditions of instability such as Ehlers-Danlos. Additionally, hip arthroscopy has been used in removal of loose bodies following total hip arthroplasty and as an adjunct for management of extra-articular conditions such as snapping psoas tendon, bursectomy, and soft tissue releases. The indications will be discussed individually below.

Labral Tears

Labral tears occur most commonly in the anterior superior quadrant of the acetabulum. When present, a labral tear can produce functionally limiting symptoms typically characterized as catching or occasionally popping. Arthroscopic visual inspection can delineate areas of degenerative tearing that are amenable to resection and/or stabilization techniques. Acetabular labral stabilization, although inherently appealing, is technically challenging and is typically reserved for acute traumatic tears of the acetabular labrum. Arthroscopy provides excellent visualization and access to the acetabular labrum (Fig. 8-2A, B).

Loose Bodies

Loose bodies are commonly associated with catching or locking presentation. They may be ossified but commonly are cartilaginous. These loose bodies within the hip are notoriously difficult to visualize with either plain x-ray views or other radiographic studies. Synovial osteochondromatosis can result in accumulation of dozens of loose bodies within the hip joint. Arthroscopic techniques are particularly helpful in the management of loose bodies because removal is associated with a high degree of symptom relief.

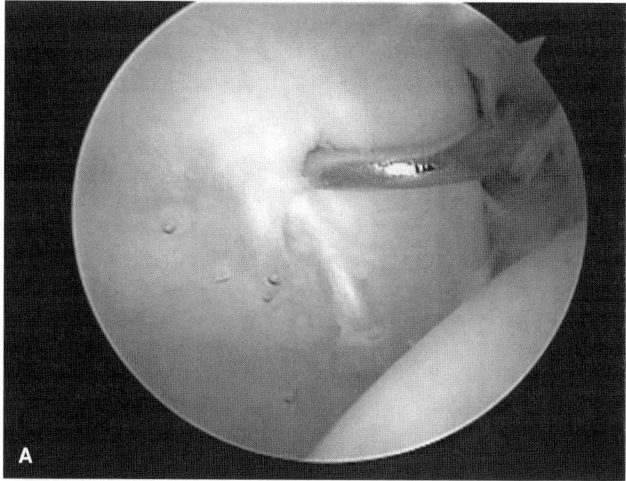

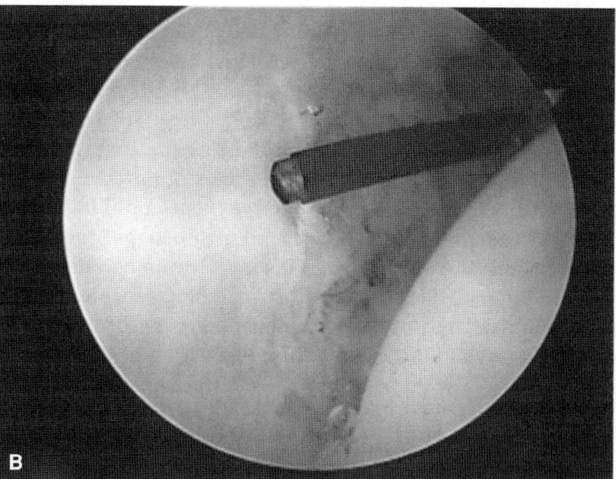

Figure 8-2 A: Tears of the acetabular labrum often occur at the junction of the labrum and the articular cartilage of the acetabulum. The distracted femoral head is visible at the right of the field. B: Flexible thermal ablation probes are quite useful in resection of degenerative labral tears.

Chondral Lesions of the Acetabulum or Femoral Head

Full-thickness chondral lesions often present in association with loose bodies. These lesions are distinguished from degenerative wear within the hip, which results in a widespread thinning of the articular cartilage and exposure of subchondral bone. Full-thickness osteochondral lesions may occur as a result of impact injury but more commonly are associated with the delamination of the chondral surface in association with other entities, including labral tears and femoro-acetabular impingement (Fig. 8-3). Resection of chondral flap injury to stable margins is associated with a high degree of symptom resolution. Clinical outcome is predicated on the size and location of the articular cartilage injury. The prognosis is typically poor when full-thickness chondral injury is present on both the acetabulum and femoral head. Additionally, when acetabular chondral lesions exceed 1 cm square, the shouldering effect of the cartilage is diminished and the prognosis is more guarded.

Figure 8-3 Chondral delamination is often seen at the anterior origin of the acetabulum in association with labral tears.

Ligamentum Teres—Rupture or Impingement

Clinical subluxation of the hip as a result of trauma may result in tearing and degenerative change within the ligamentum teres. The tendinous ligament, when avulsed from the fovea of the femoral head, may result in impingement or a catching/locking pain pattern. Arthroscopic resection of the ligamentum teres from the fovea typically results in near complete pain relief.

Synovial Abnormalities

Inflammation of the hip synovium can result from several pathologic conditions including crystalline arthropathy, collagen vascular disease, mechanical irritation, or viral cause. An effusion of the hip joint can be quite painful and is visible on T2-weighted MRI. When diagnostic uncertainty exists, aspiration of the hip is not conclusive, and other serum-based testing fails to yield a diagnostic conclusion, hip arthroscopy may be used for lavage as well as for synovial biopsy. Additionally, for conditions that are synovium based, such as synovial chondromatosis, which result in synovial tissue production of chondral or osteochondral loose bodies, arthroscopic excision of the loose bodies and thermal ablation of the visible synovial tissues can lead to symptom resolution.

Other synovium-based pathologies such as pigmented villonodular synovitis may be treated in a temporizing manner or even potentially eradicated with arthroscopic techniques. Collagen vascular diseases such as lupus, juvenile rheumatoid arthritis, or rheumatoid arthritis may manifest first with hip pain. Synovial biopsy can prove diagnostic when these patients are seronegative.

Infection

Hip arthroscopy has been used effectively in lavage and management of acute pyarthrosis of the hip. Clinical series in the literature support use of hip arthroscopy in both the adult and pediatric population following the early onset of symptoms, and good results have been reported in patients with favorable host parameters and susceptible bacteria. After lavage of the hip joint and arthroscopic assessment of the cartilaginous surfaces, a small drain can be left within the hip capsule temporarily to facilitate decompression. Obviously, arthroscopic management is performed in conjunction with appropriate antibiotic treatment.

Femoral Acetabular Impingement

The role for hip arthroscopy in femoral acetabular impingement is evolving. There are reports of patients in whom the offending femoral neck impingement is adequately decompressed arthroscopically. However, no large series to date substantiates these findings. Hip arthroscopy also can be used as an adjunct to open arthrotomy for more involved femoral acetabular impingement. Arthroscopy allows a more intimate and detailed evaluation of the acetabular labrum in the area of impingement as well as an assessment of the articular cartilage prior to initiation of a surgical dislocation of the hip for femoral neck contouring procedures.

SURGICAL TECHNIQUES

Patient positioning can be either lateral or supine. Most hip arthroscopists use a distraction apparatus specifically designed for hip arthroscopy or a fracture table (Fig. 8-4). To adequately visualize the inner aspects of the acetabulum and to assess intra-articular pathology, the femoral head must be distracted from the acetabulum. The orientation of the traction must affect a resultant force parallel to the femoral neck. This is typically achieved with a peroneal post and longitudinal distraction. The hip is slightly flexed and slightly externally rotated to relax the anterior hip capsular structures. Image intensification is used to assess joint distraction, and these cases are typically performed under general anesthesia with skeletal muscle relaxation to reduce the distraction force (Fig. 8-5).

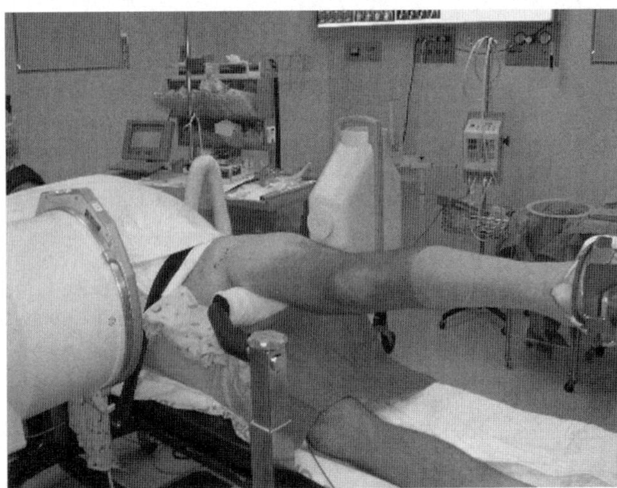

Figure 8-4 A fracture table is useful to assist with distraction of the hip. Note the positioning of fluoroscopy, which is draped within the surgical field.

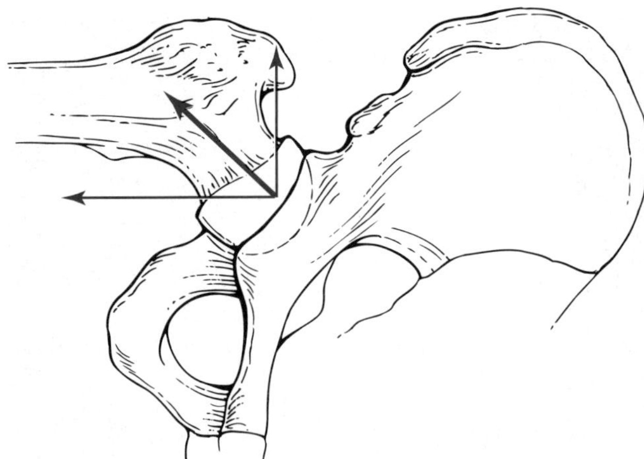

Figure 8-5 Axial traction is accompanied by lateral traction via the peroneal post. The resultant traction vector is in line with the femoral neck, allowing the femoral head to lift out of the acetabulum.

Modern arthroscopy sets contain 14-gauge 6-inch spinal needles that can be advanced into the hip capsule. A small nitinol wire is passed through the needle, then various cannula and sleeves can be advanced safely over the wire into the hip joint.

Portal Placement

Typically three working portals are used in hip arthroscopy. These include the anterior and posterior peritrochanteric portals and a direct anterior portal. The location of the peritrochanteric portal is approximately 1 to 2 cm proximal to the bony tip of the greater trochanter and located at the anterior and posterior margins of the trochanteric profile. The direct anterior portal typically is localized by drawing a vertical line from the anterior superior iliac spine down on the anterior thigh and a horizontal line from the top of the greater trochanter intersecting the anterior superior iliac spine (ASIS) line. From this point on the horizontal, the portal is lateralized to the junction of the middle third and medial third of the horizontal line from the tip of the trochanter. This location will avoid injury to the superficial femoral cutaneous nerve. The anterior and posterior peritrochanteric portals provide excellent visualization of the entire intra-articular hip. The direct anterior portal facilitates a working portal in the anterior inferior quadrant of the hip (Fig. 8-6A, B).

Both 30-degree and 70-degree arthroscopes are used. Most hip arthroscope sets provide longer instrumentation, scope cannulae, and lenses. Flexible and maneuverable thermal ablation probes provide the ability to manipulate synovial and chondral structures, and a combination of

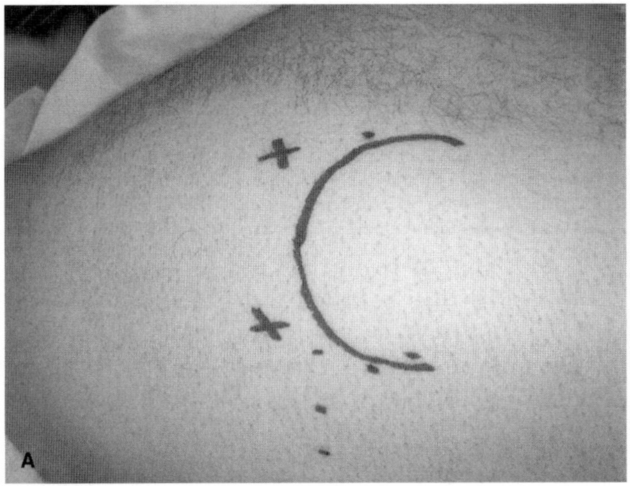

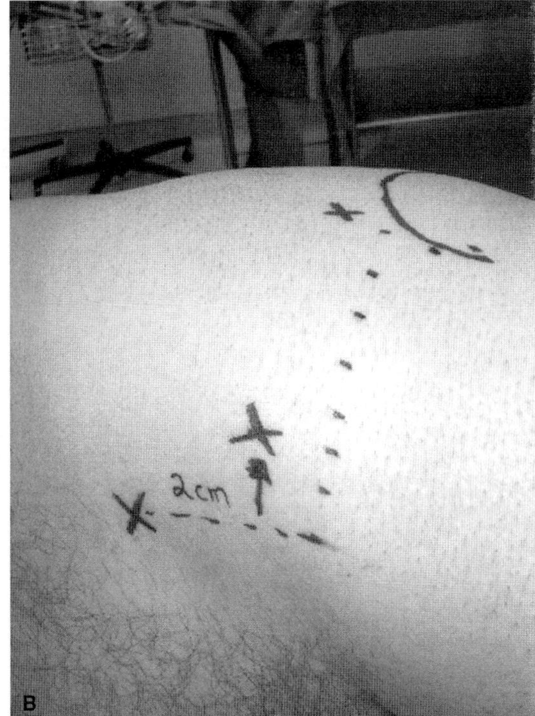

Figure 8-6 A: The trochanteric outline is used to localize the anterior and posterior peritrochanteric portals. B: The anterior portal is typically lateral to the anterior superior iliac crest.

shavers and burrs are used to assist with contouring and loose body removal.

The inferior sulcus of the hip capsule, in the region of the zone orbicularis, can be accessed for loose body removal via the anterior peritrochanteric and direct anterior portals. The femoral head is allowed to reduce into the acetabulum as traction is released. The hip joint is flexed approximately 45 degrees with slight adduction, which provides increased patulence in the inferior recess of the hip capsule. Fluoroscopy is helpful in achieving cannula positioning.

COMPLICATIONS AND CONTRAINDICATIONS

Hip arthroscopy has been shown in a large series to be a relatively safe operative intervention. The complication rate in the largest series reported to date by Villiar was 1.4%, which included transient sciatic palsy, transient femoral palsy, vaginal tear, and hematoma. Avoiding major complications including severe neurovascular injury requires exacting techniques on the part of the surgeon and fluoroscopic assistance in portal placement. The surgeon should carefully pad the perineum and the ankle as considerable distraction forces are applied during the course of the surgical procedure. Distraction time should be limited, typically to <2 hours.

Conditions that preclude distraction of the joint such as ankylosis; severe petrusio or heterotrophic ossification should discourage attempted arthroscopy due to the risk of injury from distraction and obstruction at typical portals from the surrounding bone. Because of the depth of the hip joint, morbid obesity remains a relative contraindication.

SUMMARY

Hip arthroscopy provides excellent visualization of the articular surfaces of the acetabulum and femoral head. Modern arthroscopy techniques facilitate management of a myriad of pathologic conditions within the hip joint and permit modulation of early hip disease. Refinement of indications for hip arthroscopy will continue as longer-term outcome studies emerge.

SUGGESTED READINGS

Blitzer CM. Arthroscopic management of septic arthritis of the hip. *Arthroscopy*. 1993;9(4):414–416.

Byrd JW, Thomas, Jones KS. Diagnostic accuracy of clinical assessment, magnetic resonance imaging, magnetic resonance qrthrography, and intra-articular injection in hip arthroscopy patients. *Am J Sports Med*. 2004;32:1668–1674.

Clarke MT, Arora A, Villar RN. Hip arthroscopy: complications in 1054 cases. *Clin Orthop Relat Res*. 2003;406:84–88.

Dinauer PA, Murphy KP, Carroll JF. Sublabral sulcus at the posteroinferior acetabulum: a potential pitfall in MR arthrography diagnosis of acetabular labral tears. *AJR Am J Roentgenol*. 2004;183:1745–1753.

Dorfmann H, Boyer T. Arthroscopy of the hip: 12 years of experience. *Arthroscopy*. 1999;15(1):67–72.

Elsaidi GA, Ruch DS, Schaefer WD, et al. Complications associated with traction on the hip during arthroscopy. *J Bone Joint Surg Br*. 2004;86-B:793–796.

Gray AJ, Villar RN. The ligamentum teres of the hip: an arthroscopic classification of its pathology. *Arthroscopy*. 1997;13:575–578.

Griffin DR, Villar RN. Complications of arthroscopy of the hip. *J Bone Joint Surg Br*. 1999;81:604–606.

Harris WH. Etiology of osteoarthritis of the hip. *Clin Orthop Relat Res*. 1986;213:20–33.

Hyman JL, Salvati EA, Laurencin CT, et al. The arthroscopic drainage, irrigation, and debridement of late, acute total hip arthroplasty infections: average 6-year follow-up. *J Arthroplasty*. 1999;14:903–910.

Kim SJ, Choi NH, Kim HJ. Operative hip arthroscopy. *Clin Orthop Relat Res*. 1998;353:156–165.

McCarthy JC. Hip arthroscopy: when it is and when it is not indicated. *Instr Course Lect*. 2004;53:615–621.

McCarthy JC, Lee JA. Arthroscopic intervention in early hip disease. *Clin Orthop Rel Res*. 2004;426:157–162.

Pryor GA, Villar RN, Ronen A, et al. Seasonal variation in the incidence of congenital talipes equinovarus. *J Bone Joint Surg Br*. 1991;73: 632–634.

Seldes RM, Tan V, Hunt T, et al. Anatomy, histologic features, and vascularity of the adult acetabular labrum. *Clin Orthop Relat Res*. 2001;382:232–240.

Singleton SB, Joshi A, Schwartz MA, et al. Arthroscopic bullet removal from the acetabulum. *Arthroscopy*. 2005;21(3):360–364.

Tanzer M, Noiseux N. Osseous abnormalities and early osteoarthritis: the role of hip impingement. *Clic Orthop Rel Res*. 2004;429:170–177.

Wiese M, Ruberthaler F, Willburger RE, et al. Early results of endoscopic trochanter bursectomy. *Int Orthop*. 2004;28:218–221.

9

HEAD-SPARING PROCEDURES FOR OSTEONECROSIS OF THE FEMORAL HEAD

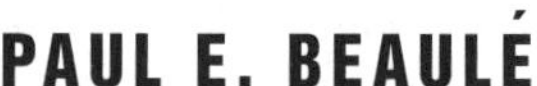
PAUL E. BEAULÉ

It is estimated that 300,000 to 600,000 people have osteonecrosis in the United States and that osteonecrosis (ON) of the femoral head accounts for approximately 10% of the more than 250,000 total hip replacements performed annually.[1] Patients with osteonecrosis of the femoral head are commonly in their 30s and 40s at the time of onset, and nearly 50% have bilateral disease. Results of total hip arthroplasty in this patient group have been inferior to other diagnostic groups.[2] These factors have led to the development of conservative surgical methods aimed at sparing the femoral head. However, the efficacy and the proper indications for these surgical interventions such as core decompression (with or without grafting), osteotomy, and hemiresurfacing arthroplasty are still debated. The preferred treatment varies according to the severity, extent of the disease, condition of the acetabular articular cartilage, and age of the patient.[2]

ETIOLOGY AND PATHOPHYSIOLOGY

Eighty percent of patients with osteonecrosis have one or more risk factors known to predispose patients to developing this disorder. Table 9-1 provides a list of the known risk factors, leaving only about 20% of patients within the idiopathic group. There is a high prevalence of underlying thrombophilia or hypofibrinolysis in patients with osteonecrosis.[3] With the increasing number of etiologic associations, it is important to delineate between these associations and pathogenesis. Mont and others have proposed that the etiology of ON is multifactorial and either there exists an accumulated tissue threshold whereby a number of hits by various etiologic factors eventually meets the threshold for disease or there are certain at-risk patients in whom some other factors trigger the pathologic response.[4]

Ficat[5] emphasized that bone necrosis is the end result of severe and prolonged ischemia, which may involve various mechanisms at different sites in extraosseous and/or intraosseous vessels. This blockage of the osseous microcirculation leads to intramedullary stasis, increasing compartmental pressure, metabolic disturbance, anoxia, and eventually death of osteocytes. The osteocytic death is eventually followed by the reparative phase, at which time the femoral head is at greatest risk of collapse when bone resorption exceeds production.[6] Because the bone most susceptible to vascular compromise is closest to the joint space, the articular surface of the femoral head can become incongruous after collapse owing to structural failure of the underlying bone. More important, the time lapse between diagnosis and severe joint deterioration of the joint leading to a major surgical procedure is about 3 years in 50% of cases.[7]

DIAGNOSIS

Clinical Features

The average age at presentation is less than 40 years old. Males are more likely to be affected than females by a ratio of 8 to 1.[5–8] The most common symptom, seen in 50% of cases, is sudden pain in the groin area, which may be progressive and associated with radiation to the thigh. The pain is often worse at night.[5] The pain is usually triggered by weight bearing or by moving the affected limb. Fifteen percent of patients will have occurrence of osteonecrosis in other joints.[4]

TABLE 9-1 RISK FACTORS ASSOCIATED WITH OSTEONECROSIS

Corticosteroid intake
Trauma
Alcohol abuse
Hypercoagulable states
Pancreatitis
Gaucher disease
Systemic lupus erythematosus
Radiation therapy
Caisson disease
Myeloproliferative diseases
Hypercholesteremia
Sickle Cell Anemia
? Smoking

On physical examination the patient may have a limp and pain with internal hip rotation, but not uncommonly the exam will fail to uncover any striking abnormalities. Thus a high index of suspicion should be maintained. Further investigations to confirm the diagnosis include plain radiographs and magnetic resonance imaging. Sufficient plain radiographs must be ordered to permit evaluation of the contour of the femoral head in more than one plane. In addition to the anteroposterior and frog lateral radiographs, an anteroposterior pelvis radiograph with the hip flexed at 45 degrees will show the anterior contour and a 40-degree caudad view will show the posterior contour.

Classification

Femoral head collapse and size and location of the osteonecrotic bone segment are recognized to be the most important prognostic factors. Ficat and Arlet's original classification scheme had four stages and was based on anteroposterior and frog lateral radiographs. Stages II and III represented the distinction between precollapse and postcollapse disease, and this classification system established the premise for staging osteonecrosis and subsequent classification systems.[5,7] Later on a stage 0 was added and qualified as the silent hip as first described by Marcus.[9] Standard radiographs show only the shadow of the mineralized portion of a bone; consequently early bone necrosis has no specific radiographic appearance, and a normal radiograph does not necessarily mean a normal hip. On the MRI, a single-density line on the T1-weighted image demarcates the normal ischemic bone interface, and a double-density line on the T2-weighted image represents the hypervascular granulation tissue.[6] On plain radiographs, the crescent sign originally described by Ficat[5] is characterized by the pathognomic appearance of a sequestrum on the radiograph within which occurs a subchondral fracture, i.e., crescent line.

Although not included in the Ficat classification, the size of the necrotic segment has been shown to influence the outcome of head-sparing procedures and was first quantified by Kerboull et al.[10] His sum included angles of the necrotic segment measured on the anteroposterior (AP) and lateral radiographs, and found a sum of angles greater than 200 degrees represented a worse prognosis.[2] (Fig. 9-1). The more recently developed University of Pennsylvania system incorporates size of lesion and magnetic resonance imaging findings (Table 9-2) and therefore represents a valuable classification system that aids in management.[11]

Osteonecrosis of the femoral head is associated with secondary involvement of the acetabular cartilage owing to mechanical damage caused by collapse of the femoral head, as demonstrated by both Steinberg[12] and Beaulé.[13] Thus acetabular cartilage must be carefully evaluated at the time of the operative procedure, and when there is severe damage, total hip replacement may be the preferred method of treatment, especially when patients are older than 40 years of age.[2]

Nishii et al.[14] reviewed 54 hips to determine the risk of collapse and progression in hips with osteonecrosis. At a mean followup of 6 years, only 31% of hips went on to collapse when the necrotic area was less than two-thirds of the weightbearing area compared to 68% with the larger areas.

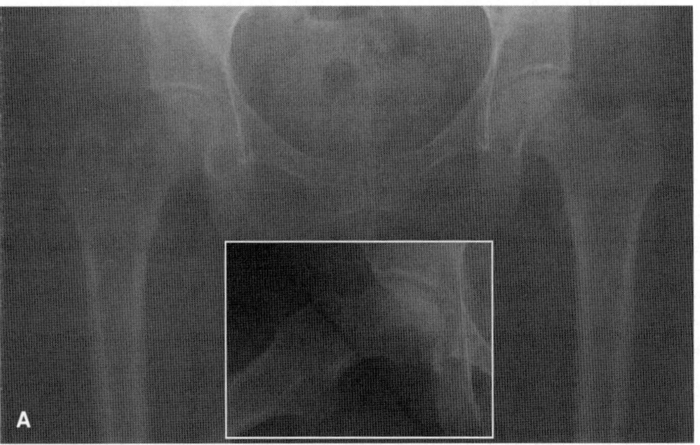

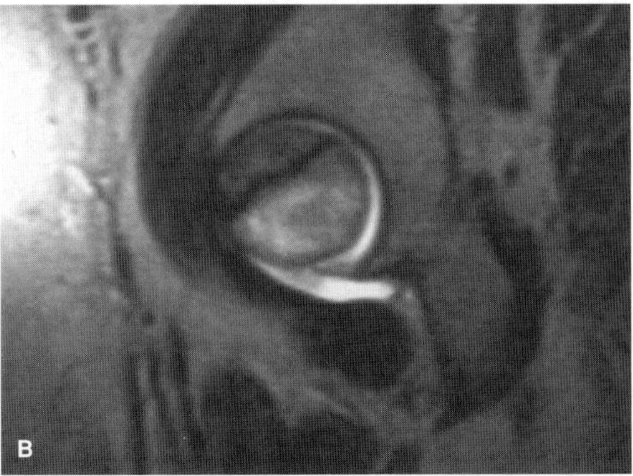

Figure 9-1 A 45-year-old female presents with an 8-month history of bilateral hip pain. **A:** Plain radiographs show bilateral collapse of femoral heads: stage IVC. **Inset** is the frog lateral of the right hip. **B:** Magnetic resonance imaging of the left hip shows the extent of necrotic lesion.

TABLE 9-2 UNIVERSITY OF PENNSYLVANIA STAGING SYSTEM FOR OSTEONECROSIS OF THE FEMORAL HEAD[11]

Stage I: **Normal radiographic findings: Abnormal MRI**

Stage II: **Cystic and sclerotic changes in the femoral head**

Stage III: **Subchondral collapse (crescent sign) without head flattening**

For stages I to III, femoral head involvement is quantified on MRI and subdivided into:

A: Mild (<15%)
B: Moderate (15%–30%)
C: Severe (>30%)

Stage IV: **Flattening of femoral head**

A: Mild (<15% of surface and >2-mm depression)
B: Moderate (15%–30% of surface or 2–4-mm depression)
C: Severe (>30% of surface or >4-mm depression)

Stage V: **Joint narrowing/acetabular changes**

Stage VI: **Advanced degenerative joint disease**

In addition, the percentage of hips that went on to arthritic changes once collapsed was 92% with necrotic areas greater than two-thirds compared to 11% with the smaller area. All hips with >2 mm of initial collapse continued to collapse. Impending femoral head collapse is seen on radiographs as a crescent sign, which represents a fracture of the bone and probably the cartilage as well, which will become further depressed depending on the size of the lesion and joint loading forces.

OPERATIVE TREATMENT OPTIONS

The age of the patient at presentation should be considered carefully; the younger the patient, the more strongly a joint- or bone-preserving procedure should be favored because it is probable that he or she may require another operative procedure. Because with osteonecrosis the acetabular cartilage of the hip is secondarily mechanically damaged after the femoral head has collapsed and this phenomenon is progressive, the duration of symptoms (pain) provides some indication of the quality of the acetabular cartilage. The extent of acetabular damage will ultimately affect the outcome of joint and bone preserving procedures, i.e., osteotomy, free vascularized fibular graft, hemiresurfacing arthroplasty, and the trapdoor procedure. With respect to the cause and risk factors of osteonecrosis, the continued use of high-dose steroids, alcohol, and/or systemic lupus erythematosus is usually associated with a poorer outcome with certain head-sparing procedures.[15] The judicious selection of the best treatment option is dependent on careful analysis of patient demographics and cause, the extent of head involvement, and articular cartilage damage of the acetabulum. The goal of treatment is to optimize outcome while simultaneously minimizing morbidity and maintaining treatment options for potential subsequent secondary procedures.

Core Decompression With or Without Grafting

The role of core decompression is for precollapse stages of osteonecrosis. The best outcomes are for lesions with <15% involvement with a 78% survivorship at an average of 63 months[16] and in those hips with sclerosis with a 95% survivorship at 10 years.[17] The value of bone grafting in addition to core decompression is uncertain. Aaron and associates[18] reported on 28 hips treated with demineralized bone matrix compared with another group without grafting, and there was no significant difference in success rate between these two groups for stage III with survivorships of 83% and 72%, respectively. More recently, Hernigou and Beaujean[19] presented their midterm results of autologous bone marrow grafting after core decompression using a 3-mm-diameter trephine. Hips with a lesion <25% in stages I and II had the best outcome with only 9 out of 145 hips requiring a total hip replacement versus 25 out of 44 hips for the rest of the stages.

Although we continue to use core decompression alone in some patients with Steinberg stage III, it has no role in the treatment of stage IV and V disease because it cannot restore articular sphericity or remove the collapsed segment from the weight-bearing area, and further cartilage degeneration is inevitable. Smith et al.[20] reported a 0% survivorship following core decompression at average follow-up of 3 years for stage IV with all patients requiring another operative procedure. Mont et al.[21] reviewed the radiographic predictors of outcome for 68 Ficat stage III (Steinberg stage IV) hips following core decompression with mean follow-up of 12 years. Only 29% had a satisfactory outcome. If core decompression is combined with grafting in patients with Ficat stage II/Steinberg stage III lesions, satisfactory results have been reported for both nonvascularized and vascularized grafts.[22,23]

Free Vascularized Fibular Graft

Free vascularized fibular graft techniques have been used to support the subchondral surface and enhance revascularization in combination with core decompression and osteoinductive cancellous bone. These grafting procedures have a role in the precollapse stages, but have inferior results in the postcollapse stages because of articular cartilage involvement and the inability to restore femoral head sphericity. For stages IV and V, several authors have reported survivorships <75% at 5 years with surviving patients having Harris hip scores <80.[20,22,24] The best results have been with earlier-stage lesions with a survivorship of 89% at 50 months for stage III compared with 65% for core decompression alone. However, one must carefully consider the potential disadvantages of this surgery such as donor site morbidity at 24%[25] and a 2.5% incidence of subtrochanteric fracture.[26]

Open Grafting of the Femoral Head

Another grafting technique, the trapdoor procedure, first described by Merle D'Aubigné,[27] has been used. In this procedure, an arthrotomy is performed to dislocate the hip anteriorly, the necrotic segment of the head is curetted out, and iliac crest bone graft is packed inside. This is done through a cartilage window of the femoral head. Mont et al.[28] reported on a series of 24 hips with Ficat stage III (Steinberg stage IVA) disease and 6 hips with early stage IV (Steinberg IVB) disease treated with this procedure. At a mean duration of follow-up of 56 months (range 30 to 60 months), 73% had good to excellent results. Of the eight hips with poor results, five had undergone subsequent operative procedures. All of the poor results had combined necrotic angles greater than 200 degrees. The results are encouraging, but the procedure has limited indications because of the difficulty in restoring the sphericity of the femoral head. Further study with longer duration of follow-up will be required to assess the utility of this procedure.

Proximal Femoral Osteotomy

The clinical results of proximal femoral osteotomy for osteonecrosis have been variable and sometimes disappointing because of the difficulty rotating the necrotic segment out from the weight-bearing zone of the hip, especially when the lesion is large. Langlais and Forestier[29] reported their results with either the Sugioka (anterior) or Kempf (posterior) rotational osteotomy in 20 patients with Ficat stages II and III (Steinberg III and IV). The Kempf osteotomy was used for the atypical case where the necrotic zone extended >30 to 40 degrees posteriorly. Patients older than 45 years and patients with either steroid- or alcohol-induced osteonecrosis were excluded from their study because of predictably poor results. They recommended the Sugioka procedure only for Steinberg stage III and the Kempf procedure for stages III and IV where the depth of the necrosis was not more than one third of the head diameter and located posteriorly.

Others advocate an intertrochanteric osteotomy because it avoids the need for a greater trochanteric osteotomy and does not risk compromising the blood supply to the femoral head. Mont et al.[30] reported on this technique in 31 hips with Ficat stage III (Steinberg IV) disease at a mean follow-up of 11.5 years. Good to excellent results were obtained in 74% of the hips. Poor results were associated with age older than 45 years, a combined necrotic angle >200 degrees, and Dinulescu et al.[31] reported similar findings with survivorship of 70% at 5 years and 45% at 10 years in 50 stage II and stage III hips. One of the main disadvantages to intertrochanteric osteotomy is the apparent negative effect on the complication rate and subsequent total hip arthroplasty, both of which are probably related to the femoral deformity created by the osteotomy.[30,32,33] Nevertheless, for surgeons with experience with the procedure, a proximal femoral osteotomy is a reasonable head-sparing operation in patients younger than 45 years of age, with Kerboull angle <200 degrees, and no continuing steroid use.

Hemiresurfacing Arthroplasty

Hemiresurfacing hip arthroplasty with cement fixation was first preformed in the early 1980s as a custom device in the young, active population to preserve femoral bone stock and permit conversion to a total hip replacement with minimal morbidity.[34–38] (Fig. 9-2). The results of this procedure have varied in different reports. Beaulé et al.[13] reviewed a series of 37 hips with a mean follow-up of 6.5 years (range 2 to 18 years), in which the acetabular cartilage involvement was photographed at the time of the operative procedure and subsequently graded. It was found that the longer duration of preoperative symptoms the more severe the acetabular damage, and that hips that had been converted to total hip replacement had a longer duration of symptoms prior to their hemiresurfacing arthroplasty than the ones that were still functioning (17 versus 12 months, respectively). The survivorship in this series was 79% at 5 years, 62% at 10 years, and 45% at 15 years. Other centers using different hemiresurfacing designs have reported comparable survivorship (i.e., 80% at 5 years and 60% at 10 years) and pain relief for osteonecrosis of the hip with Ficat stage III and early IV disease (Steinberg IVA and IVB). However, as shown by Mont et al.,[40] the pain relief is not as predictable as that following a total hip replacement: In their patients a hemiresurfacing arthroplasty had a mean Harris hip score of 88 compared with 93 for patients with a total hip resurfacing (THR). Proper component sizing and acetabular cartilage quality are probably the two most important factors affecting outcome. A remaining challenge is durability of the articular cartilage against the hemiresurfacing component.

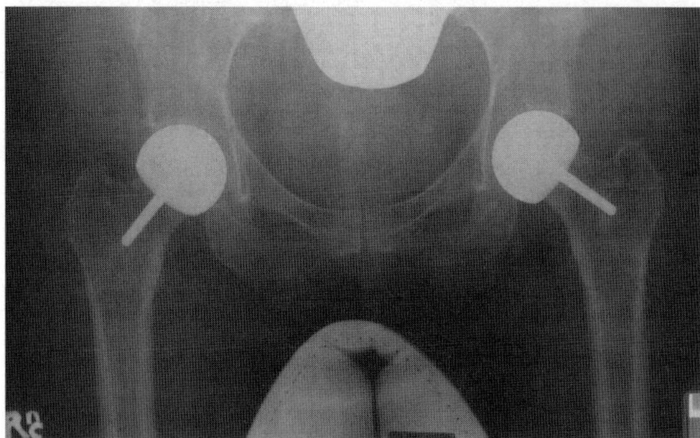

Figure 9-2 Radiograph of patient shown in fig. 9-1 after bilateral hemiresurfacing arthroplasty.

CONCLUSION AND RECOMMENDATIONS

The treatment of patients with osteonecrosis remains controversial; however, it is generally believed that the size of the lesion, as well as the stage of the disease at the time of treatment, determine the outcome of head-sparing procedures. Core decompression and or bone grafts have a role in the precollapse stages of osteonecrosis. The size of the necrotic segment plays a critical role in the outcome of proximal femoral osteotomies. Thus, unless a relatively small lesion (Kerboull angle <200 degrees) is present, hemiresurfacing arthroplasty provides a better clinical outcome compared with other head-sparing procedures with the caveat that the predictability of the pain relief is not that of a total hip replacement. Because the acetabular cartilage damage increases over time once collapse has occurred, early surgery is recommended for any type of head-sparing procedure. In the presence of notable acetabular involvement or advanced Steinberg V disease, total hip replacement offers the most predictable outcome.

REFERENCES

1. Mankin HJ. Nontraumatic necrosis of bone (osteonecrosis). *N Engl J Med*. 1992;326:1473–1479.
2. Beaulé PE, Amstutz HC. Treatment of Ficat stage III and IV osteonecrosis of the hip. *J Am Acad Orthop Surg*. 2004;12:96–105.
3. Glueck CJ, Frieberg R, Tracey T, et al. Thrombophilia, hypofibrinolysis and osteonecrosis. *Clin Orthop*. 1997;334:43–56.
4. Mont MA, Jones LC, Sotereanos DC, et al. Understanding and treating osteonecrosis of the femoral head. In: Price CT, ed. *Instructional Course Lectures*, 49. Rosemont, IL: American Academy of Orthopaedic Surgeons; 2000:169–188.
5. Ficat RP. Idiopathic bone necrosis of the femoral head. Early diagnosis and treatment. *J Bone Joint Surg*. 1985;67B:3–9.
6. Lieberman JR, Berry DJ, Mont MA, et al. Osteonecrosis of the hip: management in the 21st century. *J Bone Joint Surg*. 2002;84:834–853.
7. Arlet J. Nontraumatic avascular necrosis of the femoral head. *Clin Orthop*. 1992;277:12–21.
8. Allison GT, Bostrom MP, Glesby MJ. Osteonecrosis in HIV disease: epidemiology, etiologies, and clinical management. *AIDS*. 2003;17:1–9.
9. Marcus ND, Enneking WF, Massam RA. The silent hip in idiopathic aseptic necrosis. Treatment by bone-grafting. *J Bone Joint Surg*. 1973;55A:1351–1366.
10. Kerboull M, Thomine J, Postel M, et al. The conservative surgical treatment of idiopathic aseptic necrosis of the femoral head. *J Bone Joint Surg*. 1974;56B:291–296.
11. Steinberg ME, Hayken GD, Steinberg DR. A quantitative system for staging avascular necrosis. *J Bone Joint Surg*. 1995;77B:34–41.
12. Steinberg ME, Corces A, Fallon M. Acetabular involvement in osteonecrosis of the femoral head.*J Bone Joint Surg*. 1999;81A:60–65.
13. Beaulé PE, Schmalzried TP, Campbell PA, et al. Duration of symptoms and outcome of hemiresurfacing for hip osteonecrosis. *Clin Orthop Rel Res*. 2001;385:104–117.
14. Nishii T, Sugano N, Ohzono K, et al. Progression and cessation of collapse in osteonecrosis of the femoral head. *Clin Orthop Rel Res*. 2002;400:149–157.
15. Mont MA, Hungerford DS. Non-traumatic avascular necrosis of the femoral head. *J Bone Joint Surg*. 1995;77A:459–474.
16. Steinberg ME, Larcom PG, Strafford B, et al. Core decompression with bone grafting for osteonecrosis of the femoral head. *Clin Orthop*. 2001;386:71–78.
17. Bozic KJ, Zurakowski D, Thornhill TS. Survivorship analysis of hips treated with core decompression for nontraumatic osteonecrosis of the femoral head. *J Bone Joint Surg*. 1999;81A:200–209.
18. Aaron RK, Ciombor DM, Lord CF. Core decompression augmented with human decalcified bone matrix for osteonecrosis of the femoral head. In: Urbaniak JR, Jones JP Jr, eds. *Osteonecrosis: Etiology, Diagnosis, Treatment*. Rosemont, IL: American Academy of Orthopaedic Surgeons; 1997:301–307.
19. Hernigou P, Beaujean F. Treatment of osteonecrosis with autologous bone marrow grafting. *Clin Orthop*. 2002;405:14–23.
20. Louie BE, McKee MD, Richards RR, et al. Treatment of osteonecrosis of the femoral head by free vascularized fibular grafting: an analysis of surgical outcome and patient health status. *Can J Surg*. 1999;42:274–283.
21. Mont MA, Jones LC, Pacheco I, et al. Radiographic predictors of outcome of core decompression for hips with osteonecrosis stage III. *Clin Orthop*. 1998;159–168.
22. Urbaniak JR, Coogan PG, Gunneson EB, et al. Treatment of osteonecrosis of the femoral head with free vascularized fibular grafting. A long-term follow-up study of one hundred and three hips. *J Bone Joint Surg Am*. 1995;77:681–694.
23. Buckley PD, Gearen PF, Petty W. Structural bone-grafting for early atraumatic avascular necrosis of the femoral head. *J Bone Joint Surg*. 1991;73A:1357–1364.
24. Sotereanos DC, Plakseychuk AY, Rubash HE. Free vascularized fibula grafting for the treatment of osteonecrosis of the femoral head. *Clin Orthop Rel Res*. 1997;344:243–256.
25. Vail TP, Urbaniak JR. Donor-site morbidity with use of vascularized autogenous fibular grafts. *J Bone Joint Surg*. 1996;78-A:204–211.
26. Aluisio F, Urbaniak JR. Proximal femoral fractures after free vascularized fibular grafting to the hip. *Clin Orthop Rel Res*. 1998;356:192–201.
27. Merle D'Aubigne R, Postel M, Mazabraud A, et al. Idiopathic necrosis of the femoral head in adults. *J Bone Joint Surg*. 1965; 47B:612–633.
28. Mont MA, Einhorn TA, Sponseller PD, et al. The trapdoor procedure using autogenous cortical and cancellous bone grafts for osteonecrosis of the femoral head. *J Bone Joint Surg*. 1998;80B:56–62.
29. Langlais F, Fourastier J. Rotation osteotomies for osteonecrosis of the femoral head. *Clin Orthop Rel Res*. 1997;343:110–123.
30. Mont MA, Fairbank AC, Krackow KA, et al. Corrective osteotomy for osteonecrosis of the femoral head [see comments]. *J Bone Joint Surg*. 1996;78A:1032–1038.
31. Dinulescu I, Stanculescu D, Nicolescu M, et al. Long-term follow-up after intertrochanteric osteotomies for avascular necrosis of the femoral head. *Bull Hosp Jt Dis*. 1998;57:84–87.
32. Ferguson GM, Cabanela ME, Ilstrup DM. Total hip arthroplasty after failed intertrochanteric osteotomy. *J Bone Joint Surg*. 1994;76B:252–257.
33. Boos N, Krushell R, Ganz R, Muller ME. Total hip arthroplasty after previous proximal femoral osteotomy. *J Bone Joint Surg*. 1997;79B:247–253.
34. Meulemeester FR, Rosing PM. Uncemented surface replacement for osteonecrosis of the femoral head. *Acta Othop Scand*. 1989;60:425–429.
35. Nelson CL, Walz BH, Gruenwald JM. Resurfacing of only the femoral head for osteonecrosis. Long-term follow-up study. *J Arthroplasty*. 1997;12:736–740.
36. Scott RD, Urse JS, Schmidt R. Use of TARA hemiarthroplasty in advanced osteonecrosis. *J Arthroplasty*. 1987;2:225–232.
37. Amstutz HC, Grigoris P, Safran MR, et al. Precision-fit surface hemiarthroplasty for femoral head osteonecrosis. Long term results. *J Bone Joint Surg*. 1994;76B:423–427.
38. Hungerford MW, Mont MA, Scott R, et al. Surface replacement hemiarthroplasty for the treatment of osteonecrosis of the femoral head. *J Bone Joint Surg*. 1998;80A:1656–1664.
39. Langlais F, Barthas J, Postel M. Les cupules ajustées pour nécrose idiopathique. Bilan radiologique. *Rev Chir Orthop Reparatrice Appar Mot*. 1979;65:151–155.
40. Mont MA, Rajadhyaksha AD, Hungerford DS. Outcomes of limited femoral resurfacing arthroplasty compared with total hip arthroplasty for osteonecrosis of the femoral head. *J Arthroplasty*. 2001;16(suppl 1):134–139.

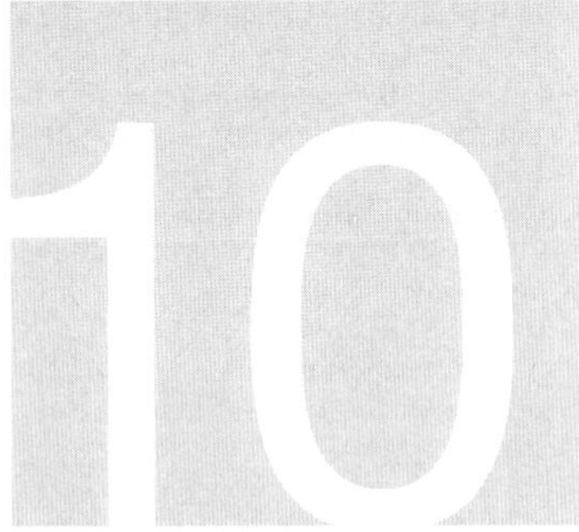

OSTEOTOMIES AROUND THE HIP

JOHN C. CLOHISY
PERRY L. SCHOENECKER

Over the past decade there has been a renewed focus on joint preservation surgery of the hip. This is owing to an enhanced understanding of the pathogenesis of degenerative hip disease, improved diagnostic imaging modalities, refined patient selection criteria, and more sophisticated surgical techniques. Perhaps most important is an appreciation of the significance of prearthritic and early arthritic hip symptoms that commonly occur before irreversible joint deterioration. These early symptoms provide a window of opportunity for surgical intervention to remedy the underlying hip abnormality and to improve the prognosis of early hip disease. The goals of joint preservation surgery are to alleviate hip symptoms, improve the functional capacity of the hip, and delay or prevent the biologic cascade of degenerative hip disease. Osteotomy surgery about the hip is one of the mainstay joint preservation strategies and will continue to play a major role in the expanding field of hip preservation surgery. Nevertheless, optimal clinical results of osteotomy surgery are realized only through careful patient selection, detailed preoperative planning, accurate surgical procedures, and supervised patient rehabilitation. The goal of this chapter is to summarize the essential concepts of hip osteotomy surgery. The fundamentals of patient evaluation and the basics of osteotomy procedures will be presented for the most common structural disorders of the hip.

PATHOGENESIS

Advanced hip osteoarthritis is a common condition in the United States as evidenced by the approximately 200,000 total hip arthroplasties performed annually. The cause of hip osteoarthritis is complex and multifactorial and continues to be an area in need of investigation. Patient characteristics including age, gender, genetic makeup, race, occupation, and activity level have all been identified as factors that impact the pathophysiology of this disease. Most relevant to hip joint preservation surgery is the known correlation between structural hip disorders and secondary osteoarthritis. Harris emphasized that over 90% of patients with osteoarthritis had an underlying deformity of the joint that was present at the cessation of growth. This concept underscores the theory that osteoarthritis of the hip is very commonly associated with a pre-existing, mechanical disorder. In the mechanically compromised hip, instability, abnormal joint loading, and/or impingement can produce abnormal shear forces and excessive loads per unit area at the articular surface and induce premature degeneration of the involved articular cartilage. If left untreated, progressive degenerative articular disease ensues and secondary osteoarthritis can develop.

Development dysplasia of the hip (DDH) is the most common structural deformity associated with secondary osteoarthritis and serves as a model of this pathophysiologic cascade. The dysplastic acetabulum is abnormally inclined in the superolateral direction and does not provide adequate anterolateral femoral head coverage. This leads to hip instability and anterolateral acetabular rim overload. As a result of localized overload, labral disease ensues and adjacent articular cartilage deterioration is initiated. Persistent instability and localized joint overload accelerate articular cartilage degeneration and secondary osteoarthritis.

DIAGNOSIS

Patient History and Physical Exam

The patient history is initially focused on determining the cause of the problem and establishing whether the hip joint is the true source of symptoms. Referred pain from other anatomic regions, most commonly the lumbar spine, needs to be excluded. The interview should then elicit any history of childhood or adolescent hip disease, previous hip surgery, hip trauma, risk factors for osteonecrosis, or a history consistent with inflammatory arthritis. If the patient has authentic hip symptoms, the duration, character, and location of pain are determined. The examiner should question about episodes of snapping, popping, or locking that may suggest soft tissue pathology about the hip or a mechanical intra-articular component to the disease. Activities that exacerbate symptoms should be noted. It is important to delineate whether the patient experiences activity-related hip pain consistent with abductor fatigue (lateral hip discomfort or tiring) or instability and associated joint overload (anterior or groin discomfort). Alternatively, the symptoms may be more consistent with anterior impingement disease (anterior or groin discomfort) and exacerbation with hip flexion activities and prolonged sitting. The severity of symptoms and functional limitations should also be discussed as patients with early and less advanced symptoms are usually better candidates for osteotomy surgery. The social history should establish the occupation, activity level, and tobacco and alcohol use habits of the patient. The overall medical condition and patient capacity to comply with surgical treatment and rehabilitation are other factors that need to be considered when contemplating osteotomy surgery. The patient should understand the goals of treatment and must be willing to actively participate in a relatively involved postoperative rehabilitation program.

Physical examination findings are of utmost importance in evaluating a patient for hip osteotomy surgery. The general physical status, including body height, weight, and apparent conditioning, is noted. During examination, sitting posture and gait pattern are observed. The hip is inspected with specific attention to the presence and position of surgical scars. The Trendelenburg test and side-lying abduction testing indicate the integrity of hip abductor strength. Abductor weakness is a common finding in patients with early hip disease. Leg-length determination is made with the patient standing, noting the presence or absence of a balanced pelvis. Functional leg-length inequality can be measured by noting the height of a block placed under the short leg necessary to balance the pelvis. Alternatively, measurement of true leg-length inequality can be made with the patient supine, measuring from the anterior superior iliac spine to the medial malleolus and comparing the measurement to the contralateral side. The neurovascular status of the extremity should also be determined, especially in patients with a history of previous hip trauma and/or surgery.

Range of motion of the hip is carefully assessed as is the presence of pain and hip joint irritability during the motion examination. When assessing hip range of motion it is important to steady the pelvis with one hand while the examiner's other hand ranges the ipsilateral hip. This determines motion end points more accurately because the examiner better appreciates forced motion of the pelvis through the hip. With this technique hip flexion, abduction, adduction, and rotation are recorded. Hip internal and external rotation both in extension and flexion are measured. Restricted flexion and internal rotation in flexion should be appreciated as this finding is common in patients with anterior femoroacetabular impingement. Again, careful appreciation of motion end points is important to accurately assess true hip joint motion and to judge the joint suitability for osteotomy surgery. The surgeon must verify that the hip has adequate range of motion to accommodate the proposed reconstruction, because a hip with inadequate motion may respond poorly to an osteotomy procedure. In general, at least 90 degrees of hip flexion should be present. One exception is the patient with a severe slipped capital femoral epiphysis (SCFE) or a posttraumatic deformity in which restricted hip flexion may be secondary to malalignment rather than degenerative changes. In contrast, a patient being evaluated for acetabular reorientation to correct classic acetabular dysplasia must demonstrate adequate hip flexion (≥105 degrees) to tolerate the osteotomy, because improved anterior coverage of the femoral head achieved with the osteotomy will reduce hip flexion motion. Thus, during evaluation the surgeon must determine that a functional motion (at least 90 degrees of flexion) will be maintained postoperatively. Similarly, hip abduction motion will be reduced with a varus-producing proximal femoral osteotomy. Therefore, preoperative hip abduction motion must be adequate (>30 degrees) to accommodate the surgical correction and to maintain adequate clinical abduction postoperatively.

Specific physical exam tests can be helpful in characterizing the underlying hip disease. The impingement test (combined flexion, adduction, and internal rotation) is performed to check for groin discomfort that may indicate labral pathology or the presence of anterior femoroacetabular impingement. This test is also an excellent screening maneuver for any intra-articular disease process and can be extremely helpful in distinguishing an intra-articular from an extra-articular disorder. Additionally, an apprehension test (extension, adduction, and external rotation) evaluates anterior stability of the hip. This maneuver elicits hip (groin) pain in the setting of an unstable dysplastic hip with insufficient anterior coverage and associated anterior instability. A positive test is common with moderate to severe acetabular dysplasia, yet hips with mild acetabular dysplasia may not be sensitive to anterior stability testing.

Radiographic Evaluation

The radiographic evaluation defines the structural anatomy of the hip in a comprehensive fashion, determines the severity of secondary osteoarthritis, and provides information regarding the effect of osteotomy correction (congruency and joint space alteration). A thorough radiographic examination of the hip is extremely important in optimizing patient selection for surgery, preoperative planning, and accurate surgical technique. To accomplish this, we obtain a full hip series including a standing anteroposterior pelvis and false profile. Frog and cross-table laterals of the hip are taken supine. When considering an osteotomy, functional radiographs are obtained to check congruency in a position mimicking the osteotomy. These radiographs are performed with the surgeon or assistant holding the extremity and are used to confirm clinical comfort in a position of radiographic congruency. For example, a flexion-abduction view is obtained to assess the hip articulation in anticipation of acetabular reorientation for treatment of classic acetabular dysplasia. This radiograph mimics the joint congruency and improved anterolateral femoral head coverage to be achieved by the osteotomy. Similarly, an abduction functional view is performed to assess the hip for a varus-producing proximal femoral osteotomy. These functional radiographs should demonstrate joint congruency without hinging and ideally show an improvement or at least maintenance of the joint space. If congruency or the optimal joint reorientation position is questionable with functional radiographs, a hip exam with fluoroscopy can provide additional information regarding the joint suitability for osteotomy surgery. With more complicated deformities, fluoroscopic examination can be extremely informative regarding congruency of the articulation and for planning an optimal osteotomy correction.

Adjunctive imaging tests are frequently obtained to thoroughly evaluate and define the disease pattern of the hip being considered for surgery. Magnetic resonance arthrogram may be indicated to assess acetabular labral disease, articular cartilage integrity, acetabular rim pathology, and femoral head and femoral neck anatomy. Alternatively, a CAT scan of the hip can be useful for more detailed characterization of osseous abnormalities and can facilitate preoperative planning. Sources of bony impingement, femoral head/neck junction anatomy, version of the acetabulum, and osteonecrotic lesion size and location are also better defined with CAT scan images. Clearly, preoperative assessment of all disease components (both acetabular and femoral) enables the surgeon to develop a comprehensive treatment plan and optimize the results of the procedure.

TREATMENT

Indications and Contraindications

The general indications and contraindications for hip osteotomy surgery are summarized in Table 10-1. It is extremely important to emphasize that several patient-related variables are considered when selecting patients for surgery and when devising a specific treatment plan. Osteotomy surgery has distinct indications, contraindications, and goals when compared with total joint replacement surgery.

Young and middle-aged patients who present with authentic hip symptoms and have an associated structural abnormality should be considered for osteotomy surgery. Typically, an optimal surgical candidate is relatively young (physiologically less than 50 years old), well-conditioned, and active. The hip has a correctable deformity, sufficient range of motion, adequate congruency, and has not progressed to advanced secondary osteoarthritis. The patient should have an understanding of the hip problem and the proposed surgical procedure and should be willing to comply with the postoperative rehabilitation protocol. Nonoperative measures, including physical therapy, activity restriction, and nonsteroidal anti-inflammatory medicines, can be used to minimize symptoms, although a long-term benefit from these modalities is unlikely. Nonsurgical measures as a primary treatment are reserved for patients who are marginal or poor candidates for an osteotomy and for patients not interested in a major hip surgery.

Various structural hip disorders can present with prearthritic or early arthritic hip symptoms prior to the development of advanced joint deterioration. In general, prearthritic conditions predispose the hip to dynamic instability, localized joint overload, impingement, or a combination of these factors. If these disorders are diagnosed early, the effects of corrective osteotomy surgery can be extremely beneficial (Tables 10-2 and 10-3). The goals of this type of surgery are to correct the underlying structural abnormality of the hip, relieve the patient's discomfort, enhance hip function and activity, and delay or prevent the progression of hip joint deterioration. Osteotomy correction can improve the structure and biology of the joint in various ways. Surgical correction can normalize the structural anatomy of the hip, enhance stability, relieve or prevent

TABLE 10-1 GENERAL INDICATIONS AND CONTRAINDICATIONS FOR HIP OSTEOTOMY SURGERY

Indications
- Structural hip abnormality
- Young (physiologically less than 50 years old)
- Adequate hip motion
- Adequate hip joint congruency
- Absence of advanced secondary osteoarthritis

Contraindications
- Inflammatory arthritis
- Advanced secondary osteoarthritis
- Inadequate hip motion
- Severe hip joint incongruency

Relative contraindications[a]
- Morbid obesity
- Tobacco use
- Major medical comorbidities

[a]Patient factors that may compromise osteotomy results are considered on an individual case basis.

TABLE 10-2 OSTEOTOMY PROCEDURES FOR SPECIFIC HIP DISORDERS

Hip Disorder	Osteotomy Options[a]
DDH	1) Acetabular reorientation (PAO) 2) Proximal femoral varus osteotomy (alone or in combination with PAO) 3) Femoral head/neck junction osteoplasty (prevent secondary impingement)
Perthes-like deformity	1) Acetabular reorientation (PAO) 2) Proximal femoral valgus osteotomy 3) Femoral head/neck osteoplasty
SCFE	1) Intertrochanteric femoral osteotomy 2) Femoral neck osteotomy 3) Femoral head/neck osteoplasty
Osteonecrosis	1) Intertrochanteric femoral osteotomy (realignment orientation dependent on lesion location)
Posttraumatic problems	1) Proximal femoral valgus (Pauwel) osteotomy (femoral neck nonunion) 2) Intertrochanteric femoral osteotomy (realignment orientation dependent on initial deformity)

[a]It must be emphasized that the optimal osteotomy procedure for each patient is based on the specific disease characteristics and will vary accordingly. Frequently, a combination of techniques (acetabular osteotomy, femoral osteotomy, and/or osteoplasty) are performed in collaborative fashion to optimize the reconstruction.
DDH, developmental dysplasia of the hip; PAO, periacetabular osteotomy; SCFE, slipped capital femoral epiphysis.

TABLE 10-3 CLINICAL RESULTS OF HIP OSTEOTOMY SURGERY (SELECTED STUDIES)

Hip Disorder	Procedure	No. Hips	Follow-up (years)	Good/Excellent[a]	Reference
DDH	PAO	75	11.3	73%	Siebenrock et al., 1999
Perthes-like Deformity	PAO (PFO)[b]	27	3.4	85%	Beck and Mast, 1997
Osteonecrosis	PFO (varus)	37	11.5	76%	Mont et al., 1996
SCFE	PFO (flexion, rotation, valgus)	39	23.4	77%	Kartenbender et al., 2000
Femoral neck nonunion	PFO (Pauwel valgus)	50	7.1	80%	Marti et al., 1989

[a] Good/excellent clinical result at follow-up.
[b] Femoral procedures performed on individual case basis.
DDH, developmental dysplasia of the hip; PAO, periacetabular osteotomy; PFO, proximal femoral osteotomy; SCFE, slipped capital femoral epiphysis.

impingement, optimize congruency, decrease localized articular surface overload, and improve the biomechanics of the joint. It is important to emphasize that joint instability and impingement can be simultaneous problems. Reconstructive techniques must aim to improve joint function by optimizing the dynamic balance between joint stability and impingement.

Distinct types of hip disease have unique pathophysiologic mechanisms of joint deterioration. Thus, the techniques of osteotomy reconstruction must be individualized to the underlying structural abnormality of the hip and to the specific disease characteristics of each case. The most common conditions amenable to joint preservation surgery include classic developmental dysplasia (DDH), Perthes-like deformities, SCFE, osteonecrosis, and posttraumatic deformities.

Developmental Dysplasia of the Hip and Techniques of Hip Osteotomy

Classic DDH is the most common indication for joint preservation osteotomy surgery of the hip. This disease is characterized by deficient anterolateral femoral head coverage, superolateral inclination of the acetabular articular surface, a lateral position of the hip center, and variable version abnormalities of the acetabulum. On the femoral side, coxa valga, excessive anteversion, and a nonspherical femoral head are common. This combination of abnormalities can result in joint instability, localized anterolateral joint overload, acetabular labral disease, and eventual secondary arthrosis. In the presence of a congruent joint and in the absence of advanced secondary osteoarthritis, symptomatic DDH is an excellent indication for a reconstructive acetabular osteotomy.

Although various acetabular osteotomy techniques have been described, the Bernese periacetabular osteotomy (PAO) has gained worldwide popularity over the past decade. This is our preferred technique because the osteotomy is performed with an abductor-sparing approach, uses orthogonal osteotomy cuts, and preserves the posterior column. It enables major multiplanar corrections, preserves acetabular fragment blood supply, provides reliable healing, and enables accelerated rehabilitation. The procedure is most commonly performed through a modified Smith-Peterson approach, and four periacetabular cuts are made to enable acetabular mobilization. The first cut is an infra-acetabular osteotomy that starts just below the inferior lip of the acetabulum, aims toward the middle of the ischial spine, and extends to the level of a trajectory bisecting the posterior column (approximately 1 cm anterior to the posterior cortex of the posterior column). The inferior osteotomy is followed by the superior pubic ramus cut, which is made just medial to the iliopectineal eminence and angled away from the joint. The third cut is made at the anterior superior iliac spine directly towards the sciatic notch. The fourth and final osteotomy cut is made with a goal of bisecting the posterior column between the articular surface anteriorly and the posterior cortex. This osteotomy meets the first infra-acetabular cut posteroinferior to the acetabulum. The acetabular fragment is then mobilized and repositioned with internal rotation, forward tilt, and medial translation. The internal rotation component of the reduction provides lateral coverage and maintains anteversion of the acetabulum. The acetabulum is fixed provisionally with k-wires, the reduction is assessed with intraoperative radiographs, and definitive fixation is then performed. Final radiographs are obtained to confirm an osteotomy correction that improves anterolateral femoral head coverage (lateral center-edge angle 20 to 30 degrees, anterior center-edge angle 15 to 25 degrees), reduces the superolateral inclination of the acetabular articular surface (0 to 15 degrees), restores a more medial position of the hip joint center (medial aspect of the femoral head 5 to 10 mm lateral to ilioischial line), and maintains anteversion of the acetabulum (Fig. 10-1A, B).

Version is assessed by the relative positions of the anterior and posterior lips, and it is important that the acetabulum not be overreduced or retroverted, as this can result in secondary anterior femoroacetabular impingement. Slight undercorrection is preferred over excessive

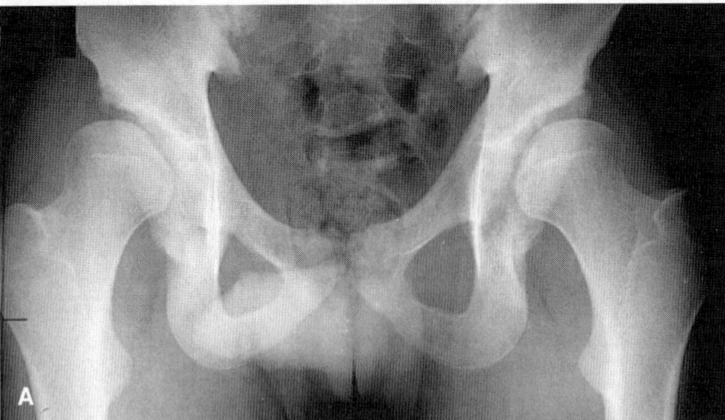

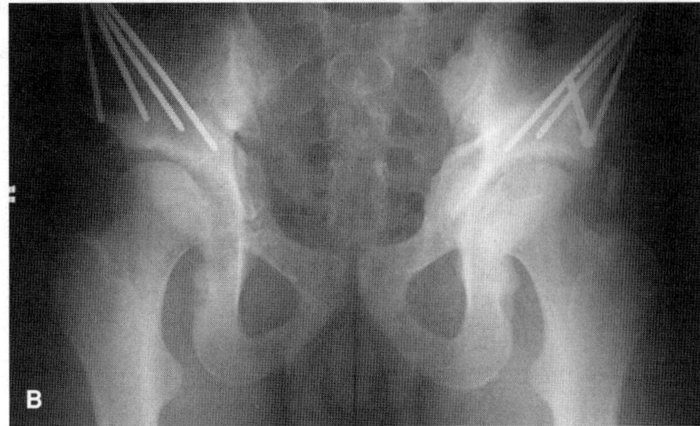

Figure 10-1 Standard periacetabular osteotomy (PAO) for developmental dysplasia of the hip (DDH). Preoperative (**A**) and postoperative (**B**) anteroposterior pelvic radiographs in a 19-year-old male collegiate athlete with hip pain and instability symptoms. He was treated with staged bilateral periacetabular osteotomies. Note the enhanced lateral coverage, decreased superolateral inclination of the acetabular articular surface, maintained anteversion, and medial translation of the hip center achieved with the osteotomy. The patient returned to full sport activities without restrictions and an excellent clinical outcome.

correction to avoid creating an femoroacetabular impingement. Additionally, hip flexion and abduction motion is checked clinically, and it is imperative that at least 90 degrees of passive hip flexion and 30 degrees of abduction are achieved on the operating room table. After range of motion evaluation, we perform an arthrotomy to inspect the integrity of the acetabular labrum and to assess for anterior femoroacetabular impingement. Large, unstable labral tears are repaired with suture anchors, whereas stable tears are left untreated. Lack of femoral head/neck offset can result in anterior femoroacetabular impingement postoperatively and can be treated with osteoplasty if found to be a source of impingement. In cases with an associated major femoral deformity, a proximal femoral osteotomy may be necessary. In severely dysplastic hips, a valgus proximal femoral deformity may have to be treated with a varus-producing intertrochanteric osteotomy to optimize the reconstruction. Long-term clinical results of the Bernese periacetabular osteotomy, as reported by Siebenrock et al., have demonstrated good to excellent results in 73% of patients followed for an average of 11.3 years. These data are derived from the learning curve experience with this osteotomy. It is likely that with contemporary patient selection criteria and refined surgical techniques, the good clinical results of this procedure will be longer lasting and more predictable.

As noted previously, the major deformity in classic DDH is usually on the acetabular side of the joint, and currently, most surgeons prefer to address the disease with acetabular reorientation. Uncommonly, the acetabular deformity is very mild and the most profound deformity is femoral-based. It consists of coxa valga with lateral joint overload. In these occasional cases a varus-producing proximal femoral osteotomy can be considered. Perhaps more commonly, a varus-producing proximal femoral osteotomy is indicated to augment the acetabular procedure in severe cases. The varus correction can be combined with extension (apex anterior correction) to enhance hip stability by containing the femoral head anterolaterally and can decrease the load per unit surface area along the anterolateral acetabular rim.

For proximal femoral osteotomies, we prefer a no-wedge technique to obtain correction and minimize the distortion of the proximal femur (Figs. 10-2, 10-3). A varus-producing realignment is performed with a transverse osteotomy at the superior aspect of the lesser trochanter and a 90-degree blade plate for reduction and fixation of the osteotomy fragments. The angle of the chisel and blade insertion dictates the amount of varus correction obtained. For example, if the blade is inserted at a 110-degree angle to the femoral shaft in the frontal plane, a 20-degree correction will be obtained when the 90-degree blade plate is inserted and the osteotomy is reduced. The blade length is estimated with templates and the blade plate offset (10, 15, or 20 mm) is determined to maintain the horizontal offset between the center of the femoral head and the longitudinal axis of the femoral shaft. Specifically, offset is maintained by medial displacement of the femoral shaft for varus osteotomies and lateral displacement for valgus osteotomies. A varus osteotomy shortens the extremity, and the preoperative plan determines the amount of shortening to be produced. For valgus-producing osteotomies, an angled blade plate (110, 120, or 130 degrees) is used. The amount of valgus correction is determined by the angle of insertion and the blade plate angle. For example, a 20-degree correction is obtained by inserting a 110-degree blade plate at a 90-degree angle to the femoral shaft in the frontal plane. With reduction of the osteotomy and fixation of the plate, a 20-degree correction is obtained. Valgus osteotomies lengthen the extremity, and resection of bone may be required to maintain equal leg lengths.

The patient is positioned supine, and a standard lateral approach to the proximal femur is performed. The Watson-Jones interval can be used for access to the anterior hip joint, acetabular labrum, femoral head, and femoral neck if

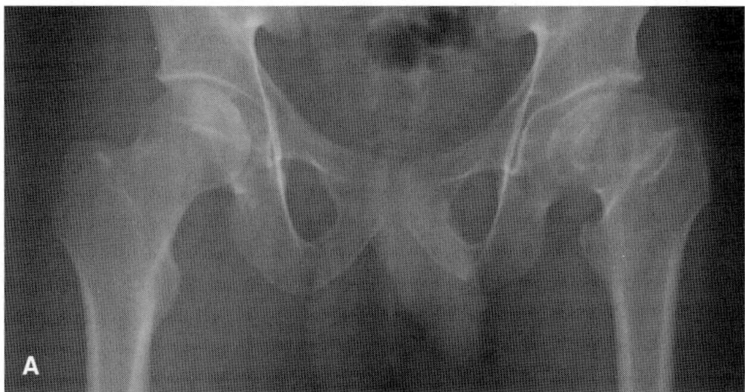

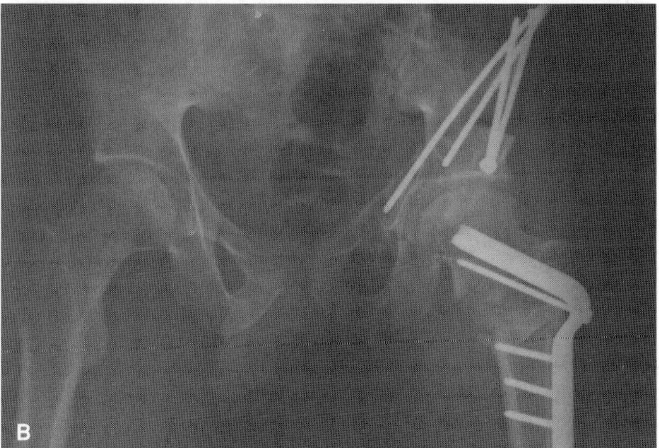

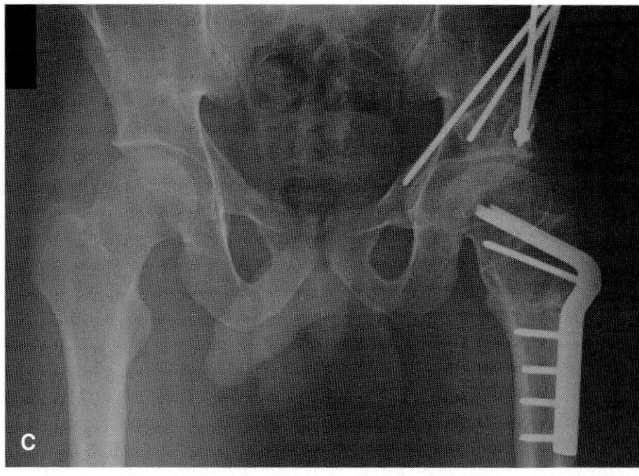

Figure 10-2 Periacetabular osteotomy/proximal femoral osteotomy (PAO/PFO) for Perthes/no wedge technique. Preoperative anteroposterior pelvic radiograph (**A**) of a 21-year-old male with a history of Perthe disease in childhood, leg-length discrepancy and a 2-year history of progressive lateral hip pain. A Perthe deformity of the proximal femur is noted, and secondary acetabular dysplasia is present. This patient was treated with a combined periacetabular osteotomy and a valgus proximal femoral osteotomy (**B**). The femoral osteotomy lengthened the extremity, enhanced the congruency of the joint, improved clinical abduction, and improved abductor function. This patient had an excellent clinical result 4 years later (**C**).

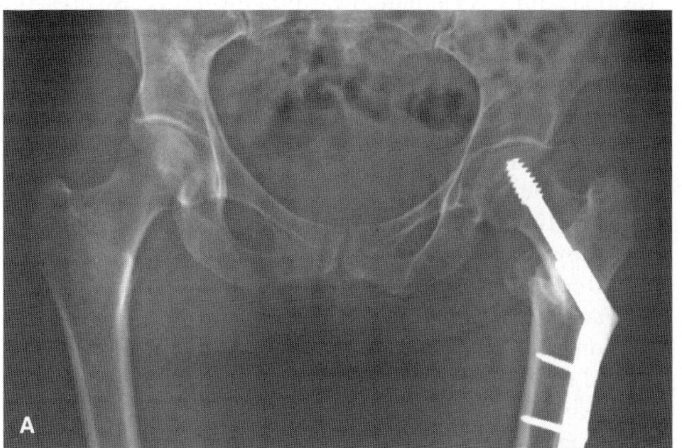

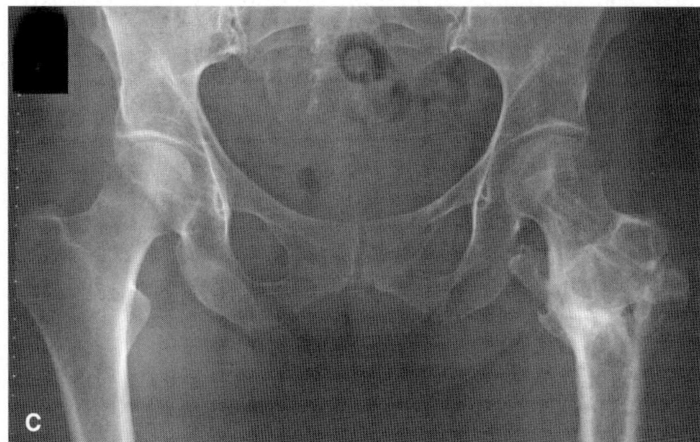

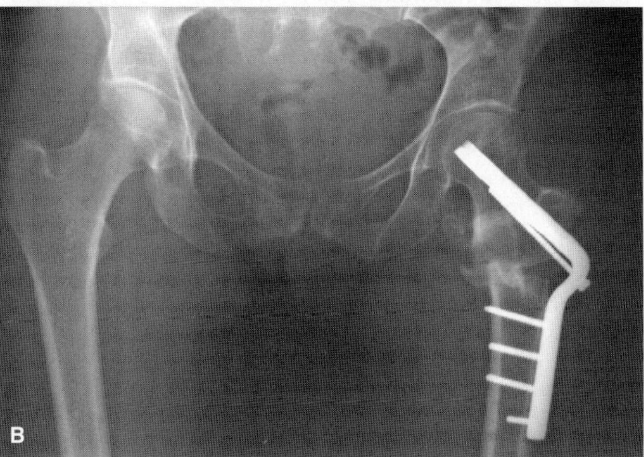

Figure 10-3 Proximal femoral osteotomy (PFO) for posttraumatic malunion. Standing anteroposterior pelvis (**A**) of the left hip in a 39-year-old female referred for evaluation of persistent hip pain after treatment of an intertrochanteric femoral fracture. Prior to fracture, the patient was an active recreational runner. She presented complaining of lateral hip pain, leg-length discrepancy, and lack of internal rotation of the left hip. On examination she had a severe limp, profound abductor weakness, a 2-cm leg-length discrepancy, and malrotation with <10 degrees of internal rotation. This proximal femoral malunion was treated with a valgus-derotation femoral osteotomy (**B**). She had an excellent clinical result and was asymptomatic at 5-year follow-up (**C**).

necessary. K-wires are placed to guide the osteotomy cut and the blade insertion. To place the blade centrally in the femoral neck, it must be inserted in the anterior half of the lateral greater trochanter owing to the posterior overhang. The insertion site should provide a 1.5- to 2.0-cm bony bridge of lateral femur cortex between the blade entry point and the osteotomy site. This minimizes the risk of fracture in this location. In general, varus and flexion/extension osteotomies are performed with a 90-degree blade plate whereas valgus corrections are obtained with blade plates ranging from 110 to 130 degrees, depending on the magnitude of correction. The chisel is advanced with a K-wire guiding the direction of insertion in the frontal plane and centrally in the femoral neck. If flexion (apex posterior) or extension (apex anterior) of the osteotomy is desired, this is incorporated by adjusting the anterior/posterior angulation of the chisel with respect to the femoral shaft. Rotation of the femur is then marked and the transverse osteotomy is made with an oscillating saw at the upper level of the lesser trochanter. The blade chisel is removed from the proximal fragment and the blade plate inserted along the prepared track. The blade plate is further secured to the proximal fragment with a 4.5-mm cortical screw. The proximal and distal osteotomy fragments are then mobilized, and the osteotomy is reduced by approximation of the lateral femur to the plate. The rotation line is used to facilitate the reduction, and care should be taken to align the two fragments without a major step-off in the anteroposterior plane. Final reduction and fixation of the osteotomy is assessed with radiographs or fluoroscopy in the anteroposterior and lateral planes, and hip range of motion (flexion and rotation) is checked by clinical examination.

Perthes Deformities

Legg-Calve-Perthes disease of childhood commonly alters the development of the femoral head and acetabulum, resulting in residual deformities that can be associated with hip symptoms in adulthood and can lead to secondary osteoarthritis. Perthes abnormalities are most remarkable on the femoral side (coxa magna, coxa plana, coxa breva, and relative trochanteric overgrowth), but can also encompass a secondary acetabular dysplasia. Generally, these abnormalities are very complex and must be evaluated carefully to optimize the surgical treatment plan. Labral disease, instability and joint overload, joint incongruence, abductor fatigue, and femoroacetabular impingement can all contribute variably to patient symptoms and should be considered.

The primary goals of treating Perthes deformities are to enhance joint stability, decrease localized joint surface overload, and relieve intra-articular impingement. Additional treatment goals may include equalization of leg lengths and repositioning of the greater trochanter. The specific characteristics of the deformity dictate the type of osteotomy correction. Hips with a femoral deformity and an associated secondary acetabular dysplasia (the most common scenario for patients who present with a prearthritic or early arthritic Perthes-like deformity) are most reliably treated with a combined acetabular reorientation and proximal femoral valgus osteotomy (Fig. 10-2A–C). With this comprehensive approach, the acetabular and femoral deformities can be addressed to optimize the hip reconstruction. This treatment strategy has been reported by Beck and Mast with good to excellent clinical results in 85% of cases at an average 3.4-year follow-up. At surgery, we now perform an arthrotomy to inspect the integrity of the acetabular labrum and to assess anterior femoroacetabular impingement from the large, nonspherical femoral head. Osteoplasty of the prominent anterior femoral head in the setting of coxa magna can minimize femoroacetabular impingement after acetabular reorientation.

For patients with a major, primary femoral deformity, a valgus osteotomy can be effective in improving congruency, relieving intra-articular impingement, lengthening the extremity, improving abductor function, and enhancing clinical hip abduction. Osteoplasty of the femoral head/neck junction may also be indicated in conjunction with the femoral osteotomy to completely address impingement disease. For Perthes hips with a less severe femoral deformity and a primary impingement problem, a femoral head/neck junction osteoplasty alone may be considered.

Slipped Capital Femoral Epiphysis

Another cause of hip dysfunction in the young patient, and premature osteoarthritis in adulthood, is a residual deformity from a SCFE. The SCFE deformity most commonly involves posteromedial displacement of the epiphysis, resulting in an extension and retroversion deformity of the proximal femur. An apparent varus deformity is also present. These patients most commonly complain of restricted hip flexion and symptoms from anterior femoroacetabular impingement combined with an external rotation deformity of the involved lower extremity. Direct correction of this deformity can be performed at the level of the femoral neck, although the risk of osteonecrosis makes this technique less attractive. Alternatively, a transverse intertrochanteric osteotomy can adequately address the deformity with less risk of osteonecrosis. A flexion and derotation osteotomy can correct the deformity and markedly improve clinical symptoms. The flexion correction should aim to place the femoral shaft perpendicular to the epiphysis in the sagittal plane. Slight valgus can be incorporated into the osteotomy but is frequently obtained with the flexion correction alone. An anterior capsulotomy should also be performed to ensure unrestricted postoperative hip extension and to inspect for residual femoroacetabular impingement. If present, the prominent anterolateral femoral head/neck junction should be resected. Severe SCFE deformities can require major deformity corrections (>50 degrees). In these cases it is particularly important to align the proximal and distal fragments by combining anterior translation and flexion of the distal fragment. This preserved alignment facilitates future total hip arthroplasty surgery.

Long-term results of intertrochanteric osteotomy for the treatment of SCFE deformities support continued use of these procedures. One recent follow-up study of the Imhauser osteotomy demonstrated good to excellent results in 77% of patients followed for an average of 23.4 years. This osteotomy provides a multiplanar correction consisting of flexion, internal rotation, and valgus that is dictated by resection of a three-dimensional intertrochanteric bone wedge. A similar multiplanar realignment can also be achieved with the no-wedge osteotomy technique discussed previously.

Osteonecrosis of the Femoral Head

The surgical management of osteonecrosis of the femoral head is a controversial topic, and there are many acceptable treatment options depending on patient characteristics, stage, size, and location of the lesion. The literature does support the intertrochanteric osteotomy as an effective strategy for the treatment of very specific disease patterns. It is imperative that these patients are carefully selected, and various factors must be considered when contemplating an intertrochanteric osteotomy for the diagnosis of osteonecrosis. Patients with a subchondral fracture and/or femoral head collapse without significant joint space narrowing can be evaluated as potential candidates for osteotomy surgery. The ideal candidate is a compliant, healthy patient not on corticosteroids who has a lesion with a combined osteonecrotic angle on the anteroposterior and lateral radiographs of <200 degrees. Such patients represent a relatively small subgroup of the patient population with osteonecrosis. In general, anterolateral lesions that can be delivered away from the weight-bearing surface of the femoral head are treated with a flexion-valgus osteotomy. This repositions the healthier posteromedial femoral head articular cartilage and subchondral bone into the weight-bearing zone. Anteromedial lesions that cannot be delivered away from the weight-bearing zone with a valgus osteotomy are managed with a varus flexion osteotomy to use the healthy posterolateral femoral head as the primary weight-bearing surface. In well-selected candidates treated with sound surgical technique, proximal femoral osteotomy can be very effective. Mont et al. reviewed 37 varus osteotomies (26 with a combined flexion or extension component) in the treatment of Ficat stage II and III disease. At 11.5 year follow-up, they noted 76% good or excellent clinical results.

Posttraumatic Hip Disorders

Selected posttraumatic disorders of the proximal femur can be excellent indications for osteotomy surgery. For example, nonunions of the femoral neck are associated with profound clinical symptoms and can be effectively managed with a valgus-producing proximal femoral osteotomy in appropriate patients. With the Pawuel technique, a laterally based closing wedge osteotomy at the intertrochanteric level achieves valgus correction. This converts the tension and shear forces across the nonunion (secondary to varus displacement) to a compressive force that facilitates healing. Marti et al. reviewed 50 cases of femoral neck nonunion treated with the Pawuel valgus-producing osteotomy at an average 7.1-year follow-up. They observed 86% of the nonunions to be healed, whereas 14% had been converted to total hip replacements.

Proximal femoral malunions may also present as a source of hip dysfunction, especially in active young patients. Such deformities must be carefully characterized, and the corrective osteotomy is planned to address the specific malunion pattern of each case. In the intertrochanteric region, a transverse osteotomy at the superior aspect of the lesser trochanter and the no-wedge technique can be used to correct multiplanar deformities and obtain predictable healing (Fig. 10-3).

Postoperative Management

Patients treated with a periacetabular osteotomy or proximal femoral osteotomy are mobilized on the first or second postoperative day. For the first 6 weeks, patients bear 30 pounds partial weight and perform isometric exercises only. At 6 weeks, active strengthening exercises are initiated with an emphasis on abductor strengthening, and weight-bearing status is advanced to 5% for an additional 4 weeks. Ten to 12 weeks postoperatively patients advance to full weight bearing depending on the details of the case and radiographic signs of healing. Aggressive hip strengthening is then permitted at this phase of rehabilitation. Unrestricted activity is allowed when radiographic healing of the osteotomy is evident. In general, we recommend hardware removal 1 to 2 years after the osteotomy to facilitate future conversion to total hip arthroplasty if required. Removal of proximal femoral blade plates also reduces the risk of trochanteric bursitis symptoms associated with the retained hardware.

Complications

Potential complications of osteotomy hip surgery include infection, nonunion, fixation failure, neurovascular injury, thromboembolic disease, and perioperative medical problems. A learning curve is known to contribute to the incidence of complications for most surgeons. Unique to acetabular osteotomy surgery are the potential complications of intra-articular fracture and overcorrection. Intra-articular fracture has a poor prognosis and usually leads to rapid joint deterioration. Overcorrection can cause secondary impingement disease and must be kept in mind when planning and performing acetabular reorientation. Persistent hip symptoms and progression of secondary osteoarthritis are additional problems that can occur; they underscore the limitations of joint preservation surgery in the setting of major degenerative changes and emphasize the importance of careful patient selection.

SUGGESTED READINGS

Beck M, Mast JW. The periacetabular osteotomy in Legg-Perthes–like deformities. *Semin Arthroplasty*.1997; 8(1):102–107.

Clohisy JC, Barrett SE, Gordon JE, et al. Periacetabular osteotomy for the treatment of severe acetabular dysplasia. *J Bone Joint Surg Am*. 2005;87(2):254–259.

Diab M, Hresko MT, Millis MB. Intertrochanteric versus subcapital osteotomy in slipped capital femoral epiphysis. *Clin Orthop Relat* Res. 2004;427:204–212.

Ganz R, Klaue K, Vinh TS, et al. A new periacetabular osteotomy for the treatment of hip dysplasias. Technique and preliminary results. *Clin Orthop*. 1988;232:26–36.

Harris WH. Etiology of osteoarthritis of the hip. *Clin Orthop.* 1986;213:20–33.

Kartenbender K, Cordier W, Katthagen BD. Long-term follow-up study after corrective Imhauser osteotomy for severe slipped capital femoral epiphysis. *J Pediatr Orthop.* 2000;20:749–756.

Leunig M, Siebenrock KA, Ganz R. Rationale of periacetabular osteotomy and background work. *J Bone Joint Surg Am.* 2001;83:438–448.

Marti RK, Schuller HM, Raaymakers EL. Intertrochanteric osteotomy for non-union of the femoral neck. *J Bone Joint Surg Br.* 1989;71:782–787.

Millis MB, Kim YJ. Rationale of osteotomy and related procedures for hip preservation: a review. *Clin Orthop Relat Res.* 2002;405:108–121.

Mont MA, Fairbank AC, Krackow KA, et al. Corrective osteotomy for osteonecrosis of the femoral head. *J Bone Joint Surg Am.* 1996;78:1032–1038.

Myers SR, Eijer H, Ganz R. Anterior femoroacetabular impingement after periacetabular osteotomy. *Clin Orthop Relat Res.* 1999;363:93–99.

Siebenrock KA. Scholl E, Lottenbach M, et al. Bernese periacetabular osteotomy. *Clin Orthop.* 1999;363:9–20.

Trousdale RT, Ekkernkamp A, Ganz R, et al. Periacetabular and intertrochanteric osteotomy for the treatment of osteoarthrosis in dysplastic hips. *J Bone Joint Surg Am.* 1995;77(1):73–85.

HIP HEMIARTHROPLASTY

KEITH R. BEREND

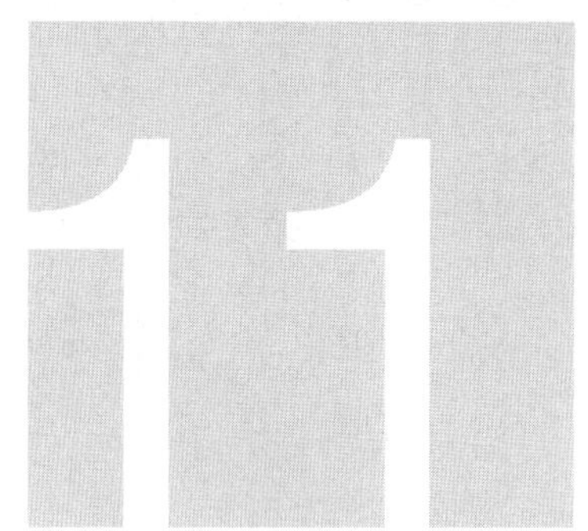

With historical roots dating back nearly a century, hip hemiarthroplasty remains one of the most commonly performed orthopedic operations still in use today. Most hip hemiarthroplasty procedures are carried out for femoral neck fractures in elderly patients. Over the decades, however, hemiarthroplasty has been used for many other indications including initial usage for osteoarthritis and as a temporizing measure for the young patient with osteonecrosis. Hemiresurfacing procedures have been used to provide a conservative alternative to total hip arthroplasty in young patients. As longer-term data have become available, the future trends in the use of hip hemiarthroplasty and more specifically hemiresurfacing arthroplasty remain to be seen. This chapter outlines three categories of indications and patient types in which hemiarthroplasty is widely used. First is the use of hemiarthroplasty for the treatment of acute femoral neck fracture. Second, the use of hip hemiarthroplasty for indications other than femur fracture is reviewed. Third, the history and continued use of hemiresurfacing techniques will be analyzed. The future of this technique for indications other than proximal femur fracture will be written by long-term studies comparing and contrasting the effectiveness of hemiarthroplasty with the now available long-term results of total hip arthroplasty in these three patient groups.

PATHOGENESIS

Hemiarthroplasty and Femoral Neck Fracture

The prevalence of femoral neck fracture is rising. As the population ages, and the larger middle-age generation reaches elderly ages, this trend will no doubt continue. Optimal treatment of nondisplaced fractures includes internal fixation with bone screws and has been described as successful in multiple reports. Treatment of nondisplaced fractures with hemiarthroplasty has been associated with increased mortality; hemiarthroplasty and should be reserved for displaced fractures, which carry a higher rate of failure when treated with internal fixation. Once fracture displacement has occurred, the optimal treatment for the fracture has not been defined. Current controversy revolves around the use of cemented versus cementless femoral stem fixation, unipolar versus bipolar articulations, and the use of acute total hip arthroplasty (THA) versus hemiarthroplasty.

TREATMENT

Internal Fixation versus Hemiarthroplasty

The results of so-called "low-demand" monoblock uncemented unipolar hemiarthroplasty, such as the Austin Moore hemiarthroplasty (Fig. 11-1), have been reported to be inferior to those of other treatment options. Blomfeldt et al.[1] examined the functional outcomes of internal fixation and monoblock uncemented unipolar arthroplasty in a series of 60 patients with an average age of 84 years. In this group with displaced fractures, the overall mortality and complication rates were not statistically different between treatment options. There was a trend toward more reoperations in the internal fixation group, however, with 33% of the internal fixation group and 13% of the hemiarthroplasty group requiring subsequent surgery. The quality of life outcomes measures used in this study did demonstrate a clear superiority in those patients who lived longer than 2 years after index surgery and had undergone internal fixation. The authors concluded that when compared with internal fixation, there are few data to recommend the use of a low-demand uncemented monoblock unipolar design in elderly patients. This view has been supported elsewhere. In a randomized controlled series, El-Abed et al.[2] demonstrated superior functional results in their group of patients treated with internal fixation when compared with hemiarthroplasty. No difference in revision rates was seen, but both the patients' and the physicians' perception of outcome was better in the internal fixation group. The superiority of internal fixation seen in some studies should be tempered by the high rates of failure seen in other series. In the hands of experienced trauma surgeons, the failure rate and subsequent surgical rate is as high as 35% with only 67% of fractures achieving bony union without avascular necrosis at 2 years following surgery. In a separate report, nonunion is reported to occur in up to 30% of cases with an additional rate of avascular necrosis occurring in up to 30% of

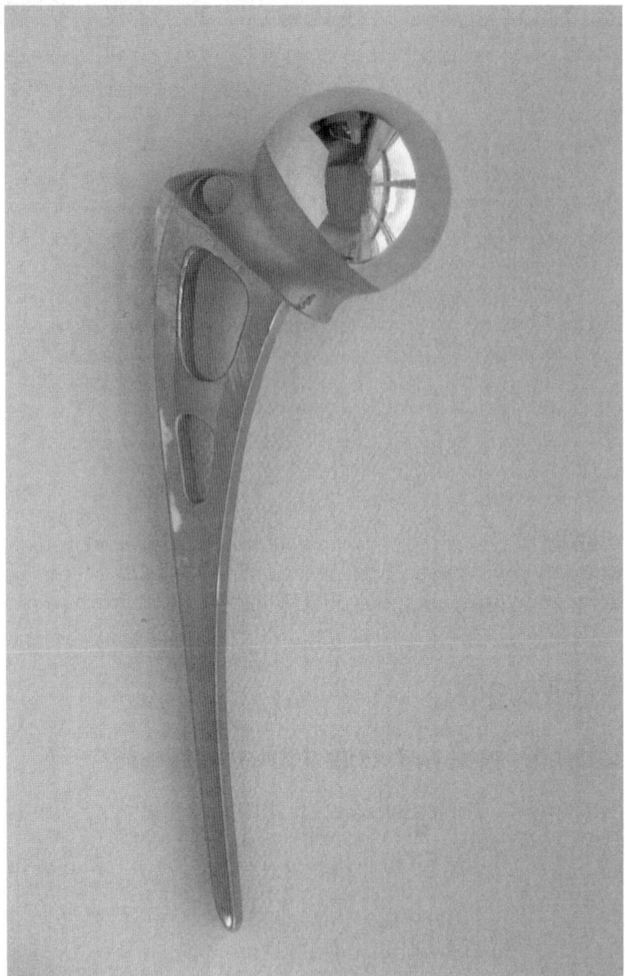

Figure 11-1 Photograph of an Austin-Moore hemiarthroplasty femoral component.

displaced femoral neck fractures treated with internal fixation.

Yau and Chiu,[3] using the same implant design concluded that its use should be avoided in younger active patients. Taken together, these data raise the question of the utility of either internal fixation or this type of uncemented monoblock unipolar design in the treatment of femoral neck fractures. Instead, other more durable designs and surgical options are indicated.

Cemented Femoral Fixation versus Cementless Fixation

Bezwada et al.[4] reviewed the clinical and radiographic outcomes of 256 cemented hemiarthroplasty devices inserted for acute femoral neck fracture over a 2-year period. All of the patients were older than 65 years of age. At an average of 3.5 years after surgery, there were two stem revisions and six cases converted to THA for recalcitrant groin pain. They concluded that cemented hemiarthroplasty is a viable treatment option with good midterm results in these elderly patients. Clearly, this 97% success far outweighs even the best reports of internal fixation or Austin Moore–type hemiarthroplasty for displaced femoral neck fractures. The use of a cemented device for hemiarthroplasty has been demonstrated to provide earlier and superior pain relief and return of function in some series. Further support for the use of a cemented hemiarthroplasty is provided by Dixon and Bannister.[5] In a review of 53 cemented bipolar hemiarthroplasties, they report that almost 70% of patients who were able to walk 1 mile before fracture were able to do the same at the time of final follow-up. Moreover, only two failures were noted in the series with 32-month follow-up. Nearly three decades ago, Beckenbaugh et al.[6] concluded that cemented hemiarthroplasty is indicated in the treatment of acute femoral neck fracture in the elderly. The cemented hemiarthroplasty still appears to be the standard to which other treatment options for displaced femoral neck fractures should be compared.

Caution is warranted, however, as the use of a cemented femoral device in the treatment of femoral neck fractures has been associated with an increased risk of death within 30 days of the surgery. Other risk factors associated with increased mortality following hip fracture treatment include female gender, advanced elderly age, pre-existing heart and lung conditions, and intertrochanteric-type fractures. It would seem prudent to weigh the possible increased risk of mortality with the benefit of earlier functional recovery when considering the use of cemented or cementless devices. Unfortunately, many of the low-demand, fracture-type stems are designed to be implanted either with or without cement, are made of cobalt-chrome, and do not have the same porous coatings that have proven to provide longevity in cementless applications. When these types of stems are implanted in a cementless fashion, the results will probably be inferior to those of cemented designs or modern porous coated stems (Fig. 11-2).

By avoiding revision for stem loosening into the second decade, primary femoral components with long-term excellent results should be the implant of choice when hemiarthroplasty is carried out for fracture. Certainly, in the younger, more active patient, this holds true.

Unipolar versus Bipolar Hemiarthroplasty

Several variables interplay in the decision between a unipolar and a bipolar prosthesis for use in hemiarthroplasty. The theoretical decrease in articular cartilage wear and increased range of motion with the bipolar device are frequently cited as the benefits obtained by choosing a bipolar design. Most frequently, cost containment is cited as the primary indication for use of a unipolar device.

Unipolar arthroplasty is a simple and cost effective approach to the surgical treatment of a displaced femoral neck fracture. More than 70% of people regain prefracture levels of ambulation, and 80% report mild or no pain at 1 year following surgery. Up to 80% survivorship at 7 years has been published with unipolar arthroplasty. There have been indications that stiffness, groin pain, cartilage degeneration, and acetabular protrusio are more frequent with unipolar designs compared with bipolar designs.

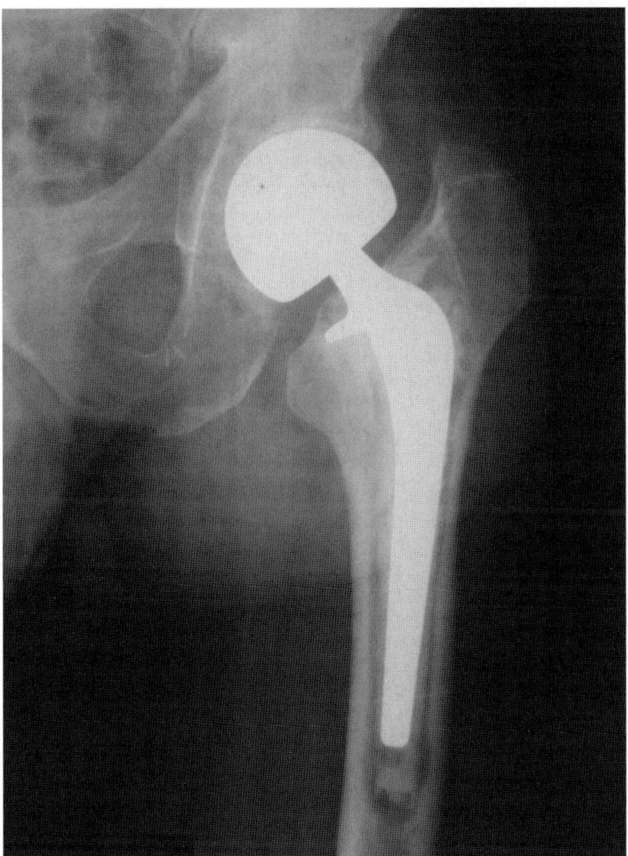

Figure 11-2 Radiograph of a 62-year-old man who presented with a left hip cemented hemiarthroplasty for treatment of fracture that had failed after 3 years secondary to stem loosening and subsidence.

In older patients who are active, higher demands place increased stresses on the implant and articular surfaces leading to lower satisfaction with the surgical results in these cases.

Bipolar hemiarthroplasty has proven slightly superior to unipolar designs in some series. Although groin pain can and does still occur in some patients, a large meta-analysis of the literature revealed that 85% of patients report mild or absent pain and 85% regain functional mobility in the first 2 years after surgery. In a separate prospective series, no advantage to bipolar over unipolar designs was seen in elderly patients treated for femoral neck fracture.

As noted, an increase in stability may be conferred by the bipolar design, and this remains a significant motivator for its use. When the bipolar does dislocate, it more frequently requires open reduction than does unipolar hemiarthroplasty. In addition, there are several reports of wear, osteolysis, and loosening associated with the polyethylene articulation in bipolar arthroplasty. Taking the above noted information into account, it would appear that a well-designed cemented or porous coated femoral stem combined with a unipolar articulation would be the treatment of choice for the elderly, low-activity patient with a displaced femoral neck fracture. Total hip arthroplasty in the treatment of these fractures has been suggested to be the ideal treatment in younger patients and may eventually prove to be the ideal treatment for all patients with displaced fractures.

In addition to the standard application of a bipolar arthroplasty for femoral neck fracture, some investigators have attempted to use these devices as a conservative option when treating young patients with osteonecrosis (ON) of the femoral head. It is believed by some that not preparing the acetabulum and placing an acetabular component may be a beneficial option in these cases. This philosophy has been tested for several decades. In 1977 Beckenbaugh et al.[6] reported inferior results using the Thompson femoral endoprosthesis and cemented fixation in cases of ON. Again in the 1980s Lachiewicz and Desman[7] reported 52% fair and poor results using a bipolar endoprosthesis as a conservative option in young patients with ON. They further noted that younger age and increasing severity of the ON carried increased risk for failure.

Cabanela[8] repeated these negative results in a small meta-analysis highlighting the long-term results of cemented and uncemented bipolar hemiarthroplasties in contrast to THA. He noted that femoral loosening was not prevented by a bipolar design and that the results of THA in ON were far superior to those of the bipolar device. There were higher rates both of complications and reoperations in the hemiarthroplasty group. Lee et al.[9] prospectively compared the results of bipolar hemiarthroplasty versus THA using an identical modern cementless femoral component. They noted a significantly better pain score in the THA group. Groin pain occurred significantly more often in the bipolar group as did buttocks pain. In addition, 23% of the bipolar group demonstrated superior head migration and acetabular degeneration. Interestingly, the incidence of dislocation, thought to be a concern with THA for acute fracture, was the same in both groups. The conclusion of this series was that THA is a better procedure in patients with ON.

Better results have been reported by Grevitt and Spencer,[10] who studied hemiarthroplasty in renal transplant patients suffering from ON. In their series of 22 cemented bipolar hemiarthroplasties, all patients had improvements in pain and 21 of the 22 had good to excellent results. One case of aseptic loosening and one acetabular complication necessitated revision at an average of 40 months follow-up. Takaoka et al.[11] echoed these acceptable results at early follow-up with the use of a bipolar device in ON. In a comparison of bipolar hemiarthroplasty with contralateral THA in the same patient, satisfactory results were equal between the sides. No statistical differences were noted in any of the clinical outcomes measured. The authors concluded that in young patients with Ficat stage III disease, a bone in-growth stem and bipolar arthroplasty is the treatment of choice. Excellent results have also been shown with the use of a bipolar device and an uncemented stem in young active patients with ON associated with sickle cell disease. Caution should be used in these cases and any scenario where acetabular bone stock may be involved because protrusion can occur, complicating conversion to THA when necessary. It appears that in selected cases of young patients with AVN, a bipolar articulation combined with a modern cementless femoral component can provide acceptable results for several years.

Surface Replacement Hemiarthroplasty

Total articular resurfacing arthroplasty procedures have gained and lost popularity several times in the relatively short history of hip arthroplasty. With more advanced bearing options, improved implantation techniques, and stringent patient selection, these procedures are enjoying a tremendous resurgence of interest worldwide. As total resurfacing initially fell from favor, owing to thin polyethylene acetabular surfaces and fixation issues, hemiresurfacing has remained a viable option in young patients with ON.

Although the theory of hemiresurfacing is quite attractive in the young active patient with ON, there have been negative reports in the literature. Cuckler and Tamarapalli[12] reported poor results but recommended this procedure in patients with ON if younger than 30 years of age as the conversion to THA is straightforward. Adili and Trousdale[13] reported similar poor results with overall survivorship of 76% at 3 years. Only 62.5% of cases reported satisfaction and good pain relief with this procedure.

As alternative bearings have become available, the role of selected hemiresurfacing has been questioned. Total resurfacing hip arthroplasty in ON has enjoyed renewed interest as results of this procedure are now being reported in a more favorable light. Beaulé et al.[14] have reported better functional results and better pain relief with the use of a metal-on-metal resurfacing than with hemiresurfacing alone.

CONCLUSIONS

Hemiarthroplasty continues to hold a strong position in the treatment of displaced femoral neck fracture in the elderly patient. Although some authors believe that total hip arthroplasty may be a better option, complications such as dislocation and increased operative time and blood loss may outweigh these benefits in the elderly low-demand patient. Both cemented and cementless fixation have shown good long-term results as have unipolar and bipolar designs. Advantages and drawbacks to each combination should stimulate personal investigation by the orthopedic surgeon as to his or her own outcomes. Hemiresurfacing arthroplasty has attractive theoretical advantages, but with alternative bearings and improved implant fixation options this procedure has decreasing and now very limited application.

REFERENCES

1. Blomfeldt R, Tornkvist H, Ponzer S, et al. Internal fixation versus hemiarthroplasty for displaced fractures of the femoral neck in elderly patients with severe cognitive impairment. *J Bone Joint Surg Br*. 2005;87(4):523–529.
2. El-Abed K, McGuinness A, Brunner J, et al. Comparison of outcomes following uncemented hemiarthroplasty and dynamic hip screw in the treatment of displaced subcapital hip fractures in patients aged greater than 70 years. *Acta Orthop Belg*. 2005;71(1):48–54.
3. Yau WP, Chiu KY. Critical radiological analysis after Austin Moore hemiarthroplasty. *Injury*. 2004;35(10):1020–1024.
4. Bezwada HP, Shah AR, Harding SH, et al. Cementless bipolar hemiarthroplasty for displaced femoral neck fractures in the elderly. *J Arthroplasty*. 2004;19(7 suppl 2):73–77.
5. Dixon S, Bannister G. Cemented bipolar hemiarthroplasty for displaced intracapsular fracture in the mobile active elderly patient. *Injury*. 2004;35(2):152–156.
6. Beckenbaugh RD, Tressler HA, Johnson EW Jr. Results after hemiarthroplasty of the hip using a cemented femoral prosthesis. A review of 109 cases with an average follow-up of 36 months. *Mayo Clin Proc*. 1977;52(6):349–353.
7. Lachiewicz PF, Desman SM. The bipolar endoprosthesis in avascular necrosis of the femoral head. *J Arthroplasty*. 1988;3(2):131–138.
8. Cabanela ME. Bipolar versus total hip arthroplasty for avascular necrosis of the femoral head. A comparison. *Clin Orthop Relat Res*. 1990;261:59–62.
9. Lee SB, Sugano N, Nakata K, et al. Comparison between bipolar hemiarthroplasty and THA for osteonecrosis of the femoral head. *Clin Orthop Relat Res*. 2004;424:161–165.
10. Grevitt MP, Spencer JD. Avascular necrosis of the hip treated by hemiarthroplasty. Results in renal transplant recipients. *J Arthroplasty*. 1995;10(2):205–211.
11. Takaoka K, Nishina T, Ohzono K, et al. Bipolar prosthetic replacement for the treatment of avascular necrosis of the femoral head. *Clin Orthop Relat Res*. 1992;277:121–127.
12. Cuckler JM, Tamarapalli JR. An algorithm for the management of femoral neck fractures. *Orthopedics*. 1994;17:789–792.
13. Adili A, Trousdale RT. Femoral head resurfacing for the treatment of osteonecrosis in the young patient. *Clin Orthop Relat Res*. 2003;417:93–101.
14. Beaulé PE, Amstutz HC, Le Duff M, et al. Surface arthroplasty for osteonecrosis of the hip: hemiresurfacing versus metal-on-metal hybrid resurfacing. *J Arthroplasty*. 2004;19(8 suppl 3):54–58.

SUGGESTED READINGS

Beaulé PE, Amstutz HC, Le Duff M, et al. Surface arthroplasty for osteonecrosis of the hip: hemiresurfacing versus metal-on-metal hybrid resurfacing. *J Arthroplasty*. 2004;19(8 suppl 3): 54–58.

Bezwada HP, Shah AR, Harding SH, et al. Cementless bipolar hemiarthroplasty for displaced femoral neck fractures in the elderly. *J Arthroplasty*. 2004;19(7 suppl 2):73–77.

Bhandari M, Devereaux PJ, Swiontkowski MF, et al. Internal fixation compared with arthroplasty for displaced fractures of the femoral neck: a meta-analysis. *J Bone Joint Surg*. 2003;85A:1673–1681.

Grecula MJ. Resurfacing arthroplasty in osteonecrosis of the hip. *Orthop Clin North Am*. 2005;36:231–242.

Healy WL, Iorio R. Total hip arthroplasty: optimal treatment for displaced femoral neck fractures in elderly patients. *Clin Orthop Relat Res*. 2004;429:43–48.

Lu-Yau GL, Keller RB, Littenberg B, et al. Outcomes after displaced fractures of the femoral neck. A meta-analysis of one-hundred and six published papers. *J Bone Joint Surg*. 1994;76A:15–25.

Wathne RA, Koval KJ, Aharonoff GB, et al. Modular unipolar versus bipolar prosthesis: a prospective evaluation of functional outcomes after femoral neck fracture. *J Orthop Trauma*. 1995;9:298–302.

TOTAL HIP ARTHROPLASTY

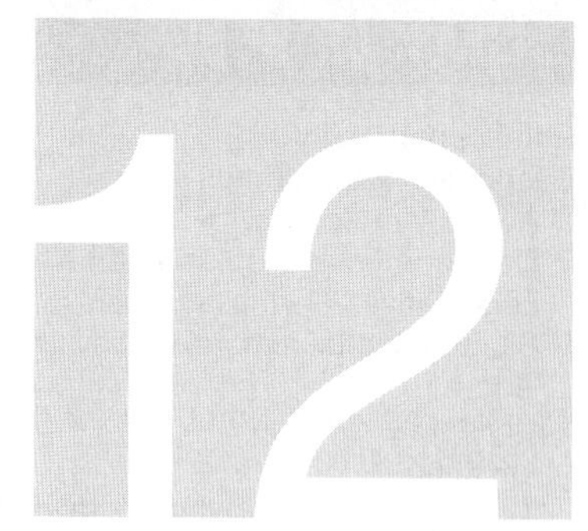

ANDREW I. SPITZER

Total hip arthroplasty (THA) is one of the most successful modern surgical procedures, eliminating the debilitating pain associated with arthritis and restoring function to the disabled patient. It provides a reliable, durable, and predictable excellent result and is generally regarded as one of the most significant advances in the management of the end-stage degenerative hip by rheumatologists, orthopaedic surgeons, the general medical community, and patients alike. Since its original introduction by Sir John Charnley at Wrightington Hospital in the United Kingdom in the late 1960s, the annual number of primary total hip arthroplasties performed has steadily increased. In addition, although originally applied to a predominantly elderly population, the technology has been extended to younger and more active patients. An aging population, improved wear properties and fixation of implants, and techniques designed to provide more rapid and complete recovery of function all have combined to increase current and anticipated future demand for total hip arthroplasty.

PATHOGENESIS

Etiology and Epidemiology

Osteoarthritis is the most common indication for total hip arthroplasty. It afflicts an estimated 21 million adults in the United States in at least one joint and may involve the hip in as many as 1.5% of the American adult population. Osteoarthritis is either primary, without identifiable cause, or secondary, owing to another systemic disease, congenital malformation, or structural abnormality of the hip joint. Joint destruction also can result from inflammatory arthropathies and rheumatologic disease (Table 12-1).

Pathophysiology

Although the actual mechanism of articular cartilage damage differs among the various causes of the arthritic hip, the final common pathway is one characterized by destruction of the smooth articular cartilage, resulting in a high friction articulation. Bone begins to grind directly on bone, generating debris, joint effusions, and in some cases frank inflammation and synovitis. The actual source of pain is unknown but may be capsular distention, synovitis, or irritated pain receptors within the bone or surrounding tissues. Motion of the joint becomes painful, especially with weight bearing, and limits mobility and function of the patient.

DIAGNOSIS

History and Physical Examination

Clinical Features

Patients suffering from an arthritic hip joint complain of pain located in the groin, buttock, or lateral hip, often radiating along the anterior thigh toward, but usually not beyond, the knee. The pain typically is worse with activity, although start-up stiffness followed by early relief with light activity may occur. Barometric and weather changes also affect the pain, with damp and cold weather usually exacerbating the symptoms. Although the pain may wax and wane, the clinical course is usually progressive. The pace of progression, however, is unpredictable and multifactorial.

As the arthritic symptoms worsen, patients complain of a limp, ipsilateral limb shortening, stiffness, and limitation in mobility and vocational and avocational tasks. Even activities of daily living, such as toenail care, donning and doffing socks and shoes, short-distance ambulation, rising from or assuming a seated position, negotiating stairs, and sleeping, become challenging and impaired. The impact of the arthritis often becomes overwhelming as each hip cycle, of which a normal individual experiences roughly a million per year, causes pain.

On physical examination the patient may demonstrate a depressed affect, frustration, and anger. Abductor weakness from involuntary guarding and subsequent atrophy, and from laxity of the abductor muscles from limb shortening, manifests in several gait abnormalities. The Trendelenburg gait occurs as the pelvis drops to the opposite side with ipsilateral single limb stance. The gluteus medius is unable to pull the body weight over the femoral head. Patients will compensate for this weakness with an abductor lurch, in which the body is thrust over the ipsilateral limb during single-limb stance, positioning the center of body mass

TABLE 12-1 CAUSES OF DEGENERATIVE DISEASE OF THE HIP

Primary osteoarthritis
Secondary osteoarthritis
- Avascular necrosis
- Developmental dysplasia of the hip
- Legg-Calves-Perthes disease
- Slipped capital femoral epiphysis
- Trauma
- Crystalline disease
- Infection
- Multiple or spondyloepiphyseal dysplasia
- Prior surgery
- Paget disease
- Acromegaly
- Hypothyroidism
- Hyperparathyroidism
- Ehlers-Danlos syndrome
- Sickle cell disease
- Thalassemia
- Hemophilia
- Gaucher disease
- Ochronosis
- Wilson disease
- Hemochromatosis

Rheumatologic disease
- Rheumatoid arthritis
- Lupus
- Psoriatic arthritis
- Spondyloarthropathies
  - Ankylosing spondylitis
  - Reiter disease

directly over the femoral head and minimizing the lever arm and resulting torque imposed by body weight, a so-called Duchenne gait (Fig. 12-1). The gait will also typically become antalgic, with the patient minimizing the time spent weight bearing on the involved hip because of the pain. Finally, shortening of the limb because of loss of the joint space and bony collapse or penetration may also impact gait, resulting in a rise and fall of the ipsilateral shoulder with each step.

Additional physical findings include diminished range of motion, with hip flexion and internal rotation most commonly affected. Flexion contracture may be present. This is measured as an inability to fully extend the hip while the other hip is flexed, fixing the pelvis and preventing pelvic hyperextension to achieve hip extension (Thomas test) (Fig. 12-2). Adduction contracture, which may require correction at the time of surgery to prevent dislocation of the total hip arthroplasty, can occur as well, with an inability to passively abduct the limb. Limb-length discrepancy is common and should be accurately measured. Actual limb length is measured between two bony prominences with a fixed relationship to one another, such as the anterior superior iliac spine and the lateral or medial malleolus. Measurement between points without such a fixed relationship, such as the pubic symphysis or umbilicus and a malleolus, will result in erroneous and unreliable values that vary with pelvic obliquity and abduction of the hip. Pelvic obliquity causing apparent, accentuated, or pseudonormalized limb-length inequality should also be recognized to warn patients about what their perceptions of limb length may be postsurgery.

Finally, a thorough examination of both lower extremities and spine should be performed, including an assessment of the neurologic and circulatory status of the limbs. Other causes of pain and factors that may compromise the outcome of total hip arthroplasty should be identified.

Radiologic Features

A low anteroposterior (AP) pelvis radiograph, taken from the level of the anterior superior iliac spine to distal, will usually provide adequate visualization of the acetabulum and the length of the femur in which the prosthesis will sit. A full AP pelvis may be necessary if significant bone erosion or abnormality exists. A true lateral hip radiograph ("shoot-through" lateral) allows evaluation of the anterior and posterior hip joint space. A frog-limb lateral (Löwenstein) will normally complete the films required for a thorough evaluation. On occasion, additional pelvic views—inlet, outlet, obturator and iliac oblique, and false profile—or longer views of the femur in multiple planes may be useful.

The hallmark of an arthritic hip is loss of the cartilage-containing joint space, with bone articulating directly against bone. An osteoarthritic hip also may demonstrate subchondral sclerosis, bony cysts, and marginal osteophytes. Inflammatory arthropathy tends to be less hypertrophic, with global joint space loss and in some cases a minimum of periarticular reaction. Avascular necrosis is characterized by prominent sclerosis and/or cysts of the femoral head, femoral head collapse, and secondary acetabular arthritic change. Residual findings from childhood disease may include persistent uncoverage of the femoral head, acetabular dysplasia, subluxation, coxa magna, and deformity of the femoral head from slipped capital femoral epiphysis. Posttraumatic deformity can assume almost any configuration.

Important factors to observe, in addition to the arthritic joint and the bony reaction, include bone quality, which may affect fixation choice, and any anatomic variants that may present challenges at the time of surgery, such as unusually tall or short stature, excessive coxa vara or coxa valga, unusually large and potentially structurally significant cysts, and extremely small or large femoral or acetabular anatomy.

Lines, angles, and measurements that may help to define the anatomic abnormalities either causing or resulting from the arthritis include Shenton's line, Klein's line, Kohler's line, the center-edge angle, acetabular index, neck-shaft (CCD) angle, and the femoral cortical index. Assessment of the radiographs with these tools may facilitate surgical planning and enhance the surgeon's appreciation of the unique reconstructive challenges of each hip.

Diagnostic Workup

Although the history, physical examination, and radiographs will be adequate to establish the diagnosis and cause of arthritis in most cases, additional studies may be necessary. An MRI may differentiate intrinsic articular pathology from periarticular soft tissue irritation and will make the

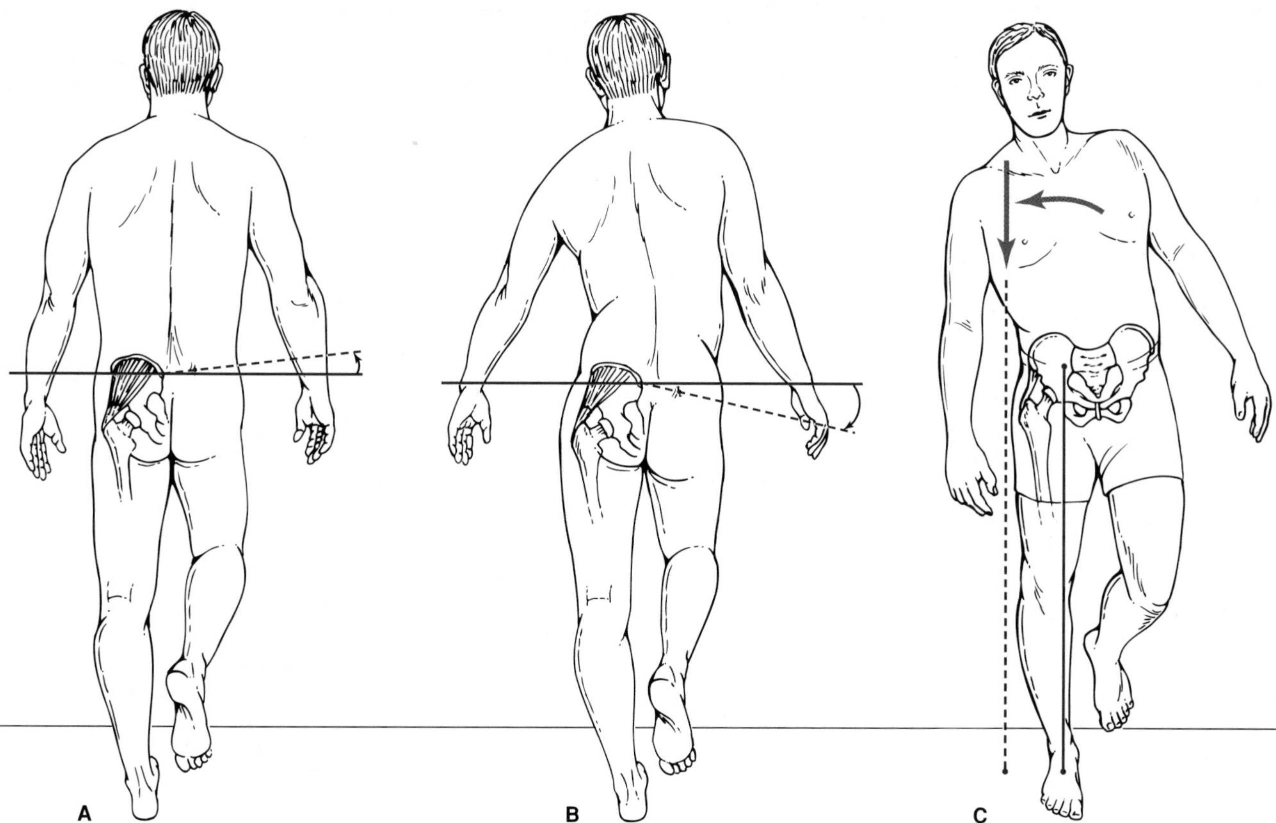

Figure 12-1 A: Normal gluteus medius function. **B.** Weak gluteus medius causing a positive Trendelenburg sign with the pelvis dropping on the contralateral side. **C:** Abductor lurch or Duchenne gait.

diagnosis of early avascular necrosis (AVN) prior to radiographic findings. CT scans will define complex bony abnormalities, and three-dimensional reconstructions can improve the surgeon's three-dimensional understanding of complex deformities. Nuclear scintigraphy may be useful to assess metastatic disease when suspected or other sites of disease that may be primary sources of pain. Laboratory studies assessing inflammatory disease markers such as rheumatoid factor, anti–nuclear antibodies, lyme titers, and others can help to define systemic disease. Complete blood count, sedimentation rate, and C-reactive protein measurements may be useful to evaluate for local or systemic infection. Aspiration of the joint, when clinical suspicion for infection is present, yields fluid that should be an-

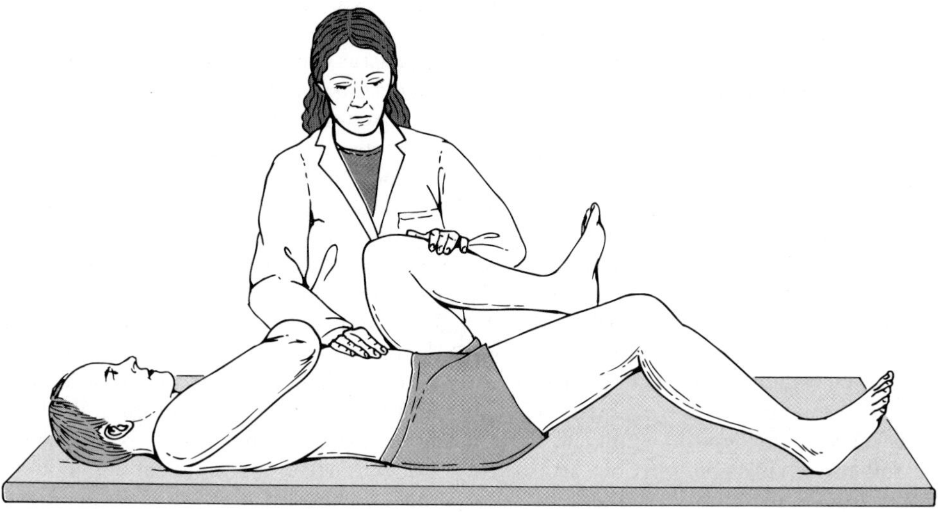

Figure 12-2 Thomas test for hip flexion contracture.

alyzed with cell count and differential; glucose level; microscopic review with appropriate stains for bacteria, fungi, and acid-fast bacilli; and formal culture for these organisms as well.

In many arthritic patients, concurrent pain from other arthritic anatomic locations can confuse the clinical picture. The hip can be the primary pain generator but can refer pain to the knee or cause a gait abnormality that exacerbates underlying spinal disease or ipsilateral or contralateral lower-extremity arthritic joints. Despite pain in these other areas, the severely arthritic hip should be addressed primarily. For example, it is generally advisable to replace the arthritic hip before undertaking spinal surgery, because the persistent gait abnormality may compromise the results of spine surgery. Similarly, hip replacement should precede an ipsilateral knee replacement when both joints are symptomatic and arthritic, because the referred pain from the hip and hip stiffness can compromise outcome and rehabilitative efforts after knee surgery. Furthermore, the new center of rotation of the hip should be used to establish a neutral mechanical axis (a factor critical in total knee arthroplasty longevity) prior to embarking on the knee reconstruction. When a true differential diagnosis dilemma exists as to the actual source of pain, diagnostic injections of local anesthetic with or without corticosteroid may help to define the primary source of pain.

In the absence of radiographic evidence for significant arthritis, alternative sources of pain must be sought. An MRI with and without arthrography along with diagnostic aspiration and injection may be useful to distinguish intra-articular from extra-articular pathology. A further workup may include evaluation of other anatomic locations and the neurologic and metabolic status of the patient (Table 12-2). Pain that is only presumptively located in the hip is not an indication for total hip arthroplasty in the absence of proven articular pathology that warrants such a major intervention.

TABLE 12-2 ALTERNATIVE SOURCES OF HIP PAIN

Location	Condition
Intra-articular	Stress fracture
	Impingement
	Labral tear
	Synovitis
	Infection
	Tumor
	Avascular necrosis
	Dysplasia and bone overload
Periarticular	Bursitis
	Tendinitis
	Nerve entrapment
	Strain
	Sprain
Extra-articular	
Abdomen/pelvis	Hernia
	Ovarian pathology
	Testicular pathology
	Sacroiliac disease
	Pubic symphysis instability
Spine	Herniated nucleus pulposus
	Degenerative disc or facet disease
	Spinal stenosis
	Instability
Systemic	Metabolic bone disease
	Osteoporosis
	Other
	Inflammatory/rheumatologic disease

TREATMENT

Nonoperative Management

The goals for treating the arthritic hip are to eliminate pain and, when possible, to restore motion to the joint and mobility to the patient. Often this requires surgery, but conservative, nonoperative treatment should be exhausted before proceeding directly to the operating theatre. The American College of Rheumatology publishes guidelines for the management of Osteoarthritis. These guidelines can be used as a paradigm for treating the degenerative hip of any cause. Simple analgesics, nonsteroidal anti-inflammatory drugs, and disease modifying agents when available may be offered as a first line of treatment. These all may be combined with physical therapy and judicious use of adaptive aids and assistive devices for both ambulation and other activities of daily living. Intra-articular injections of corticosteroids may diminish the intensity of acute inflammatory flares in the joint. Local application of ointments and compounds are usually not useful around the hip because of the depth of the joint beneath the often robust soft tissue envelope. Other adjuncts such as the use of nutraceuticals and intra-articular injections of viscosupplements may be useful but at present have not been scientifically proven to be effective. When these modalities fail, surgical intervention becomes appropriate to consider.

Operative Treatment

Indications and Contraindications

The indications for total hip arthroplasty include pain unresponsive to nonoperative management along with radiographically proven severe degenerative disease. The patient must also have a realistic expectation relative to activity level, with a willingness to minimize impact loading activities and excessive exercise. Active infection either locally, systemically, or at a distant location is an absolute contraindication to joint arthroplasty. In addition, pain about the hip without documented cause or radiographically proven degenerative disease in the absence of compelling symptoms should not be treated with hip arthroplasty.

The list of relative contraindications is more controversial. Younger males with osteoarthritis, for instance, are a cohort that has a documented higher failure rate after total hip arthroplasty, presumably because of activity level and intensity. Counseling with appropriate caution and warning must be given to these patients contemplating total hip arthroplasty. Other relative contraindications include the very elderly, those medically at risk for perioperative morbidity or mortality, immunocompromised status increasing risk of infection, and unwillingness or inability to comply with recommended precautions or restrictions.

Surgical Goals

The goals of total hip arthroplasty are straightforward and intuitive. The reconstruction must re-establish normal anatomy, as closely as possible, with regard to limb length and femoral offset, and preserve soft tissue tension to ensure stability. Immediate and long-term fixation of the components along with bearing surfaces that are optimized to reduce wear are critical to reliable and durable service. Perioperative complications should be minimized with careful preoperative planning and vigilant perioperative management. And, most important, the patient's pain should be relieved and mobility and function should be restored.

Preoperative Planning

The preoperative planning process helps ensure intraoperative achievement of the surgical goals of total hip arthroplasty. The process begins with a thorough medical evaluation, identifying and treating sources of infection, and optimizing the patients' cardiovascular, pulmonary, and general health status. The orthopaedic evaluation includes history, examination with an assessment of gait disorder, range of motion, limb lengths, neurovascular status and skin integrity, radiographic imaging, and, if necessary, special studies. Ideally, with an understanding of the underlying pathology, the surgeon can use templates on the radiographs to size and place the components, appreciate the biomechanical alterations of both the diseased hip and the proposed reconstruction, mentally rehearse the procedure, and anticipate pitfalls. Patient education regarding precautions and expectations facilitates postoperative rehabilitation and discharge planning. Finally, the process culminates in the operating room with choice of anesthesia and patient preparation including perioperative antibiotics, urinary bladder management, careful patient positioning, and meticulous sterile technique.

Surgical Approaches and Exposures

There are numerous surgical approaches, each with certain benefits and risks, that enable the hip surgeon to accomplish the goals of total hip arthroplasty. In addition, modifications of each of these approaches, some of which have been published and others that remain technical pearls of master hip surgeons, have evolved over time. In choosing a surgical approach, the surgeon should carefully consider familiarity, skill, and the idiosyncrasies and characteristics of each approach. There is no single best or worst methodology, but a measured analysis should reveal the right combination of surgeon, patient, and surgical approach to optimize the outcome.

Charnley first performed his low frictional torque arthroplasty through a trochanteric osteotomy, which allowed for wide exposure of the hip and offered the opportunity to adjust abductor tension when reattaching the trochanter. Unfortunately, nonunion of the osteotomy occurred in as many as 25% of patients in some series. Although still useful in complex primary and revision surgery, this approach has largely been abandoned for exposure of the straightforward primary total hip arthroplasty.

The posterior approach, which classically centers a posteriorly directed incision over the trochanter, incises the iliotibial band laterally and splits the fibers of the gluteus maximus muscle. The gluteus medius is elevated, the short external rotators are detached from their trochanteric insertion, and a posterior capsulotomy and dislocation are performed. Although this approach provides the most extensile exposure, higher dislocation rates have been reported. However, with a more truncated exposure, repair of the soft tissue, and with the use of larger bearing surfaces, that dislocation rate should be significantly reduced.

Anterolateral approaches use a vertical incision centered over the trochanter. The iliotibial band is split distally, and the fibers of the tensor fascia lata are split proximally. In the direct lateral approach, the surgeon detaches the anterior portion of the gluteus medius and a portion of the vastus lateralis as a soft tissue sleeve, sometimes with a wafer of bone attached. In the anterolateral approach, the surgeon detaches the anterior third of the gluteus medius, often with a wafer of trochanteric bone as well. Anterior capsulotomy and dislocation are performed. The acetabulum is well visualized in these approaches, and the dislocation rate has been reported to be lower. However, these exposures are not as easily extensile, often require postoperative weight bearing and activity limitations while the soft tissue/bony abductor sleeve heals, and have been associated with a higher incidence of gluteus medius weakness and limp.

The direct anterior approach uses an anterior incision along the interval between the tensor fascia lata and the sartorius muscles. Splitting this interval allows direct visualization of the anterior capsule, which can be incised, enabling anterior dislocation. Although this muscle-splitting approach provides good acetabular exposure and improved hip stability, it is not extensile, and exposure of the femur can be challenging. Management of intraoperative complications may necessitate a second, more extensile approach. In addition, the use of a specialized fracture table for patient positioning is a prerequisite.

There has been a great deal of interest recently in total hip arthroplasty performed through miniaturized incisions using so-called minimally invasive techniques. Most agree that these techniques carry with them a steep learning curve, and significant complications have been reported. Most also agree, though, that more rapid rehabilitation may be facilitated and that less invasive surgery has forced hip surgeons to refine and improve surgical technique. The critical lesson learned from this recent process is that any incision through which a total hip arthroplasty is performed should be large enough and at a suitable site to enable proper positioning of the components with a minimum of soft tissue and bony injury.

Implant Choice

The proper choice of implants requires a basic understanding of the various options available and their design features. Both cemented and cementless femoral and acetabular components are available. Multiple bearing surface options also exist and can significantly affect the longevity of the hip reconstruction.

Acetabulum. Although metal-backed cemented acetabular components with inner polyethylene liners have been used in the past, cemented acetabular components today consist of all-polyethylene designs of varying outer and inner diameters. The backside normally is textured to enhance fixation by promoting cement interdigitation and interlock. Although these components are generally less expensive, they have proven to have higher loosening rates than uncemented cups in most series. This is also probably owing in part to the technical demands of adequately cementing an acetabular component into a bleeding cancellous acetabular bed and the difficulty of achieving proper cement interdigitation into the bone.

Cementless acetabular components have become the implant of choice in most primary total hip arthroplasties for North American surgeons. They consist of a metal outer shell of varying diameter, which is textured on its bone-opposing surface with either sintered beads, plasma spray, fiber mesh, or tantalum to create pores of optimum size of 150 to 400 nm to promote bone ingrowth. The shape of this shell is either less than a hemisphere, hemispheric, or with a peripheral flare designed to increase the interference fit between the shell and the bone. Additional features of the metal shell include optional holes for screw fixation to bone, a locking mechanism for the inner liner, and the ability to accommodate multiple modular liners with varying offsets, lips, orientations, inner diameters, and materials, including in some cases metal, ceramic, and polyethylene. The versatility of these cups accommodates widespread application and has led to an outstanding clinical track record of excellent fixation.

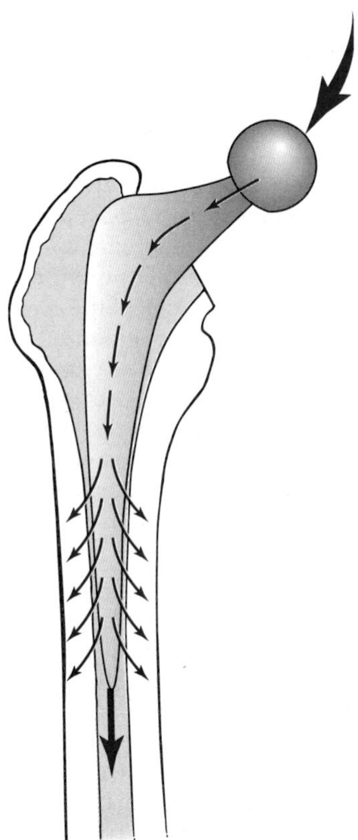

Figure 12-3 Force transmission in a composite beam cemented stem reconstruction.

Femur. Both cemented and uncemented femoral components of successful design can produce excellent long-term results when implanted with excellent surgical technique.

There are two disparate cemented femoral stem fixation philosophies, which have influenced their respective stem designs. Both philosophies rely on proper cement technique to achieve a strong bone/cement bond. This technique is based on an understanding of bone cement not as an adhesive, but rather as a grout requiring intrusion into and interdigitation within the cancellous bone of the inner femur. The composite beam philosophy and design strives also to achieve a perfect bond of the cement to the stem, by texturing, precoating with methacrylate monomer, or otherwise roughening the surface of the stem. This bonding of prosthesis to cement and cement to bone can lead to stress shielding of the proximal bone, with most of the load transmitted through the stiffer stem, bypassing the periprosthetic bone (Fig. 12-3). Debonding from the cement or the bone can occur, which signals loosening and can cause abrasive production of wear debris and subsequent osteolysis. In contrast, the taper-slip philosophy and design strives to engage a multitapered, polished, collarless stem into the cement mantle, exploiting the viscoelastic property of cement and its ability to creep. The stem never achieves a bond with the cement, but rather continues to engage the cement, often with a small amount of subsidence. The engaging taper generates hoop stresses that are transmitted radially to the surrounding bone, favorably loading the periprosthetic bone (Fig. 12-4). Although the success of some cemented stems from both philosophies has been outstanding, problems from the loosening of rough surface stems, leading to extensive periprosthetic bone osteolysis caused by the wear particles liberated by cement abrasion, dampened enthusiasm for cemented stems in North America. Nevertheless, the taper-slip philosophy with its potential for positive bone remodeling and its proven durability has gained popularity worldwide.

Cementless femoral stems, similar to cementless acetabular cups, rely on bone ingrowth into a textured surface to achieve durable fixation. There are a myriad of designs with variability of material, surface texture and length of coating, fixation concept (fit and fill versus taper fit), bone preparation recommendations (broached versus machined), modularity, and stiffness-reducing features such as coronal slots, and hollowed stems. Each design feature has potential distinguishing merit, but the clinical performance of many cementless stems of many designs has been outstanding. With bone ingrowth, however, comes stress shielding, to some degree, potential for thigh pain from modulus mismatch and micromotion concentration at the stem tip, intraoperative femoral fracture risk, and challenging revisions. Nevertheless, the straightforward implantation techniques, the potential for permanent biologic implant fixation, and reliability and predictability of cementless femoral stems have stimulated enthusiastic use for many patient demographic groups, particularly in the United States.

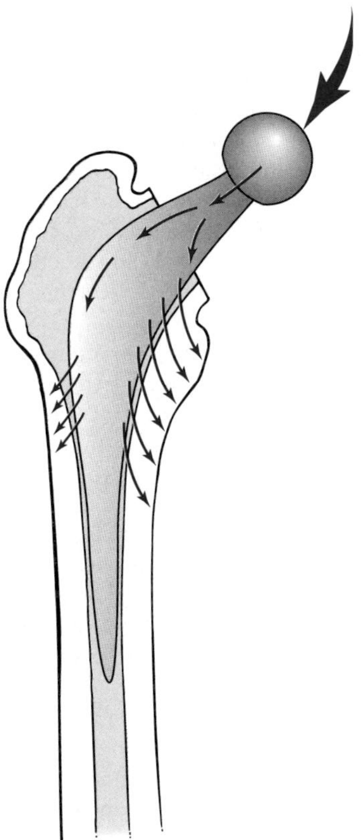

Figure 12-4 Force transmission in a taper slip cemented stem reconstruction.

Bearing Surface. The choice of bearing surface has taken on extraordinary importance in recent years owing to the pervasive problem of periprosthetic osteolysis resulting from polyethylene wear in metal head on conventional high-molecular-weight polyethylene bearing surfaces. Recently cross-linking of polyethylene, which provides dramatically improved wear properties in vitro and reduced oxidation potential, has been introduced. Early critical studies demonstrate reduced wear compared with conventional polyethylenes. The mechanical properties of these new polyethylenes are moderately reduced however. The very low wear rate, the opportunity to use large femoral head sizes, and improved materials have led to renewed interest in metal against metal and ceramic against ceramic. In contrast to polyethylene bearings, where boundary lubrication predominates and where increasing the head size increases the frictional torque and volumetric wear, with hard on hard bearing couples, larger-diameter heads favor fluid film lubrication and reduce the number of wear particles while imparting the associated benefits of improved stability and range of motion.

Both commonly used hard on hard bearing couples have some potential problems. Metal on metal couples are associated with increases in serum cobalt and chromium metal ion levels. The significance of increased ion levels is unclear, and to date no major clinical problems have been identified. Carcinogenesis or distant organ toxicity remain theoretical concerns. It is advisable to avoid the use of metal-on-metal implants in women of childbearing age, patients with significant kidney disease, and those with documented metal allergy. Ceramic-on-ceramic couples carry a risk of fracture despite material improvements that reduce this risk. Ceramics are also sensitive to impingement between the femoral head and the prosthetic liner; thus accurate implant positioning is especially important for these implants. A squeaking noise may occur in a few patients with ceramic-on-ceramic bearings.

Implant Choice Summary. In summary, the hip replacement surgeon has a vast array of implant options, most of which seem to provide at least very good short-term results. Nuances of differences, which may not emerge until long-term follow-up is available, may eventually help surgeons individualize implants to patients based on age, activity level, bone quality, expectations, longevity, and metabolic status. In the meantime, an understanding of the design principles of the various implants, along with their theoretical and proven risks and benefits must suffice to guide implant choice.

Surgical Technique

Acetabulum. Once the surgical exposure of choice has been performed, full 360-degree visualization of the acetabulum must be achieved. To facilitate this, the remaining acetabular labrum is removed along with the transverse acetabular ligament inferiorly. The fatty remnant of the pulvinar is resected to identify the fovea and thus the usual limit of medial reaming. In some cases a large medial osteophyte will need to be removed to reveal the pulvinar remnant. In addition, capsular resection or release, based on the preoperative deformities, may be necessary to enable adequate retraction of the femur for full acetabular exposure. Retractor placement is entirely dependent on surgical approach and should be individualized to maximize visualization.

Acetabular reaming commences with medialization to the appropriate depth, followed by reaming (in the intended orientation of the actual implant) to proper size. Reamer size is increased stepwise until subchondral bleeding bone is identified in a hemispheric shape, maintaining constant vigilance to central reaming and remaining wall thicknesses.

For cementless cups, underreaming by 1 to 2 mm ensures a strong interference press fit, which should be tested with an appropriately sized trial. Depending on the appearance of the prepared acetabulum, a cup size is chosen, with or without fixation holes. Cysts or defects are bone grafted with autogenous morcellized bone graft as necessary. The actual shell is impacted into place, with screw holes positioned superoposterior to avoid the neurovascular structures at risk in the anterior hemisphere of the acetabulum. Orientation of 10 to 30 degrees of anteversion and 40 to 50 degrees of abduction should be achieved by use of either a positioner guide or intra-articular landmarks. A useful pearl is to orient the inferiormost portion of the cup at the level of the teardrop and the posterior edge of the cup at the level of the ischium. Stability of the cup is tested with the inserter in place, and full seating is verified. Screws are placed, if desired. Overhanging osteophytes that can cause impingement and dislocation are removed, especially in the anterosuperior and posteroinferior quadrants. A trial liner can be placed for subsequent trial reduction.

For cemented cups, line-to-line reaming is usually recommended, as the many polyethylene cups provide for a cement mantle of 1 to 4 mm. Additional cement fixation holes are drilled into the ilium, ischium, and pubis. The acetabulum is irrigated of debris, which could compromise cement interdigitation into the cancellous bone. Cement is introduced in a doughy phase and pressurized. The cup is inserted, with meticulous attention to positioning. Excess cement is removed, and the cup is held in place until the cement is fully cured.

Femur. During the initial exposure of the hip, prior to femoral head resection, the position of the current center of rotation is identified and measured relative to other bony landmarks such as the lesser or greater trochanters. Additional aids to ensure limb-length equalization and to minimize excessive lengthening may be used at this point as well. The neck resection level and orientation is established based on preoperative templating. With the head resected, preparation of the canal commences. The Pyriformis Fossa, which is lateral and posterior, must be clearly identified. A box or round osteotome may be used to remove any retained superolateral femoral neck or any other obstructing portion of the trochanter preventing access to the Pyriformis Fossa. Vigilance is necessary to maintain a lateral position and avoid varus alignment of reamers, broaches, or actual implants.

Cement technique is critical to the success of any cemented stem. Indeed, it is useful to conceive of the femoral stem and the cement as two distinct implants that must optimally interact to achieve the best result. Therefore, the idiosyncrasies of each component must be understood. Cement itself is a grout, not an adhesive, requiring intrusion into and interdigitation with the dense cancellous bone on the endosteal surface. As it is introduced, it must be in a viscous enough phase to resist any back bleeding, which creates laminations and weakened areas in the cement, and to withstand pressurization without running out of the canal. Of course, the bony substrate must be prepared properly to accept the cement, occluding the medullary canal to enable pressurization and retaining the endosteal adjacent cancellous bony structure.

For cemented stems, the medullary canal may be opened with a canal finder but should not be reamed vigorously, which could remove the cancellous bone, burnish the endosteum, and significantly compromise the shear strength at the bone/cement interface by eliminating the cancellous structure into which cement must intrude for strength. Serial broaching establishes the size of the stem that achieves stable fixation. Calcar reaming is performed for a collared stem and may be performed for a collarless stem. Trial reduction should be performed with trial neck segments and trial heads of varying neck lengths. Range of motion, limb length, and soft tissue tension assessment should be carried out at this point, along with a careful evaluation of stability in the at-risk positions, determined by the surgical approach. Biomechanical parameters can be modified by choosing different cup liner options, such as lipped, face-changing, or extra-offset liners, or stem options including offset, neck length, and head size. Proper component orientation should be verified. A useful technique to ensure a combined cup and stem anteversion of 30 to 60 degrees is to rotate the fully extended femur until the transverse plane of the head matches the face of the acetabulum. The degree of femoral internal rotation establishes the combined anteversion angle. Limb length should also be assessed at this point, using the methodology of measuring the femoral center of rotation to a fixed anatomic landmark and comparing that with the value obtained prior to head resection as described above, or using any system or device that is reproducible for the individual surgeon.

Once the construct is satisfactory to the surgeon, the broach is removed. The canal is brushed and cleared of any loose cancellous bone. The endosteal bone covering the entrance to the lesser trochanter may be removed with a large curette without excavating the lesser trochanter to allow for cement interdigitation in that area. The canal diameter is sized for a cement restrictor, and this is placed 1 to 2 cm distal to the intended tip of the stem. The stem is assembled with any centralizers on the back table, avoiding contact of the surface of the stem with blood or other contaminants that may compromise the cement/implant interface. The canal is irrigated with pulsatile lavage and dried to provide the optimum interface for cement application. Cement is mixed, and once a doughy viscosity has been reached, is introduced in a retrograde fashion using a cement gun. Pressurization with a proximal canal occluder is held for a sustained period of time, depending on the behavior characteristics of the cement, but long enough to allow steady flow of the cement into the cancellous structure. Some advocate venting of the canal at this point to prevent the rare cardiovascular collapse reported in the literature, although most surgeons eliminate this step except in the most high risk individuals. Immediate insertion of the stem should follow release of pressurization to prevent any backflow of cement out of the interstices of the cancellous bone. Meticulous attention to alignment in the AP and medial-lateral (ML) dimensions and to proper anteversion of 10 to 20 degrees is critical. The stem, once fully seated, should be held firmly until the cement hardens, but excess cement should be removed prior to final curing. The technique for cementing a femoral stem is demanding, and each detail contributes to an ideal result.

The preparation of the canal for a cementless stem is much more idiosyncratic. The alignment issues and the methodology for lateralization and opening the medullary canal pertain to cementless stems, just as described above for cemented stems. For stems designed for fit and fill, a distal reaming process followed by a proximal reaming or broaching step establishes stable fixation. Alternatively, tapered stems may require only serial broaching, exploiting the richly vascularized cancellous bony structure, which can be compacted to support a stem in three-point fixation. Trial reduction is performed exactly as described for a cemented stem. The actual cementless stem is slightly larger than the broaches or trials; therefore, it should be inserted firmly but carefully, particularly as it begins to seat. One must resist the urge to pound harder on the implant as resistance is met. Rather, multiple lighter taps gently seat the implant while avoiding an intraoperative fracture. Circumferential inspection around the visible proximal femur is advisable.

If a fracture is identified, the prosthesis should be removed enough to effect complete reduction. Cerclage of the intertrochanteric and, if necessary, the subtrochanteric region can restore the integrity of the proximal femur and its ability to resist the hoop stresses imparted by the implant. The implant is reinserted and stability is verified.

Once the femoral implant is inserted, a final trial reduction may be performed. Minor adjustments in the neck length can correct any soft tissue laxity or tightness resulting from the final implant seating at a location slightly different from the broach or trial. Any areas of bony or soft tissue impingement should be relieved. The actual head is then impacted over the clean and dry neck. The hip is articulated, soft tissue or bony repair is completed, depending on the chosen surgical approach, and the fascia, subcutaneous tissues, and skin are closed in a routine fashion.

Postoperative Management

Rapid mobilization has become routine. Weight bearing is usually as tolerated, unless an intraoperative complication requiring protection has occurred. Walking assistive devices such as walker, crutches, or cane are recommended for support and to avoid falls. They may be gradually discontinued over 3 to 6 weeks, and sometimes even sooner. Although some controversy exists about the utility of instructing patients in dislocation precautions, conventional wisdom suggests that patients should be warned to avoid the at-risk positions, determined by the surgical approach.

Perioperative pain management is critical to rapid mobilization. There is a general shift away from parenteral narcotics because of their associated complications, especially sedation, confusion, and postoperative nausea and vomiting. A multimodal approach is preferred by many, including elements such as regional anesthetic and block techniques, preoperative and postoperative long-acting oral analgesics, intraoperative wound infiltration, and all supplemented with immediate-release narcotics and or intramuscular or subcutaneous narcotics for breakthrough pain.

Complications

Intraoperative Complications. Most but not all intraoperative complications or their sequelae can be eliminated by vigilance. Preoperative medical evaluation and clearance along with expert anesthesia will substantially reduce the risks associated with anesthesia. Careful surgical technique along with a thorough knowledge of the anatomy reduces risk of neurologic or vascular injury. Intraoperative fractures occurring during implant insertion should be identified and fixed as described in the technique section above. Infection is perhaps the most dreaded complication for both surgeon and patient alike. Antibiotics, usually from the first-generation cephalosporin family, administered preoperatively and continued for 24 hours postoperatively are the single most effective prophylaxis against infection. Additional interventions that may further reduce the incidence of infection include meticulous sterile technique, operating in a laminar flow environment or under ultraviolet lights, the use of body exhaust systems, Betadine-impregnated adhesive skin drapes, antibiotic irrigation, gentle handling of the soft tissues, and careful wound management.

Postoperative Complications. Early postoperative complications are uncommon, but can dramatically impair early rehabilitation and recovery; therefore, prophylaxis is appropriate. There is a risk of deep vein thrombosis following total hip arthroplasty. Pharmacologic prophylaxis using a low-molecular-weight heparin, pentasaccharide, or Coumadin is appropriate for most patients, and usually is continued for 10 days to 3 months, depending on the chosen agent and the individual patient risk factors. Mechanical adjuncts include pneumatic compression devices, compression stockings, and rapid mobilization. Rapid mobilization enhances return of pulmonary, bowel, and bladder function and reduces complications such as pneumonia, urinary tract infection, severe constipation, and skin breakdown. Additional aids such as urinary bladder catheterization, stool softeners, pulmonary toilet, and cushioned mattresses or pressure-point protectors can be helpful. Total hip arthroplasty can be associated with two to three units of blood loss from intraoperative and postoperative bleeding. Routine blood count monitoring should continue during hospitalization, and sometimes even after discharge, to avoid anemia-related complications. In addition, perioperative use of marrow stimulants such as Erythropoietin may minimize overall exposure to blood transfusions, and autologous predonation may reduce exposure to allogeneic blood.

Long-Term Complications. The risk of infection exists beyond the perioperative period. Any bacteremia can potentially cause infection in a prosthetic joint. Because nonsurgical treatment of infected prostheses is notoriously unsuccessful, and because the operative treatment is often associated with morbidity and even mortality, vigilant prophylaxis is mandated. Any systemic or distant infection should be treated aggressively. The choice of prophylaxis against bacteremia induced by other surgery should be guided by the organisms most likely present at the surgical site. Controversy exists regarding prophylaxis before routine dental care and other less invasive procedures such as endoscopy. Some would argue that the risk of antibiotic resistance and adverse reactions increases with prophylaxis, and therefore it should not be routine, at least after 2 years from surgery except in the immunocompromised host. However, it is the opinion of the author that the benefits of any reduction in the likelihood of infection following even these minor procedures more than outweigh the minimal risks of resistance or adverse reaction to antibiotic use, particularly in the elderly population in whom joint replacement is most common and who are more likely to be immunocompromised from chronic disease. The risk of dislocation reduces dramatically after 3 months; however, there is a lifelong cumulative risk. Wear-induced periprosthetic osteolysis is a significant long-term challenge. Modern bearing surfaces, which reduce particulate wear and its sequelae, should reduce the incidence of this periprosthetic osteolysis. Aseptic loosening is primarily related to the service life of the prosthesis. The cumulative risk of loosening increases over time, but even at 25 to 30 years of follow-up remains low at or about 1% per year total. Unfortunately, the only definite solution is surgical revision. Catastrophic failure of the implant itself is rare, because metallurgic modifications stimulated by fracture of early-generation prostheses have been implemented.

SUGGESTED READINGS

Arthritis Foundation Web site. http://www.arthritis.org/default.asp. Accessed December 2006.

Barrack R, Booth R, Lonner J, et al., eds. *Orthopaedic Knowledge Update: Hip & Knee Reconstruction* 3. Rosemont, IL: American Academy of Orthopaedic Surgeons; 2006.

Berry DJ, Von Knoch M, Schleck CD, et al. The cumulative long-term risk of dislocation after primary Charnley total hip arthroplasty. *J Bone Joint Surg Am*.2004;86-A:9–14.

Callaghan J, Rosenberg A, Rubash H. *The Adult Hip*. 2nd ed. Philadelphia: Lippincott Williams & Wilkins; 2007.

Dorr L. *Hip Arthroplasty*. Philadelphia: Saunders Elsevier; 2006.

Dunlop DJ, Masri BA, Greidanus NV, et al. Tapered stems in cemented primary total hip replacement. *Instr Course Lect*. 2002;51:81–91.

Geerts W, Pineo G, Heit J, et al. Prevention of venous thromboembolism. *Chest*. 2004;126:338S–400S.

Lieberman J, Berry D, eds. *Advanced Reconstruction Hip*. Rosemont, IL: American Academy of Orthopaedic Surgeons; 2005.

Mahomed NN, et al. Rates and outcomes of primary and revision total hip replacement in the United States medicare population. *J Bone Joint Surg Am*. 2003;85-A:27–32.

Morrey B, ed. *Joint Replacement Arthroplasty*. 3rd ed. Philadelphia: Churchill Livingstone; 2003.

Osteoarthritis of the hip: a compendium of evidence-based information and resources. http://www.aaos.org/Research/documents/oainfo_hip.asp. Accessed December 2006.

Phillips CB, Barrett JA, Losina E, et al. Incidence rates of dislocation, pulmonary embolism, and deep infection during the first six months after elective total hip replacement. *J Bone Joint Surg Am*. 2003;85-A:20–26.

Recommendations for the medical management of osteoarthritis of the hip and knee: 2000 update. American College of Rheumatology Subcommittee on Osteoarthritis Guidelines. *Arthritis Rheum*. 2000;43:1905–1915.

Sharkey PF, Parvizi J. Alternative bearing surfaces in total hip arthroplasty. *Instr Course Lect*. 2006;55:177–184.

Shen G. Femoral stem fixation. *J Bone Joint Surg*. 1998;80B:754–756.

Spitzer A. The cemented femoral stem: selecting the ideal patient. *Orthopedics*, 2005;28(suppl): s841–s848.

COMPLICATIONS OF TOTAL HIP ARTHROPLASTY: PREVENTION AND MANAGEMENT

VAISHNAV RAJGOPAL
DOUGLAS D. R. NAUDIE

Total hip arthroplasty (THA) is extremely successful for the restoration of function and relief of pain resulting from arthritic conditions of the hip. However, complications can and do occur after THA. This chapter reviews the major complications associated with THA, which include (but are not limited to) the following: infection, neurovascular injury, thromboembolism, instability, heterotopic ossification, leg-length discrepancy, component fracture or failure, and the possibility of systemic complications. Each of these complications will be reviewed and methods of prevention and management will be discussed.

INFECTION

Infection in the setting of THA has a major impact on patient satisfaction, morbidity, and mortality and places a large financial burden on the healthcare system. The incidence of infection after THA has remained relatively constant, 1% to 2%, for primary THA and 3% to 5% for revision THA. The development of a periprosthetic infection depends on the number and virulence of the bacteria, the status of the wound environment, and the host's ability to eliminate the bacteria. *Staphylococcus aureus* and *Staphylococcus epidermidis* account for >50% of the pathogens in patients with a THA infection; Gram-negative aerobic and facultative organisms for 11% of pathogens, and anaerobic bacteria 12% of pathogens. Pathogens that cause infection originate from the patient's skin (most frequent), blood, or the operating room environment. The wound environment is important and often suboptimal in patients who have advanced vascular disease, a history of multiple operative procedures, extensive scarring, or a history of wound infection. Increased risks of infection have been shown to occur in patients with rheumatoid or psoriatic arthritis, those on immunosuppressive medication, or those with diabetes mellitus, hemophilia, obesity, and malnourishment.

Classification

Periprosthetic infections around a THA are classified based on mode and timing of presentation (Table 13-1). *Acute postoperative infections* (type I) may be caused by wound colonization, infected hematomas, or superficial infections spreading to the periprosthetic space and usually present during the first postoperative month. *Late chronic infections* (type II) originate at the time of surgery, but owing to either a small inoculum or low virulence of the organisms, onset of presentation is often delayed to between 1 and 24 months. *Acute hematogenous infections* (type III) are the least common and characterized by deterioration in a previously well-functioning joint; these may be associated with a history of an acute illness or recent dental work. *Positive intraoperative cultures* (type IV) was added as a fourth type to include patients with two out of five positive intraoperative cultures without any other features of obvious infection.

Prevention

The factors that are important in the prevention of periprosthetic THA infection include proper identification of risk factors, surgical technique, and operating room environment. Prophylactic antibiotic use is the most important factor for reducing the incidence of deep periprosthetic

TABLE 13-1 CLASSIFICATION OF INFECTED TOTAL JOINT REPLACEMENTS

Type	Presentation	Treatment
I. Acute postoperative infection	Acute infection within first month	Attempt debridement and prosthetic retention
II. Late chronic infection	Chronic indolent infection presenting after first month	Prosthetic removal
III. Acute hematogenous infection	Acute onset of symptoms in a previously well-functioning total hip arthroplasty	Attempt debridement and prosthetic retention or prosthetic removal
IV. Positive intraoperative Culture	Two or more positive intraoperative cultures	Extended (6 weeks) organism-specific antibiotics

infection. The optimal time for its administration is just before the skin is incised, and current recommendations are that systemic antimicrobial prophylaxis be given 30 to 60 minutes before the skin incision is made. Prolonged procedures require an additional intraoperative dose of antibiotic. Other measures designed to reduce the incidence of infection include the use of body exhaust suits, laminar flow (vertical laminar airflow units generally reduce airborne contamination better than horizontal units), ultraviolet lights (which destroy airborne bacteria), proper sterilization of instruments, careful preparation of the operative site, the use of double gloves, and reduction of traffic flow in the operating room. Characteristics of the prosthesis have also been found to predispose a patient to infection: cobalt-chromium surfaces have been found to be more conducive to infection than titanium surfaces; porous surfaces have been found to be more conducive to infection than polished surfaces.

Postoperative urinary tract infections occur in approximately 7% to 14% of patients. No correlation has been found, however, between bacteria isolated from urine and those isolated from deep infections. Late hematogenous (type III) infections have been reported following dental, gynecologic, urologic, and gastroenterologic procedures. *Streptococcus viridans* is the predominant bacteria in the human oral flora but accounts for a low percentage of late infection around prosthetic joints. Dental procedure prophylaxis (associated with gingival hemorrhage) includes amoxicillin 2 g PO (or clindamycin 300 mg PO) administered 1 hour prior to procedure. The American Society of Colon and Rectal Surgeons and the American Society for Gastrointestinal Endoscopy do not recommend prophylactic antibiotics for colonoscopy, sigmoidoscopy, or endoscopy.

Diagnosis

Infection should be suspected in the presence of a warm, erythematous, swollen wound with persistent drainage, unremitting pain, and an irritable range of motion. Night or rest pain is also worrisome. Radiographic evidence of early failure should also raise concern for septic loosening. Investigations to rule out infection include erythrocyte sedimentation rate (ESR), C-reactive protein (CRP), aspiration, frozen section, and intraoperative cultures.

Management

Treatment options for an infected THA include suppressive antibiotics, irrigation and debridement with prosthetic retention, prosthetic exchange (one- or two-stage), resection arthroplasty, arthrodesis, and very rarely amputation. Management is ultimately dictated by timing of the diagnosis, medical presentation, and patient comorbidities. The goals of treatment are eradication of infection and restoration of function of the affected limb. Antibiotic therapy and operative debridement remain the mainstays of treatment. Cephalosporins are the most commonly used antibiotics in the setting of THA infection and have a broad spectrum of activity against the most common pathogens involved in THA infection. They also have low toxicity to patients and high soft tissue and bone concentrations. Since the late 1990s, however, several strains of resistant bacterial flora have emerged.

The presence of a foreign body (implant) makes the eradication of infection without operative debridement almost impossible. In addition, bacteria can adhere to the surface of a biomaterial and form a biofilm, or glycocalyx, that protects the bacteria from antibiotics and host defenses. Surgical debridement should include excision of all infected and necrotic tissue and the removal of cement, wires, cables, plates, screws, nonabsorbable sutures, and prostheses. Patients who present with an acute (type I or III) infection can be treated with surgical debridement, polyethylene liner exchange, and component retention (if well fixed) followed by intravenous antibiotics. The optimal treatment for patients with chronic infections (type II) is surgical debridement, removal of components, insertion of an antibiotic spacer, and administration of intravenous antibiotics under the direction of an infectious disease specialist (usually about 6 to 8 weeks). The use of a PROSTALAC (prosthesis of antibiotic-loaded acrylic cement) offers the advantages of better mobilization, control over limb-length discrepancy, and antibiotic delivery.

Reimplantation should be considered depending on wound healing, antibiotic effectiveness, soft tissue and bone quality, and potential for rehabilitation. Antibiotic suppression is reserved for those patients who are too sick or refuse surgery, when the organism is identifiable and sensitive to an appropriate oral antibiotic, the prosthesis is well fixed, and there are no signs of systemic sepsis. Long-term suppression is reported to have about a 30% success rate, with the outcome being retained implants. In select patients who may not be able to tolerate a second surgery, a one-stage exchange can be used with the advantages of a single hospitalization and avoidance of interim instability, disuse atrophy, and limb shortening. Two-stage exchange with the use of antibiotic-loaded cement has the lowest overall reinfection risk and a success rate approaching 90%. Resection arthroplasty is an uncommon salvage procedure for an infection around a THA and is most indicated for patients who are not candidates for staged reimplantation or who are unable to comply with postoperative rehabilitation protocols. Arthrodesis is recommended in young patients with unilateral hip infections. Disarticulation of the hip is performed only in the face of life-threatening infection, severe loss of soft tissue and bone stock, and vascular injury.

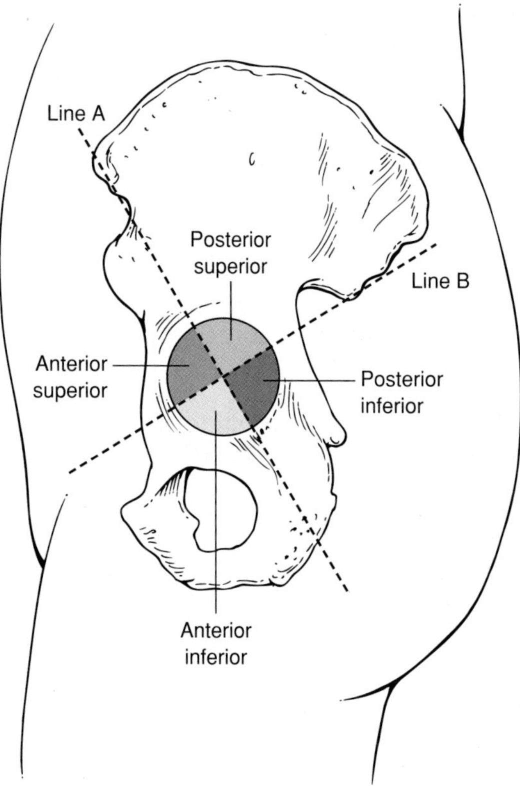

Figure 13-1 Diagram of the four acetabular quadrants created by two intersecting lines from the anterior and posterior superior iliac spines. (Reproduced with permission from Wasielewski RC, Cooperstein LA, Kruger MP, et al. Acetabular anatomy and the transacetabular fixation of screws in total hip arthroplasty. *J Bone Joint Surg Am.* 1990;2[4]:501–508.)

NEUROVASCULAR INJURY

Neurologic and vascular injuries are among the most distressing complications of THA for both patient and surgeon. The prevalence of nerve palsy after THA has been reported as between 0.6% and 3%; this incidence increases up to around 5% for revision THA or for THA done for congenital dysplasia. The sciatic, femoral, obturator, and gluteal nerves can be injured. The prevalence of vascular injury is extremely rare, ranging from 0.2% to 0.3%. Nonetheless, vascular injuries to the iliac, femoral, obturator, and gluteal arteries have been described. The proposed causes of nerve or vascular injury include direct trauma, traction or pressure from retractors, extremity positioning, excessive tensioning (often from lengthening the extremity), ischemia, thermal injury from cement, constriction by wire or suture, or dislocation of the components. The placement of acetabular screws into major intra-abdominal vascular cavities has also been reported with catastrophic results.

Prevention

A thorough knowledge of the neurovascular structures about the pelvis helps the surgeon to avoid injury to these vital structures. Extreme care must be undertaken during surgical dissection, retractor placement, insertion of acetabular screws, and the passing of cerclage wires. Preoperative angiography may be indicated for high-risk situations, such as those involving intrapelvic migration of a failed acetabular component or intrapelvic extravasation of cement. Anatomic studies have defined four acetabular quadrants created by the intersecting lines from the anterior and posterior iliac spines (Fig. 13-1). The posterior-superior quadrant has been shown to be the safest area for the placement of acetabular screws. Placement of screws in the anterior-superior or anterior-inferior quadrants should be avoided because of risk of vascular injury to the iliac vessels.

Management

In instances of significant intraoperative bleeding, the anesthetist and nursing staff should be immediately informed so as to have appropriate blood and instruments (vascular clips) available. All vascular injuries should be treated with prompt identification, application of pressure, proximal and distal control of the vessel, and hemostasis with direct repair, shunting, clipping, or ligation of the vessel. A vascular surgeon may be required for major vascular injuries. In instances of postoperative neurovascular compromise, a surgical exploration is warranted if there has been passage of cerclage wires around the femur, excessive lengthening of the extremity has occurred, or a large postoperative hematoma is diagnosed or suspected.

A knee immobilizer should be worn in patients with a femoral nerve injury to prevent knee buckling. Patients with sciatic or peroneal nerve injury should have the foot splinted postoperatively to prevent equinus deformity.

THROMBOEMBOLISM

Thromboembolism (TE) is the most common complication following THA and is the leading cause of postoperative morbidity. Abnormalities in coagulation that occur following THA can be related to the Virchow triad of venous stasis, endothelial damage, and hypercoagulable state. Venous stasis occurs as a result of leg positioning during the procedure, localized postoperative swelling, and postoperative immobility. Venous endothelial injury occurs with local dissection, thermal injury from cautery or bone cement, and during limb positioning for component insertion. Hypercoagulability results from the intraoperative stimulus of the clotting cascade and because blood loss can result in reduction in antithrombin III and inhibition of the fibrinolytic system. The presence of a factor V Leiden mutation (activated protein-C resistance), antiphospholipid antibody syndrome, protein C and S deficiency, and genetic abnormalities related to antithrombin III increase the risk of TE. Previous TE and active malignancy are the other most potent risk factors for postoperative TE. Use of hormone replacement or oral contraceptive therapy, pregnancy, advanced age, obesity, smoking, poor mobilization, and lengthy duration of surgery are less potent risk factors for TE.

Prophylaxis of TE disease

Without either mechanical or pharmacologic prophylaxis, asymptomatic deep vein thrombosis (DVT) will develop after 40% to 60% of THAs, proximal DVT will develop after 15% to 25% of THAs, and a fatal pulmonary embolism (PE) will develop after 1% to 3% of THAs. Prophylaxis of TE disease was recommended by the National Institutes of Health (NIH) consensus in 1986. The American College of Chest Physicians (ACCP) currently recommends the use of fractionated heparin, warfarin (target INR [international normalized ratio] 2.0 to 3.0), or fondaparinux (Table 13-2). This prophylaxis should occur even if the patient has been discharged. The ACCP also recommends that patients at high risk of TE (active malignancy, obesity, bilateral surgery) should receive extended prophylaxis for 28 to 35 days. The ACCP recommends against the use of acetylsalicylic acid (ASA), dextran, low-dose unfractionated heparin, graduated compression stockings, intermittent compression stockings, or venous foot pumps as the *only* method of prophylaxis. Under the influence of current prophylaxis, 85% to 90% of all DVTs following THA occur in the calf, and 17% to 23% of these distal thrombi extend to more proximal veins in the thigh. After 7 to 10 days of prophylaxis, the frequency of symptomatic TE within 80 days of surgery is between 2% and 3%, symptomatic nonfatal PE is 0.6%, and fatal PE is 0.06%.

Anesthetic Considerations

The use of regional anesthesia has been shown to reduce the occurrence of DVT by 40% to 50%. The proposed mechanism is probably related to a sympathetic blockade resulting in increased lower extremity blood flow mitigating the effects of stasis. The use of short-acting unfractionated heparin given intravenously following component insertion has also been found to significantly inhibit fibrin formation. Patients who receive autologous blood have demonstrated lower rates of DVT (9%) and PE (0.3%) compared with those patients who received banked blood (DVT of 13.5% and PE of 0.7%).

Pharmacologic Methods

Warfarin is the most commonly used agent for prophylaxis of TE disease following THA and exerts its anticoagulant effect by inhibiting the hepatic production of vitamin K–dependent clotting factors II, VII, IX, and X. Warfarin is administered orally but requires regular monitoring of the INR. Unfractionated heparin exerts its anticoagulant effect through a high binding affinity for antithrombin III, thereby accelerating the inhibition of thrombin, factor IX, and Xa. Fractionated low-molecular-weight heparins (LMWH) differ in their molecular weights and exert their anticoagulant effect through the inhibition of factor Xa. These offer several advantages over unfractionated heparin because they have better bioavailability, prolonged circulating half-life, and a lower frequency of development of thrombocytopenia. However, in 1997 the United States Food and Drug Administration (FDA) issued a public health advisory on the use of fractionated heparin with epidural or spinal anesthesia. This was owing to reports of epidural and spinal hematomas causing permanent neurologic injury following the use of neuraxial anesthesia and LMWH. Fondaparinux is a synthetic pentasaccharide that acts as a specific inhibitor of factor Xa with no direct inhibition of thrombin. Although an effective prophylactic agent, it causes an irreversible change to the binding site for factor Xa and has been associated with an increased risk of a major bleeding episode if

TABLE 13-2 ACCP GRADE 1A RECOMMENDATIONS FOR THROMBOEMBOLISM PROPHYLAXIS IN TOTAL HIP ARTHROPLASTY

Medication	Dosage	Duration
LMWH	12h before surgery, 12–24h after surgery or 4–6h after surgery at half usual dose followed by full high-risk dose next day	At least 10 days postop; 28–35 days for high-risk patients
Warfarin	Adjusted dose (INR target 2.0–3.0) started before surgery or evening of surgery	At least 10 days postop; 28–35 days for high-risk patients
Fondaparinux	2.5 mg started 6–8h after surgery	At least 10 days postop; 28–35 days for high-risk patients

ACCP, American College of Chest Physicians; LMWH, low-molecular-weight heparin; INR, international normalized ratio.

administered within 6 hours of surgery. Aspirin limits platelet aggregation by inhibiting thromboxane A2 and offers the advantages of low cost, ease of administration without monitoring, and few bleeding complications. However, the PEP (Pulmonary Embolism Prevention) trial found that aspirin did not reduce the risk of symptomatic DVT following THA, and therefore, it is not recommended as the only means of prophylaxis.

Mechanical Modalities

External pneumatic compression devices (EPCDs) increase venous return, decrease stasis, and enhance endothelial-derived fibrinolysis without bleeding risk. Calf and thigh sleeves have been associated with a reduction in distal calf DVT but a greater prevalence of high-risk proximal DVT after THA compared with warfarin. EPCDs alone have not been shown to be more effective than pharmacologic prophylaxis after THA but may offer an advantage when used in combination.

Diagnosis

Detection of TE may be clinically obvious or subtle. The presence of calf tenderness (the Homan sign), low-grade fever, fatigue, tachycardia, and diaphoresis may or may not be present. Patients with proximal DVT may have pain or swelling in their thigh. The classic presentation of PE, consisting of shortness of breath, pleuritic chest pain, mental status changes, tachycardia, and tachypnea, is rarely present. Ascending contrast venography is the most reliable and sensitive method for detection of asymptomatic and nonocclusive venous thrombi in the THA patient; however, this is expensive, invasive, and has been associated with complications including contrast-induced nephropathy, limb edema, and contrast allergy. Doppler ultrasound is a noninvasive technique that allows visualization of venous channels but is not sufficiently sensitive for routine postoperative surveillance of the THA patient. The ACCP guidelines recommend against the routine use of Doppler ultrasound screening at the time of hospital discharge in asymptomatic patients following THA. A chest radiograph in conjunction with an electrocardiogram and ventilation-perfusion (V/Q) scan can help in the diagnosis of PE; however, PE can be more accurately diagnosed with spiral CT, MR, or pulmonary angiography.

Management of Established TE Disease

Continuous intravenous heparin administration or high-dose fractioned LMWH followed by oral anticoagulation with warfarin for 3 months is recommended for isolated cases of proximal DVT and 6 months in cases of PE. Anticoagulation prevents further thrombus formation while allowing the fibrinolytic system to dissolve clots that have already formed. An inferior vena cava filter is reserved for circumstances where full anticoagulation is absolutely contraindicated or with recurrent PE despite therapeutic anticoagulation.

INSTABILITY

Dislocation is among the most frequent and distressing complications for a patient following THA. The incidence of dislocation after THA varies widely (0.3% to 9%) with most large series averaging 2% to 3% for primary THA. Many variables can predispose to dislocation, including disease and patient, surgical, and rehabilitation factors (Table 13-3).

Risk Factors

Many risk factors for THA dislocation have been identified; however, not all studies support all risk factors. Disease conditions such as developmental dysplasia of the hip, prior hip surgery, and nonhealed fracture and disease states such as rheumatoid arthritis and prior sepsis have been identified as risk factors for dislocation following THA. Gender has also been recognized to influence the likelihood of dislocation, with dislocation reported to occur twice as frequently in females as in males in some studies. Age was not found to be important as a risk factor for THA instability in many studies; however, two studies have shown that older patients have higher dislocation rates. Factors that may decrease the patient's ability to control the hip, such as alcoholism or

TABLE 13-3 RISK FACTORS CONSIDERED TO RELATE TO DISLOCATIONS AFTER TOTAL HIP ARTHROPLASTY

Disease Factors	Patient Factors	Surgical Factors	Rehabilitation Factors
Developmental dysplasia	Female gender	Posterior approach	Flexion/internal rotation
Fracture	Age	Excessive cup version or abduction	Extension/external rotation
Prior hip surgery	Alcohol abuse	Trochanteric avulsion	Time from surgery
Rheumatoid arthritis	Height	Femoral offset	Immobilization after surgery
Prior sepsis	Weight	Cup extended wall	
Bilaterality	Emotional stability	Surgeon experience	
Arc of motion		Head size	
		Leg-length discrepancy	

Adapted from Morrey BF. Difficult complications after hip joint replacement. *Clin Orthop*. 1997;344:179–187, with permission.

neuromuscular disease, also have been shown to increase dislocation rates.

The surgical approach has been shown to influence the rate of dislocation, with the lateral and anterolateral approaches showing lower dislocation rates than the posterior approach. More recently, however, enhanced soft tissue closure after posterior approach has shown significantly reduced dislocation rates. The orientation of the acetabular component has also been related to dislocation, with retroverted components predisposing to posterior dislocation and excessively anteverted components predisposing to anterior dislocation. Vertical orientation of the acetabular component (>55 degrees) has also been considered a risk factor for dislocation (Figs. 13-2 and 13-3). Femoral head size and the avoidance of re-enforcement at the base (a "skirt") have also been studied as possible factors in dislocation, and it is believed that enlarging the size of the femoral head and avoiding the use of a skirt improves hip stability. When head size is increased and skirts are avoided, the head-to-neck ratio is increased, the range of motion required for intra-articular impingement increases, and dislocation decreases. A similar benefit can be gained by decreasing the femoral neck diameter for a given head diameter or by using a neck trunnion with a narrow anterior-posterior profile. The use of acetabular outside diameters >62 mm have also been shown to have greater dislocation rates than when components <60 mm were used. Elevated rim and lipped liners have also been shown to improve stability, provided they are used to maximize restoration of femoral offset and avoid impingement. Finally, surgeon experience influences the dislocation rate, with less experienced surgeons having a higher dislocation rate than experienced surgeons.

A recent randomized, prospective controlled trial evaluated the role of postoperative functional restrictions on the prevalence of dislocation. This study found removal of commonly used restrictions (extremes of range of motion, abduction pillows, elevated toilet seats and chairs) did not increase the prevalence of dislocation, but conversely promoted lower costs and a higher level of patient satisfaction. The postoperative time frame of dislocation has also been shown to be important in predicting future dislocations. The greatest risk of dislocation occurs within the first 3 months after surgery. Dislocations that occur beyond 5 weeks have been shown to have a higher rate of recurrent dislocation than those in patients who had their initial dislocation within the first 5 weeks.

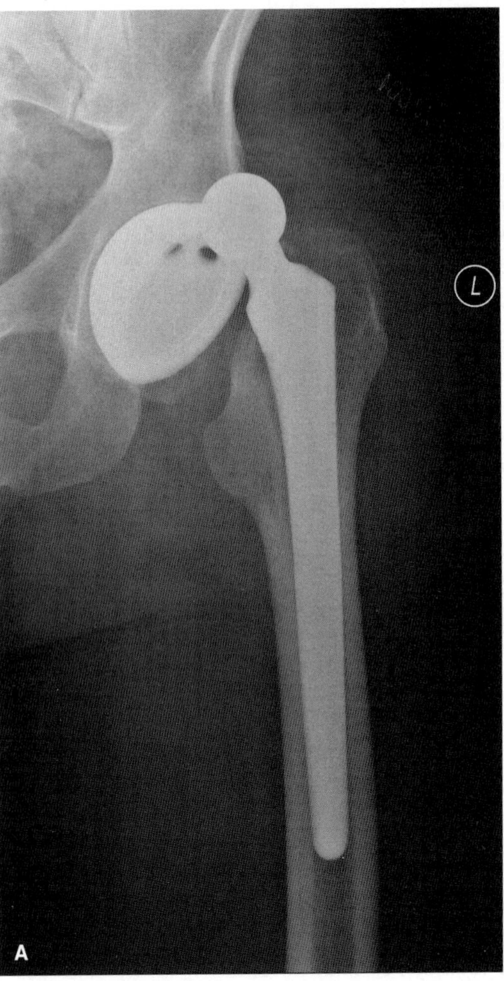

Figure 13-2 **A:** Anteroposterior radiograph of a dislocated total hip arthroplasty demonstrating a vertically positioned acetabular component and resultant hip dislocation. **B:** Anteroposterior radiograph of the same patient after revision total hip arthroplasty in which the cup was revised and repositioned and the femoral head was upsized to a 32-mm-diameter head.

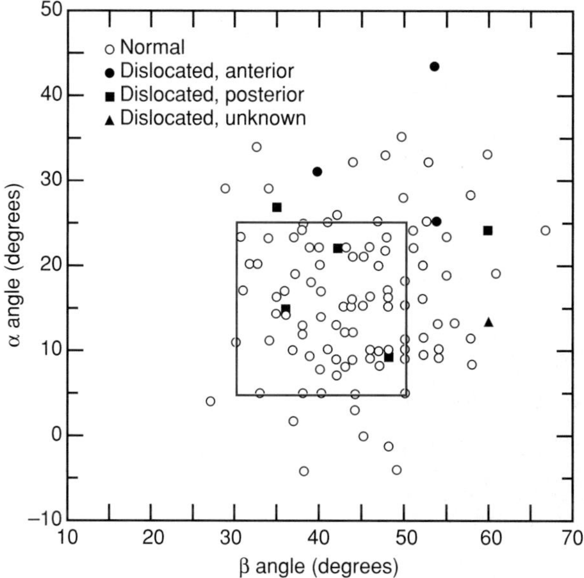

Figure 13-3 Schematic diagram illustrating the safe zone of 45 ± 10 degrees vertically and 15 ± 10 degrees of anteversion as the range of acetabular component position that will provide the highest stability. α angle represents cup anteversion; β angle represents cup abduction. (Reproduced with permission from Lewinnek GE, Lewis JL, Tarr R, et al. Dislocation after total hip-replacement arthroplasties. *J Bone Joint Surg Am*. 1978;60[2]:217–220.)

Classification

The direction of dislocation of a THA is usually posterior, with anterior dislocation being much less frequent. Dorr and associates have proposed a classification system based on increasing severity of the cause: Type I dislocations can be attributed to malposition of extremity, Type II dislocations are caused by soft-tissue imbalance, and Type III by component malposition.

Prevention and Management

The best prevention of instability following THA is to recognize all of the contributing factors that can lead to dislocation and avoid them. When a dislocated THA is encountered, the immediate treatment is closed reduction with either conscious sedation in the emergency department or general anesthesia in the operating room. The usual method of reduction is longitudinal traction with the hip in slight flexion. Care must be taken not to dislodge or dissemble a well-seated, modular component. Postreduction immobilization in the form of a brace and reinforcement of motion precautions can be used to avoid redislocation. For recurrent hip instability, the underlying cause of dislocation should be addressed (Fig. 13-3). Operative management should focus on correcting the cause of the dislocation, and surgical planning should include all possible revision options: modular liner and head exchange, trochanteric advancement, use of a constrained acetabular liner, or revision of one or both components. Patients should also be counseled regarding expectations as the results of revision surgery for recurrent instability are mixed.

HETEROTOPIC OSSIFICATION

Heterotopic ossification (HO) in the soft tissues surrounding the hip joint is a frequent complication of THA, with a reported incidence between 0.6% and 61.7%. The extent of HO may vary from slight to complete bony ankylosis (Fig. 13-4). The cause and pathogenesis of HO are not clear but are related to the duration of the surgical procedure and to the amount of soft tissue dissection. HO is associated with such conditions as ankylosing spondylitis, Forestier disease, posttraumatic arthritis, and in some males with considerable bilateral osteophytic osteoarthritis. Surgical approach may also increase the risk of HO after THA, with anterior and anterolateral approaches demonstrating an increase in the possibility of HO compared with the transtrochanteric and posterior approaches.

Classification

The most commonly used classification is that described by Brooker (Fig. 13-5): Grade 0 has no ossification, grade I represents one or two isolated areas of ossification each <1 cm in diameter, grade II represents more widespread isolated areas of ossification along the proximal femur or acetabular rim, grade III ossification covers more than half of the distance between the femur and pelvis but does not bridge the entire distance, and grade IV ossification bridges the entire distance between the femur and pelvis.

Prevention

The identification of patients at risk for HO should be a priority. Various treatment modalities have been developed to reduce the incidence of HO following THA. Low-dose radiation has been shown to help in the prevention of HO. Various radiation protocols have been described including a single preoperative or postoperative (800 cGy) dose. If irradiation is chosen for prophylaxis postoperatively, it is recommended that cementless porous implants should be adequately shielded or a cemented implant be used. Nonsteroidal anti-inflammatory drugs (NSAIDs) inhibit prostaglandin synthesis and may interfere with the inflammatory response and subsequent development of heterotopic bone. Indomethacin has been used successfully. Bisphosphonates have the ability to prevent mineralization of osteoid but have no inhibitory effect on the formation of osteoid matrix itself, and clinical trials have not shown a significant benefit in the prevention of HO formation from this treatment.

Diagnosis

HO is usually painless and rarely requires removal; however, some patients may develop local signs of inflammation such as erythema, effusion, tenderness, and loss of motion. Assessment of the extent and severity of HO is made on radiographic analysis. HO may become visible as early as 3 to 4 weeks postoperatively.

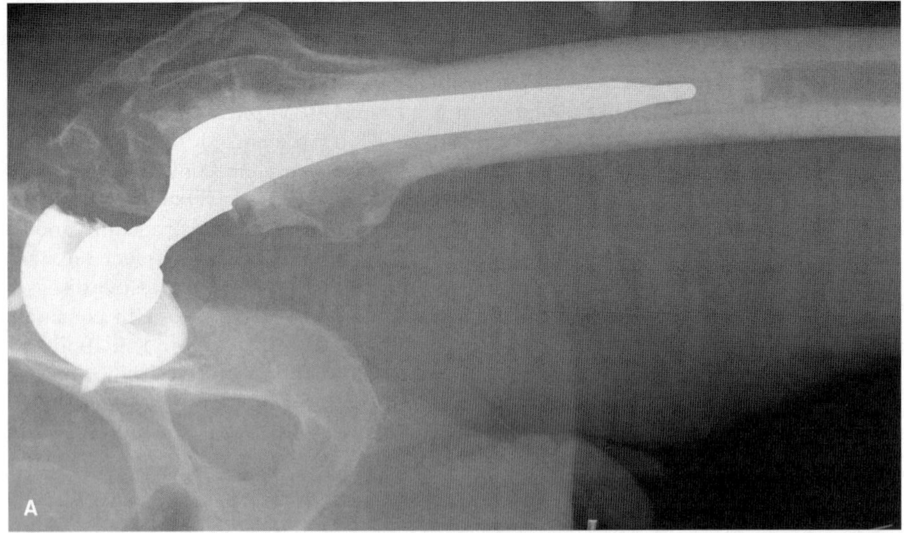

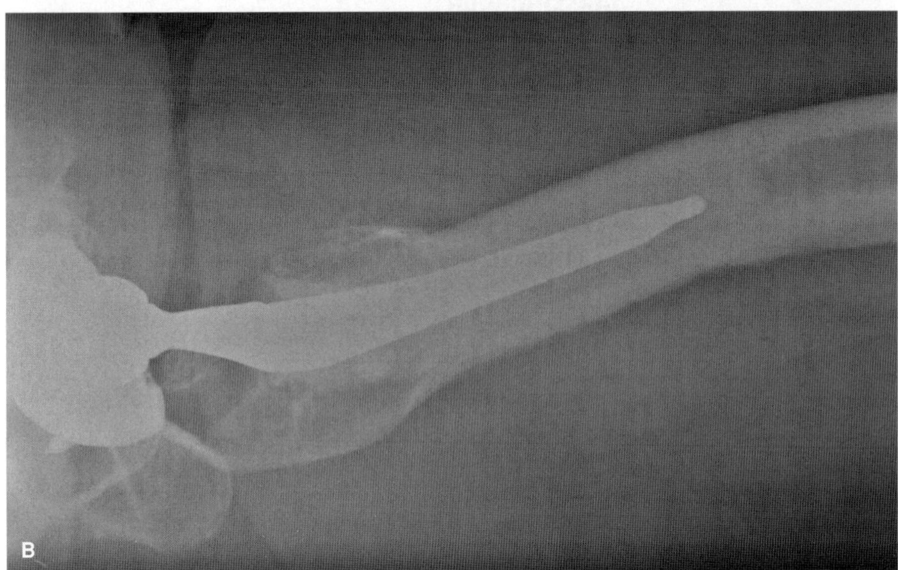

Figure 13-4 Anteroposterior (**A**) and lateral (**B**) radiographs of a patient several years after left total hip arthroplasty demonstrating severe heterotopic bone formation in the soft tissues adjacent to the left total hip arthroplasty.

Management of Established Heterotopic Ossification

Once HO becomes visible on radiographs, only surgical excision will eradicate it. If surgical excision is warranted because of limitation of motion, the procedure should be delayed until about 6 to 12 months after the index arthroplasty to permit maturation of the HO and the development of a fibrous capsule (which allows for more precise dissection of planes and reduces the amount of trauma to the surrounding tissues).

LEG-LENGTH DISCREPANCY

Limb-length discrepancy (LLD) is a potential complication following THA and can adversely affect an otherwise excellent outcome. Patient dissatisfaction from this complication is the most common cause of litigation against the orthopaedic community. The true prevalence of postoperative LLD is difficult to quantify because of marked variation in reporting methods and in the interpretation of its clinical significance.

Prevention

The frequency of LLD can be reduced by conducting careful preoperative templating from standardized radiographs and by taking intraoperative measurement of limb-length differences and offset with various measurement methods.

Management

When faced with a patient who has symptomatic postoperative LLD, it is important first to determine if the LLD is a true discrepancy or an apparent discrepancy secondary to a flexion or abduction contracture of the hip. In many cases, patients have a postoperative abduction contracture of the hip, which gives them a pelvic obliquity, resulting in an operated leg that seems too long. When these patients stand with the feet close together, the contralateral normal

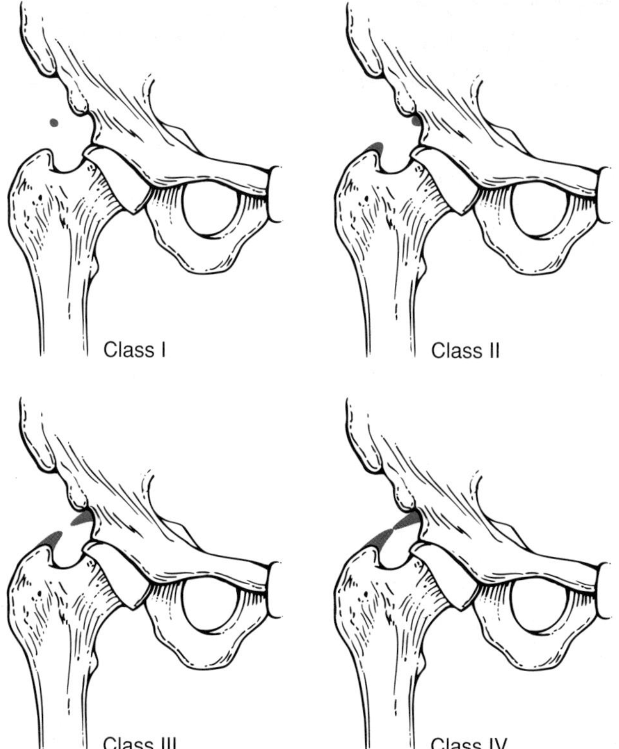

Figure 13-5 Schematic diagram outlining the Brooker classification of heterotopic bone formation around a total hip arthroplasty (Reproduced with permission from Brooker AF, Bowerman JW, Robinson RA, et al. Ectopic ossification following total hip replacement: incidence and a method of classification. *J Bone Joint Surg Am.* 1973;55:1629–1635.)

hip will be in an adducted position and will feel shorter than the leg on the operated side. These patients should be asked to stand with their feet widely separated so that both hips are equally abducted; in doing so the pelvis becomes level and the legs then seem equal in length. For these patients, an appropriate program of abductor muscle strengthening often is helpful.

When a true limb-length discrepancy exists because of overlengthening, it is important to determine the amount of true lengthening. This can be accomplished with the use of osseous landmarks or blocks under the foot. It is also important to discuss with the patient the reason for dissatisfaction and his or her expectations of treatment. Revision to correct a substantial postoperative LLD is seldom indicated because the procedure is fraught with the possibility of postoperative hip instability. As a result, although patient dissatisfaction may be great, surgery to correct true overlengthening is not frequently performed. LLD that is not associated with back or hip pain, sciatica, or recurrent dislocation should almost always be treated nonoperatively by placing a shoe lift on the short side. Revision arthroplasty is considered to be the last course of action in patients with ongoing symptoms of instability, gait dysfunction, and low back pain, and one recent study has reported success with revision for true overlengthening (although this was performed for less than one half of 1% of total hip surgery performed at their institution).

PERIPROSTHETIC FRACTURE

With the increasing number of THAs performed each year and an aging population, the rates of revision THA have been increasing. Revision THA can be undertaken for any reason, but commonly occurs as a result of periprosthetic fracture, wear, or osteolysis.

Periprosthetic Acetabular and Femoral Fractures

Periprosthetic fractures around the acetabular or femoral components of a THA are complications that a reconstructive surgeon must be able to manage. These fractures can occur intraoperatively or postoperatively. The incidence of intraoperative acetabular periprosthetic fracture has been reported to be <0.2%. The acetabulum can fracture from impaction forces incurred while employing a press-fit technique into an acetabulum that has been underreamed by 1 or 2 mm in relation to the acetabular component. Other contributing factors include osteopenia and Paget disease. Postoperative periprosthetic acetabular fractures usually occur as a result of bone loss from osteolysis but can also occur because of traumatic fracture.

Periprosthetic femoral fractures occur more frequently and can also occur intraoperatively or preoperatively. A review of the Mayo clinic joint registry demonstrated an intraoperative femoral periprosthetic fracture rate of 1% in primary THA and 7.8% in revision THA. These fractures are more common when the femoral component is inserted without cement at the time of primary THA. A similar increased prevalence of fracture with cementless femoral stems is seen in the revision setting. Revision THA with impaction grafting is associated with a higher incidence of intraoperative and postoperative fractures. Postoperative periprosthetic fractures of the femur occur in from 0.1% to 2.1%.

Classification

Callaghan described a classification system of intraoperative periprosthetic acetabular fractures that includes those occurring around the anterior wall, transverse, inferior lip, and posterior wall fractures. Peterson and Lewallen classified postoperative periprosthetic acetabular fractures into two types: Type I is a clinically and radiologically stable acetabular component, and type II is an unstable acetabular component. The Vancouver classification is the one most commonly used for periprosthetic femur fractures and considers three important factors: the site of the fracture, the stability of the implant, and the quality of the surrounding bone stock. For those that occur *intraoperatively*, type A fractures are proximal metaphyseal (not extending into the diaphysis), type B fractures are diaphyseal (not extending into the distal diaphysis and therefore not precluding diaphyseal long-stem fixation), and type C fractures are distal fractures extending beyond the longest extent of the longest revision stem and can include the distal metaphysis (Table 13-4). Each type is subclassified into subtype 1, representing a simple cortical perforation, subtype 2, representing a displaced linear crack, and subtype 3, representing a displaced, or unstable fracture.

TABLE 13-4 VANCOUVER CLASSIFICATION OF INTRAOPERATIVE AND POSTOPERATIVE FEMUR FRACTURES

Intraoperative Fracture	Subtypes	Postoperative Fracture	Subtypes
A. Proximal metaphyseal fractures not extending into the diaphysis	1. Simple cortical perforation 2. Undisplaced linear crack 3. Displaced or unstable fracture	A. Fractures around the trochanteric region	G. Around the greater trochanter L. Around the lesser trochanter
B. Diaphyseal fractures not extending into the distal diaphysis	1. Simple cortical perforation 2. Undisplaced linear crack 3. Displaced or unstable fracture	B. Fractures around or just distal to the femoral stem	1. Femoral implant well-fixed 2. Femoral implant loose but good bone stock 3. Femoral implant loose and poor bone stock
C. Distal fractures extending into the distal metaphysis	1. Simple cortical perforation 2. Undisplaced linear crack 3. Displaced or unstable fracture	C. Fractures distal to the femoral stem	

Adapted from Morrey BF. Difficult complications after hip joint replacement. *Clin Orthop*. 1997;344:179–187, with permission.

For those that occur *postoperatively*, type A fractures occur around the trochanteric region and can be subclassified into A_G (greater trochanter) and A_L (lesser trochanter). Type B fractures occur around or just distal to the femoral stem and can be subclassified into B_1 fractures in which the femoral implant is well fixed, into B_2 fractures in which the femoral implant is loose but bone stock is good, and into B_3 fractures in which the implant is loose and there is a severe loss of bone stock. Type C fractures occur distal to the stem and can be treated independently of the arthroplasty above (Fig. 13-6).

Prevention and Management

Intraoperative acetabular fractures should be assessed for stability. Stable fractures can be treated conservatively whereas unstable fractures require fixation and postoperative weight-bearing restrictions. Early postoperative acetabular fractures are treated according to their pattern. Patients with stable, minimally displaced acetabular fractures, in whom a cementless component has been augmented with screw fixation, can be treated conservatively with union expected in most cases. Late postoperative acetabular fractures are usually associated with significant osteolysis and often warrant operative intervention.

Intraoperative femoral fractures that are diagnosed at the time of surgery should be addressed at that time with simple bone grafting (type A_1), cerclage wiring (type A_2), or with the use of wires, cables, cortical strut grafts, trochanteric claw plates, and a diaphyseal-fitting stem (types A_3, B_1, B_2, and B_3). Diaphyseal fractures should be bypassed by at least two cortical diameters with a diaphyseal-fitting stem. If the fracture occurs distal to a well-impacted femoral stem (type C), the stem should be retained and the fracture should be treated with extramedullary strut and cable augmentation or formal open reduction and internal fixation. Intraoperative fractures that are identified in the immediate postoperative period should be evaluated fully with radiographs to determine extent. Most of these fractures are stable, minimally displaced, do not compromise the fixation of the prosthesis, and will unite successfully without complication.

Postoperative periprosthetic femoral fractures are treated using the Vancouver classification. Type A_G fractures are usually stable and can be treated with protected weight bearing and avoidance of abduction for 6 to 12 weeks. Internal fixation is considered if the greater trochanter has displaced >2.5 cm or if the patient has pain, instability, and abductor weakness. Type A_L fractures are rare, but if they involve a large portion of the calcar femorale, they may result in loss of implant stability and therefore revision THA is necessary. Type B_1 fractures should be treated with open reduction and internal fixation with or without cortical strut grafts. B_2 fractures are treated with revision to a longer femoral stem and fracture fixation with cerclage wires with or without cortical strut grafts. Patients with B_3 fractures often require structural allograft replacement of the proximal femur with an allograft-prosthetic-composite revision, tumor prosthesis, or a custom implant. Patients with type C fractures are treated with standard open reduction and internal fixation.

WEAR AND OSTEOLYSIS

Patients with polyethylene wear and pelvic osteolysis following total hip arthroplasty present a difficult problem because patients are usually asymptomatic and satisfied with the function of their existing hip replacement (Fig. 13-7). The problem becomes more difficult because there is a reported morbidity and risk of complications associated with surgical revision for polyethylene wear and osteolysis, and the long-term outcomes of surgical procedures done to address these problems are unknown.

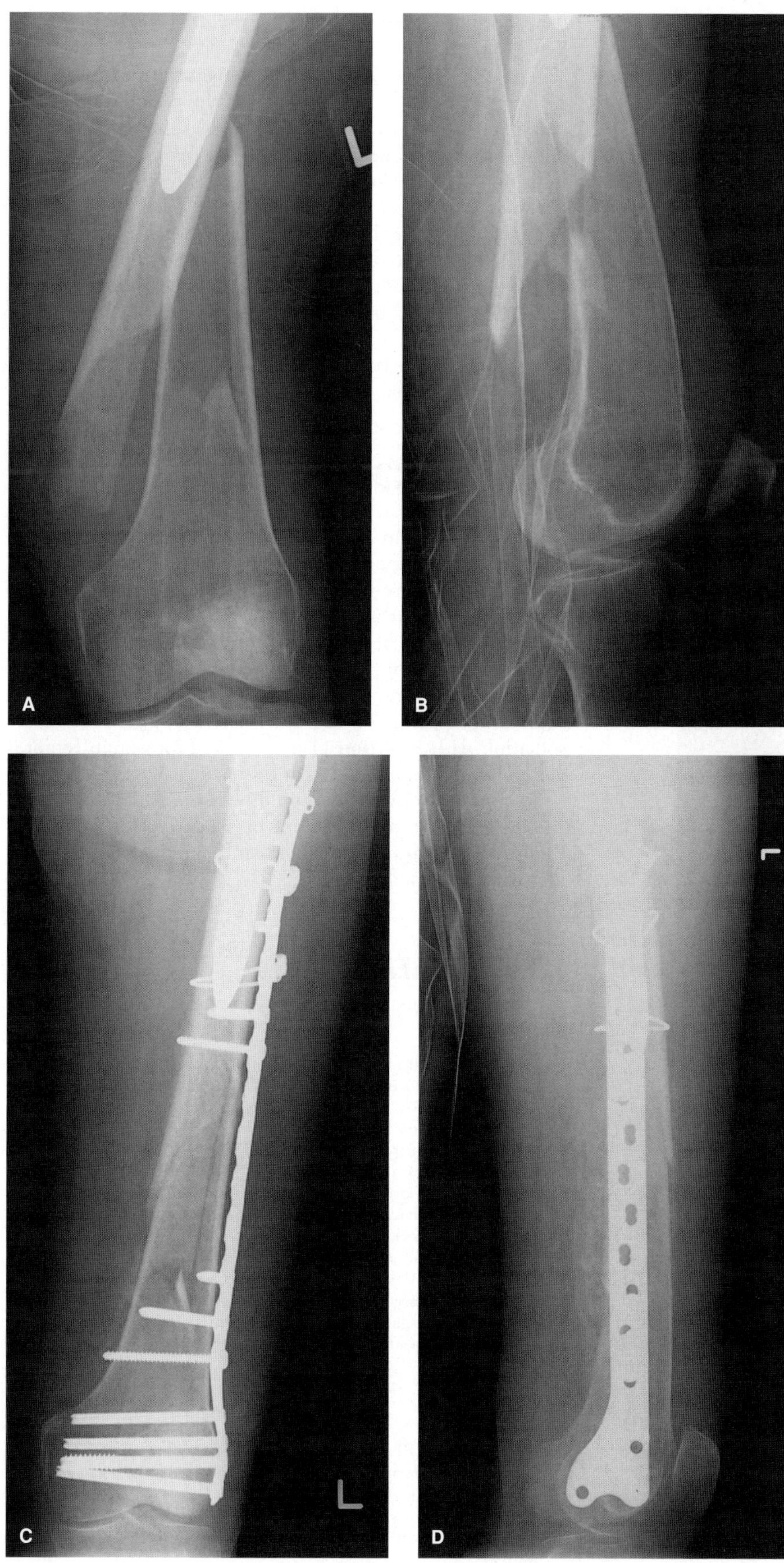

Figure 13-6 Anteroposterior (A) and lateral (B) radiographs of a patient with a Vancouver C periprosthetic fracture. Postoperative anteroposterior (C) and lateral (D) radiographs of the same patient following internal fixation with a locking condylar plate.

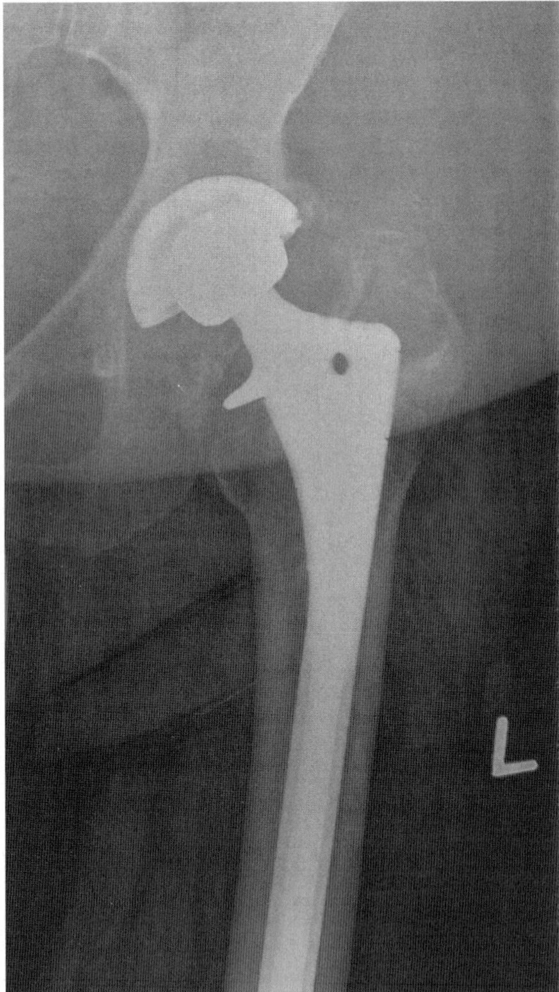

Figure 13-7 Anteroposterior radiograph of a 46-year-old woman demonstrating eccentric wear of the acetabular polyethylene component and severe periprosthetic osteolysis.

Prevention and Management

Although eccentric head position is an indication of wear, it is not by itself a reason for revision. Revision is indicated only when polyethylene wear is extensive and complete wear-through is imminent. For stable acetabular cups, exchange of the polyethylene liner is recommended. Even if the acetabular component and the locking mechanism have a bad track record with significantly increased revision rates, strong consideration should be given to cementing a polyethylene liner into the retained well-fixed shell. Revision of the acetabular shell is indicated if it is unstable or nonmodular, if hip stability cannot be achieved, or if the thickness of the replaced polyethylene liner is <6 mm thick. Modular femoral heads should be exchanged if possible when the stem is retained in a revision procedure as the degree of surface roughness of the femoral head may influence future wear and subsequent osteolysis. The rationale behind the surgical treatment of excessive wear is twofold: to prevent complete wear-through that could damage the inside of the metal shell, and to replace the debris-producing bearing surfaces with surfaces that wear less.

The decision to operate on a patient with extensive osteolysis is based on the likelihood of the patient developing complications related to the osteolysis (such as cup loosening) during his or her lifetime. An operation usually is indicated if the lesion is rapidly increasing in size or if the lesion is eroding away cortical support of the cup. Treatment is determined on a case-by-case basis; in general, revision is indicated in most but not all symptomatic patients and some but not all asymptomatic patients. Although some morbidity is associated with liner exchange (particularly instability), concern revolves around the bone loss associated with a full cup revision and uncertainty as to whether the revised cup will gain bone in-growth.

SYSTEMIC COMPLICATIONS

THA can result in morbidity related to pulmonary, cardiac, gastrointestinal, renal, or postoperative mental status changes. These are best prevented through careful preoperative assessment (often in conjunction with an internist and anesthesiologist) to identify any modifiable risk factors. Management of these problems involves addressing the system involved. Rarely, THA can result in mortality. Death from cardiac arrest during THA has been described in association with insertion of a cemented long-stem femoral component. When faced with this scenario, excessive pressurization of the cement should be avoided, consideration should be given to placement of a venting hole distal to the femoral isthmus, and invasive hemodynamic monitoring should be used.

SUGGESTED READINGS

Infection

Deacon JM, Pagliaro AJ, Zelicof SB, et al. Prophylactic use of antibiotics for procedures after total joint replacement. *J Bone Joint Surg*. 1996;78A:1755–1770.

Garvin KL, Hanssen AD. Infection after total hip arthroplasty: past, present, and future. *J Bone Joint Surg*. 1995;77A:1576–1588.

Hanssen AD, Osmon DR, Nelson CL. Prevention of deep periprosthetic joint infection. *J Bone Joint Surg*. 1996;78A:458–471.

Masterson EL, Masri BA, Duncan CP. Treatment of infection at the site of total hip replacement. *J Bone Joint Surg*. 1997;79A:1740–1749.

Salvati EA, Delle Valle AG, Masri BA, et al. The infected total hip arthroplasty. *Instr Course Lect*. 2003;52:223–245.

Spangehl MJ, Younger AS, Masri BA, et al. Diagnosis of infection following total hip arthroplasty. *J Bone Joint Surg*. 1997;79A:1578–1588.

Instability

Cobb TK, Morrey BF, Ilstrup DM. The elevated-rim acetabular liner in total hip arthroplasty: relationship to postoperative dislocation. *J Bone Joint Surg*. 1996;78A:80–86.

Lewinnek GE, Lewis JL, Tarr R, et al. Dislocation after total hip replacement arthroplasties. *J Bone Joint Surg Am*.1978 60(2):217–220.

Morrey BF. Difficult complications after hip joint replacement. *Clin Orthop*. 1997;344:179–187.

Paterno SA, Lachiewicz PF, Kelley SS. The influence of patient-related factors and the position of the acetabular component on the rate of dislocation after total hip replacement. *J Bone Joint Surg.* 1997;79A:1202–1210.

Peak EL, Parvizi J, Ciminiello M, et al. The role of patient restriction in reducing the prevalence of early dislocation following total hip arthroplasty. A randomized, prospective study. *J Bone Joint Surg.* 2005;87A:247–253.

Soong M, Rubash HE, Macaulay W. Dislocation after total hip arthroplasty. *J Am Acad Orthop Surg.* 2004;12:314–321.

Leg-Length Discrepancy

Konyves A, Bannister GC. The importance of leg length discrepancy after total hip arthroplasty. *J Bone Joint Surg Br.* 2005;87(2):155–157.

Maloney WJ, Keeney JA. Leg length discrepancy after total hip arthroplasty. *J Arthroplasty.* 2004;19:108–110.

Parvizi J, Sharkey PF, Bisset GA, et al. Surgical treatment of limb-length discrepancy following total hip arthroplasty. *J Bone Joint Surg.* 2003;85A:2310–2317.

Thromboembolic Disease

ACCP recommendations on antithrombotic and thrombolytic therapy. *Chest.* 2004;126(3 suppl):172S–696S.

Berry DJ. Venous thromboembolism after a total hip arthroplasty: prevention and treatment. *Instr Course Lect.* 2003;52:275–280.

Kearon C. Duration of venous thromboembolism prophylaxis after surgery. *Chest.* 2003;124:386–392.

Pellegrini VD, Clement D, Lush-Ehmann C, et al. Natural history of thromboembolic disease after total hip arthroplasty. *Clin Orthop.* 1996;333:27–40.

Heterotopic Ossification

Brooker AF, Bowerman JW, Robinson RA, et al. Ectopic ossification following total hip replacement: incidence and a method of classification. *J Bone Joint Surg Am.* 1973 55(8):1629–1635.

Fransen M, Neal B. Non-steroidal anti-inflammatory drugs for preventing heterotopic bone formation after hip arthroplasty (review). *Cochrane Database Syst Rev.* 2005;3:1–29.

Iorio R, Healy WL. Heterotopic ossification after hip and knee arthroplasty: risk factors, prevention, and treatment. *J Am Acad Orthop Surg.* 2002;10:409–416.

Neurovascular Injury

Barrack RL. Neurovascular injury. *J Arthroplasty.* 2004;4S1:104–107.

Pritchett JW. Nerve injury and limb lengthening after hip replacement: treatment by shortening. *Clin Orthop.* 2004;418:168–171.

Wasielewski RC, Cooperstein LA, Kruger MP, et al. Acetabular anatomy and transacetabular fixation of screws in total hip arthroplasty. *J Bone Joint Surg.* 1990;72A:502.

Periprosthetic Fracture

Della Valle CJ, Momberger NG, Paprosky WG. Periprosthetic fractures of the acetabulum associated with a total hip arthroplasty. *Instr Course Lect.* 2003;52:281–290.

Masri BA, Dominic Meek RM, Duncan CP. Periprosthetic fractures evaluation and treatment. *Clin Orthop.* 2004;420:80–95.

Mitchell PA, Greidanus NV, Masri BA, et al. The prevention of periprosthetic fractures of the femur during and after total hip arthroplasty. *Instr Course Lect.* 2003;52:301–308.

Systemic Complications

Patterson BM, Healey JH, Cornell CN, et al. Cardiac arrest during hip arthroplasty with a cemented long-stem component. *J Bone Joint Surg Am.* 1991;73(2):271–277.

Wear and Osteolysis

Engh CA Jr, Hopper RH, Engh CA Sr. Wear-through of a modular polyethylene liner: four case reports. *Clin Orthop.* 2001;383:175–182.

Jacobs JJ, Roebuck KA, Archibeck M, et al. Osteolysis: basic science. *Clin Orthop.* 2001;393:71–77.

Maloney WJ, Galante JO, Anderson M, et al. Fixation, polyethylene wear, and pelvic osteolysis in primary total hip replacement. *Clin Orthop Relat Res.* 1999;369:157–164.

Orishimo KF, Claus AM, Sychterz CJ, et al. Relationship between polyethylene wear and osteolysis in hips with a second-generation porous-coated cementless cup after seven years of follow-up. *J Bone Jt Surg Am.* 2003;85:1095–1099.

Terefenko KM, Sychterz CJ, Orishimo KF, et al. Polyethylene liner exchange for excessive wear and osteolysis: a report of 10 cases. *J Arthroplasty.* 2002;17:798–804.

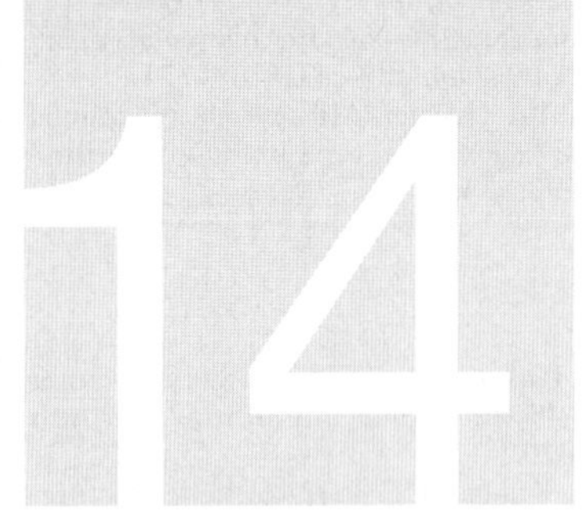

EVALUATION OF THE PAINFUL TOTAL HIP ARTHROPLASTY

CRAIG J. DELLA VALLE
KEVIN J. BOZIC

Total hip arthroplasty (THA) is among the most commonly performed and successful orthopaedic operations. In 2003 there were over 230,000 primary THAs performed in the United States alone, and in terms of quality-adjusted life years gained, THA is one of the most cost-effective health care interventions available. Despite the overwhelming success of THA for the treatment of end-stage hip disease, failures do occur, and the patient with a painful THA is one of the most difficult challenges for the orthopaedic surgeon to evaluate and treat. The purpose of this chapter is to review the workup and evaluation of the painful THA.

PATHOGENESIS

Etiology

The differential diagnosis of the painful THA is extensive (Table 14-1), and is most logically divided into causes that are intrinsic and extrinsic to the hip joint.

Intrinsic Causes of Pain

Infection should always be considered as a cause of pain because the treatment decisions rendered are fundamentally different if periprosthetic infection is identified. Mechanical loosening can occur early as a result of poor surgical technique or failure of osseointegration of a cementless implant, or it can occur late owing to failure of the cement mantle with a cemented implant. Stress fractures can be seen in the pubic rami (Fig. 14-1), are most commonly associated with female sex and osteopenia, typically occur within the first year postoperatively, and present with groin pain. Periprosthetic fractures, when not associated with obvious trauma, typically affect the greater trochanter in association with osteolysis or severe stress shielding. If a transtrochanteric approach was used for exposure, a nonunion of the greater trochanter can develop and cause pain. Osteolysis and polyethylene wear can cause pain secondary to the inflammatory response to wear debris. Occult instability or subluxation of the prosthetic hip is another potential cause of pain. Modulus of elasticity mismatch between a stiff implant (typically a large-diameter, cementless femoral stem) and the host bone can cause pain in the thigh. Trochanteric bursitis is a relatively common source of pain and has been associated with an anterolateral exposure to the hip and changes in femoral offset that occur at the time of surgery. Iliopsoas tendonitis presents as groin pain and has been associated with underanteverted, vertically oriented, and oversized acetabular components.

Extrinsic Causes of Pain

The most common cause of hip-related pain that is extrinsic to the hip joint is degenerative disease of the lumbar spine. Vascular claudication (particularly of the aortoiliac system) may also cause pain in the groin, buttock, or thigh that can be confused with pain directly related to the hip joint as can peripheral nerve dysfunction, hernias, and referred pain from intra-abdominal or genitourinary pathology. Less frequently seen causes of pain include metabolic bone disease and primary or metastatic bone cancers.

Epidemiology

Revision total hip arthroplasty accounted for approximately 15% of all total hip arthroplasties performed in 2003. With expanding indications for THA including younger and more active patients, an aging population and an ever-increasing total number of patients who have undergone THA in the past, even with improvements in surgical techniques and materials, the number of patients presenting with pain and failure following THA may rise in the future.

TABLE 14-1 DIFFERENTIAL DIAGNOSIS OF THE PAINFUL TOTAL HIP ARTHROPLASTY

Intrinsic causes

- Infection
- Mechanical loosening
  - Cemented
  - Cementless
- Stress fracture
- Periprosthetic fracture
- Nonunion
- Osteolysis
- Occult instability
- Tip of stem pain (modulus mismatch)
- Inflammatory bursitis, tendonitis (trochanteric, iliopsoas)

Extrinsic causes

- Lumbar spine disease
  - Stenosis (neurogenic claudication)
  - Disc herniation (radiculopathy)
  - Spondylolysis/spondylolisthesis
- Peripheral vascular disease
- Nerve injury/irritation (sciatic, femoral, meralgia paresthetica)
- Hernia (femoral, inguinal, obturator)
- Intra-abdominal or genitourinary pathology
- Metabolic disease (Paget disease, osteomalacia)
- Malignancy/metastases

DIAGNOSIS

A thorough history and physical examination can provide critical information that allows the evaluating surgeon to narrow the differential diagnosis and is the basis for a focused workup of the patient with a painful THA.

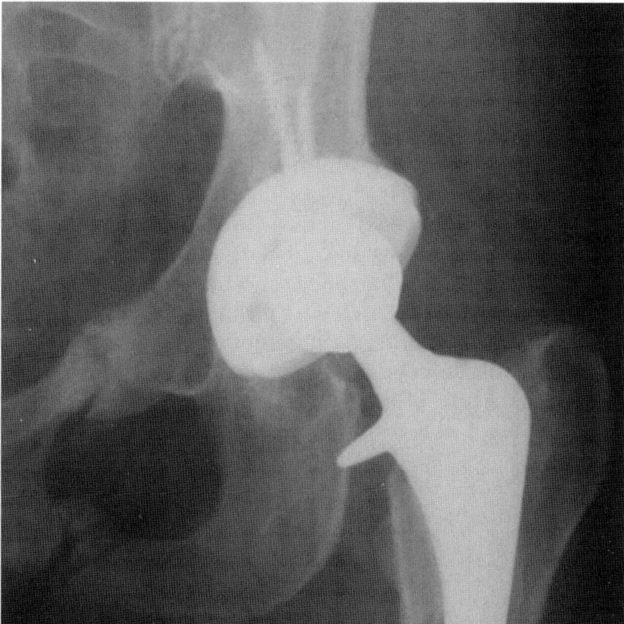

Figure 14-1 Healed stress fractures of the pubic rami that occurred subsequent to the THA.

The temporal onset, duration, severity, site, and character of the pain provide important clues in determining the cause of the painful THA. Persistent pain since surgery, without a painfree interval, is suggestive of infection (particularly if the pain experienced now is of a different nature than that prior to surgery), failure to obtain initial implant stability, or misdiagnosis of the original cause of the patient's pain when seeking total hip arthroplasty in the first place (particularly if the pain is unchanged when compared with preoperatively).

When interviewing patients with a painful THA, it is important to ask about any abnormal or persistent wound drainage that occurred after surgery and to determine if the patient was placed on antibiotics for an extended period of time or if he or she was returned to the operating room shortly after surgery as each of these factors should raise the suspicion for chronic infection. Acute pain following systemic illness, dental or gastrointestinal procedures, or a distant site of infection suggests the possibility of an acute hematogenous infection. Infection should also be considered more likely in patients with predisposing risk factors such as diabetes mellitus, inflammatory arthritis, immunocompromised states, renal failure, and skin disorders. Later onset of pain after a painfree interval suggests aseptic loosening, periprosthetic stress fracture, osteolysis, or late infection.

Activity-related pain that is severe but is improved by rest suggests loosening, fracture, and neurogenic or vascular claudication. Constant pain, pain at rest, or pain at night can be indicative of infection or malignancy. Pain that begins when a patient starts to walk after sitting or resting (often referred to as "start-up pain") has been associated with loosening, micromotion, iliopsoas tendonitis (particularly groin pain when rising out of bed or out of a car), or lumbar spine disease. The onset of pain after a traumatic fall may be caused by fracture or traumatic loosening. Patients with both lumbar spine and hip disease may find that their symptoms of neurogenic claudication worsen after successful THA, secondary to increased activity levels.

Pain localized to the groin or the deep buttock often is associated with acetabular component loosening. Buttock pain that radiates below the knee suggests a neurogenic cause, such as lumbar disc disease or spinal stenosis. Thigh pain has been linked to femoral component loosening or a modulus mismatch as previously described. Localized pain over the greater trochanter is indicative of trochanteric bursitis or nonunion.

Physical Examination

A thorough physical examination of the patient with a painful THA should include a comprehensive musculoskeletal examination focusing on the ipsilateral and contralateral hip, knee, and spine and starts with a patient who is dressed in a gown for examination. Inspection of the skin to look for scars and signs of infection, including warmth, erythema, fluctuance, wound drainage, or sinus tracts is helpful and surprisingly oftentimes overlooked. The surgeon also should look for obvious muscle wasting around the hip or in the lower extremity. The patient's gait should be observed for evidence of antalgia, limb-length discrepancy, muscle weakness, or a Trendelenburg gait. A Trendelenburg gait is indicative of abductor muscle weakness and is more common after the use of an anterolateral approach to the hip. True and apparent leg lengths should be measured using graduated blocks as patients with lumbar spine disease and/or fixed pelvic obliquity may present with notable differences between their true and apparent leg lengths.

A detailed neurovascular examination also should be done to rule out neurogenic and vascular causes of pain. Peripheral nerve injuries involving the sciatic or femoral nerve may result in distal muscle weakness such as a foot drop. Surgeons must be sure to establish the temporal relationship of the muscle weakness and limb-length inequality in relation to the time of surgery. Progressive limb shortening after THA documented on serial examinations suggests mechanical failure of fixation.

Palpation can be useful in the diagnosis of trochanteric bursitis, inguinal hernia, and stress fractures of the pelvic ring. Range of motion (ROM) should be assessed carefully to determine which (if any) positions reproduce the patient's pain. Pain with active ROM or at extremes of motion is indicative of loosening, whereas pain with passive ROM may indicate occult infection. Pain with passive straight leg raising should raise suspicion of sciatic nerve irritation. Pain or apprehension in certain reproducible positions, particularly at extremes of motion, is indicative of instability or impingement. Pain with resisted hip flexion and passive extension often is associated with iliopsoas tendonitis.

TABLE 14-2 DEFINITIONS OF RADIOGRAPHIC LOOSENING OF CEMENTED FEMORAL STEMS

Definite loosening

- Subsidence of the component
- Fracture of the stem
- Cement mantle fracture
- Radiolucent line between the stem and cement mantle not present on the immediate postoperative radiograph

Probable loosening

- Radiolucent line at the bone/cement interface that is either continuous or >2 mm wide at some point

Possible loosening

- Radiolucent line at the cement/bone interface between 50% and 100% of the total bone/cement interface

From Harris WH, McGann WA. Loosening of the femoral component after use of the medullary-plug cementing technique. Follow-up note with a minimum of five-year follow-up. *J Bone Joint Surg.* 1986;68A:1064–1066, with permission.

Radiographic Evaluation

Plain Radiographs

A thorough radiographic evaluation of the patient with painful THA begins with a critical review of serial plain radiographs that are of high enough quality to identify subtle changes and to evaluate for signs of loosening or migration of the prosthesis. Care should be taken to note differences in radiographic technique, including orientation, penetration, and rotation.

The most widely accepted criteria for radiographic loosening of cemented femoral stems have been proposed by Harris and McGann. This classification includes criteria for definite, probable and possible loosening (Table 14-2). Major signs of osseointegration of a cementless femoral component were identified by Engh et al. and include the absence of reactive, radiodense lines around the porous-coated portion of the implant and presence of endosteal spot-welds. Minor signs of osseointegration include calcar atrophy, a stable distal stem, and the absence of a pedestal. Major signs of failure of osseointegration are extensive reactive lines around the porous-surfaced portion of the implant, whereas the absence of endosteal spot-welds is considered a minor sign of failed osseointegration.

Similar to cemented femoral components, the stability of a cemented acetabular component has been divided into definite loosening (migration of >5 mm or a fracture of the cement mantle), probable loosening (100% radiolucent line at the bone/cement interface) and possible loosening (radiolucent line of 50% to 99% at the bone/cement interface). Criteria for loosening of a cementless acetabular component include migration (of >5 mm), the presence of broken screws (if present), and a complete radiolucent line around the component. Udomkiat et al. reported radiolucent lines that progressed after 2 years postoperatively, radiolucent lines of ≥ 1 mm in thickness that appeared after the second postoperative year, and a radiolucent line of >2 mm in any zone were particularly useful predictors of cementless acetabular component loosening.

Although plain radiographs are not very sensitive for the evaluation of infection, certain radiographic findings are highly indicative of infection including periosteal new bone formation and endosteal scalloping. Component loosening that occurs within the first 5 years in an otherwise well-performed THA is particularly suggestive of infection.

Aspiration and Arthrography

Preoperative aspiration of the hip, with fluoroscopic guidance, to diagnose infection should be performed on a selective basis as this test has been associated with a high rate of false-positives and is time consuming, expensive, and uncomfortable for the patient. It is typically recommended when the clinical suspicion for infection is high (based on the history or presence of risk factors), when the erythrocyte sedimentation rate (ESR) and/or C-reactive protein (CRP) are elevated, or when failure occurs <5 years postoperatively. When fluid is obtained, specimens should be sent for aerobic, anaerobic, acid-fast bacilli and fungal cultures as well as a cell count with differential. The precise cutoff for identifying infection with a cell count is controversial; however, the use of >50,000 white blood cells (WBC) as would be applicable to a native hip is associated with a high rate of false-negatives. At our own centers, >3,000 WBC has been found to be highly suggestive of infection, and similar values have been identified for evaluating infection at the site of a total knee arthroplasty; we typically use cell counts intraoperatively as an adjunct to or instead of an intraoperative frozen section as a screening tool for infection. Similarly, the cutoff value for the differential is somewhat unclear, with different authors suggesting values of between 65% and 90% neutrophils. In contrast to an aspiration for identifying infection, aspiration arthrography of the hip to delineate component loosening has been found to have a low sensitivity and specificity, especially for uncemented implants, and has been abandoned at most centers.

Anesthetic Injection

Local anesthetic injections can be useful in localizing the origin of pain in a patient with a painful THA and provide information as to whether the source of pain is intracapsular or extracapsular. Braunstein et al. reported that 10 of 11 patients with an identifiable intracapsular cause for pain obtained complete relief of pain within 20 minutes of an intraarticular bupivacaine injection. If a patient does not experience relief of symptoms after intra-articular injection, extra-articular sources of pain should be sought. Similarly, if a patient is suspected of having pain derived from the lumbosacral spine, relief from a local anesthetic injection at this site can assist in ruling out pain arising from a THA.

Nuclear Medicine Studies

Nuclear medicine studies occasionally may be helpful in evaluating the patient with a painful THA in whom the history, physical examination, and plain radiographic studies are unclear and revision surgery is not otherwise indicated (Fig. 14-2). Although a highly sensitive indicator of bone turnover and activity, this technique has a low specificity and the results are generally not considered accurate within 2 years of prosthetic implantation. Increased uptake on ^{99}Tc MDP can be seen with various conditions, including loosening, infection, heterotopic bone formation, stress fractures, modulus mismatch, tumors, metabolic bone disease, and reflex sympathetic dystrophy. Lieberman et al., in a series of 54 hips that subsequently were revised, reported that bone scans were not more helpful than serial radiographs in determining component stability; the authors recommended a bone scan only if plain radiographic studies are inconclusive.

Gallium citrate (^{67}Ga), which preferentially is taken up by leukocytes, has been used in combination with technetium bone scans to differentiate between septic and aseptic loosening. Both sensitivity and accuracy have been reported as poor, however, and this testing modality has been abandoned in most centers.

The use of indium-111–labeled leukocyte scans to identify deep infection also has yielded disappointing results that have been reported to be only slightly better than with gallium citrate scans. Scher et al. studied 143 hips and knees that had a reoperation for a painful or loose total joint arthroplasty or a prior resection arthroplasty. The positive predictive value only was 54%; however, the negative predictive value was 95%, suggesting that a negative scan is useful in predicting the absence of infection in a patient who is being evaluated for a painful total joint arthroplasty. The addition of technetium-99m–labeled sulfur colloid marrow scanning has been used at some centers in an attempt to decrease the high rate of false-positive indium scans secondary to physiologic marrow packing that can cause an accumulation, slowing, or retardation of flow of (indium-labeled) leukocytes around a prosthesis. The method provides some improvements; however, sensitivity has remained low and thus all of these tests are used only as a second line of investigation when the results of other testing modalities are unclear.

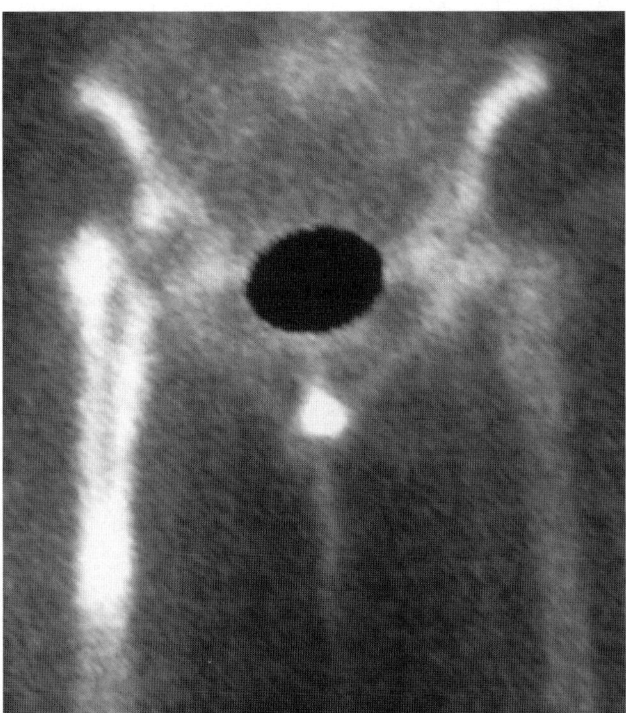

Figure 14-2 Three-phase bone scan showing diffuse uptake around the femoral component indicative of loosening.

Computed Tomography

Computed tomography (CT) has been described as a useful adjunct, when used selectively, for evaluating the painful THA. Specific software packages are required to compensate for artifact generated by metallic prosthesis, and a preprocedure direct consultation with a radiologist is recommended to optimize the result. Its greatest utility seems to be in identifying and quantifying periprosthetic osteolysis and for evaluating component positioning that may be contributing to instability; it can also be useful for identifying iliopsoas tendonitis (Fig. 14-3).

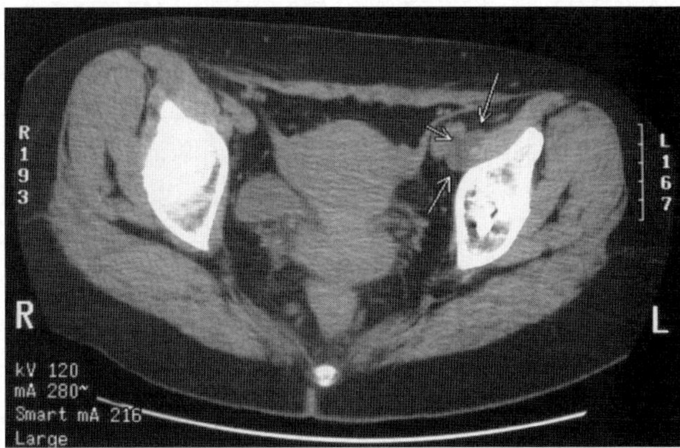

Figure 14-3 CT scan of the pelvis showing enlarged iliopsoas tendon (*arrows*).

Magnetic Resonance Imaging

Magnetic resonance imaging (MRI) is another potentially useful tool for evaluating the painful THA; however, the input of a radiologist is imperative to ensure that appropriate pulse sequences and software are used to decrease metallic artifact. MRI has been found to be useful in evaluating the soft tissues to identify iliopsoas tendonitis, incompetence of the hip capsule, and damage to the abductor musculature; for identifying and quantitating osteolysis; and for evaluating the adjacent neurovascular structures; it has also been suggested as a potential way to evaluate for infection and component loosening or fracture.

Laboratory Tests

An erythrocyte sedimentation rate (ESR) and C-reactive protein (CRP) should be obtained from any patient being evaluated for a painful THA. If these values are elevated, deep periprosthetic infection must be suspected and additional evaluation with preoperative or intraoperative testing (e.g., intraoperative frozen section or intraoperative cell count) should be done. In one series of 202 revision THAs, all patients with a deep infection had an elevated ESR (>30 mm/hour) or CRP (>1 mg/dL). In this series, the combination of a normal ESR and CRP reliably predicted the absence of infection (100% specificity). It is important to

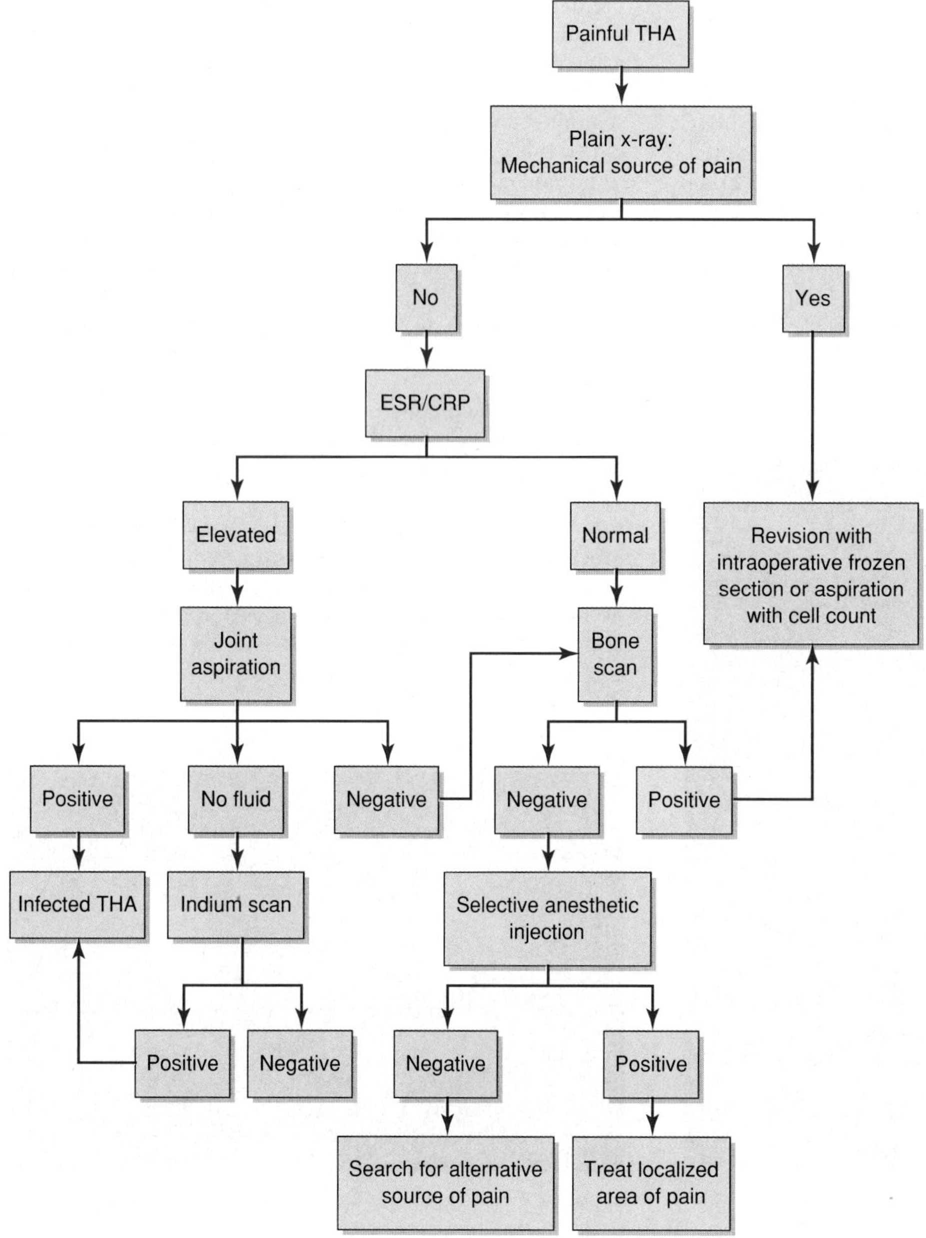

Figure 14-4 Algorithm for evaluation of the painful total hip arthroplasty. ESR/CRP, erythrocyte sedimentation rate/C-reactive protein.

recognize, however, that the ESR and CRP are nonspecific markers of inflammation and may be elevated by chronic inflammatory conditions (such as rheumatoid arthritis), recent surgical intervention, or systemic illness. The ESR, although usually normal by 6 months postoperatively, may be elevated for as much as 1 year after uncomplicated THA.

Diagnostic Workup Algorithm

Evaluation of the patient with a painful THA is a complex task that requires diligence and patience on the part of the surgeon and the patient (Fig. 14-4). After a thorough history and physical examination, a focused and careful radiographic and laboratory workup can be done at a reasonable cost and with a high degree of accuracy.

TREATMENT

Surgical Indications/Contraindications

When considering revision surgery for the patient with a painful THA, a clear diagnosis of the condition that is responsible for the patient's symptoms must be sought prior to further operative intervention as the risks of revision THA can be substantial; also, repeat surgery without a clear diagnosis of a condition that can be remedied by surgical intervention may be met with a high rate of persistent pain and an unsatisfied patient. Patients must be clearly counseled on the cause of their problem, the treatment options, and the risks of operative intervention. Nonoperative measures and observation are the mainstays of treatment until a definitive and treatable diagnosis can be confirmed.

Definite indications for revision surgery in the patient who is a reasonable risk medically for elective operative intervention include chronic infection and loose implants. Patients with a diagnosis of infection should be revised to prevent both worsening of infection and the associated bone loss that can ensue if treated nonoperatively. Similarly, patients with loose implants may sustain periprosthetic bone loss if the problem is neglected, which in turn can lead to greater operative complexity, a higher risk of complications and a poorer clinical result when revision surgery finally is performed. Further details regarding revision of surgical technique, results, and postoperative management are covered in Chapter 15.

SUGGESTED READINGS

Barrack RL, Harris WH. The value of aspiration of the hip joint before revision total hip arthroplasty. *J Bone Joint Surg*. 1993;75A:66–76.

Bohl W, Steffee A. Lumbar spinal stenosis: a cause of continued pain and disability in patients after total hip arthroplasty. *Spine*. 1979:4:168–173.

Bourne RB, Rorabeck CH, Ghazal ME, et al. Pain in the thigh following total hip replacement with a porous-coated anatomic prosthesis for osteoarthrosis. *J Bone Joint Surg*. 1994;76A:1464–1470.

Braunstein EM, Cardinal E, Buckwalter KA, et al. Bupivacaine arthrography of the post-arthroplasty hip. *Skeletal Radiol*. 1995;24:519–521.

Della Valle CJ, Zuckerman JD, DiCesare PE. Periprosthetic sepsis. *Clin Orthop*. 2004;420:26–31.

Engh CA, Massin P, Suthers KE. Roentgenographic assessment of the biologic fixation of porous-surfaced femoral components. *Clin Orthop*. 1990;257:107–128.

Harris WH, McGann WA. Loosening of the femoral component after use of the medullary-plug cementing technique. Follow-up note with a minimum of five-year follow-up. *J Bone Joint Surgery*. 1986;68A:1064–1066.

Lieberman JR, Huo MH, Schneider R, et al. Are technetium bone scans necessary? *J Bone Joint Surg*. 1993;75B:475–478.

O'Neill D, Harris WH. Failed total hip replacement: Assessment by plain radiographs, arthrograms, and aspiration of the hip joint. *J Bone Joint Surg*. 1984;66A:540–546.

Potter HG, Nestor BJ, Sofka CM, Ho, et al. Magnetic resonance imaging after total hip arthroplasty: evaluation of periprosthetic soft tissue. *J Bone Joint Surg*. 2004;86A:1947–1954.

Scher DM, Pak K, Lonner JL, et al. The predictive value of indium-111 leukocyte scans in the diagnosis of infected total hip, knee, or resection arthroplasties. *J Arthroplasty*. 2000;15:295–300.

Spangehl MJ, Masri BA, O'Connell JX, et al. Prospective analysis of preoperative and intraoperative investigations for the diagnosis of infection at the sites of two hundred and two revision total hip arthroplasties. *J Bone Joint Surg*. 1999;81A:672–683.

Udomkiat P, Wan Z, Dorr LD. Comparison of preoperative radiographs and intraoperative findings of fixation of hemispheric porous-coated sockets. *J Bone Joint Surg*. 2001;83:1865–1875.

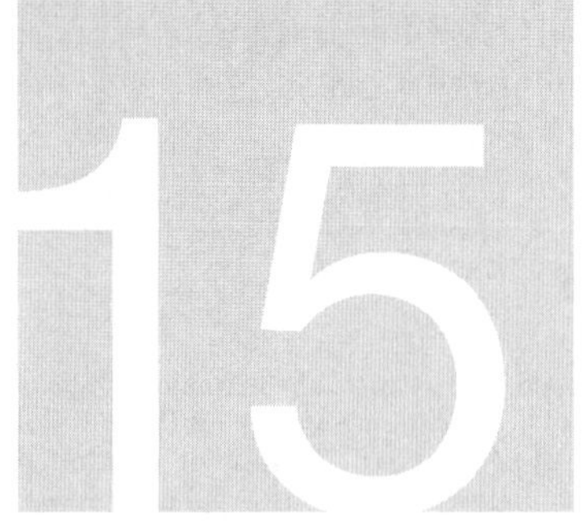

REVISION TOTAL HIP ARTHROPLASTY

JAVAD PARVIZI
KANG-IL KIM

Currently over 20,000 revision hip arthroplasties are performed in North America per year. Longer life expectancy, implantation of prosthetic hips in younger and active patients, and the increase in the number of patients with hip arthroplasty in place for decades are some of the reasons for the rise in the incidence of revision THA. Hip arthroplasty may fail and necessitate revision for many reasons (Table 15-1). The goal of revision THA, as for primary surgery, is to relieve the patients' symptoms and restore function. The main challenge of revision surgery, however, is to accomplish these objectives in the setting of compromised bone stock, poor soft tissue, and the possible presence of infection. Hence, both planning and execution of revision hip arthroplasty can be very different and in many occasions much more difficult than primary arthroplasty. Extensile surgical approaches, more sophisticated prosthetic devices, and more restricted postoperative protocols are common in revision arthroplasty. Because of the above noted challenges, the outcome of revision arthroplasty in terms of improvement in function (as measured by validated instruments), complication rate, and longevity of the prosthesis are inferior compared with primary THA.

MANAGEMENT OF FAILED HIP ARTHROPLASTY

Pain is usually the main symptom of patients presenting with failed hip arthroplasty. Other modes of presentation can include mechanical symptoms (such as subluxation) and dysfunction owing to hip stiffness or limp. Wear and osteolysis may be asymptomatic. Regardless of the mode of presentation, all patients with presumed failure of hip arthroplasty need a detailed clinical and radiographic evaluation.

Clinical Evaluation

The duration of symptoms, intensity, and the degree of patient disability imparted by the symptoms may be elicited from detailed history. The cause of pain that has been present since primary THA is likely to be different from symptoms that commenced many years after the initial arthroplasty. Evaluation of patient comorbidities such as diabetes predisposing to infection, history of spinal disease that can masquerade as hip pain, medications that may cause muscular pain, and previous surgical history in the affected hip as well as other joints is also critical. Detailed examination to confirm suspected cause, measurement of limb length, assessment of abductor strength and gait, and detection of neurovascular insufficiency are also necessary.

Diagnostic Evaluation

Routine anteroposterior and lateral radiographs can be very informative and are likely to demonstrate the cause of failure in most cases. Gross component malpositioning, severe osteolysis, wear, radiolucent lines indicative of loosening, fractures, limb-length discrepancy, and occasionally signs of infection can be discerned from the initial radiographs. A full-length femur radiograph is valuable if long-stem femoral fixation is anticipated. On occasion other imaging modalities such as long-leg standing radiographs to assess limb length, computerized tomography (CT) to better assess component positioning or the degree of osteolysis, or MRI to evaluate coexistence of spinal conditions may need to be performed. Furthermore, nuclear imaging and aspiration of the joint to confirm or rule out periprosthetic infection may also need to be considered. On very rare occasions specialized tests such as intravenous pyelography or angiography may be performed in patients with intrapelvic components or intrapelvic cement that may need to be removed.

Preoperative Planning

Revision THA can vary from a relatively simple procedure (such as the change of acetabular liner) to a very complex surgery (such as revision of well-fixed acetabular and femoral components). Preoperative planning is paramount to ensure appropriate provisions are in place during revision surgery. Although the decision to

TABLE 15-1 INDICATIONS FOR REVISION HIP ARTHROPLASTY

Common reasons for revision
Aseptic loosening
Instability
Infection
Periprosthetic fracture
Osteolysis
Wear
Uncommon reasons for revision
Limb-length discrepancy
Thigh pain
Material failure (stem fracture, dislodgement of acetabular liner)
Impingement
Noisy hip (ceramic-on-ceramic bearing surface)

perform revision of one or both components can be made in most cases prior to surgery, sometimes unrecognized loosening, malpositioning, or damage to the bearing surface of a nonmodular femoral stem necessitates revision of a component that was not anticipated preoperatively. Furthermore, removal of well-fixed and well-positioned monolithic femoral components, to allow better visualization of the acetabulum, may be necessary during revision surgery. Hence, it is essential for the reconstructive surgeon to have studied the previous operative records of the patient to ensure that appropriate components, instruments, and support teams will be available during revision THA.

INDICATION FOR REVISION ARTHROPLASTY

Aseptic Loosening

Prosthesis loosening is one of the most common indications for revision THA. Aseptic loosening can present with radiolucent lines at the prosthesis/bone, cement/bone, or cement/prosthesis (debonding) interfaces. Radiolucent lines indicative of definite loosening are usually progressive (i.e., developed over time) or circumferential (covering the entire prosthesis surface) and usually >2 mm wide. Diagnosis of aseptic loosening of an uncemented femoral stem can be challenging (Fig. 15-1A). Engh et al. have described major and minor radiographic signs of stem loosening: The presence of reactive lines (white lines around the stem), stem subsidence (Fig. 15-1B), and distal pedestal not in contact with the tip of the stem are some of those radiographic signs. Component subsidence or change in position, if subtle, can be ascertained only by evaluation of serial radiographs. Further imaging studies such as oblique radiographs may be required to confirm aseptic loosening that is suspected clinically but cannot be confirmed on conventional radiographs. A clinical history of start-up pain usually is present with a loose femoral stem. Revision of loose femoral components often can be done without the need for extensile approaches (Fig. 15-1C) unless the component subsides under the greater trochanter, making extraction without a fracture difficult. Revision of a loose acetabular component can also be performed with minimal bone loss if careful exposure of the acetabulum is performed. Exposure of the

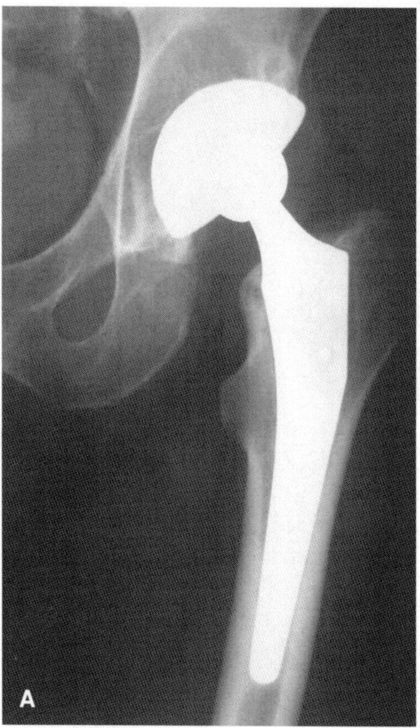

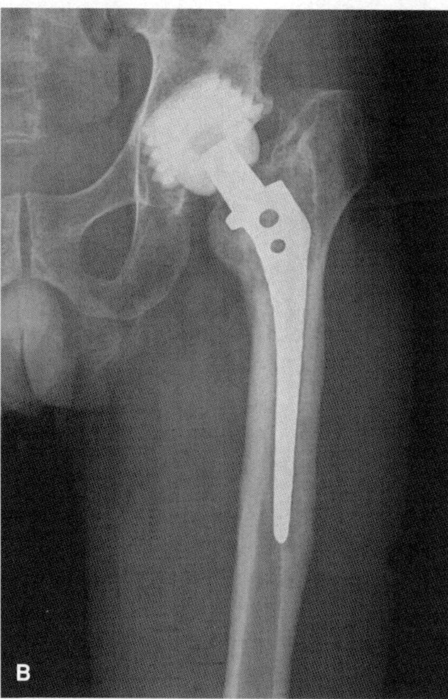

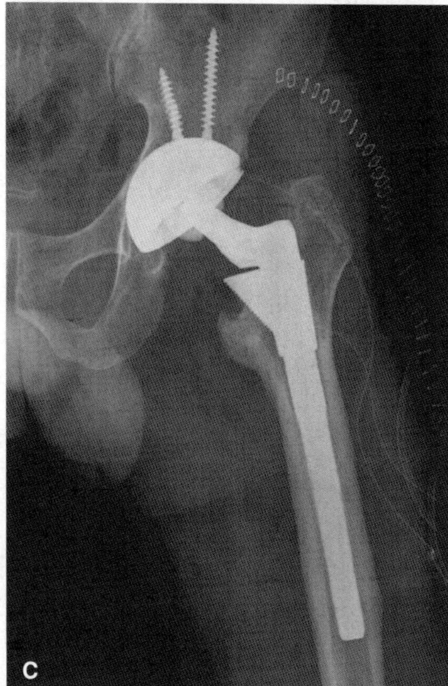

Figure 15-1 Anteroposterior radiograph (**A**) of a proximally coated stem in a patient with severe thigh pain. Aseptic loosening of the femoral stem was suspected but obscure to confirm based on the radiographs. Note the reactive lines around the proximally coated region of the stem and the lack of osteointegration. Anteroposterior radiograph of the hip in a patient with gross loosening and subsidence of the femoral stem (**B**). Revision in which modular femoral stem was used (**C**).

acetabulum in the presence of a well-fixed femoral stem can be challenging.

Periprosthetic Osteolysis

Osteolysis denotes loss of focal bone mass over time (Fig. 15-2). Around hip implants, the process is usually the result of activation of macrophages and osteoclasts that can occur with generation of wear particles or with infection. Osteolysis without component loosening can be asymptomatic and forms the main rationale for periodic evaluation of patients with joint arthroplasty, particularly those at specific risk for this problem. Active patients with high demand on their prosthetic hip are in this category. Conventional radiography underestimates the degree of osteolysis. In recent years the use of CT scans to assess the extent and location of osteolysis has been described.

The indications for intervention, and the optimal type of surgical procedure for patients with asymptomatic osteolysis is currently in evolution and not universally agreed on. There is, however, no dispute in that surgical intervention should be considered for patients with extensive osteolysis and impending periprosthetic fracture, particularly in younger patients in whom bone mass is critical, and for symptomatic patients. Options available for treatment of osteolysis around well-fixed acetabular components include isolated periacetabular bone grafting through a trapdoor or through access points around the cups or through screw holes, replacement of the bearing surface with or without bone grafting of the lesion (done through screw holes), or revision of the acetabular component. Osteolysis associated with loose acetabular or femoral components is addressed by revision arthroplasty. Frequently particulate or bulk allograft bone is used in an effort to restore the bone mass and allow mechanical fixation of the components.

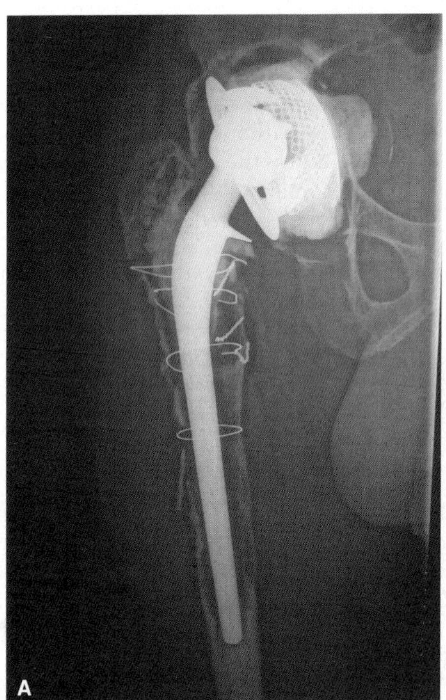

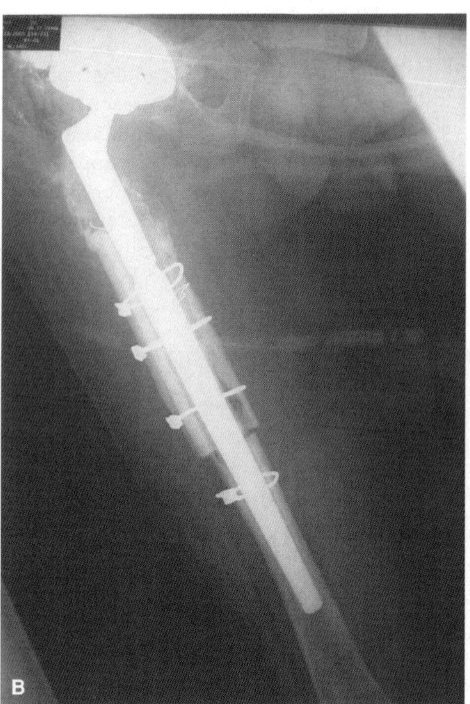

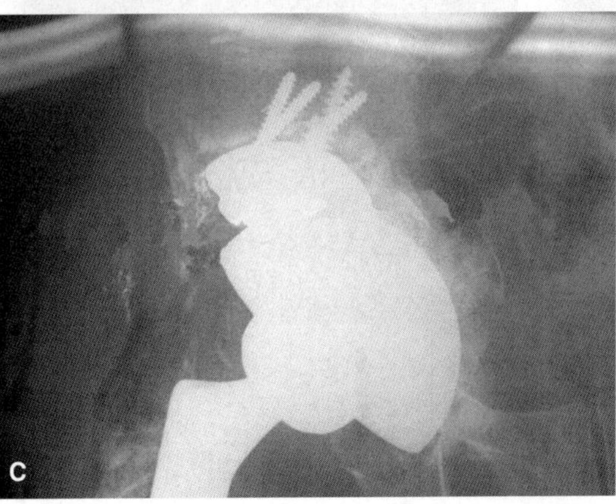

Figure 15-2 Anteroposterior radiograph of the hip in a 69-year-old patient with polyethylene wear and extensive osteolysis (**A**). The revision of both the acetabular and femoral component was performed (**B**). Trabecular metal augments were used to fill the defect in the acetabulum (**C**).

Instability

Instability following THA is not an uncommon complication. The incidence of dislocation following THA varies between 0.3% and 10% after primary and up to 28% after revision arthroplasty. It is well accepted that dislocation is more common after THA in patients with impaired cognition, soft tissue laxity or deficiency, underlying diagnosis of hip fracture, and female gender. Furthermore, technical factors such as the use of a small-diameter femoral head and performing the surgery through a posterolateral approach without capsular repair seem to adversely influence the risk of instability. Other technical factors such as the use of elevated acetabular liners, femoral component neck geometry, and femoral component offset may also influence the risk of instability. As our understanding of the causes of dislocation has evolved over the last decade, refinements in surgical techniques have been introduced that probably will result in a decline in this complication.

Dislocation following THA can occur at any time. However, most reported dislocations occur within the first few months after the index surgery. About two thirds of dislocations can be treated by closed reduction without a need for further intervention. Recurrent instability, which often necessitates reoperation, can occur owing to many reasons. The most common include component malpositioning and soft tissue laxity. However, two important points need to be mentioned. First is that the cause of recurrent instability in many cases may be multifactorial. Second, the exact cause for recurrent instability in some cases cannot be discerned with certainty. The surgical treatment options available to address recurrent instability consist of revision of malpositioned components, use of a larger-diameter femoral head, bipolar arthroplasty, greater trochanteric advancement, soft tissue re-enforcement, and the use of constrained liners.

The type of surgical strategy elected to address recurrent instability depends on the cause. Revision arthroplasty for recurrent instability in general is much more likely to be successful when a discernible cause for instability can be identified.

Revision of the malpositioned component is one of the most common of surgical interventions for dislocation (Fig. 15-3). Although definitions of malpositioning vary, the optimal positioning for acetabular component is thought to be 10 to 30 degrees of anteversion and 35 to 50 degrees of inclination or abduction. When components are positioned outside this zone, instability is more likely to result. The position of the acetabular component in relation to the anatomic landmarks (the teardrop on the radiographs) is also important. Cross-sectional studies such as CT may be needed to accurately assess component position (Fig. 15-3B).

If soft tissue laxity or deficiency is deemed to be the main cause of instability, then the use of a larger femoral head, bipolar arthroplasty, or more commonly a constrained liner is advocated (Fig. 15-4). One of the main attractions of constrained liners is that they may be used without the need to revise a well-fixed and well-positioned acetabular components.

Periprosthetic Infection

Despite all the recent advances, periprosthetic infection (PPI) continues to occur following THA. The incidence of PPI is reported to be between 0.5% and 3%. Several factors adversely influence the incidence of PPI, including revision surgery and compromised immune status of the patient.

Total joint arthroplasty infections are sometimes categorized based on the presumed mechanism and timing of infection. *Acute postoperative infections* are thought to result from infecting organisms that gained access to the joint during surgery or soon after from overlying skin or a draining wound. Infections of this type generally become symptomatic within a few days or weeks of the arthroplasty. *Late chronic infections* may result from proliferation of organisms inoculated during surgery, either from the air, surgical instruments, or the implant itself. The lag period is the time taken for the organisms to proliferate and declare deep infection. *Hematogenous infections* represent seeding of an arthroplasty site by organisms carried by the blood stream from a different site (e.g., urinary tract infection, cutaneous or mucosal ulcer, and so on). The distinction between these types may be difficult and is somewhat arbitrary.

Although diagnosis of florid PPI can be reached without much difficulty, the detection of occult infection using the current methods for diagnosis can be challenging. A high degree of suspicion for PPI should be entertained in patients with early loosening of components. Serologic tests such as C-reactive protein, erythrocyte sedimentation rate, and white cell count may be used to screen for infection. Aspiration of the joint is the most definitive test for ongoing PPI. A few nonspecific changes suggestive of infection may be apparent on plain radiographs (Fig. 15-5A). These include periosteal reaction, scattered foci of osteolysis, and generalized bone resorption in the absence of wear. However, most patients with PPI, especially those presenting acutely, do not have obvious radiographic findings suggestive of infection, or have radiographic features indistinguishable from those seen in aseptic loosening. The use of additional imaging such as the bone scan (particularly labeled white blood cell scans), and recently, positron emission tomography (PET) may occasionally be useful (Fig. 15-5B).

The possible treatment of PPI includes irrigation and debridement of the hip with retention of the components, one-stage exchange arthroplasty, or resection arthroplasty with delayed reimplantation. PPI occurring early (within 4 weeks) after index arthroplasty or hematogenous infection presenting acutely may be treated with irrigation and debridement without resection of the components as long as the components are well positioned and fixed. The reported success rate of this method varies but probably is about 50%. Two-stage exchange is the most common method of treating prosthetic infection in North America. An antibiotic-impregnated bone cement spacer frequently is placed in the hip after the initial resection, and the patient usually is treated with 4 to 8 weeks of intravenous antibiotics. On rare occasions one-stage exchange arthroplasty may be considered for patients infected with a low-virulence organism that is sensitive to most antibiotics. Resection arthroplasty may be the treatment of choice for a select group of patients

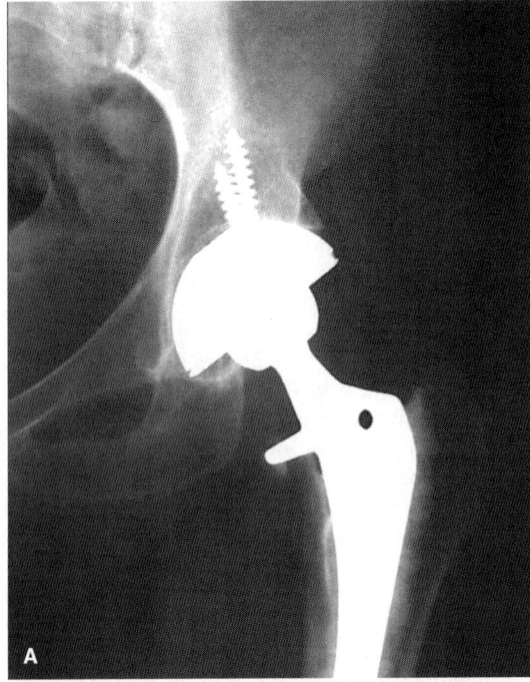

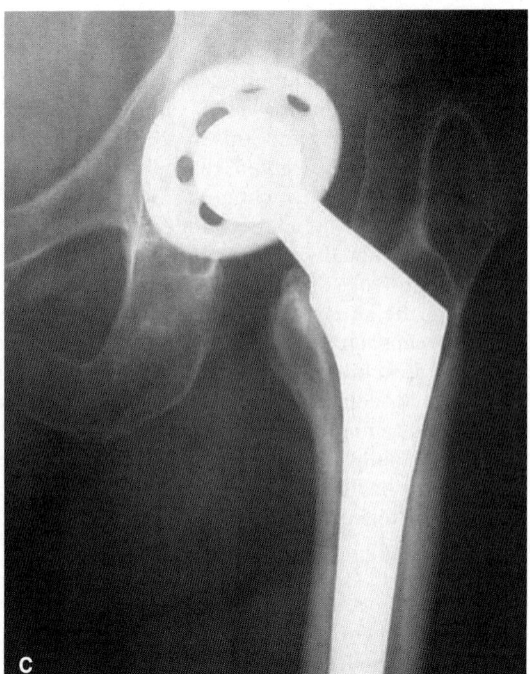

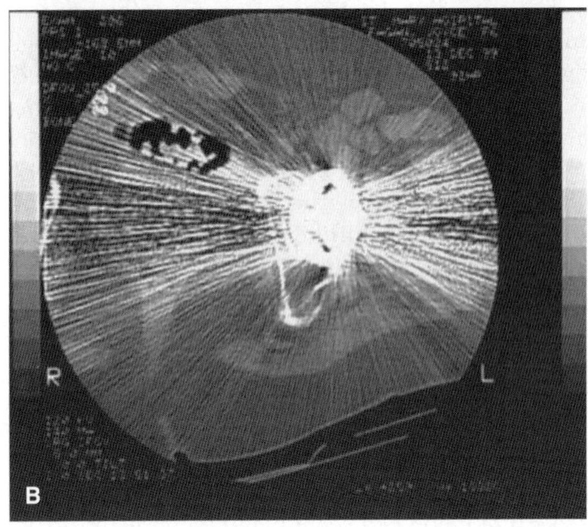

Figure 15-3 Anteroposterior radiograph of a patient with component malpositioning and instability (**A**). The computed tomography clearly showed malposition of the acetabular component as retroversion (**B**). The retroverted cup was repositioned during revision surgery (**C**).

with inadequate bone stock or soft tissues precluding reimplantation or recalcitrant infection.

Polyethylene Wear

Wear of the bearing surfaces is the most important factor limiting the longevity of the hip arthroplasty. Age and activity level are among the most important predictors of bearing wear rate. Polyethylene wear per se is usually not an indication for revision THA unless it results in polythene fracture, wear-through, osteolysis, or pain (owing to synovitis from wear debris). In recent years great strides in the design of articulation materials have been made with promising prospects. The introduction of highly cross-linked polyethylene is one such improvement that has resulted in reduction of wear both *in vitro* and *in vivo*. Other alternative bearing surfaces that are currently in use include alumina ceramic-on-ceramic and metal-on-metal articulations.

Periprosthetic Fracture

Various classifications for periprosthetic fractures around the hip have been proposed. The Vancouver periprosthetic fracture classification system is widely used and lends itself to devising a treatment strategy. This classification system takes into account the site of fracture, the status of the femoral component, and the proximal femoral bone quality. Type A fractures are around the proximal femur involving the greater trochanter or the lesser trochanter. The stability of the stem is not usually compromised. These fractures often are associated with osteolysis of the proximal femur. Treatment is directed toward management of underlying osteolysis. The fracture itself does not usually require fixation

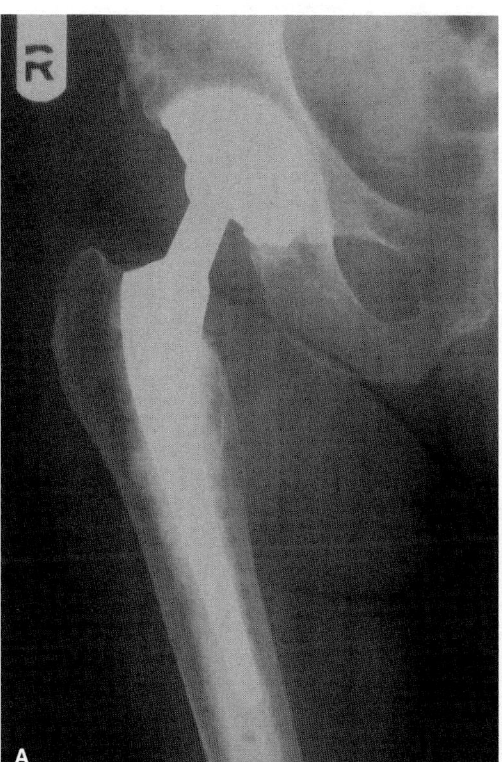

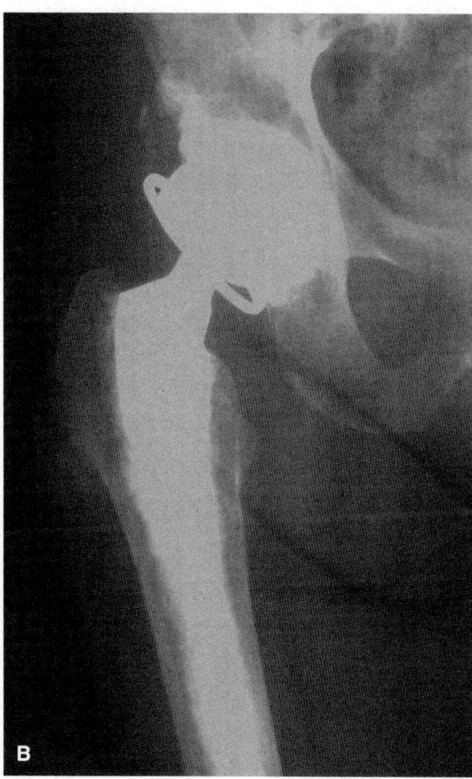

Figure 15-4 Anteroposterior radiograph of a patient with recurrent instability that was deemed secondary to inadequate soft tissue (abductor) envelope (**A**). The acetabular component, although slightly vertical, was found to be well fixed during surgery. A constrained liner with a larger femoral head was used to address the problem in this patient (**B**).

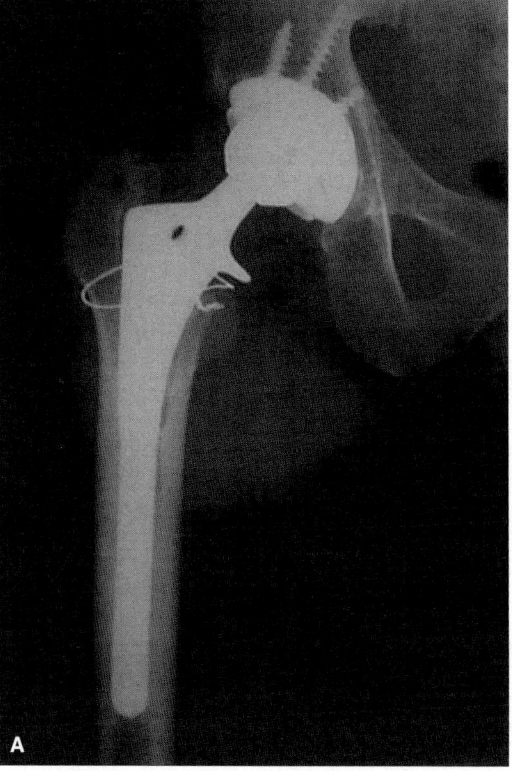

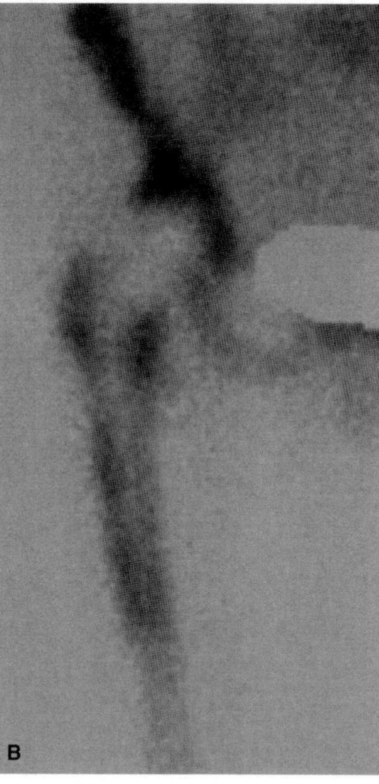

Figure 15-5 Plain radiograph showing area of focal osteolysis (scalloping) around the midportion of a well-fixed uncemented stem (**A**). This appearance is highly suggestive of periprosthetic infection. Increased uptake in the corresponding area of infection in the right femur was noted on the PET scan (**B**).

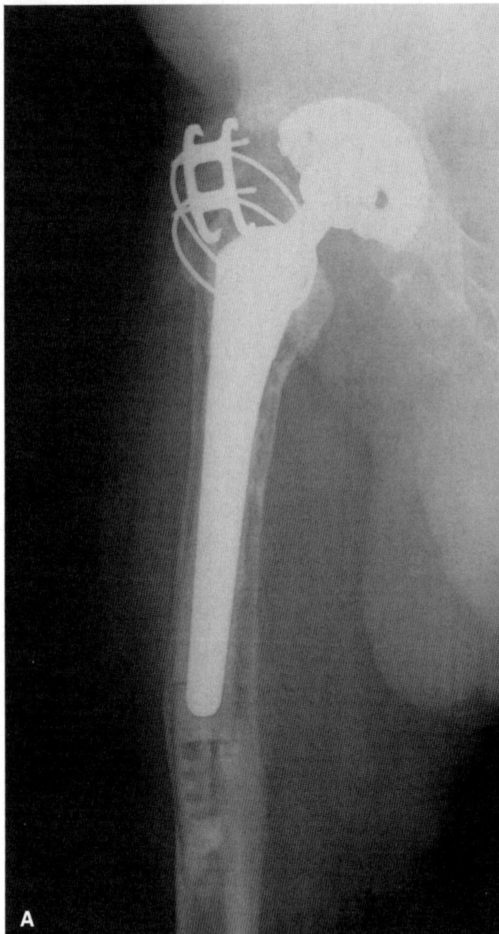

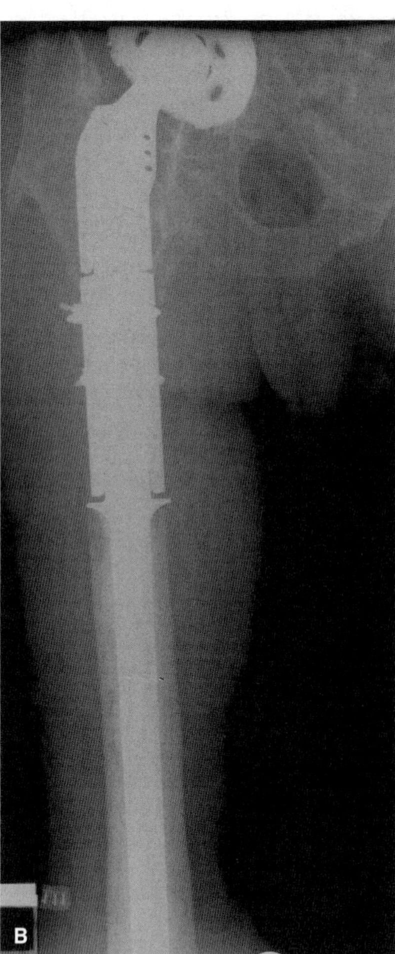

Figure 15-6 Anteroposterior radiograph of a patient with Vancouver type B3 periprosthetic fracture (**A**). Proximal femoral replacement was used for reconstruction of this fracture (**B**).

unless the greater trochanter is displaced to compromise abductor function. Type B fractures are those occurring around the femoral stem. In type B1 fractures the femoral stem is stable. Most can be treated with internal fixation of the fracture using plates, screws, cerclage cables, and strut grafts while retaining the well-fixed stem. Fractures associated with loosening of the femoral stem (types B2 and B3) are treated with revision of the femoral component and simultaneous fracture fixation (Fig. 15-6).

Leg-Length Discrepancy

Limb-length discrepancy (LLD) following total hip replacement is not uncommon and can be bothersome to the patient. Patients frequently complain of LLD in the early postoperative period, and in most instances the LLD is functional and the symptoms resolve with time. However, there remains a small subset of patients who continue to be symptomatic. Most can be treated with shoe lifts to compensate for the problem; further surgery is performed only in rare instances (Fig.15-7).

Material Failure

Fracture of the femoral stem was not infrequent with early prostheses made of stainless steel or cast cobalt chromium that were susceptible to fatigue fracture. Improvements in engineering and metallurgy have enabled manufacturers to produce arthroplasty components that are extremely strong and resilient. Fractures of modern monolithic femoral stems are exceedingly rare. Fracture of the femoral stem, in the rare occasions that may occur, usually involves modular components (Fig. 15-8). Poor proximal bone support in a stem that is well fixed distally can lead to cantilever loading of the stem and subsequent fatigue fracture.

With increasing use of modular acetabular components, dissociation or dislodging of the acetabular liner has also been reported. This problem was more common particularly with some designs of acetabular components that did not have sophisticated locking mechanisms.

CLASSIFICATION OF BONE DEFICIENCY

One of the major challenges of revision THA is the management of bone loss. Depending on the extent and location of bone loss, different surgical strategies are used.

There are two commonly used acetabular bone deficiency classification systems. The American Academy of Orthopaedic Surgeons (AAOS) system can be used in both primary and revision arthroplasty. It categorizes bone loss as segmental or cavitary defects along with pelvic discontinuity and arthrodesis. *Segmental defect* describes full-thickness

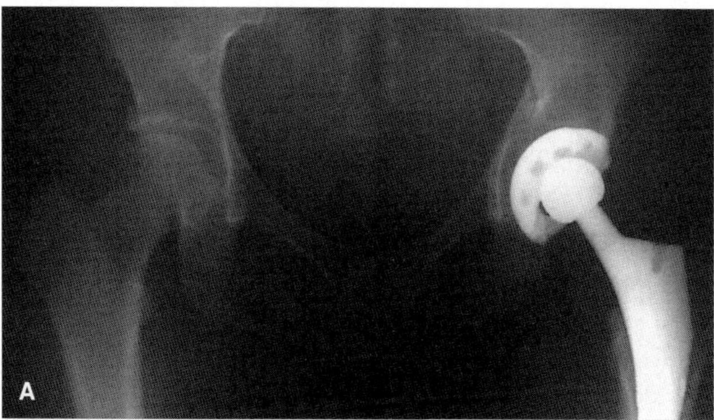

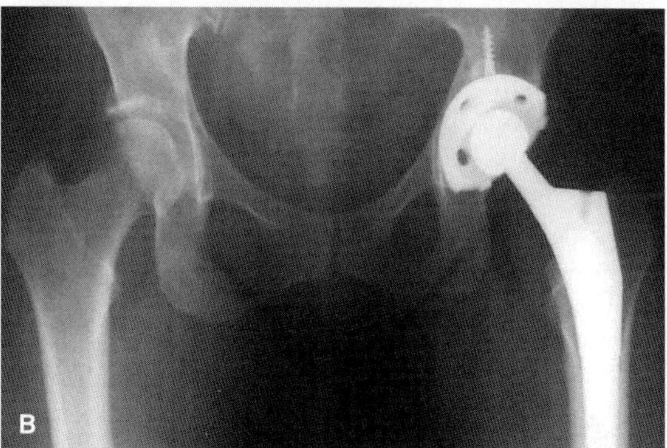

Figure 15-7 The anteroposterior radiograph (A) of the hip in a 54-year-old patient in whom the acetabular component has been placed inferior to the anatomic position (teardrop), with the revised hip radiograph (B) demonstrating proper positioning of the cup that addressed the limb lengthening.

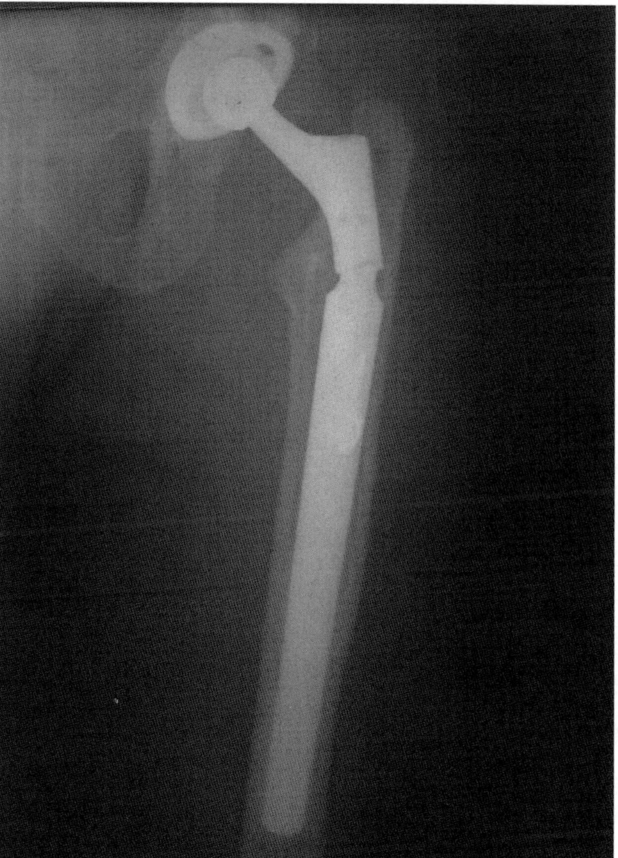

Figure 15-8 Anteroposterior radiograph of the pelvis demonstrating fatigue fracture of the modular conical femoral stem.

loss of bone in the supporting rim of acetabulum or the medial wall. *Cavitary defect* describes volumetric loss of bone within the acetabular cavity. Complete transverse disruption of the supporting anterior and posterior columns of acetabulum constitutes *pelvic discontinuity*. Another classification system proposed by Paprosky is based on the severity of bone loss and helps predict the surgeon's ability to achieve implant stability with a hemispheric cup. The system describes four radiographic landmarks to evaluate the extent of bone loss, which are the following: proximal migration of acetabular component (migration of joint center), integrity of the teardrop, ischial bone loss, and violation of the Köhler line by prosthetic migration.

Femoral Bone Loss

Several classification methods for periprosthetic femoral bone loss have been proposed. Most define the severity of proximal bone loss by the amount of cancellous bone loss, the amount of cortical bone loss, and the distal extent of this bone loss. These classification methods can be used to choose necessary revision implants.

SURGICAL EXPOSURE

An essential element of successful revision arthroplasty is obtaining adequate exposure of the hip. If possible, the old incision should be used or incorporated into the new incision. In many revisions a conventional anterolateral or posterolateral approach may be used. The advantages of anterolateral or direct lateral approaches include excellent acetabular exposure, decreased rate of sciatic nerve palsy, and reduced incidence of postoperative dislocations. Disadvantages of the anterolateral approach include difficulty of accessing the posterior column for cage implantation or bone grafting, increased risk of heterotopic ossification, reduced visualization of the proximal femur, and the higher incidence of postoperative limp. Advantages of the posterolateral approach are good visualization of the posterior column and entire acetabulum, preservation of the abductor mechanisms, and lower incidence of heterotopic ossification. Disadvantages include difficult acetabular exposure when the femoral component is in situ, and a higher dislocation rate compared with anterior or lateral approaches.

Extensile exposures not infrequently are required during revision arthroplasty. One of the most common extensile exposures is the extended trochanteric osteotomy (ETO). ETO is considered the exposure of choice for removal of well-fixed stems. It is also particularly useful for removal of a well-fixed cement mantle, particularly in infected cases. Another extensile exposure is the Wagner osteotomy in which the proximal femur is split in the coronal plane. Finally, conventional trochanteric osteotomy, or so-called trochanteric slide (in which the abductors, greater trochanter, and vastus lateralis are kept in continuity), also are useful in selected complex revisions. Extensile exposures allow better visualization of both the femur and the acetabulum while minimizing soft tissue damage. Fixation of extended osteotomies can be performed with the use of cables or wires. The osteotomy fragment can sometimes be advanced to modulate soft tissue tension and enhance hip stability.

Removal of Acetabular Component

Good exposure of the acetabulum is key for removal of the acetabular component while avoiding bone loss. Removal of a loose acetabular component usually can be performed with relative ease. In recent years acetabular extraction systems have been introduced; these consist of thin curved osteotomes that can be inserted behind the cup and rotated around a ball placed inside the liner. It is crucial that the osteotome be placed at the interface between the cup and the cement mantle or the bone as opposed to being inserted into the substance of retroacetabular bone.

Removal of Femoral Component

Extraction of a loose femoral component usually can also be performed after obtaining good exposure of the femur. Extended exposures may be needed for removal of a well-fixed femoral stem or cement mantle. In cases where a portion of cement mantle remains, particularly in the distal femur, the use of an anterolateral window in the cortex may be most appropriate for complete removal of the remaining cement. It is important to remember that any such defect in the cortex will need to be bypassed by a stem spanning at least two cortical diameters distal to the defect. In most cases the cement mantle can be removed with the use of a combination of ultrasonic or mechanical extraction systems.

ACETABULAR REVISION

An acetabular component may be revised for loosening, infection, malposition, or wear. The objective of the procedure should be restoration of the hip center of rotation, remedy of deficient bone, and secure component fixation in optimal orientation.

Cementless Acetabular Revision

A cementless hemispheric cup can be used in acetabular revisions. Several large series report excellent mid- to long-term survivorship of their techniques. The outcome is good even with limited acetabular bone grafting including morselized grafting of cavitary defects. The prerequisite for a successful outcome is obtaining appropriate press fit and adequate surface area of contact between the cementless cup and the host bone. The use of newer high-friction, highly porous metals such as tantulum may allow successful reconstruction using this method even when the bone loss is severe. It is important to note that the location of the contact area is a critical factor. Deficiencies of the superior weight bearing dome at the socket may be filled with structural allograft or metallic component augments. Many defects may be obliterated by reaming of the cavity to allow insertion of a jumbo acetabular cup. The advantage of using a jumbo cup is that it allows restoration of the hip center of rotation and improved cup contact against the host bone.

Options for Reconstruction of Bone Defects

Type I: Segmental Deficiency

Most segmental defects that involve a small area of acetabular rim can be treated using a cementless hemispheric cup. The defect is usually reamed away prior to insertion of the uncemented cup. Defects remaining after reaming can be treated with particulate bone grafting. The bone graft is packed into the defect using the reamer in a reverse direction. For larger defects with intact columns, structural graft or metal augments may be used.

Type II: Cavitary Deficiency

Most cavitary defects also can be managed with cementless hemispheric components. In most cases the rim area is intact allowing press-fit insertion of the cementless component. Larger defects can be filled with particulate bone grafting. For larger defects, especially in the medial wall region, impaction bone grafting with wire mesh can be considered.

Type III: Combined Segmental and Cavitary Deficiency

There are several different options for treating these defects. Cementless jumbo cups, with bone grafting, can be used in most cases as long as adequate surface area of contact between the porous acetabular cup and the host bone can be achieved. For cases with a small surface area of contact and a large defect, proper fixation of an uncemented component may not be possible. For these cases cemented cups with impaction grafting or reconstruction cages may be more appropriate.

Type IV: Pelvic Discontinuity

One of the most challenging problems in revision THA is acetabular reconstruction for pelvic discontinuity with complete separation of inferior and superior regions as a result of transverse defects and/or fractures. In spite of all preoperative radiographic assessments, pelvic discontinuity may be recognized or detected only during surgery. Hence, it is crucial for reconstruction surgeons to ensure that appropriate acetabular components are in place to deal with this problem during complex revisions. Pelvic discontinuity should be suspected in patients with massive bone loss. Any defects leading to disruption of the posterior column should also lead the surgeon to suspect pelvic discontinuity. When detected, appropriate reduction and fixation of the "fracture," usually by plating of the posterior column, typically is performed prior to insertion of an acetabular component.

FEMORAL REVISION

The main principles for femoral reconstruction are to obtain rigid fixation for the femoral component,to restore limb length and hip stability, and when possible to restore bone stock.

Cementless Femoral Revision

Proximally Coated Stems

Although proximally coated femoral stems are used commonly during primary THA, the results of revision THA using this stem design are disappointing. The main reason is that after removal of a previous femoral stem, little to no bone may exist to allow proper fixation of this stem design and subsequent biologic integration in the metaphyseal region of the proximal femur. Hence, proximally coated femoral stems are not commonly used during revision surgery.

Extensively Coated Stems

Fully porous-coated femoral stems are commonly used for revision hip arthroplasty. The extensively coated stems bypass the sclerotic and often weakened proximal femur to achieve secure fixation in the relatively healthy femoral diaphysis. The implant's initial rotational stability and subsequent biologic fixation are excellent in most cases. To optimize the outcome, these stems should be implanted in femoral canals with adequate (>5 cm) diaphyseal length for scratch fit. The stem should bypass any defects in the cortex by at least two canal diameters. An onlay cortical allograft may be used for larger defects (more than one third of the canal diameter) of the cortex. All cement in the femoral canal should be removed before reaming the canal. A curved stem, conforming to the anatomy of the canal, should be used when longer components are being implanted. Depending on the design, reaming of the femoral canal to an appropriate diameter to allow good press fit without causing fracture should be carried out. In cases with high likelihood for fracture of the femur or in cases in which longitudinal fracture of the femur occurs, cerclage cables or wires may be used. Although extensively coated stems are reported to have excellent outcomes in revision surgery, some problems are associated with this femoral component design, one of which is stress shielding.

Modular Femoral Stems

Fluted, tapered modular cementless femoral stems also can be used to gain diaphyseal fixation. Modular femoral stems provide intraoperative versatility to allow adjustment of limb length, offset, and version.

Proximal Femoral Replacement

After the initial success of the megaprosthesis in patients with neoplastic conditions, the indications for this type of reconstructive procedure were expanded to include patients presenting with failed THA and massive proximal femoral bone loss. With refinements in design, namely introduction of modular prostheses, megaprostheses have been used in cases of proximal femoral bone deficiency.

Megaprotheses currently are reserved for use mostly in elderly or sedentary patients with massive proximal bone loss. In younger patients in whom bone loss of high magnitude is encountered that cannot be reconstructed by conventional means, an allograft-prosthetic composite would be preferred over femoral prosthetic replacement.

Allograft-Prosthetic Composite

Allograft bone used may be in the form of strut grafts placed against defects in the femoral cortex or an allograft-prosthetic composite (APC). The type and length of allograft used depend on various factors, particularly the extent of bone loss and the status of the soft tissues. An important prerequisite for the use of APC is the availability of sufficient distal femoral length for secure fixation of the femoral stem. The advantages of using an APC (besides its ability to restore bone mass) are that it allows transmission of normal load to the distal host bone and prevents further distal bone loss. The soft tissue in the proximal region of the femur also can be attached to the allograft bone with some potential for healing and integration. The major disadvantages of using an APC are the higher incidence of infection, graft fracture, nonunion of the allograft with the host bone, technical difficulty of fashioning the composite, and the relatively long operation time.

Cemented Femoral Revision

Although cementless femoral stems are the most commonly used revision femoral components, cemented stems also may be used in selected cases. Cemented femoral revision generally is indicated in patients with good bone stock and available cancellous bone for interdigitation. Following removal of a previous femoral component, usually little if any cancellous bone remains; thus the mechanical bond of cement to bone in revision typically is reduced, particularly if the previous component was cemented. Hence, the use of cemented femoral components during revision surgery is limited. Femoral impaction allografting and revision with allograft-prosthesis composite are two scenarios in which cemented femoral stems need to be used. Another occasion is when a well-fixed prior cement mantle is left in place and another femoral component is either impacted into the mantle or cemented into the previous cement mantle, the so-called cement-within-cement technique. If this strategy is to be used, some important steps needs to be taken. The mantle is dried, then multiply scratched and roughened to increase the contact surface area and improve interdigitation for the new cement mantle. The cement is injected during a relatively liquid stage.

Impaction Allograft with Cemented Stem Revision

This difficult technique is most commonly considered for femora with cavitary metaphyseal or diaphyseal deficiencies and an intact cortical envelope. Small segmental deficiencies also can be treated with the use of a wire mesh or cortical strut graft. The technique involves compression of particulate cancellous bone allograft into the cavitary defects to reconstruct the osseous architecture of the femur and concomitant use of a polished cemented femoral stem. Before insertion of the grafts, the inner surface of the femur should be cleaned thoroughly. A cement plug is inserted to restrict the bone graft. The recommended graft size is generally as small as 4 to 6 mm^3. Special instruments are used to obtain optimal graft impaction. The stem is cemented into the graft mantle. The major advantage of using femoral impaction allograft is the restoration of bone stock. This technique, however, is challenging. Subsidence of the stem, either with or without the graft mantle, have been reported in a few series, emphasizing that the results are dependent on technique and patient selection. A high incidence of periprosthetic fracture also has been reported at the tip of the femoral stem when short-stemmed implants were used routinely.

Selection of Fixation Method

Although there are no hard-and-fast rules with regard to which stem design or type should be used during revision surgery, some general rules apply. The first goal should be a good long-term clinical outcome, and a secondary goal should be restoration or maintenance of bone mass. The first objective usually precludes the use of conventional monoblock proximally coated uncemented stems in almost all cases and also the use of cemented stems in most cases. The use of both aforementioned stem designs necessitate good quality and volume of bone in the metaphysis and the canal, which is rarely the case during revision surgery. Hence, uncemented distally fixed stems are used more commonly. When extensively coated stems are being used, it is crucial to ensure that adequate diaphyseal fixation is achieved. This minimizes the possibility of stem subsidence, pain, instability, and limb shortening. For patients with extensive bone loss, proximal femoral replacement in older and less active patients and allograft-prosthesis composite in younger patients are preferred. Regardless of which stem design and type are used, revision surgery can be a challenging experience and should be undertaken only by those familiar with all the intricacies. Attention to detail and delivery of optimal surgical care are essential for a predictable and good outcome of any surgical procedure, particularly revision arthroplasty.

SUGGESTED READINGS

Berry DJ. Antiprotrusio cages for acetabular revision. *Clin Orthop*. 2004;420:106–112.

Daly PJ, Morrey BF. Operative correction of an unstable total hip arthroplasty. *J Bone Joint Surg Am*. 1992;74:1334–1343.

D'Antonio JA, Capello WN, Borden LS, et al. Classification and management of acetabular abnormalities in total hip arthroplasty. *Clin Orthop*. 1989;243:126–137.

D'Antonio JA, McCarthy JC, Barger WL, et al. Classification of femoral abnormalities in total hip arthroplasty. *Clin Orthop*. 1993;296:133–139.

Duncan CP, Masri BA. Fractures of the femur after hip replacement. *Instr Course Lect*. 1995;44:293–304.

Engh CA, Culpepper WJ 2nd, Kassapidis E. Revision of loose cementless femoral prostheses to larger porous coated components. *Clin Orthop*. 1998;347:168–178.

Mardones R, Gonzalez C, Cabanela ME, et al. Extended femoral osteotomy for revision of hip arthroplasty: results and complications. *J Arthroplasty*. 2005;20:79–83.

Parvizi J, Sharkey PF, Bissett GA, et al. Surgical treatment of limb-length discrepancy following total hip arthroplasty. *J Bone Joint Surg Am*. 2003;85:2310–2317.

Schreurs BW, Bolder SB, Gardeniers JW, et al. Acetabular revision with impacted morselized cancellous bone grafting and a cemented cup. A 15- to 20- year follow-up. *J Bone Joint Surg Br*. 2004;86:492–497.

Zimmerli W, Trampuz A, Ochsner PE. Prosthetic-joint infections. *N Engl J Med*. 2004;351:1645–1654.

PHYSICAL EVALUATION OF THE KNEE

16

JASON R. HULL

The primary goals of any patient encounter are formulation of the correct diagnosis and initiation of an appropriate course of treatment. Despite many advances in laboratory and imaging technology, a thorough history and physical examination remains the most effective instruments in achieving these goals. The clinician may establish a provisional diagnosis early in the patient encounter after hearing only the patient's presenting complaint and history of present illness. A detailed history will direct the focus and extent of the physical examination and aid in refining the diagnosis. Close interaction with the patient during the history and physical examination promotes accurate assessment of the patient's level of disability and formulation of an individualized treatment plan appropriate for their expectations and goals for recovery.

HISTORY

Details of the patient's presenting symptoms should be explored in a clear, systematic fashion and include discussion of location, timing, quality, severity, and aggravating/relieving factors. Pain is the most common complaint that drives orthopaedic patients to seek medical evaluation. Asking the patient to point to the most painful area of the knee is a simple way to determine the anatomic location of the symptoms. The timing of onset should be explored, because symptoms may start insidiously and slowly progress with a waxing and waning course, or may start suddenly after a major or minor traumatic event. The pattern of symptoms may provide immediate insight regarding a presumptive diagnosis. For example, initially osteoarthritis may cause aching pain that localizes to one area of the knee, occurs only after prolonged weight-bearing activities, and is relieved by short periods of rest. This may be differentiated from early pain owing to inflammatory arthritis, which may be more diffuse, constant, and unrelieved by rest. Besides pain, the presence of mechanical symptoms and subjective instability should be reviewed. Locking, catching, and popping are suggestive of a meniscal tear, loose body, or focal lesion of the articular surface. Instability can be caused by true ligamentous insufficiency or may be owing to reflex inhibition of the quadriceps from knee pain or effusion. It is important to inquire about past events specific to the joint, as patients may not readily recall childhood illnesses or conditions that affected the knee, and they may not mention previous minor surgical interventions such as arthroscopy.

Ascertaining the patient's level of dysfunction is paramount. Informed discussions regarding risk-benefit ratios of potential conservative and surgical treatment options cannot take place until this is established. Functional deficits should be evaluated in the context of the patient's baseline level of physical activity including activities of daily living, occupational and work-related activities, and leisure activities (Table 16-1). As symptoms worsen patients typically exhibit progressive activity modification and adaptive mechanisms, such as using assistive devices for ambulation (cane, walker), using the hands to assist in rising from a chair, and altering stair climbing technique or avoiding stairs altogether. Standardized physician-administered (e.g., Knee Society Clinical Rating System) and patient-administered (e.g., Western Ontario and McMaster University Osteoarthritis Index) rating scales can be useful in evaluating patients' functional deficits. Perceptions regarding level of disability may vary greatly between patients with different occupations or cultural backgrounds. Because of the physical demands of his work, a laborer may perceive himself to be disabled earlier in the disease process than a sedentary office worker. Some patients tolerate lifestyle changes more effectively than others and may be willing to change careers or give up favorite leisure activities to avoid surgical treatment.

All previous medical and therapeutic interventions, both prescribed and unprescribed, should be discussed. Patients will often fail to mention treatments such as over-the-counter nonsteroidal anti-inflammatory medications and self-directed therapeutic exercise. Discovering the

TABLE 16-1 HISTORY: ASSESSING FUNCTIONAL DEFICITS AND DISABILITY

Do you have pain
—at rest?
—with activities only?
—that wakens you at night?
How do you go up and down stairs?
Can you rise from a chair without assistance?
Do you have difficulty with your own shoes and socks?
Do you walk with a
—cane?
—crutches?
—walker?
How far can you walk?
Can you do your own grocery shopping?
Have you had to leave work early because of pain?
Have you had to give up any leisure activities that you enjoy?

frequency, duration, and efficacy of all prescribed interventions, including activity modification, orthotics, physical therapy, pain and anti-inflammatory medications, and injections, is important for determining the next step in treatment.

A review of systems is essential for a complete history and may be included in the history of present illness. Specific inquiry regarding constitutional symptoms may uncover fever, anorexia, weight loss, fatigue, and generalized morning stiffness, which are indicative of an inflammatory condition such as rheumatoid arthritis or infection. The review of systems should also cover other possible sources of knee symptoms, including the neurovascular system, spine, and adjacent joints. The hip and spine are common sources of referred pain to the knee (Fig. 16-1). The review of systems should also be used to identify medical issues that require attention prior to any surgery, such as undiagnosed cardiac or respiratory disease and recent or ongoing infections, particularly of the genitourinary tract and oropharynx.

The patient's past medical, past surgical, family, and social histories will offer diagnostic clues as well as information that dictates available treatment options and the manner in which they are executed. The medical history may reveal an underlying systemic inflammatory condition as the cause for the knee condition and preclude nonarthroplasty surgical options. An extensive medical history, especially cardiac, may eliminate surgical options altogether. A review of the patient's medications may identify active medical conditions the patient failed to discuss previously. In addition, make note of any medications that should be discontinued perioperatively, such as nonsteroidal anti-inflammatory agents, anticoagulants, and disease-modifying antirheumatic drugs. The social history should include details of the patient's current living conditions and whether the patient will have adequate assistance at home after hospital discharge. The patient's use of alcohol, tobacco, or illicit substances must be documented accurately, as these agents may necessitate alterations in perioperative medical management or possibly disqualify the patient from surgical intervention.

PHYSICAL EXAMINATION

As with collection of a complete history, the physical evaluation of the patient presenting with knee symptoms must be completed in a systematic fashion. The order and organization of the exam is a matter of personal preference, but in general must include inspection, palpation, range of

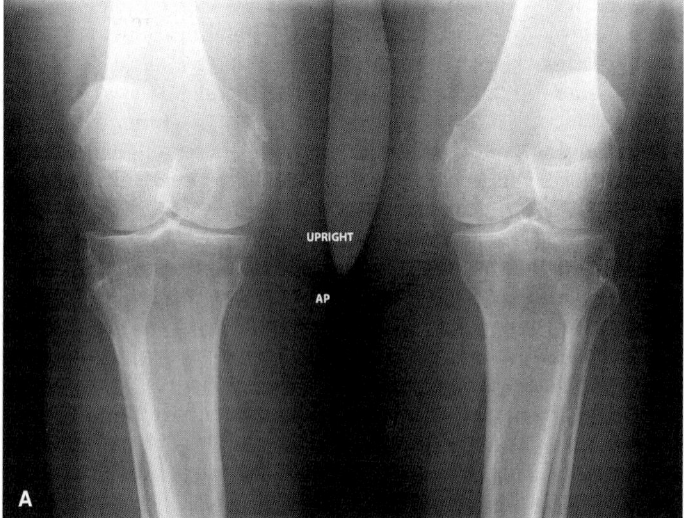

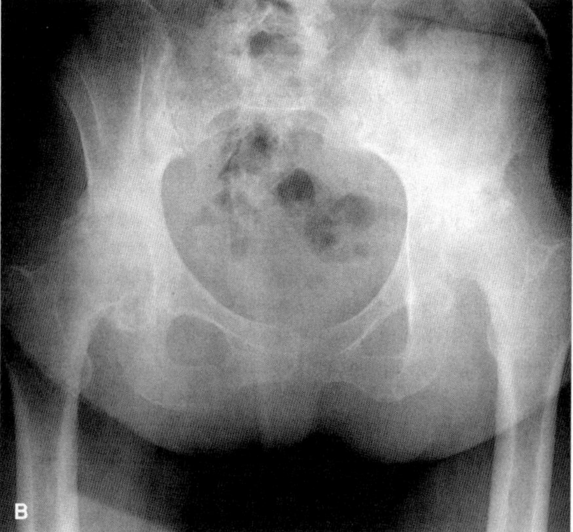

Figure 16-1 Radiographs of a 54-year-old patient referred for treatment of severe bilateral knee pain. **A:** Standing anteroposterior radiograph of both knees demonstrates mild to moderate osteoarthritis. Note the oblique view of both knees, as the patient could not internally rotate her hips to neutral for the study. **B:** Anteroposterior radiograph of the pelvis demonstrates severe arthrosis of both hip joints. Staged bilateral total hip arthroplasty resulted in complete resolution of her symptoms.

motion, ligamentous exam, and neurologic and vascular evaluation. The examination should include evaluation of both knees. Normal findings are most frequently symmetrical, so asymmetry may indicate the presence of pathology. To minimize guarding during examination of the affected knee, examine the uninvolved knee first. Avoid areas of known tenderness and exacerbating maneuvers until as late in the exam as possible.

Inspection, Palpation, and Range of Motion

The physical examination may begin the first time the clinician lays eyes on the patient. Briefly observing how the patient moves on the way to the examination room may provide a more candid glimpse of the patient's gait and reliance on assistive devices than when he or she is asked to ambulate during the formal exam. Much can be learned regarding a patient's level of physical dysfunction and disability by general observation during the interview as well as during the formal examination. General appearance and body habitus must be noted. Observe the patient's posture of the spine, hips, and knees while seated. While removing shoes and socks and getting on and off the exam table, the patient may exhibit abnormal movement to compensate for pain or stiffness. Watch carefully for facial expressions and wincing that indicate pain.

The formal examination may begin with the patient standing. Inspection of the spine may reveal a scoliosis or alteration of normal lumbar lordosis with associated paravertebral spasm. Check the range of motion of the lumbar spine with flexion, extension, side bending, and rotation. Patients with osteoarthritis of the lumbar spine often experience lumbar pain with extension. The bony landmarks of the pelvis can be palpated to assess for pelvic obliquity. A fixed pelvic obliquity owing to lumbosacral disease will not correct when a block is placed under the apparently short limb. Abductor weakness, often associated with hip pathology, can be recognized with the Trendelenburg test. During a single leg stance, the abductor muscles on the supporting extremity contract to maintain a level pelvis. A positive test occurs when the abductors are not strong enough to support the body's weight and the hemipelvis opposite the supported limb drops toward the floor.

Gross limb alignment in the standing position provides some indication of the location of the knee pathology. Genu varum suggests involvement of the medial compartment, whereas genu valgum suggests involvement of the lateral compartment. During gait these deformities may prove to be dynamic, with worsening of the varus and valgus deformities during stance phase observed as lateral and medial thrusts at the knee, respectively. The presence of a thrust in the setting of osteoarthritis has prognostic implications, as these knees demonstrate a propensity for disease progression. A dynamic recurvatum deformity during stance phase should alert the clinician to the possibility of an underlying neurologic condition, extensor mechanism dysfunction, or significant ligamentous laxity. Posture of the ankles and feet should not be overlooked. Hindfoot bracing for a flexible planovalgus deformity of the foot and ankle may provide symptomatic relief for an ipsilateral valgus knee.

Assessment of the patient's gait pattern is an essential component of the examination. The patient's effort to reduce joint load at the knee can result in many compensatory gait changes. Pain during weight bearing causes the patient to limit the amount of time spent in stance phase of gait, producing an antalgic gait (classic limp), which is the most common adaptive gait pattern. Decreased cadence may be observed, which effectively reduces all external moments on the affected knee. Reduced stride length results from a decrease in forward reach of the involved extremity in late swing phase, which diminishes the external sagittal plane moment at the knee during heel strike. An out-toeing gait may be observed in patients with painful varus osteoarthritis of the knee, which reduces the adduction moment at the knee by shortening the moment arm. Likewise, patients may lean the trunk toward the affected weight-bearing extremity to reduce the moment arm between their center of gravity and the limb's mechanical axis. This should not be confused with the Trendelenburg lurch observed with hip pathology and concurrent abductor weakness and dysfunction.

The remaining components of an abbreviated hip and spine exam can be completed with the patient lying supine before focusing on the knee. Patients with a lumbar radiculopathy may exhibit tenderness in the region of the sciatic notch. The clinician should perform maneuvers that place the sciatic nerve under tension, including the straight leg raise and contralateral straight leg raise tests. Examine the hips, starting with palpation of the greater trochanter. Localized tenderness suggests greater trochanteric bursitis, which can present with referred pain to the lateral thigh and occasionally the lateral aspect of the knee. The ability to perform an active straight leg raise against gravity and added resistance should be tested. Groin and anterior hip or thigh pain with this maneuver may suggest intra-articular hip pathology. Active side-lying hip abduction may produce similar symptoms, and patients with advanced hip disease may not be able to overcome gravity. Passive hip motion may also produce groin and thigh pain. Loss of hip motion, especially flexion and internal rotation, is a strong indicator for the presence of advanced hip pathology.

As the examination moves toward the knee, global inspection of the lower extremities should be performed. Muscle tone, atrophy, and defects in the thigh and calf should be noted. Recording thigh and calf circumference at fixed distances above and below the patella allows objective measurement of muscle atrophy. The presence and severity of peripheral edema should be noted, along with any pretibial skin changes or varices associated with chronic venous stasis.

The overall alignment of the extremity should be reassessed. In thin patients, varus and valgus alignment can be quantified with a goniometer centered on the anterior aspect of the patella. Deformities of the thigh and lower leg should not be overlooked. Many patients will fail to mention remote trauma and surgery in their history. Healed scars should be discussed with the patient, because they may indicate the presence of posttraumatic or surgical deformities that are not outwardly visible, especially in overweight and obese patients. Scars about the knee may provide insight regarding the underlying diagnosis and should be accurately documented for preoperative planning. Skin rashes may suggest a systemic cause for the patient's knee pathology. When present over the knee, rashes are associated with increased risk of surgical site infection and should be treated prior to operative intervention.

Diffuse and localized soft tissue swelling should be assessed with the patient supine and the knee in extension and in flexion. Knee effusions can be assessed by compressing the suprapatellar pouch and assessing ballottement of the patella. Effusions must be differentiated from synovial thickening or bogginess, which suggests inflammatory arthritis. Although nonspecific, slight skin warmth over the knee relative to the adjacent calf and thigh can indicate the presence of a generalized synovitis. Localized swelling may represent the site of isolated pathology or may be an indicator of a more remote or generalized process. For example, localized medial joint line swelling may be identified in the presence of a meniscal cyst with an underlying meniscal tear. In contrast, swelling and fullness in the popliteal fossa at or medial to the midline commonly represents a popliteal (Baker) cyst. A popliteal cyst can be associated with any process that produces a chronic effusion, such as a remote, isolated process that results in synovitis, or a generalized condition such as inflammatory arthritis.

A thorough understanding of the topical and underlying gross anatomy of the knee joint is imperative for diagnosing underlying knee pathology. The normal anatomic landmarks of the anterior knee may be obscured by a large knee effusion or diffuse soft tissue swelling. Bony landmarks should be identified and palpated, including the femoral epicondyles, fibular head, tibial tubercle, patellar margins, and medial and lateral joint lines. Bony thickening at the joint line suggests the presence of osteophytes. Note areas of localized tenderness. Soft tissue structures adjacent to or crossing the knee joint, such as the pes anserine bursa and hamstring tendons, are often significant pain generators and should not be ignored. The integrity of the extensor mechanism can be checked with an isometric quadriceps contraction and straight leg raise.

Knee range of motion can be assessed in the supine position. By convention, full extension is 0 degrees, with up to 10 degrees of hyperextension considered normal. Flexion in the normal adult knee is to approximately 135 or 140 degrees, with 105 degrees required for normal performance of activities of daily living in Western societies. Comparison of active and passive range of motion is necessary to distinguish between joint contracture and extensor lag. A flexion contracture is identified by the inability to passively position the knee in full extension. Causes include soft tissue contracture such as hamstring and gastrocnemius tightness, and mechanical block from a meniscus tear, loose body, or osteophyte formation. A discrepancy in active and passive extension represents an extensor lag and may be attributable to pain or extensor mechanism dysfunction from weakness or disruption. A knee with a large joint effusion assumes a 15- to 25-degree resting position and can cause loss of both active and passive flexion and extension. During range of motion assessment, crepitus is a common finding and may be localized to a particular compartment by palpation of the knee.

Evaluation of the patellofemoral joint should begin with the patient standing. The Q-angle (quadriceps angle), which is the acute angle formed by intersecting lines drawn from the center of the tibial tubercle to the center of the patella and from the center of the patella to the anterior-superior iliac spine, is a measure of the lateral pull of the quadriceps on the patella. A Q-angle >15 to 17 degrees is associated with altered patellofemoral mechanics and anterior knee pain. Complex torsional deformities of the lower extremity, most commonly increased femoral anteversion, can be associated with an increased Q-angle and should be evaluated during assessment of hip motion. Tracking of the patella in the femoral sulcus should be observed during gait and with both active and passive knee extension. Excessive lateral movement of the patella as it exits the femoral sulcus during terminal knee extension is known as the J-sign. Typically the patella does not articulate with the femoral sulcus until the knee is flexed 25 to 30 degrees, so patellar tilt and medial-lateral patellar glide should be assessed with the knee in a slightly flexed position. Lack of patellar mobility, as well as lateral tracking with crepitus as the knee flexes past 30 degrees, may indicate the presence of patellofemoral arthritis. Patella alta and baja can be assessed clinically with the knee flexed 90 degrees over the end of the exam table. Tenderness of the medial and lateral facets of the patella can be evaluated, but may be falsely positive in the presence of interposed synovitis.

Evaluation of the menisci should begin with palpation of the medial and lateral joint lines. Tenderness at the apex of a meniscal tear is a common finding owing to its peripheral nerve fibers and localized synovitis. Numerous provocative tests exist for evaluation of the menisci, most of which attempt to reproduce pain or palpable clicks by trapping the abnormally mobile or torn meniscus between two joint surfaces. Of these, the McMurray test is probably the most widely used. With the patient supine, the knee is brought into deep flexion and maximal external rotation with one hand on the foot. The opposite hand is placed on the knee with the fingers over the posteromedial joint line, and the knee is brought into extension while a varus force is applied to the knee. Posteromedial pain and a palpable or audible click indicate a positive test. The maneuver can be repeated for the posterolateral meniscus by internally rotating the tibia and applying a valgus force as the knee is passively extended.

Ligamentous Evaluation

Determination of knee joint stability is important for establishing a diagnosis and formulating potential conservative and operative treatment plans. The clinician must be able to distinguish isolated ligament deficiency from complex and rotational instability patterns. However, exhaustive review of the many specific tests for ligament integrity and complex instability patterns of the knee are beyond the scope of this chapter. Simple evaluation of the cruciate and collateral ligaments is presented here. The reader should refer to a comprehensive source for a complete review of the ligamentous examination of the knee.

The anterior cruciate ligament is the primary restraint to anterior movement of the tibia on the femur. Its integrity is best evaluated with the Lachman and anterior drawer tests.

The Lachman test is performed with the knee in 30 degrees of flexion. With one hand stabilizing the femur, anteriorly directed pull is applied to the tibia. A positive test results in excessive anterior translation of the tibia with a soft end point. In knees that are difficult to examine, such as those of obese patients, or in the setting of acute pain or swelling, the anterior drawer test may be useful. With the hip flexed 45 degrees and the knee flexed 90 degrees, the foot is stabilized on the exam table and again anteriorly directed pull is applied to the tibia. The posterior cruciate ligament is the primary restraint to posterior movement of the tibia on the femur. It is best evaluated with the posterior drawer test, performed with the extremity in the same position used for the anterior drawer test. A positive test is marked by posterior subluxation of the tibia on the femur when a posteriorly directed force is applied to the anterior tibia.

Evaluation of the collateral ligaments is performed by applying simple varus and valgus stresses to the knee in both full extension and again with the knee flexed 30 degrees. In full extension, the collateral ligaments, posterolateral capsule, and posteromedial capsule are all in a taut position. Therefore, varus and valgus stresses applied with the knee in full extension tests the integrity of the collateral ligaments as well as the posterolateral and posteromedial capsular structures. The posterior capsular structures relax when the knee is flexed 30 degrees, better isolating the collateral ligaments in resisting varus and valgus stresses. The cruciate ligaments are also taut in extension, so the presence of significant laxity to varus or valgus stress in full extension suggests cruciate ligament disruption in addition to collateral ligament disruption.

In knees with coronal plane deformities that exhibit varus-valgus instability, the clinician must distinguish true ligamentous insufficiency from pseudolaxity. For example, varus knees with osteoarthritis typically exhibit articular cartilage and bone loss in the medial compartment. Laxity to varus stress could represent lateral collateral ligament insufficiency or rotation of the tibia into varus as the medial femoral condyle settles into the defect in the medial tibial plateau. Conversely, laxity to valgus stress may represent correction of varus alignment as the tibia rotates back to neutral position. Inability to passively correct a coronal plane deformity may indicate the presence of long-standing disease with secondary medial or lateral soft tissue contracture that requires release at the time of reconstruction.

Neurologic and Vascular Evaluation

The neurovascular status of the affected extremity must not be neglected. Neurologic evaluation should include muscle testing, sensory examination, and assessment of deep tendon reflexes. Prior inspection should have identified atrophy or loss of muscle tone in the thigh and leg. Strength testing is performed by resisted isometric contraction of all major muscle groups, including hip flexion, extension, and abduction; knee flexion and extension; and ankle dorsiflexion and plantarflexion. Sensation can be evaluated by testing light touch, paying special attention to deficits in a dermatomal distribution. Deep tendon reflexes can be tested at the knee and ankle. The patellar reflex is predominantly an L4 reflex, and the Achilles reflex is an S1 reflex. Vascular assessment must include examination of the skin for signs of peripheral vascular disease, such as smooth shiny skin with hair loss, skin and subcutaneous soft tissue atrophy, and ulcerations. Palpation of peripheral pulses should include femoral, popliteal, posterior tibial, and dorsalis pedis pulses.

SUGGESTED READINGS

Bellamy N, Buchanan WW, Goldsmith CH, et al. Validation study of WOMAC: a health status instrument for measuring clinically important patient relevant outcomes to antirheumatic drug therapy in patients with osteoarthritis of the hip or knee. *J Rheumatol*. 1988;15:1833–1840.

Clark JP, Hudak PL, Hawker GA, et al. The moving target: a qualitative study of elderly patients' decision-making regarding total joint replacement surgery. *J Bone Joint Surg Am*. 2004; 86:1366–1374.

Insall JN, Dorr LD, Scott RD, et al. Rationale of the Knee Society clinical rating system. *Clin Orthop Relat Res*. 1989;248:13–14.

Liorzou G. *Knee Ligaments: Clinical Examination*. Berlin: Springer-Verlag; 1991.

Mundermann A, Dyrby CO, Andriacchi TP. Secondary gait changes in patients with medial compartment knee osteoarthritis. *Arthritis Rheum*. 2005;52:2835–2844.

Reider B. Knee. In: Reider B, ed. *The Orthopaedic Physical Examination*. 2nd ed. Philadelphia: Elsevier; 2005;201–246.

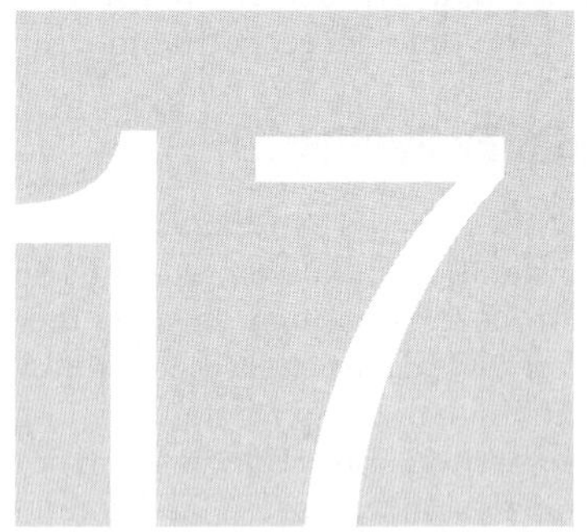

IMAGING OF THE KNEE

JASON R. HULL

Although the history and physical examination are the most important instruments in evaluating joint pain, musculoskeletal imaging remains an essential adjunct. Multiple imaging modalities are available to confirm a provisional diagnosis or narrow the differential diagnosis. Because many imaging techniques are costly and require radiation exposure for the patient, they should be used judiciously. Imaging should begin with a standard set of plain radiographs, with special radiographic views and more elaborate modalities used if indicated. Once a diagnosis is established and a treatment plan initiated, imaging also can be used to monitor disease progression or response to treatment.

PLAIN RADIOGRAPHY

Plain radiography is the modality of choice for initial confirmatory or screening imaging. Modern equipment and techniques have reduced the amount of ionizing radiation required for routine radiography. The equipment and processing are relatively inexpensive and widely accessible compared with other modalities. The osseous anatomy of the knee is simple and easily understood, making interpretation of the images straightforward.

Initial Radiographic Evaluation

To some degree the images included in a screening examination are a matter of preference and may even be tailored to answer specific questions raised during the history and physical examination. However, the initial radiographic examination should include the least amount of radiation necessary to adequately visualize the essential anatomic features of the knee:

- Osseous structures of the distal femur, proximal tibia, and patella
- Alignment of the knee joint
- Joint space
- Periarticular soft tissues

The author prefers four views for the initial radiographic examination: (i) standing weight-bearing anteroposterior (AP) view, (ii) standing weight-bearing posteroanterior (PA) flexion view, (iii) lateral view, and (iv) axial view of the patella.

The standing AP view of the knee (Fig. 17-1A) is obtained with the patient standing with equal weight on both lower extremities, knees fully extended, and toes pointing straight ahead. The beam is positioned horizontally at the level of the distal pole of the patella. Inclusion of both knees on one image allows for careful side-to-side comparison for subtle abnormalities. Like a standard non–weight-bearing AP radiograph, the standing AP view allows inspection of many osseous landmarks of the knee, including the distal surfaces of the femoral condyles, medial and lateral epicondyles, medial and lateral tibial plateaus, tibial spines, and the head of the fibula. However, the weight-bearing radiograph more accurately represents the condition of the articular surface and is more likely to exhibit tibiofemoral joint space narrowing if pathology is present. With no mechanical load through the knee, non–weight-bearing technique allows relaxation through the joint and may project artificial widening of the joint space. In addition, much like physical evaluation, assessment of tibiofemoral alignment on a weight-bearing radiograph better illustrates the functional alignment of the joint.

With the exception of stationary standing, few weight-bearing activities occur with the knee in full extension. In addition, tibiofemoral contact area decreases and contact force increases as the knee flexes, making the posterior weight-bearing surfaces of the femoral condyles susceptible to early degeneration under pathologic conditions. The addition of a weight-bearing 45-degree PA flexion view allows for assessment of the posterior weight-bearing surfaces of the femoral condyles and provides a tangential view of the medial and lateral weight-bearing surfaces of the tibial plateau (Fig. 17-1B). This view is also obtained with the patient standing with equal weight on both lower extremities and toes pointing straight ahead, but the knees are flexed 45 degrees with the patellae touching the vertically oriented radiograph cassette. The beam is directed posteroanterior, angled 10 degrees caudad, and centered at the level of the distal pole of the patella. An additional advantage of this view is visualization of the intercondylar notch of the femur, similar to that observed with a traditional tunnel view.

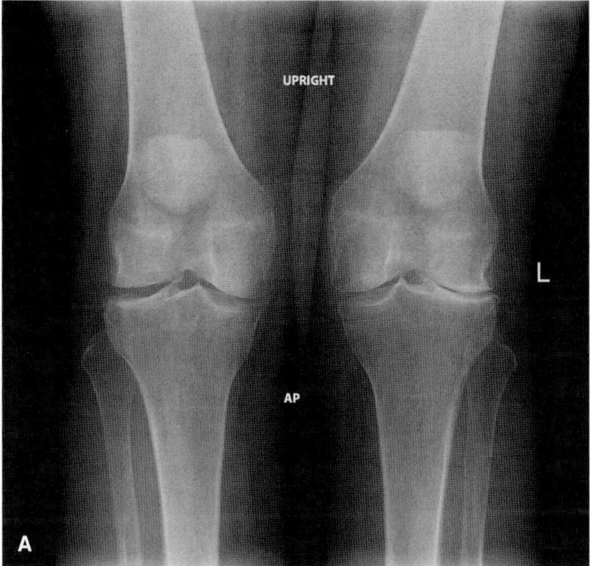

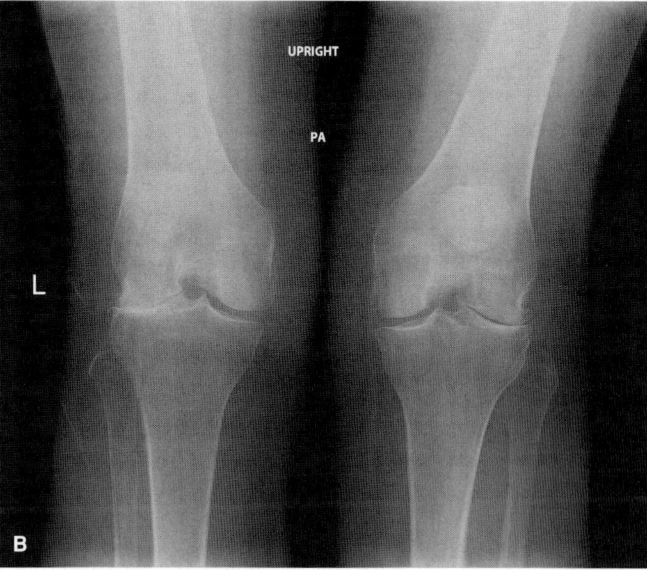

Figure 17-1 A: Standing anteroposterior view of the knees demonstrates significant narrowing of the lateral compartment joint space in the left knee with a well-maintained joint space of the contralateral right knee. B: Weight-bearing 45-degree posteroanterior flexion view reveals complete loss of the lateral compartment joint space in both knees.

The lateral view of the knee (Fig. 17-2) is obtained with the patient lying with the lateral aspect of the affected knee against the radiograph table. With the knee flexed approximately 30 degrees, the x-ray beam is directed tangential to the surfaces of the tibial plateau, perpendicular to the radiograph cassette under the lateral aspect of the knee. The lateral view also visualizes most landmarks of the distal femur, proximal fibula, and proximal tibia, adding an orthogonal view for complete evaluation of osseous architecture. Additionally, the proximal and distal poles of the patella and relationships of the patellofemoral articulation can be assessed, as well as the soft tissues of the extensor mechanism.

A tangential axial view of the patella (Fig. 17-3) must be obtained to visualize the medial and lateral facets of the patella, alignment of the patella within the femoral sulcus, and the status of the patellofemoral joint space. Multiple techniques have been described for obtaining the axial view, differing only by angle of knee flexion at which the image is obtained. The Merchant view is probably the most popular and widely used method, owing to its clear representation of the medial and lateral patellar facets, patellofemoral joint space, and alignment. The view is obtained with patient's knees flexed 45 degrees over the end of the exam table. The x-ray beam is directed caudally through the patella, at an angle 30 degrees below horizontal, at a film cassette resting on the patient's shins in a position perpendicular to the x-ray beam.

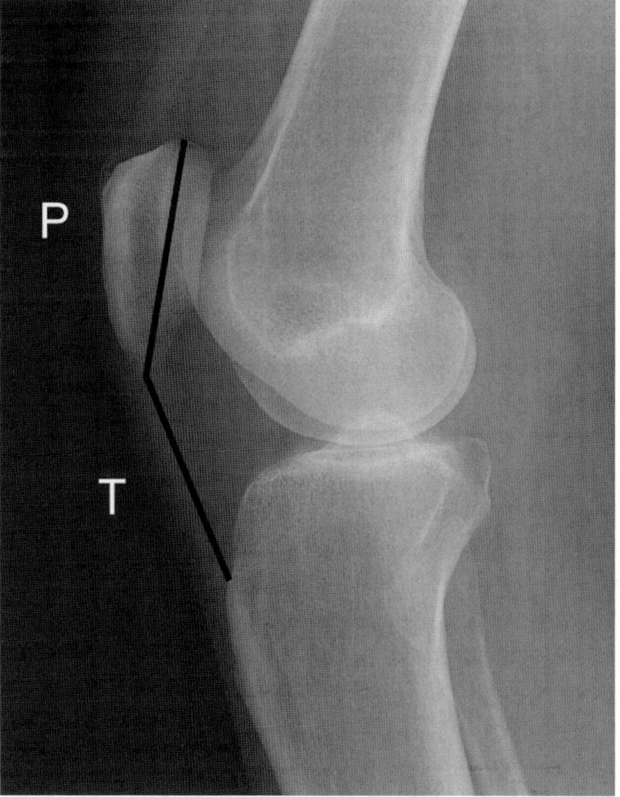

Figure 17-2 Lateral view of the knee. The Insall-Salvati ratio (T/P) can be used to determine the height of the patella relative to the sulcus of the distal femur. The ratio of the length of the patellar tendon (T) to the diagonal length of the patella (P) should differ by no more than 20%.

Image Interpretation

Evaluation of any plain radiograph must be performed in a routine, systematic fashion. The patient's name, date of examination, and laterality (right versus left) of the image

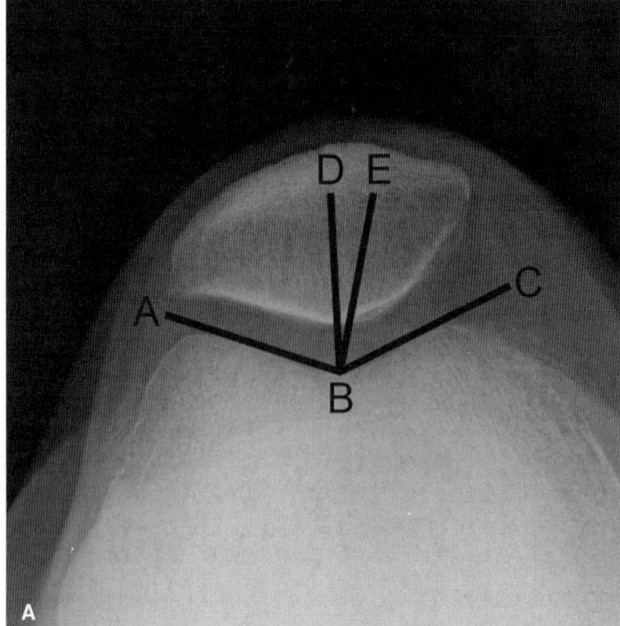

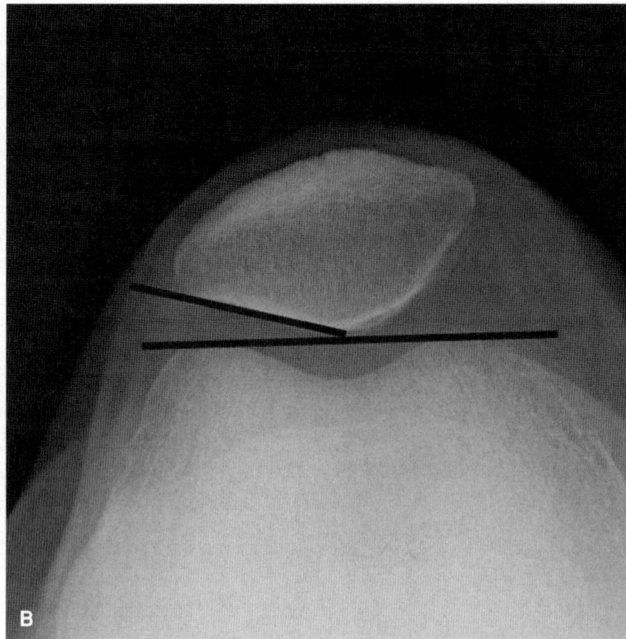

Figure 17-3 Merchant view of the knee. **A:** To measure the congruence angle, line DB is established as a reference line that bisects the sulcus angle ABC. A second line is drawn from the apex (ridge) of the patella to the center of the sulcus. Congruence angle DBE is positive if it opens lateral to reference line DB, and measurements greater than approximately 15 degrees indicate lateral patellofemoral subluxation. **B:** The lateral patellofemoral angle is formed by a tangent across the medial and lateral condyles and a line parallel to the lateral facet of the patella. An angle that opens medially represents excessive lateral patellar tilt.

must be verified. The clinician should briefly review the image for quality control to make sure all pertinent anatomy is visualized, paying particular attention to image penetration, joint position, and orientation of the x-ray beam.

The clinician must review the extent of the patient's soft tissue and osseous anatomy visible on an image. Like the components of a thorough history, the findings peripheral to the knee joint may provide valuable diagnostic clues and historical data that could alter the diagnosis or treatment plan. The presence of significant vascular calcification indicates the presence of peripheral vascular disease and may preclude the use of a tourniquet should surgical intervention be warranted. Evidence of posttraumatic or postsurgical changes may be evident in the femoral or tibial diaphyses near the margins of the image, requiring additional images for complete evaluation. Rarely, occult soft tissue masses and neoplasms may be identified as subtle soft tissue densities adjacent or peripheral to the knee joint. Likewise, osseous neoplasms may be identified, either as an incidental finding or as the primary source of the patient's symptoms.

Osseous Structures

Evaluation of the osseous structures of the knee begins with identification of all major osseous landmarks (Table 17-1) and assessment of general architecture. The lateral femoral condyle is normally smaller than the medial condyle and exhibits a more acute radius of curvature posteriorly. The medial and lateral tibial plateaus are also asymmetric, with the larger medial plateau demonstrating a concave contour on the lateral projection and the lateral plateau exhibiting slight convexity. Both tibial surfaces slope posteriorly approximately 10 degrees. The patella, best visualized on the axial view, consists of asymmetric medial and lateral facets.

TABLE 17-1 RADIOGRAPHIC LANDMARKS AND ANATOMY OF THE KNEE

Femur

- Medial and lateral condyles
- Intercondylar notch
- Medial and lateral epicondyles
- Physeal scar

Tibia

- Medial and lateral tibial plateaus
- Tibial spines
- Tibial tubercle
- Physeal scar

Fibula

- Upper end (head)

Patella

- Medial and lateral facets
- Proximal and distal poles

The medial facet is smaller and slightly convex, and the larger lateral facet is concave in the coronal plane. Gross abnormalities in size, shape, contour, or spatial relationships of major osseous structures may indicate the presence of congenital, developmental, or posttraumatic pathology.

Osseous structures must be inspected for intraosseous abnormalities indicative of metabolic or neoplastic processes. Bone quality and mineralization can provide diagnostic clues, with generalized osteopenia present in the setting of inflammatory arthritides as a result of intense regional hyperemia. Conversely, degenerative conditions are associated with increased mineralization in the subchondral region as a result of increased local stresses. All joint surfaces should be examined for focal defects, wear patterns, and other signs of remodeling such as osteophyte formation.

Alignment

The anatomic axis of the knee is represented by the intersection of lines drawn parallel to the long axes of the femur and tibia and is typically between five and seven degrees of valgus. In most patients, the standing AP view allows for adequate assessment of tibiofemoral alignment in the coronal plane. However, patients with pre-existing congenital, posttraumatic, or postsurgical deformities of the femur or tibia require an AP long-leg hip to ankle radiograph for accurate assessment of the anatomic axis (Fig. 17-4). The mechanical weight-bearing axis of the knee, illustrated by a straight line drawn from the center of the femoral head to the center of the ankle joint, can also be determined on the long-leg radiograph. A line passing through the middle third of the proximal tibia represents a neutral mechanical axis, whereas lines passing through the medial third and lateral third represent varus and valgus mechanical axes, respectively.

The relationship of the patella to the distal femur must be evaluated on both the lateral and axial images of the knee. The height of the patella relative to the distal femur is evaluated on the lateral radiograph using the Insall-Salvati ratio (Fig. 17-2). Normal patellar height is represented by a ratio of one, whereas ratios of 0.8 and 1.2 represent patella baja and patella alta, respectively. The relationship of the patella to the sulcus of the distal femur is evaluated on the axial view of the patella. Patellofemoral subluxation can be evaluated objectively by calculating the congruence angle (Fig. 17-3A). When the apex of the patella lies lateral to the center of the femoral sulcus and the congruence angle is >15 degrees, lateral patellofemoral subluxation is present. The lateral patellofemoral angle assesses patellar tilt (Fig. 17-3B) and opens medially in the presence of abnormal lateral tilt.

Articular Cartilage and Joint Space

Erosion of articular cartilage, expressed as joint space narrowing on plain radiographs, is the final common pathway for many disease processes of the knee joint and must be accurately assessed in the medial, lateral, and patellofemoral compartments. Many disease processes produce predictable patterns of joint space narrowing. For example, inflammatory conditions result in generalized enzymatic destruction of articular cartilage and diffuse joint space narrowing on plain radiographs. Conversely, osteoarthritis begins as a localized mechanical process that leads to focal cartilage loss and joint space narrowing.

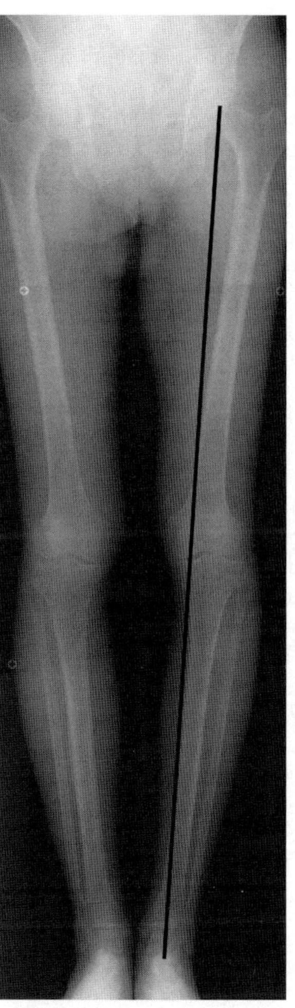

Figure 17-4 Anteroposterior long-leg hip-to-ankle radiograph. The mechanical axis of the limb is determined by a line between the center of the femoral head and the center of the ankle.

As stated previously, a standing AP radiograph is more predictive of tibiofemoral articular cartilage loss than a non–weight-bearing view. However, the weightbearing 45-degree PA flexion view is the most sensitive plain radiographic method for detection of tibiofemoral joint space narrowing (Fig. 17-1). With this technique, the x-ray beam is tangential to the weight-bearing surfaces of the femoral condyles and tibial plateau and perpendicular to the desired joint space measurement, therefore providing accurate assessment of the actual joint space. Because the patella does not enter the femoral sulcus until the knee is flexed 30 degrees, axial views of the patellofemoral joint must be obtained at flexion angles >30 degrees to visualize the patellofemoral articulation. The traditional skyline view is obtained with the knee flexed >90 degrees, and in this degree of flexion the patella contacts the femur distal to the femoral sulcus. The patellofemoral joint space is well visualized on the Merchant view, obtained at 45 degrees of knee flexion (Fig. 17-3).

Soft Tissues

Differential absorption of the x-ray beam by adjacent tissues of varying composition allows visualization of many peripheral soft tissue features. The extensor mechanism is the only normal periarticular soft tissue structure routinely visualized on plain radiographs. On the lateral view, adjacent adipose tissue delineates the linear soft tissue densities of the quadriceps and patellar tendons proximal and distal to the patella, respectively. Many pathologic processes can be diagnosed by their characteristic appearance as soft tissue densities. On the lateral image, joint effusion is an easily identified soft tissue mass deep to the quadriceps tendon. Popliteal cysts are also fluid-filled masses occasionally identified as soft tissue densities on the lateral radiograph. Intra-articular and extra-articular soft tissue structures are commonly visualized secondary to calcification. Intra-articular findings include chondrocalcinosis from deposition of calcium pyrophosphate dihydrate crystals in articular cartilage and menisci. Osteocartilaginous loose bodies are associated with many conditions affecting the articular surface, including trauma, chondromalacia patella, osteochondritis desiccans, and osteoarthritis. They may be identified anywhere within the knee joint including the femoral notch, suprapatellar pouch, medial and lateral gutters, and the posterior recesses of the knee. Extra-articular soft tissue calcifications commonly occur in tendinous and ligamentous structures. Calcification at the origin of the medial collateral ligament (Pellegrini-Stieda sign) signifies prior injury to the medial collateral ligament. Notable soft tissue calcifications in the region of the popliteal vessels may suggest need for further evaluation with ultrasonography to rule out aneurysm and pseudoaneurysm of the popliteal artery.

MAGNETIC RESONANCE IMAGING

Magnetic resonance imaging (MRI) has become a powerful complement to plain radiography for evaluation of the painful knee. Although costly, MRI has many advantages over other imaging modalities and has supplanted many older imaging techniques. MRI provides multiplanar capability and unrivaled image contrast with spatial resolution comparable with that of computed tomography (CT). The ability to enhance tissue contrast by variation of scanning parameters allows for comprehensive evaluation of all osseous and soft tissue structures of the knee, including articular cartilage, without exposing the patient to ionizing radiation.

The utility of MRI for evaluation of overuse and acute injuries to soft tissue structures of the knee, including tendons, capsuloligamentous structures, and the menisci, is unrivaled and is well documented in the orthopaedic and sports medicine literature. The reader is referred to other sources for a comprehensive review of these topics.

MRI can be particularly useful in the early diagnosis of many pathologic processes of bone before they are detectable by plain radiography. Osteonecrosis, stress fracture, osteomyelitis, and neoplasm may all share a stage when patients present with significant symptoms but normal plain

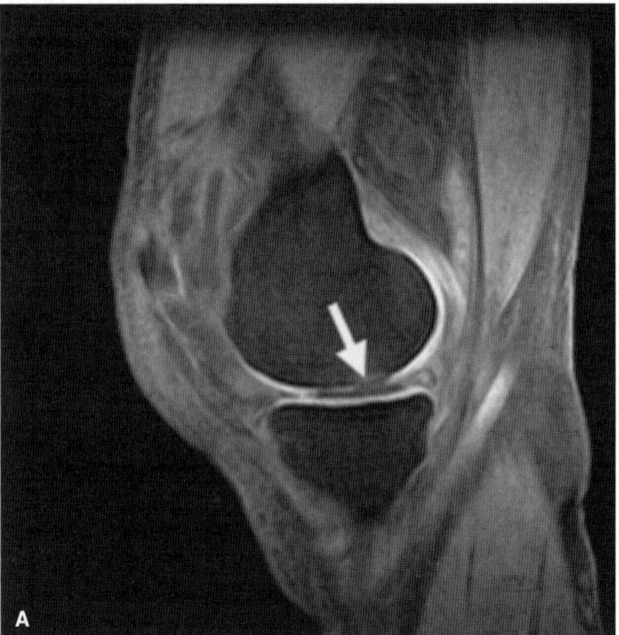

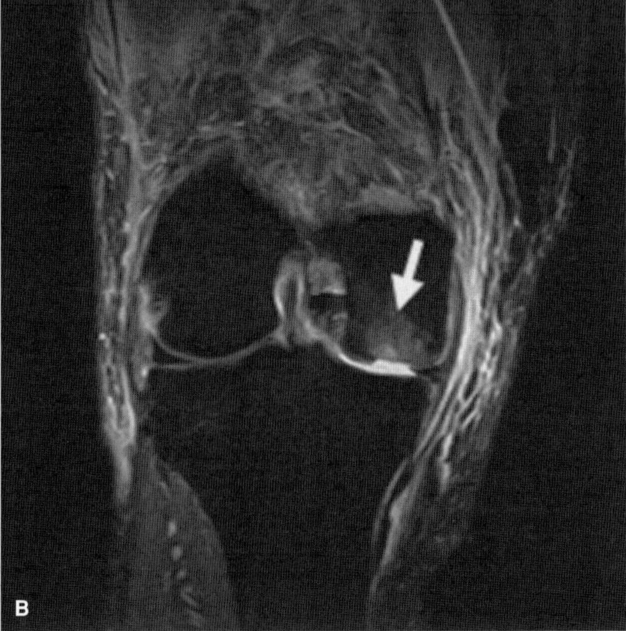

Figure 17-5 Images depicting a high-grade articular cartilage defect in the distal weight-bearing surface of the medial femoral condyle. **A:** Sagittal fat-suppressed three-dimensional spoiled gradient-echo image demonstrating fluid, which is low signal intensity, within the lesion (*arrow*). **B:** Coronal short time inversion recovery (STIR) image of the same lesion. Note the adjacent edema in the subchondral bone (*arrow*).

radiographs. All of these conditions cause early accumulation of marrow edema at the site of the lesion. MRI capitalizes on these early changes in local tissue characteristics, which are manifested as areas of high signal on T2-weighted images.

Assessment of isolated articular cartilage injuries has improved with the implementation of imaging sequences designed specifically for articular cartilage. The two most commonly used sequences are the T1 fat-suppressed three-dimensional (3D) spoiled gradient-echo technique and the T2 fast spin echo technique. The 3D gradient echo sequence displays articular cartilage as a smooth band of hyperintense tissue along the cortical margin of the articular surface (Fig. 17-5A). On the T2 fast spin echo sequence, articular cartilage is a smooth band of intermediate signal intensity. Articular defects in this sequence are visualized much as an arthrogram, with hyperintense fluid filling the defect and interrupting the normally smooth contour. Both techniques exhibit a high degree of accuracy, with the best results in the patellofemoral joint where the hyaline cartilage is thickest. The short time inversion recovery (STIR) sequence is also a commonly used sequence and produces images similar to the fast spin echo technique (Fig. 17-5B).

Interest in MRI evaluation of articular cartilage of the knee has increased in recent years, mostly because of the development of articular cartilage restoration procedures. The improved imaging techniques help identify appropriate candidates for reconstruction, aid in preoperative planning, and provide a reliable method for following postoperative progress and response to treatment without the need for repeat arthroscopy. Imaging of the articular surface can also help with patient selection for corrective osteotomies about the knee, with or without the need for cartilage restoration. Imaging can offer preoperative prognostic information to patients undergoing arthroscopy for other reasons, as the presence of articular surface defects has a negative impact on clinical outcome.

SUGGESTED READINGS

Ahlback S. Osteoarthrosis of the knee. A radiographic investigation. *Acta Radiol*. 1968;277(suppl):7–72.

Elias DA, White LM. Imaging of patellofemoral disorders. *Clin Rad*. 2004;59:543–557.

Gold GE, Hargreaves BA, Stevens KJ, et al. Advanced magnetic resonance imaging of articular cartilage. *Orthop Clin North Am*. 2006;37:331–347.

Jungius KP, Schmid MR, Zanetti M, et al. Cartilaginous defects of the femorotibial joint: accuracy of coronal short inversion time inversion-recovery MR sequence. *Radiology*. 2006;240:482–488.

Leach RE, Gregg T, Siber FJ. Weight bearing radiography in osteoarthritis of the knee. *Radiologica*. 1970;97:265–268.

McGrory JE, Trousdale RT, Pagnano MW, et al. Preoperative hip to ankle radiographs in total knee arthroplasty. *Clin Orthop Rel Res*. 2002;404:196–202.

Merchant AC, Mercer RL, Jacobsen RH, et al. Roentgenographic analysis of patellofemoral congruence. *J Bone Joint Surg Am*. 1974;56:1391–1396.

Rosenberg TD, Paulos LE, Parker RD, et al. The forty-five degree posteroanterior flexion weightbearing radiograph of the knee. *J Bone Joint Surg Am*. 1988;70:1479–1483.

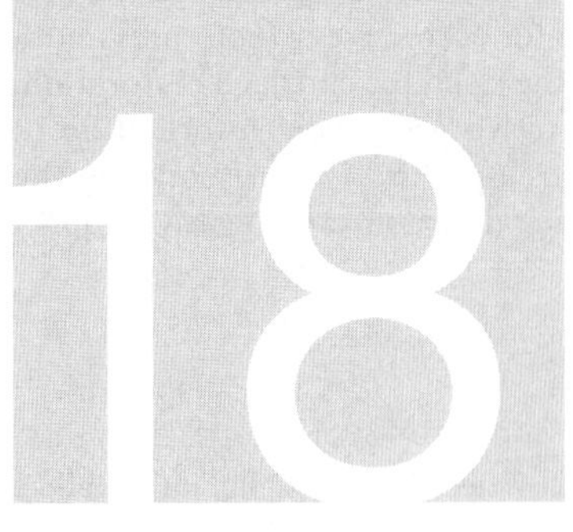

OSTEOARTHRITIS AND INFLAMMATORY ARTHRITIS OF THE KNEE

HARI P. BEZWADA
JESS H. LONNER
ROBERT E. BOOTH, JR.

In the presence of arthritis, pain is the leading reason for patients to present for medical evaluation. They may have either monoarticular or polyarticular complaints. Osteoarthritis affects >40 million people annually, and there is an association with advanced age. Rheumatoid arthritis, although far less prevalent, commonly has a younger age of onset and often is more debilitating than osteoarthritis, with polyarticular and systemic manifestations. It is important to differentiate inflammatory from noninflammatory arthritis, as the diagnosis has clear implications in terms of both treatment and prognosis.

OSTEOARTHRITIS

Osteoarthritis is the end result of various disorders that lead to structural or functional failures in one or both knees. The knee is a diarthrodial joint with bone, cartilage, and connective tissue. The subchondral bone is covered by hyaline cartilage, which is made up of type II collagen, chondrocytes, and proteoglycans. The arrangement of type II collagen along the joint surface provides tensile strength. Proteoglycans assist with water retention and provide a low-friction bearing surface and shock absorption. Normal synovial fluid provides nourishment to hyaline cartilage and has viscoelastic properties. The volume of synovial fluid increases in osteoarthritis and is high in prostaglandins, collagenases, tumor necrosis factor 1, and interleukins. Osteoarthritic synovial fluid is also low in hyaluronate.

Repetitive microtrauma is thought to create biomechanical alterations in the cartilage matrix, which leads to subsequent breakdown of both cartilage and subchondral bone. The water content within the type II collagen increases and proteoglycan synthesis increases in an attempt to promote joint repair. Chondrocytes within the cartilage matrix eventually become overwhelmed with attempting repair and release metalloproteinases. The metalloproteinases cause further destruction and thinning of the cartilage matrix. More subchondral bone becomes exposed as the cartilage thins, leading to increased stresses and subchondral sclerosis along with the development of osteophytes. Subchondral cysts form as synovial fluid is forced beneath the joint surface.

The severity of osteoarthritis is best determined by reviewing weight-bearing radiographs. Typical radiographs include weight-bearing anteroposterior and lateral views. Patellar skyline or Merchant views are best to evaluate the patellofemoral joint, patellar tracking, and patellar tilt. A weight-bearing 45-degree flexion or notch view (posteroanterior) is useful in evaluating degenerative changes mostly involving the posterior femoral condyles. Magnetic resonance imaging, nuclear scans, and computed tomography have limited utility.

INFLAMMATORY ARTHRITIS

Classic signs of inflammatory arthritis include warmth, erythema, swelling, synovitis, and pain. The presentation may involve a single or multiple joints with additional systemic complaints. The illness may have a waxing and waning course. The level of joint involvement may be symmetrical or asymmetrical and acute or chronic. The keys to diagnosis include careful history and physical examination and judicious review of appropriate laboratory and imaging studies.

Rheumatoid arthritis (RA) is the most prevalent chronic, symmetrical inflammatory polyarticular arthritis. Clinical

TABLE 18-1 DIFFERENTIAL DIAGNOSIS OF INFLAMMATORY ARTHRITIS

Lyme disease
HIV-associated arthritis
Hepatitis C
Rheumatoid arthritis
Crystal arthritis
Reiter syndrome
Acute rheumatic fever
Psoriatic arthritis
Bowel-related arthritis
Juvenile arthritis
Ankylosing spondylitis
Connective tissue disease
Viral arthritis
Mycobacterial arthritis
Fungal arthritis

findings include rheumatoid nodules, symmetrical synovitis, seropositive rheumatoid factor, synovial fluid inflammatory findings, and radiographic changes including erosions and osteopenia. Osteophytes and sclerosis are unusual in RA.

Lyme disease may have either a monoarticular or polyarticular presentation, and there is typically a history of a tick bite and a target skin lesion (erythema chronicum migrans). However, both the history and presence of constitutional symptoms are variable. Serologies (Lyme titers) are useful in confirming the diagnosis; synovial fluid analysis may show an elevated white blood cell count with a preponderance of neutrophils.

Other inflammatory arthropathies include Reiter disease, psoriatic arthritis, and seronegative rheumatoid arthritis. Various rheumatologic tests, such as rheumatoid factor, antinuclear antibody, and HLA B-27, can help establish the diagnosis. Arthritis may also be associated with HIV infection, hepatitis C infection, inflammatory bowel disease, crystal deposition, and connective tissue disorders (Table 18-1).

SYNOVIAL ANALYSIS

Synovial fluid analysis is a useful adjunct in differentiating inflammatory, noninflammatory, and septic arthritis. Aspiration should be performed with caution in patients with overlying cellulitis or soft tissue infection because of the risk of direct inoculation of the joint. Normal knee synovial fluid has a volume of several milliliters and a white blood cell count <200. Synovial fluid also contains hyaluronate (glycosaminoglycan) produced by synoviocytes and is typically transparent with a straw color.

Abnormal synovial fluid has increased volume, decreased viscosity, diminished clarity, and a change in color. Microscopic analysis for the numbers and types of cells as well as the presence of crystals is important. Synovial fluid culture, serologic analysis, and immunologic evaluations should be performed as necessary (Table 18-2).

TREATMENT

Nonoperative Treatment

The first line of treatment for arthritis of the knee includes both physical modalities and pharmacologic interventions. The goals are simply to decrease pain and improve function. Presently, little can be done to reverse the degenerative process (Tables 18-3, 18-4).

Physical Therapy

Physical therapy can improve and maintain the patient's functional level. Physical therapy programs should consist of stretching, proprioceptive exercise, strengthening, and conditioning. Range of motion and stretching are critical parts of a therapy program as they help to maintain function. The quadriceps atrophy that occurs with knee arthritis may be both rapid and dramatic. Most exercise and strengthening programs are focused on the quadriceps mechanism, although hamstring strengthening may be important for balancing the quadriceps/hamstrings ratio. Patients with knee arthritis who undergo quadriceps strengthening show

TABLE 18-2 SYNOVIAL FLUID ANALYSIS

	Noninflammatory	Inflammatory	Septic
Color	Straw-colored	Yellow	Variable
Clarity	Transparent	Translucent	Opaque
Total WBC	200–3,000	2,000–75,000	Usually >100,000
Differential			
PMNs	<25%	>50%	>75%
Lymphocytes	<25%	<25%	<10%
Monocytes	None	25%	<10%
Crystals	None	May be present	None
Protein	Usually normal	>32 g/dL	>3 g/dL
Glucose	90% of blood	75% of blood	50% of blood
Culture	Negative	Negative	Positive

WBC, white blood count; PMNs, leukocytes (polymorphonuclear).

TABLE 18-3 MEDICAL TREATMENT OF INFLAMMATORY ARTHRITIS

Nonsteroidal anti-inflammatory drugs (NSAIDs)
- Salicylates
- Cyclooxygenase-1 inhibitors
- Cyclooxygenase-2 inhibitors

Disease-modifying antirheumatic drugs ((DMARDS)
- Gold
- Antimalarials (hydroxychloroquine, chloroquine)
- Sulfasalazine
- Penicillamine
- Azathioprine
- Methotrexate
- Cyclosporine
- Leflunomide
- Etanercept
- Corticosteroids

improvements in quadriceps strength, knee pain, and function. Isometric exercises are generally best tolerated. General aerobic conditioning from low-impact exercises improves both patients' overall health and arthritic symptoms. Water therapy is especially useful in obese patients as the force of gravity is virtually eliminated. Warm water hydrotherapy raises body temperature, causes superficial vasodilatation, increases peripheral circulation, has a sedative effect on nerve endings, and causes muscle relaxation.

Biomechanical Devices

Valgus-producing unloader knee braces may be helpful in varus gonarthrosis especially when there is instability and lateral thrust. These braces use a three-point pressure system to decrease the deformity and off-load the affected compartment. Brace-wear compliance is variable, as unloader braces tend to be uncomfortable and less effective in the obese. Orthotics, namely lateral heel wedges, may also be helpful in varus gonarthrosis. Patients with valgus knee deformities in association with a planovalgus foot may benefit from a foot-ankle orthosis. Assistive devices such as a cane or walker substantially reduce forces across the affected joint.

External Energy

Therapeutic heat may produce analgesia of the free nerve endings and subsequent muscle relaxation. The obligatory increase in blood flow from local heat may also wash out inflammatory mediators. Ultrasound is a deep heat modality that may have efficacy in relieving arthritis pain. It also has mechanical effects that create fluid movements around cells, which in turn alters cell permeability, promotes collagen synthesis, and alters painful nerve fibers. The use of transcutaneous electrical neuromuscular stimulation (TENS) has been controversial. Cryotherapy may reduce pain by reducing muscle spindle activity and raising the pain threshold.

Weight Loss and Activity Modification

Modest weight loss may have dramatic effects on arthritis pain. Joint reactive forces may reach three to four times body weight across the knee. This factor increases to sevenfold to eightfold across the patellofemoral joint in deep flexion. The increased joint forces from body weight are also affected by cyclical loading, i.e., number of steps taken. Activity modification also may be chondroprotective. Excessive impact loading of the knee should be avoided as it may have a deleterious effect on knee function and arthritis.

Pharmacologic Interventions

The most commonly used nonnarcotic analgesic is acetaminophen, which can be effective, particularly in milder cases, when used frequently as a first-line treatment for arthritis. The risks include hepatotoxicity and interstitial nephritis in large regular doses. Narcotic analgesics may be effective for temporary pain relief, but have well-known side effects on the central nervous system and gastrointestinal system.

TABLE 18-4 TREATMENT OF THE ARTHRITIC KNEE

I. Nonoperative treatment
  A. Physical therapy
    1) Exercise
    2) Water therapy
  B. Biomechanical
    1) Bracing/orthotics
    2) Assistive devices (cane, crutches)
  C. External energy
    1) Heat
    2) Ultrasound
    3) Transcutaneous electrical neuromuscular stimulation (TENS)
    4) Cryotherapy
  D. Education
    1) Weight loss
    2) Activity modification
  E. Alternative treatments
    1) Acupuncture
    2) Biofeedback
  F. Pharmacologic intervention
    1) Analgesics
    2) Nonsteroidal anti-inflammatory drugs (NSAIDs)
    3) Viscosupplementation
    4) Injectable corticosteroids
  G. Nutraceuticals/dietary supplements
    1) Glucosamine/chondroitin
  H. Topical agents
    1) Capsicin
    2) Aspercreme
II. Operative treatment
  A. Arthroscopy
  B. Osteotomy
    1) High tibial osteotomy
    2) Distal femoral osteotomy
  C. Unicompartmental knee arthroplasty
  D. Total knee arthroplasty

Nonsteroidal Anti-inflammatory Drugs (NSAIDs). One of the first-line therapies in the medical management of inflammatory arthritis is nonsteroidal anti-inflammatory drugs (NSAIDs). Salicylates were among the first NSAIDs used with typical doses of 300 to 600 mg three to four times a day. Salicylates should not be used in gout as they have been implicated in increasing serum uric acid levels. The main side effects are gastrointestinal, hematologic, hepatic, and renal.

Most NSAIDs inhibit the cyclo-oxygenase enzymes. The exceptions include nonacetylated salicylates such as Arthropan, Trilisate, and Disalcid. Cyclo-oxygenase is critical in producing prostaglandins. Prostaglandins have many effects in the body, including vasodilation, gastrointestinal mucosal protection, and inflammation. Prostaglandin E_2 may contribute to local inflammation within the joint space. It appears that reducing the amount of prostaglandin E_2 leads to less joint pain. The most common side effects of NSAIDs are on the gastrointestinal system; the frequency ranges from 15% to 35%. Renal toxicity also may occur as a result of interstitial nephritis or renal hypoperfusion.

Two subgroups of cyclo-oxygenase have been discovered. Cyclo-oxygenase-1 (COX-1) is found in most tissues and is important in maintaining mucosal integrity of the gastrointestinal tract and renal perfusion. Cyclooxygenase-2 (COX-2) is found mostly at the site of inflammation. Selective COX-2 inhibitors are associated with improved gastric tolerance compared with other NSAIDs. Recent evidence has suggested that there is an increase in adverse cardiac events in patients with cardiac disease treated with some COX-2 inhibitors, so the indication for their use over an extended period of time is yet to be defined.

Disease-modifying antirheumatic drugs include gold compounds, antimalarials, sulfasalazine, penicillamine, cytotoxic drugs (azathioprine, methotrexate), cyclosporine, and flunomide. Recent developments include tumor necrosis factor antagonists, examples of which include etanercept, infliximab, and adalimumab (Table 18-3).

Injectable Corticosteroids. Typical intra-articular injection combines a synthetic corticosteroid and local anesthetic. The addition of a local anesthetic reduces the incidence of postinjection symptom flare. Multiple studies have supported an improvement in symptoms over placebo 1 to 2 weeks following injection. Yet by 4 weeks, the results become very similar. Although corticosteroids are commonly administered, there is little literature to direct surgeons as to the optimal steroid preparation, dosage, frequency, and length of treatment. Systemic side effects from corticosteroid injections include allergic reactions, intra-articular infection, and potential hyperglycemia in brittle diabetics. Frequent injections over the long term are associated with local fat atrophy and cartilage degeneration from decreased collagen formation. Additionally, pain masking may lead to overuse and cartilage breakdown. Therefore most clinicians recommend that injections be given no more frequently than every 3 or 4 months.

Viscosupplementation. Hyaluronic acid is a key constituent of both cartilage and synovial fluid. Osteoarthritis is associated with a loss of hyaluronic acid from the cartilage and the production of low-molecular-weight hyaluronic acid by synoviocytes. The result is the presence of a less viscous hyaluronate in the arthritic joint. Hyaluronic acid injection may be considered for patients with symptomatic osteoarthritis that has not responded to other conservative measures.

Several products are available; the differences between them are mainly based on the molecular weight of the cross-linked hyaluronic acids. It is not clear how formulation differences impact clinical efficacy or response. Multiple studies appear to support the efficacy of each of these formulations, with a low-risk side effect profile. The most common side effect is a sterile partial inflammatory effusion, which can be difficult to distinguish from infection. Hyaluronic acid appears better than placebo, and the effect is similar to that of nonsteroidal anti-inflammatories. The analgesic effect appears to last for several months. A course of viscosupplementation may be repeated every 6 months, although the efficacy may be reduced and the risk of allergic reaction may increase.

Nutraceuticals/Dietary Supplements

Although studies are scant and poorly controlled, there has been some suggestion that certain naturally occurring dietary supplements, herbal remedies, and so-called nutraceuticals may be helpful in the management of knee arthritis. Omega-3 fatty acids may reduce the production of inflammatory mediators in the body and have been shown to reduce stiffness in patients with rheumatoid arthritis. Methylsulfonylmethane (MSM), glucosamine, and chondroitin sulphate are popular supplements that have been touted for their virtues in slowing down the progression of arthritis. Glucosamine ostensibly enhances cartilage production and reduces pain to a level similar to that of NSAIDS, although conflicting reports have suggested this to be a placebo effect. Chondroitin sulfate may inhibit proteases and thereby slow the progression of arthritis and reduce inflammation. Antioxidants, namely vitamins C, D, E, may be beneficial in cartilage formation, but further study is necessary.

Topical Agents

Aspercreme (10% trolamine salicylate cream) is absorbed percutaneously and hydrolyzed into salicylic acid. Topical application of capsaicin affects the A, delta, and C nerve fibers and secondarily leads to depletion of substance P.

Surgical Management

Arthroscopy

Arthroscopy has a limited role in the management of the osteoarthritic knee. The presence of mechanical symptoms is the main indication for arthroscopic intervention in the presence of degenerative joint disease (DJD), usually when arthritis is mild and associated with a meniscus tear. Severe or end-stage arthritis should be excluded with weight-bearing radiographs prior to arthroscopy as the likelihood of success is dependent on the degree of arthritic changes. Arthroscopic debridement in osteoarthritis has not been better than placebo. An additional role of arthroscopy may be in the case of isolated cartilage lesions or defects in which microfracture, subchondral drilling, or abrasion techniques can be used. The clinical data to support these techniques remain limited. Mosaicplasty or autologous chondrocyte transplantation can be performed in young patients with small lesions but are not presently advocated for more diffuse and advanced degenerative disease. Arthroscopic synovectomy with or without biopsy may have a role in inflammatory synovitis.

Osteotomy

Valgus-producing high tibial osteotomy is indicated in patients with varus gonarthrosis and isolated medial compartment arthritis. Varus-producing distal femoral osteotomy is indicated in patients with valgus gonarthrosis and isolated lateral compartment arthritis. Other general requirements include age younger than 50 years, intact anterior cruciate ligament, minimal flexion contracture, good motion, noninflammatory arthritis, and no dynamic thrust. Because of the apparent short-term superiority of unicompartmental arthroplasty, periarticular osteotomies are not being performed as frequently as a decade ago, except perhaps in young laborers with unicompartmental disease.

Unicompartmental Arthroplasty

The role of unicompartmental arthroplasty in the arthritic patient continues to evolve. Minimally invasive techniques are enhancing the popularity of this procedure, particularly as an alternative to periarticular osteotomy. In the past, the ideal patient was older than 60 years of age and led a sedentary lifestyle. More current indications might include active middle-aged patients undergoing a first arthroplasty as a staged procedure before total knee arthroplasty (TKA). Benefits might include less invasive surgery, less blood loss, more natural knee kinematics (retaining both cruciate ligaments), a faster recovery than with TKA, and more pronounced pain relief than osteotomy. Isolated monocompartmental arthritis of the tibiofemoral joint or patellofemoral joint remain true indications for unicompartmental arthroplasty. Degenerative changes in other compartments and inflammatory arthritis are contraindications.

Total Knee Arthroplasty

Total knee arthroplasty is the procedure of choice for most patients with severe tricompartmental arthritis and provides reliable and durable results. Inflammatory arthritis, deformity, contractures, and instability are best managed with total knee arthroplasty rather than the other surgical procedures.

SUGGESTED READINGS

Argensen JN, Chevrol-Benkeddache Y, Aubaniac JM. Modern unicompartmental knee arthroplasty with cement: a three to ten year follow-up. *J Bone Joint Surg Am.* 2002;84:2235–2239.

Behrens F, Shepard N, Mitchell N. Metabolic recovery of articular cartilage after intra-articular injections of glucocorticoid. *J Bone Joint Surg Am.* 1976;58:1157–1160.

Bradley JD, Brandt KD, Katz BP, et al. Comparison of an antiinflammatory dose of ibuprofen, an analgesic dose of ibuprofen, and acetaminophen in the treatment of patients with osteoarthritis of the knee. *N Engl J Med.* 1991;325:87–91.

Buckwalter JA, Mankin HA. Articular cartilage: degeneration and osteoarthritis, repair, regeneration, and transplantation. *Instr Course Lect.* 1998;47:487-504.

Dervin GF, Stiell IG, Rody K, et al. Effect of arthroscopic debridement for osteoarthritis of the knee on health-related quality of life. *J Bone Joint Surg Am.* 2003;85:10–19.

Ethgen O, Bruyere O, Richy F, et al. Health-related quality of life in total hip and total knee arthroplasty. A qualitative and systematic review of the literature. *J Bone Joint Surg Am.* 2004;86:963–974.

Felson DT, Zhang Y, Anthony JM, et al. Weight loss reduces the risk for symptomatic knee osteoarthritis in women. The Framingham Study. *Ann Intern Med.* 1992;116:535–539.

Goldenberg DL, Reed JI. Bacterial arthritis. *N Engl J Med.* 1985;312: 764–771.

Hanssen AD, Stuart MJ, Scott RD, et al. Surgical options for middle-aged patients with osteoarthritis of the knee joint. *Instr Course Lect.* 2001;50:499–511.

Holden DL, James SL, Larson RL, et al. Proximal tibial osteotomy in patients who are fifty years old or less. A long-term follow-up study. *J Bone Joint Surg Am.* 1988;70:977–982.

Leopold SS, Redd BB, Warme WJ, et al. Corticosteroid compared with hyaluronic acid injections for the treatment of osteoarthritis of the knee. A prospective, randomized trial. *J Bone Joint Surg Am.* 2003;85:1197–1203.

McAlindon TE, LaValley MP, Gulin JP, et al. Glucosamine and chondroitin for treatment of osteoarthritis: a systematic quality assessment and meta-analysis. *JAMA.* 2000;283:1469–1475.

Moseley JB, O'Malley K, Petersen NJ, et al. A controlled trial of arthroscopic surgery for osteoarthritis of the knee. *N Engl J Med.* 2002;347:81–88.

Nussmeier NA, Whelton AA, Brown MT, et al. Complications of COX-2 inhibitors parecoxib and valdecoxib after cardiac surgery. *N Engl J Med* 2005;352:1081–1091.

Soll AH. Nonsteroidal anti-inflammatory drugs and peptic ulcer disease. *Ann Intern Med.* 1991;114:307.

POSTTRAUMATIC RECONSTRUCTION—KNEE

GEORGE J. HAIDUKEWYCH

Fractures and ligament injuries around the knee joint are among the most common orthopaedic injuries encountered. Although contemporary methods of ligament reconstruction and open reduction and internal fixation (ORIF) can result in excellent long-term outcomes, occasionally posttraumatic arthritis can result. Reconstructive options include some form of osteotomy, arthrodesis, or arthroplasty. Challenges include stiffness, scarring, bony defects, malalignment, presence of extensive (often broken) hardware, and compromised soft tissues, Reconstructive decision making is based on patient age, activity, and the anatomic location and extent of damage to the articular surface. This chapter reviews reconstructive options for patients with posttraumatic arthritis of the knee.

DIAGNOSIS

The specifics of preoperative evaluation vary based on whether the prior injury involved fracture of the distal femur, proximal tibia, or patella or was purely ligamentous. Some guiding principles, however, are common to all such evaluations. First and foremost, careful evaluation of the patient's complaints is important. The location and quality of pain, gait disturbance, and deformity should be ascertained. Preoperative range of motion (ROM) should be documented, as multiple studies have demonstrated that postoperative ROM correlates with preoperative ROM. These knees can be quite stiff from posttraumatic arthrosis and multiple prior operations.

The location of prior scars, skin grafts, and flaps should be evaluated. The status of the extensor mechanism, any contractures, and the status of the collateral ligaments should be documented. The neurovascular status of the limb should be carefully evaluated and documented.

RADIOGRAPHIC EVALUATION

High-quality anteroposterior, lateral, and Merchant views are necessary to evaluate alignment, bony deficiency, location of hardware, and anatomic location of degenerative change. Long-standing so-called hip-to-ankle radiographs can assist the surgeon in evaluating angulatory deformity.

Occasionally there will be uncertainty regarding the status of a fracture union. In this situation, conventional or computed tomography can assist in evaluation of healing status.

PREOPERATIVE WORKUP

Preoperative medical optimization is recommended, including cessation of tobacco use, if possible. With a history of an open fracture or failed internal fixation, a complete blood count (CBC) with differential, sedimentation rate, and C-reactive protein should be obtained if there is any suspicion of infection. Aspiration of the knee may provide useful information in selected cases.

TREATMENT

The most difficult aspect of posttraumatic reconstruction around the knee is choosing the right operation for the patient. In most instances arthroplasty is chosen; occasionally the decision making is more complex (Fig. 19-1). Consider, for example, a 30-year-old overweight laborer with painful tricompartmental disease after an open knee dislocation with a prior vascular repair and free flap with current range of motion of 30 to 60 degrees. Although treatment should be individualized after a thorough discussion of various options with the patient, some general principles should be followed.

Typically, older, lower-demand patients are managed with arthroplasty and younger, more active patients are offered osteotomy or arthrodesis. In general, younger patients with single-compartment degenerative change and angular malalignment are selected for corrective osteotomy. Patient expectations, age, activity, and status of the articular

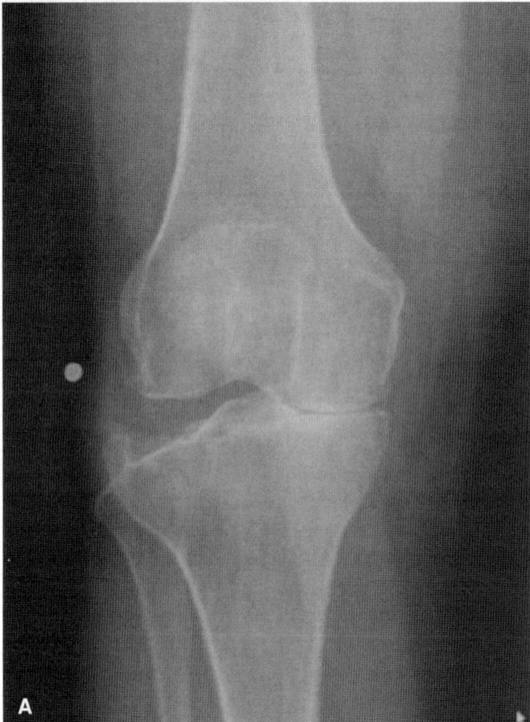

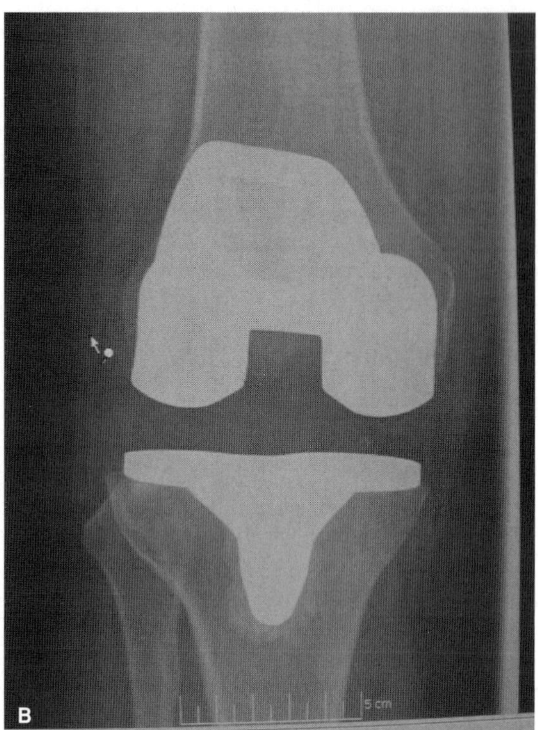

Figure 19-1 A: Posttraumatic degenerative joint disease (DJD) after tibial plateau fracture. B: Treated with total knee arthroplasty.

surface all guide decision making. The author has found that most patients are not willing to accept an arthrodesis.

The principles of osteotomy and arthrodesis are covered elsewhere in this text. Therefore, we will focus on the specific technical considerations for arthroplasty in this setting.

TOTAL KNEE ARTHROPLASTY FOR POSTTRAUMATIC DEGENERATIVE JOINT DISEASE

Dealing with Hardware

There is tremendous variability in the internal fixation implants used to treat fractures about the knee. Typically it is wise to remove hardware that is symptomatic or that will interfere with the arthroplasty. In certain situations, it may be preferable to remove only a portion of the hardware. For example, a long lateral plate on the tibia may be left in situ, simply removing the proximal screws that interfere with tibial tray implantation. This avoids the need for extensive soft tissue dissection and avoids the need to bypass multiple stress risers distally in the tibial shaft. These can be sites of cement extravasation or postoperative fracture. In situations where extensive hardware must be removed, especially through multiple incisions, it may be best to remove the hardware in a first operation, then perform the definitive reconstruction after the soft tissue has recovered. When infection is a concern, the reconstruction should be staged. The author prefers to remove hardware only if it precludes performance of the arthroplasty or if it is symptomatic.

Dealing with Skin Issues

Many patients in this setting will have an incision in a nonideal location for total knee arthroplasty (TKA). Typically the most recent or most lateral incision should be chosen that avoids the elevation of a large subcutaneous flap. A preoperative consultation with a plastic surgeon may be helpful in more complex cases. In some cases, especially those with prior skin grafts or very adherent skin over the patellar tendon or tibial tubercle, one may consider preparatory gastrocnemius flap coverage prior to arthroplasty. The TKA is then planned after flap maturation and soft tissue recovery. This may avoid a situation in which a flap is required after skin breakdown with the prosthesis already implanted.

Exposure Problems

Stiffness is common in knees with posttraumatic arthritis, and it makes exposure more difficult. General principles for safe exposure include careful protection of the patellar tendon with sequential release of scarring in the suprapatellar area, gutters, and peritendinous tissue. The so-called quadriceps snip can be a useful technique. The author prefers to perform an arthrotomy gradually traversing the quadriceps tendon and extending laterally into the vastus lateralis musculature. This leaves a long area of tissue for subsequent repair. Combined external rotation of the tibia, resection of the cruciate ligaments, and a proximal medial tibial "peel" is generally adequate. Patellar subluxation, rather than eversion, may be preferred. These typical exposure techniques are commonly used during revision arthroplasty and are covered in greater detail elsewhere in this text. The author prefers to avoid the so-called quadriceps turn down and tibial tubercle osteotomies when possible. The turn down may devascularize the tendon and patella, and the tubercle fragment may be difficult to reattach with a previously fractured tibia.

Dealing with Deformity (Malunion, Nonunion)

Angular malunion is rare with contemporary open reduction and internal fixation (ORIF) techniques and implants. However, occasionally the patient may present with a malunion that makes traditional TKA difficult or impossible. Long-standing hip-to-ankle radiographs are essential. By templating the amount of bone resection necessary to achieve a normal limb axis and horizontal joint line, the surgeon can determine whether corrective osteotomy should be performed prior to arthroplasty (Figs. 19-2A,B). If excessive bone would need to be resected to perform the arthroplasty (for example, the distal femoral resection would compromise a collateral ligament), the malunion should be corrected prior to TKA. Although rare, rotational malunion can occur, typically of the distal femur. A CT scan, including cuts through both femoral necks and both distal femoral epicondyles, can quantify the rotational deformity preoperatively. Because component rotation affects patellar tracking and long-term performance of the arthroplasty, malunions such as malrotations may be corrected prior to surgery. The author has found retrograde nailing after intramedullary osteotomy and derotation useful in this setting. This allows visualization of the epicondylar axis and simplifies hardware removal during later arthroplasty. Angular deformity of the femur and tibia are also effectively managed by oblique osteotomy and plating, especially if translation of the medullary canals precludes nailing techniques. Performing a TKA even in the case of a minor malunion can be challenging, and extra medullary alignment guides are often needed (Fig. 19-2). Alternatively, computer-assisted navigation systems may be considered when conventional jigs cannot be reliably applied. A comprehensive discussion of deformity correction about the knee is beyond the scope of this chapter.

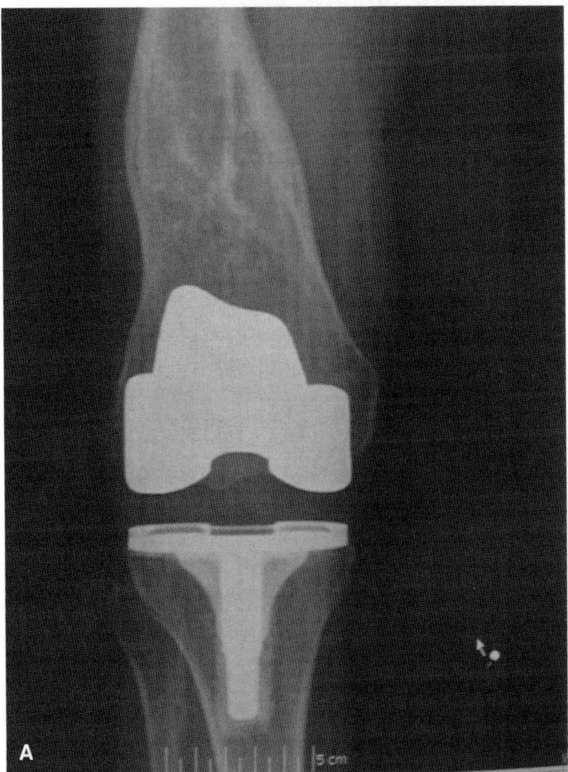

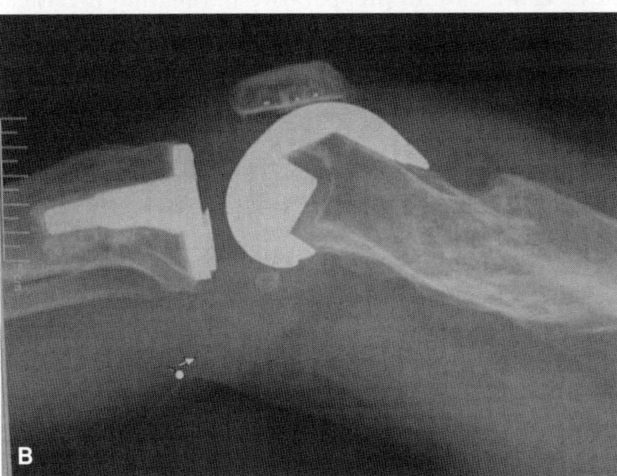

Figure 19-2 Total knee arthroplasty after distal femur malunion, anteroposterior (A) and lateral (B) views.

Dealing with Nonunions

In general, in the nonunion setting, the decision regarding TKA versus revision ORIF is based on patient age, status of the articular surface, and remaining articular bone stock. Nonunions of fractures of the proximal tibia are rare. If they occur, the options include revision ORIF and bone graft, or a TKA. No large series of TKA performed in this setting has been reported. Some have recommended bypassing the nonunion with a long stem and bone grafting the nonunion with autologous bone from the bony cuts.

Nonunions of distal femur fractures pose greater challenges and are more common. Usually it is preferable to obtain fracture union with revision ORIF if sufficient bone stock remains distally. Some authors have recommended TKA with intramedullary fixation of the nonunion using the cut bony fragments as autograft. Kress et al. reported a series of nine patients treated for periarticular nonunions with TKA and stems with excellent results. Haidukewych et al. reported a series of 17 patients undergoing TKA for failed ORIF or nonunion of the distal femur. Two of three patients treated with TKA with intramedullary stem stabilization of the nonunion healed. Anderson et al. achieved successful union in ten patients with long-stem fixation and autograft. These limited series document that TKA with stem fixation used to "nail" the nonunion can be effective in selected cases.

In older, lower-demand patients with inadequate distal bone stock for conventional arthroplasty or revision ORIF, the use of distal femoral replacements, so-called tumor

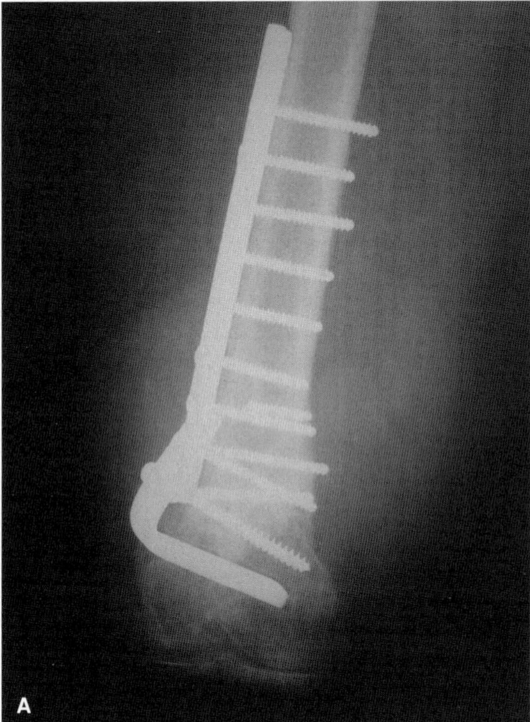

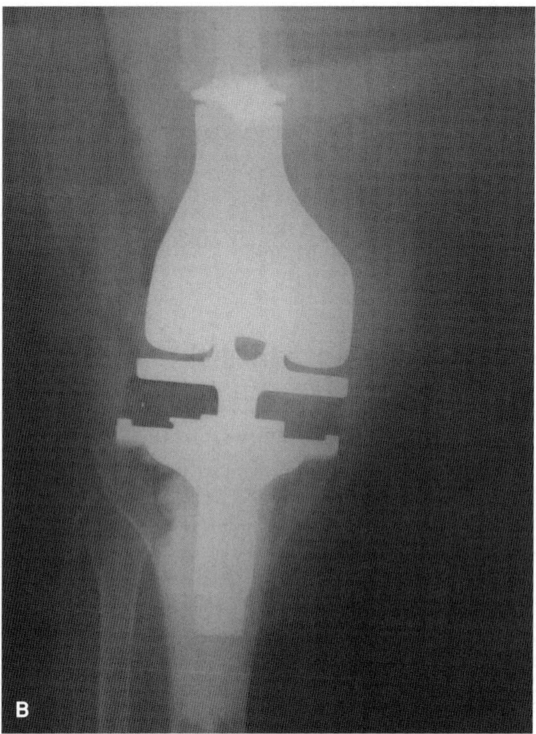

Figure 19-3 A,B: Multiply operated distal femoral nonunion with posttraumatic degenerative joint disease treated with a distal femoral replacement.

prostheses may be the most predictable option (Fig. 19-3). These offer the advantage of immediate weight bearing for the typically elderly population undergoing these surgeries. Cemented fixation in this setting allows secure initial component fixation in diaphyses that are typically capacious and osteopenic.

Dealing with Bony Deficiency

The techniques for dealing with bony deficiency in the posttraumatic setting are similar to those used during revision arthroplasty. Generally, defects are managed incrementally with techniques such as cement fill, cement and screws, metal augmentation with wedges or cones, or structural allograft as the defect size increases. Large cavitary deficiencies are rare in this setting but, if present, can be managed with commercially available metal metaphyseal cones or impaction bone grafting techniques.

The liberal use of stems should be encouraged to bypass stress risers and unload deficient periarticular bone. In general, if a metal augment is used, a stem should be used as well. Cemented and cementless stems can be used effectively, and there are advantages and disadvantages to each choice. If a long diaphyseal engaging stem is necessary (for example, to bypass empty screw holes after plate removal), cementless stems are generally preferred. Cement is used on the cut bony surfaces and exposed metaphysis, but the diaphyseal fixation is uncemented. Recent data on the use of this so-called hybrid stem fixation technique documented excellent results in the revision setting. Careful preparation of the diaphysis and intraoperative radiographs are recommended owing to the risk of iatrogenic femur fracture. Short, uncemented, metaphyseal engaging stems have demonstrated a concerning rate of failure in recent series and should not be used. If a short stem is chosen, cementing is a prudent choice.

So-called offset stems may be necessary in the setting of translational deformity to avoid component malposition. Commercially available stems exist that allow the surgeon to choose the optimum stem position. This may be most useful for diaphyseal engaging stems. Shorter, cemented stems often can be "cheated" after overreaming to afford good stability in the face of angular and translational deformities. Again, careful preoperative templating is critical to fully understand the deformity and avoid intraoperative difficulties. Very rarely, a custom component may be necessary.

Choice of Prosthesis Constraint

The posttraumatic knee with a history of knee dislocation is among the most challenging of reconstructions. Residual tibiofemoral subluxation and varying amounts of ligamentous damage can make achieving a balanced arthroplasty in this setting very unpredictable. Careful preoperative examination can alert the surgeon to ligamentous insufficiency that may require the use of more constrained implants.

In general, the implant with the least constraint necessary to provide symmetric flexion and extension gaps and

TABLE 19-1 TOTAL KNEE ARTHROPLASTY FOR POSTTRAUMATIC CONDITIONS

Author	No. Patients	Site	Success	Comments
Anderson et al. (CO, 1990)	10	Distal femur and tibia nonunion	All healed	30% complications
Kress et al. (JA, 1993)	9	Tibia and femur nonunion	All healed	All bone grafted
Freedman et al. (JOT, 1995)	5	Distal femur megaprosthesis	4 good, 1 poor	Extensor lag, 1 infection
Davila et al. (JOT, 2001)	2	Distal femur megaprosthesis	Both excellent	Case report only
Saleh et al. (JBJS, 2001)	15	Tibial plateau	HSS Knee Score 50 → 80	20% infection rate 5 of 15 "failed"
Springer et al. (CO, 2001)	69; 14 were nonunions	Distal femur megaprosthesis	Knee scores improved 40 → 77	32% overall complication rate 14.5% infection
Weiss et al. (JBJS, 2003)	62	Tibial plateau fx	77% good or excellent 22% poor or fair	10% intraop complications 29% postop complications
Haidukewych et al. (JA, 2005)	17	Distal femur nonunion	91% survivorship at 15 y	29% intraop complications 29% postop complications

CO, *Clinical Orthopaedics*; JA, *The Journal of Arthroplasty*; JOT, *Journal of Orthopaedic Trauma*; JBJS, *The Journal of Bone and Joint Surgery*; HSS, Hospital for Special Surgery.

satisfactory knee stability should be used. Although posterior cruciate ligament (PCL)–retaining designs may be used in selected situations with minimal deformity, in most posttraumatic cases substitution of the PCL will facilitate correction of deformity and accurate ligament balancing.

The use of constrained condylar implants is dictated by the status of the collateral ligaments. If these designs are chosen, consideration should be given to the use of a stem on the components owing to the increased forces the bone/implant interface will experience. The young patient with the deficient medial collateral ligament (MCL) presents perhaps the greatest challenge. Advancement of the native MCL or allograft reconstruction of the MCL may be considered in this setting. Data are limited on the optimum reconstruction in this setting. A more neutral limb axis (less overall valgus) should be considered as well.

Hinged implants and tumor prostheses are reserved for low-demand patients with global ligamentous and bony deficiency. Younger active patients may be better served with arthrodesis; however, few are willing to accept this option.

SUMMARY OF CLINICAL DATA

A summary of the recent clinical data is found in Table 19-1.

SUMMARY

Posttraumatic conditions of the knee are common, and having effective reconstruction strategies is important. Younger patients are typically candidates for joint-preserving options such as osteotomy or arthrodesis, whereas older patients typically are salvaged with TKA. Attention to specific details preoperatively and intraoperatively is necessary to minimize complications. The vast majority of published series document predictable functional improvement but higher complication rates when compared with primary TKA.

SUGGESTED READINGS

Anderson SP, Matthews LS, Kaufer H. Treatment of juxtaarticular nonunion fractures at the knee with long-stem total knee arthroplasty. *Clin Orthop*. 1990;260:104–409.

Bellabarba C, Ricci WM, Bolhofner BR. Indirect reduction and plating of distal femoral nonunions. *J Orthop Trauma*. 2002;16:287–296.

Clatworthy MG, Ballance J, Brick GW, et al. The use of structural allograft for uncontained defects in revision total knee arthroplasty. *J Bone Joint Surg Am*. 2001;83-A:404–411.

Davila J, Malkani A, Paiso JM. Supracondylar distal femoral nonunions treated with a megaprosthesis in elderly patients: a report of two cases. *J Orthop Trauma*. 2001;15:574–578.

Dennis DA. The structural allograft composite in revision total knee arthroplasty. *J Arthroplasty*. 2002;17(suppl 1):90–93.

Freedman EL, Hick DJ, Johnson EE, et al. Total knee replacement including a modular distal femoral component in elderly patients with acute fracture or nonunion. *J Orthop Trauma*. 1995;9:231–237.

Garvin KL, Scuderi G, Insall JN. Evolution of the quadriceps snip. *Clin Orthop*. 1995;321:131–137.

Haidukewych GJ, Berry DJ, Jacofsky DJ, et al. Treatment of supracondylar femur nonunions with open reduction and internal fixation. *Am J Orthop*. 2003;32:564–567.

Haidukewych GJ, Springer BD, Jacofsky DJ, et al. Total knee arthroplasty for salvage of failed internal fixation or nonunion of the distal femur. *J Arthroplasty*. 2005;20:344–349.

Honkonen SE. Degenerative arthritis after tibial plateau fractures. *J Orthop Trauma*. 1995;9:273–277.

Kress KJ, Scuderi GR, Windsor RE, et al. Treatment of nonunions about the knee utilizing custom total knee arthroplasty with press-fit intramedullary stems. *J Arthroplasty*. 1993;8:49–55.

Lonner JH, Pedlow FX, Siliski JM. Total knee arthroplasty for post traumatic arthrosis. *J Arthroplasty*. 1999;14:969–975.

Lonner JH, Siliski JM, Jupiter TB, et al. Posttraumatic nonunion of the proximal tibial metaphysis. *Am J Orthop*. 1999;28:523–528.

Roffi RP, Merritt PO. Total knee replacement after fractures about the knee. *Orthop Rev*. 1990;19:614–620.

Saleh KJ, Sherman P. Katkin P, et al. Total knee arthroplasty after open reduction and internal fixation of fractures of the tibial plateau: a minimum five-year follow-up study. *J Bone Joint Surg Am*. 2001; 83-A:1144–1148.

Springer BD, Hanssen AD, Sim FH, et al. The kinematic rotating hinge prosthesis for complex knee arthroplasty. *Clin Orthop*. 2001;392:283.

Volpin G, Dowd GS, Stein H, et al. Degenerative arthritis after intraarticular fractures of the knee. Long-term results. *J Bone Joint Surg Br*. 1990;72:634–638.

Weiss NG, Parvizi J, Trousdale RT, et al. Total knee arthroplasty in patients with a prior fracture of the tibial plateau. *J Bone Joint Surg Am*. 2003;85-A:218–221.

Wolff AM, Hungerford DS, Pepe CL. The effect of extraarticular varus and valgus deformity on total knee arthroplasty. *Clin Orthop*. 1991;271:35–51.

Wu CC, Shih CH. Distal femoral nonunion treated with interlocking nailing. *J Trauma*. 1991;31:1659–1667.

SEPTIC ARTHRITIS

M. WADE SHRADER
DAVID J. JACOFSKY

Acute bacterial infection of a joint, known as acute septic arthritis, is a serious, and can be a life-threatening, infection. Septic arthritis occurs primarily through three mechanisms: (a) direct inoculation through an open wound or penetrating object (including surgery); (b) spread from adjacent infected tissue, such as a soft tissue infection or local osteomyelitis; or (c) hematogenous seeding from bacteremia. Even with appropriate, aggressive intervention and treatment, septic arthritis can cause substantial morbidity, and a delay in diagnosis or treatment can make the consequences even more serious.

Septic arthritis most commonly affects small children and the geriatric population. Patients with any immune system compromise are especially at risk, including those patients with diabetes, rheumatoid arthritis, malnutrition, and chronic renal or liver failure. Patients using intravenous drugs and those with chronic indwelling intravenous catheters are at higher risk. Vascular insufficiency may increase the risk of infection by compromising host immune defenses and also can impair the treatment of infection by decreasing delivery of antimicrobial agents to infected tissues.

PATHOGENESIS

The incidence of septic arthritis in the general population has been estimated to be 2 cases per 100,000, although the incidence is much higher in immunocompromised populations. In patients with rheumatoid arthritis, the incidence has been estimated to be between 30 and 70 cases per 100,000. The most commonly affected joint is the knee.

The most common source of infection is hematogenous spread. Joints are at risk for hematogenous seeding because of the lack of basement membranes in the synovial tissues. Thus, bacteria that are present in the blood vessels have relatively easy access to the joint space without the barrier of the basement membrane.

The most common infectious agent in adult septic arthritis is *Neisseria gonorrhea*. This infection often occurs in sexually active young adults, is typically polyarticular, and may be associated with a papular rash. Gonococcal septic arthritis can be successfully treated with antibiotics and is the only type of joint infection that does not require surgical debridement.

The most common cause of nongonococcal septic arthritis in adults is from *Staphylococcus aureus*. Patients typically have monoarticular involvement, and bacteria are usually spread hematogenously. The hip and knee are the most common joints involved, although infections of the shoulder, elbow, wrist, and ankle also may be seen. Methicillin-resistant strains of staphylococcus (MRSA) are becoming more prevalent, with three out of four positive *S. aureus* cultures being methicillin-resistant in some centers.

Other infectious agents may be responsible for septic arthritis, depending on the patient population and the environment. Streptococci, *Salmonella*, and *Pseudomonas* are all frequently encountered organisms.

DIAGNOSIS

The clinician must maintain a high level of suspicion for septic arthritis because of the serious consequences of a missed diagnosis. Patients typically present with a swollen, red, painful joint. They often will not be able to bear weight on the affected lower extremity and will complain of decreased joint motion secondary to pain. Fevers and chills are sometimes present. Often, however, all of these complaints are not present, and the severity of the symptoms can be quite variable. A thorough history should be elicited, specifically considering any recent infections, immune compromise, social history, travel history (to exclude tick bites), and a complete sexual history. Musculoskeletal infections caused by mycobacterial or fungal organisms do not typically present with the acute, dramatic inflammatory response seen in bacterial infections. The diagnosis in these cases often is made based on a high index of suspicion of the health care provider.

Physical Exam

The physical exam should focus on determining if any signs of infection are present. Vital signs, including temperature, should be obtained. The joint should be examined for effusion, erythema, and tenderness to palpation. The most specific sign of septic arthritis is pain with passive range of motion, which should be determined in any physical exam of the extremities. In the knee, septic arthritis may be differentiated from septic prepatellar bursitis by determining if pain with range of motion is seen only in deeper flexion (bursitis) or can be elicited at near full extension as well.

Radiographic Features

Plain radiographs are recommended for most musculoskeletal complaints of the extremities. Plain films should be scrutinized to determine if there are any fractures, dislocations, or other pathologic bony processes that might explain the patient's symptoms. Plain radiographs may not always be helpful in the diagnosis of septic arthritis, although in more chronic cases erosive changes can be seen. Soft tissue swelling, loss of soft tissue planes, or effusions may be the only findings on radiographs of patients with septic arthritis. Chronic or neglected infections can progress to adjacent osteomyelitis, which often can be detected on plain radiographs.

Magnetic resonance imaging (MRI) can be helpful in some circumstances. MRI views will definitely show effusion and fluid collections that may be infectious. MRI also may demonstrate other reasons for joint swelling, such as ligament rupture or meniscal tear. Nuclear imaging with technetium bone scan or indium-tagged white blood cell scan also can be used, but often are not necessary to confirm the diagnosis.

Laboratory Workup

Screening laboratory values should be obtained in all patients, both to assist in the diagnosis of the septic arthritis and to follow the indices after treatment. A complete white blood count with differential, erythrocyte sedimentation rate (ESR), and C-reactive protein should be obtained if infection is suspected, although inflammatory disorders alone can lead to false-positive results.

The gold standard in diagnosis of septic arthritis remains arthrocentesis (joint fluid aspiration). The joint should be aspirated with a large-bore needle, and this should be done *before* empiric antibiotic treatment is begun. Fluoroscopy can be used to aid in the aspiration, if necessary for some joints (e.g., hip). The fluid should immediately be sent for Gram stain, cell count, culture, and crystal analysis. Cultures from superficial sites such as draining fistulas should be avoided, as the organisms colonizing these sites may not be the same as the deeper infecting organism. Joint fluid cultures are positive in about 85% of nongonococcal septic arthritis, but only in about 25% of cases in which gonococcus is the infecting agent.

A joint fluid aspirate analysis that shows a nucleated white blood cell count >100,000/mm^3 is indicative of septic arthritis, and counts between 50,000/mm^3 and 100,000/mm^3 are inflammatory but not necessarily infectious. The white blood cell differential count also provides valuable information to aid in the diagnosis. A differential count with an unusually high proportion of polymorphonuclear cells (>90%) is also highly suggestive of septic arthritis, whereas <50% neutrophils is unlikely to be an acute infection.

Joint fluid analysis must be performed in a timely, urgent fashion to allow treatment that will prevent the systemic spread of infection and preserve the health of the articular cartilage. Intra-articular lysosomal enzyme release, including metalloproteases and collagenases, can digest glycosaminoglycans and cause articular cartilage cell death. The release of these enzymes is mediated by cytokines such as interleukin-1 (IL-1). Cartilage softening and fissuring can be seen secondary to glycosaminoglycan depletion within 7 days from the onset of infection. Laboratory investigations in animal models have shown that joint debridement and lavage decrease the rate and magnitude of collagen breakdown, probably through the removal of leukocytes and associated destructive enzymes.

TREATMENT

The three classic principles in management of the acute septic joint are as follows: (a) thorough joint drainage and synovial debridement, (b) appropriate antibiotic therapy, and (c) joint rest in a stable position. All three of these treatment principles are crucial in the successful treatment of septic arthritis.

There are three techniques to drain a septic joint: (a) open drainage, lavage, and debridement; (b) arthroscopic drainage, lavage, and debridement; and (c) serial aspirations, lavage, and drainage. Controversy remains over which method is the most appropriate way to treat a septic joint. The gold standard remains an open arthrotomy, which allows for adequate drainage and lavage and provides the opportunity for a thorough synovial debridement, a factor that many surgeons feel is key to successful treatment. Experienced arthroscopists argue that they can provide equally efficacious drainage and lavage through the arthroscope. Proponents of arthroscopic debridement also argue that they can actually perform a more thorough synovial debridement by using posterior portals to allow for debridement of the posterior compartment of the knee. Although its indications and use are limited, serial aspirations and lavage also can be successful in treating the native septic joint, particularly if the infection is <72 hours old and the patient is not immunocompromised. It is critical, however, that if the patient does not show significant improvement within 24 to 48 hours with repeated aspirations, surgical irrigation and debridement should be performed. In general, closed suction drainage for 24 to 48 hours after operation is recommended.

The initial antibiotic should be chosen based on the patient risk factors, patient history and clinical signs, and the initial Gram stain. Culture results should dictate change to the most appropriate antibiotic, based on sensitivity data.

Typically, intravenous antibiotics are continued for 4 to 6 weeks. When nonviable tissue is encountered in the joint and when a clinical response to treatment is not seen, a "second-look" surgery and repeat debridement may be indicated.

The joint should be kept immobilized for the first 48 to 72 hours of treatment. However, once clinical improvement is noted, the patient should begin rehabilitation, including range-of-motion and strengthening exercises. Some surgeons advocate the use of continuous passive motion (CPM) devices to minimize the possibility of forming postinfectious intra-articular adhesions. Dynamic splints, passive motion exercises, and joint manipulations are used as needed but are rarely necessary.

After the septic arthritis has been successfully treated, the joint involved may develop arthritis, or suffer from decreased loss of motion. Any subsequent surgical treatment aimed at that joint (for example: capsular release, osteotomy, arthroplasty) must take into account the possibility of residual infection.

SUGGESTED READINGS

Canale ST, ed. *Campbell's Operative Orthopedics*. 9th ed. St. Louis, MO: Mosby–Year Book; 1998.

Dubost JJ, Soubrier M, Sauvezie B. Pyogenic arthritis in adults. *Joint Bone Spine*. 2000;67(1):11–21.

Kohli R, Hadley S. Fungal arthritis and osteomyelitis. *Infect Dis Clin North Am*. 2005;19:831–851.

Koval KJ, ed. *Orthopedic Knowledge Update 7, Home Study Syllabus*. Rosemont, IL: American Academy of Orthopedic Surgeons; 2006.

Leirisalo-Repo M. Early arthritis and infection. *Curr Opin Rheumatol*. 2005;17(4):433–439.

Morrissy RT, Weinstein SL. *Lovell and Winter's Pediatric Orthopedics*. 4th ed. Philadelphia: Lippincott-Raven Publishers;1996.

Perry CR. Septic arthritis. *Am J Orthop*. 1999;28:168–178.

Rice PA. Gonococcal arthritis (disseminated gonococcal infection). *Infect Dis Clin North Am*. 2005;19:853–861.

Ross JJ. Septic arthritis. *Infect Dis Clin North Am*. 2005;19:799–817.

Smith JW, Chalupa P, Shabaz Hasan M. Infectious arthritis: clinical features, laboratory findings and treatment. *Clin Microbiol Infect*. 2006;12(4):309–314.

Zimmermann B III, Mikolich DJ, Ho G Jr. Septic bursitis. *Sem Arth Rheum*. 1995;24:391–410.

MISCELLANEOUS CONDITIONS

ROBERT J. ESTHER

Osteoarthritis or the inflammatory arthropathies cause the vast majority of knee degeneration. A handful of other conditions, however, can lead to significant morbidity. It is important for the physician to be familiar with these less common entities to avoid diagnostic pitfalls and to provide appropriate care. Although this review stresses the orthopedic issues in caring for these patients, treating these conditions often is best accomplished with coordinated input from different specialties. These conditions (Table 21-1) are a heterogeneous group with various causes. Although they are uncommon, it is useful to be aware of the key features of these conditions when evaluating a patient with knee complaints.

PATHOGENESIS

Osteonecrosis

Osteonecrosis of the knee comprises an array of entities. The exact mechanism for development of this condition remains elusive. An area of the involved bone sustains an ischemic insult that initiates a process of remodeling and collapse. Depending on the location and extent of this collapse, articular surface incongruity leads to joint degeneration. Spontaneous osteonecrosis usually develops in older patients (sixth or seventh decade) without any antecedent trauma or other known risk factor. Younger patients also may develop knee osteonecrosis, usually in association with trauma or other known risk factors such as alcohol consumption or corticosteroid use.

Synovial Chondromatosis

Synovial chondromatosis is an idiopathic process in which articular (hyaline) cartilage is produced in the soft tissues around joints. These cartilaginous areas can then break free and become loose bodies. Patients develop locking, catching, and other mechanical symptoms based on the size and number of these cartilaginous lesions. As a consequence of intra-articular loose bodies, patients develop secondary degenerative changes. Most cases are monoarticular, with the knee joint involved most commonly. Men are approximately two times more likely than women to develop this disorder.

Secondary chondrosarcoma arising in synovial chondromatosis is an exceedingly rare phenomenon. If imaging or clinical findings raise even the possibility of malignancy, it is appropriate to refer the patient to an orthopedic oncologist for further management.

Hemophilic Arthropathy

Hemophilic arthropathy occurs as a consequence of recurrent intra-articular hemorrhages in patients with clotting factor deficiencies. Hemophiliac arthropathy therefore begins with intra-articular bleeding. Reaction to intra-articular blood leads to varying degrees of synovitis. This inflamed synovium is then more susceptible to further intra-articular bleeds, setting up a potential cycle in which patients have recurrent hemarthroses. The extensive chronic synovitis that ensues eventually leads to joint erosions and, over time, end-stage arthropathy.

Pigmented Villonodular Synovitis

Pigmented villonodular synovitis (PVNS) is an idiopathic proliferative condition of synovium in which there is an accumulation of giant cells and hemosiderin. PVNS does not have malignant potential but can be locally aggressive, leading to considerable synovitis that produces erosions and secondary degenerative changes. The knee joint is most commonly involved and, as in synovial chondromatosis, most cases are monoarticular. PVNS is a synovial disease but also can involve periarticular sites such as tendon sheaths and bursae.

Gout and Pseudogout

Patients with pseudogout and gout can develop intra-articular reactions to the characteristic crystals of the two conditions. The body mounts an inflammatory response to the crystals, thereby leading to secondary joint inflammation and eventually degeneration. Patients with calcium pyrophosphate deposition disease (CPPD), or pseudogout, may have a spectrum of findings from acute synovitis to a long-standing arthropathy with secondary degenerative changes. These patients also can develop deposits in hyaline

TABLE 21-1 LESS COMMON CAUSES OF KNEE DEGENERATIVE JOINT DISEASE

Osteonecrosis
Pigmented villonodular synovitis
Synovial chondromatosis
Crystal deposition
  Uric acid (gout)
  Calcium pyrophosphate deposition disease (CPPD; pseudogout)
Hemophilia

and meniscal cartilage. Gout is caused by symptomatic elevation of uric acid, also leading to an inflammatory response to crystals. A combination of dietary factors and medicines—especially thiazide diuretics—can precipitate gouty flares.

DIAGNOSIS

Physical Examination and History

As with any medical condition, the evaluation of these patients begins with a careful history. The orthopedist should inquire about onset and duration of symptoms, any antecedent of inciting events, other joints involved, and systemic conditions for which the patient requires medical treatment. Patients with hemophilia should be asked about the number of prior intra-articular bleeds.

As discussed in prior chapters, physical examination should include surface appearance, limb alignment, range of motion, tenderness, instability, presence of effusion, and a thorough neurovascular exam.

For patients with an effusion, an aspiration may be diagnostically useful and give considerable, albeit temporary, symptomatic relief. Synovial fluid in gout and pseudogout will show characteristic crystals under the microscope: Uric acid crystals will be negatively birefringent, and calcium pyrophosphate crystals will be positively birefringent. As some laboratories do not routinely examine body fluid for crystals, it is important to specify this request on the order. Synovial fluid may be bloody in patients with PVNS, but a nonbloody tap does not necessarily exclude this diagnosis. Synovial fluid should also be sent for further laboratory investigations including cell count and, when warranted, Gram stain and culture.

Radiologic Features

Although in some instances a patient may be referred having already had an MRI or other advanced cross-sectional imaging, the accepted first step in radiographic evaluation should be orthogonal plain x-ray films. In addition to these films, additional radiographs may be useful. A standing anteroposterior (AP) view of both knees affords the opportunity to evaluate the contralateral joint. A patellar view is useful for evaluating the patellofemoral articulation. In addition to the usual radiographic stigmata of joint degeneration, films should be scrutinized for loose bodies, radiolucent bony changes, effusions, and changes in the soft tissues. As noted in other chapters, concerns about limb alignment should be addressed by long-leg films that include the hip and ankle.

Although most orthopedists are comfortable with the radiographic manifestations of knee degeneration, the conditions in this chapter often require ancillary studies such as bone scan or magnetic resonance imaging (MRI). As with all medical tests, advanced imaging should be ordered to answer a specific question that will guide diagnosis or treatment. MRI is also useful in the face of unusual or unexpected findings on plain films, such as radiolucent changes on both the tibial and femoral sides of the knee joint. Magnetic resonance imaging is clearly superior to plain films for evaluating soft tissues, bone marrow, and articular cartilage. Computed tomography (CT) scanning is not usually indicated or helpful in the conditions outlined here. Although orthopedists are increasingly comfortable with different imaging modalities, a radiologist with specialized musculoskeletal training is invaluable in choosing which imaging studies are most appropriate and also in the subsequent interpretation of these studies.

Radiographic diagnosis of knee osteonecrosis may be difficult, especially in early stages. Plain films may be negative initially. Traditionally, bone scans have been used for diagnosis. More recent reports show a high sensitivity for MRI. Moreover, MRI is useful in characterizing the exact location and extent of bony and cartilaginous involvement. The classic location of knee osteonecrosis is the medial femoral condyle, but the lateral condyle and proximal tibia also may be involved.

Radiographic manifestations of synovial chondromatosis include intra-articular and periarticular cartilaginous bodies (Fig. 21-1). As these bodies contain varying amounts of mineral, not all will necessarily show up on plain films. MRI is useful in these cases to see the extent and number of loose bodies. As with PVNS, the location and extent of disease as characterized on MRI helps the surgeon plan the appropriate operative treatment.

The radiographic manifestations of PVNS may be subtle, including joint erosions that may appear on both sides of a joint. Occasionally, one may appreciate a soft tissue mass or large effusion on plain film (Fig. 21-2). Because PVNS is a soft tissue process, MRI is the best imaging method to gauge the extent of disease (Fig. 21-3). MRI is extremely useful in preparing an appropriate treatment plan for PVNS of the knee.

Calcium pyrophosphate deposition has a typical radiographic appearance termed *chondrocalcinosis*. Radiographic manifestations include calcifications of the articular cartilage and the meniscus. Unless one suspects a superimposed meniscal tear or other intra-articular pathology, MRI is not indicated as part of the workup of CPPD.

TREATMENT

Nonoperative Management

As with many musculoskeletal disorders, the first line of treatment in many of these conditions is symptomatic care

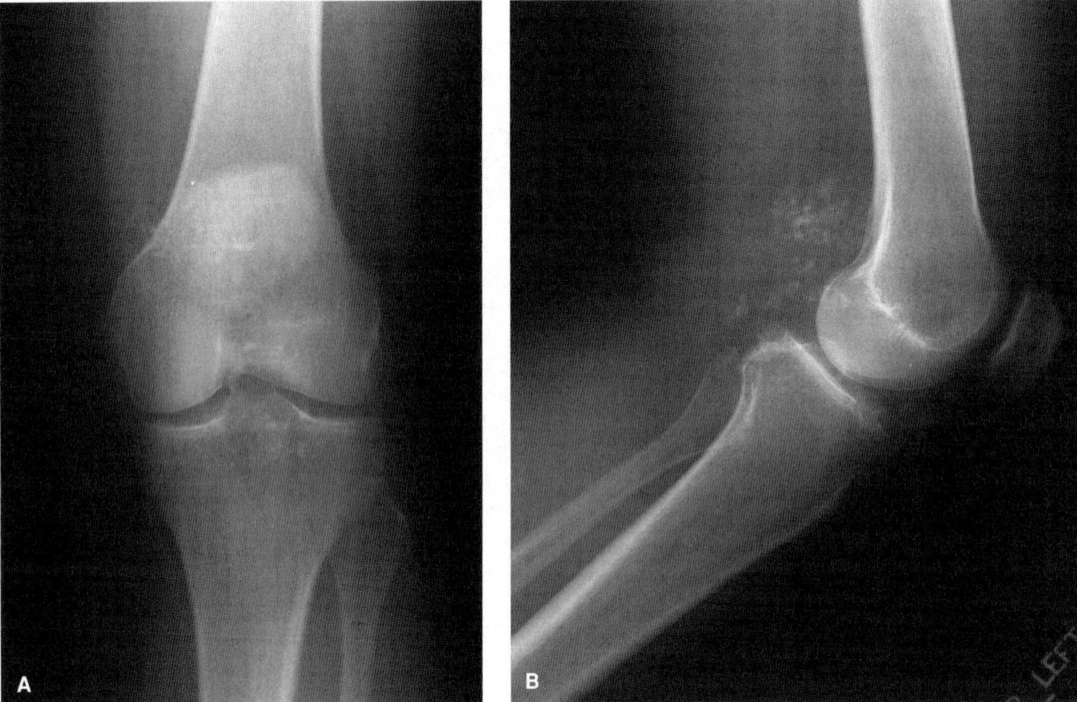

Figure 21-1 Anteroposterior (A) and lateral (B) knee x-ray views showing mineralized cartilaginous areas consistent with synovial chondromatosis.

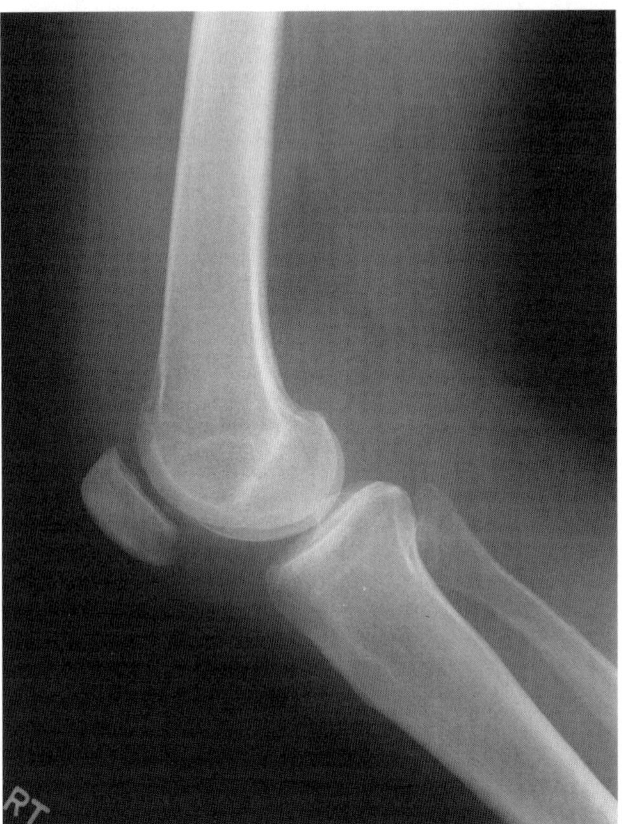

Figure 21-2 Lateral knee radiograph in a patient with pigmented villonodular synovitis. Note the considerable soft tissue mass posteriorly and the absence of significant osseous abnormalities.

including symptom modification and anti-inflammatory medication. Surgical management is indicated when nonoperative methods no longer benefit the patient.

Appropriate medical management is important in treating patients with hemophilia. Avoiding trauma and closely following clotting factor levels are two straightforward ways to minimize the number of intra-articular bleeds. Patients with recent bleeds also may benefit from a brief period of joint immobilization to allow time for soft tissues to recover. Because patients with hemophilic arthropathy tend to develop soft tissue contractures, however, immobilization should be used judiciously.

Patients with hemophilia should be treated at medical centers where the surgeon is supported by an active medical hemophilia program. Hemophiliacs undergoing invasive procedures should be screened for clotting factor inhibitors.

In hemophiliacs, operative intervention not only is potentially dangerous, but also consumes considerable resources, including the time and energy of consulting services and laboratory surveillance of factor and inhibitor levels. For this reason, P-32 radiation synovectomy is attracting increasing interest in the treatment of early arthropathy. Radiation synovectomy is especially appropriate in patients without significant joint degeneration. Although it obviously cannot reverse existing articular damage, the procedure can help break the vicious and destructive cycle of synovial irritation and intra-articular hemorrhage.

Management of gout is primarily symptomatic. Anti-inflammatory medicines and colchicine are useful in acute flares. For long-term control of high blood uric acid levels, patients should be managed in conjunction with colleagues

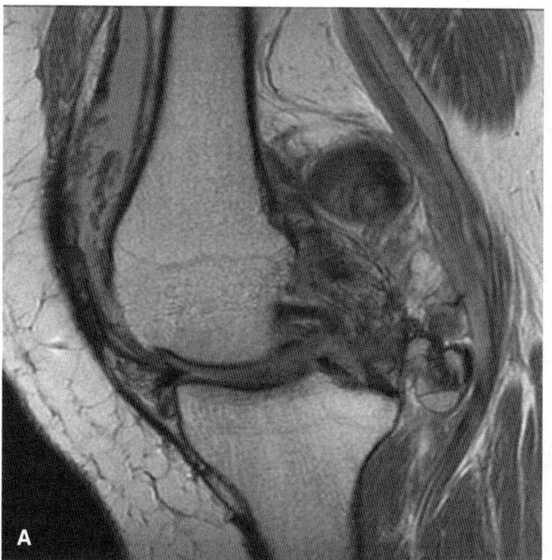

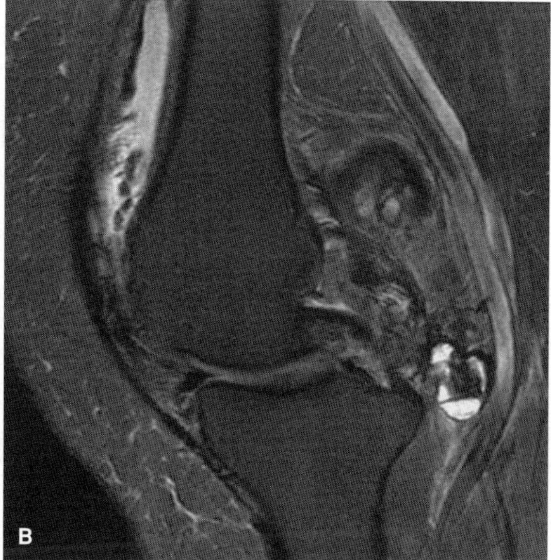

Figure 21-3 Proton density (A) and T2 (B) magnetic resonance images of the same knee as Figure 21-2 showing extensive pigmented villonodular synovitis (PVNS).

in internal medicine. Pharmacologic treatment (allopurinol) in combination with dietary modifications is recommended.

Osteonecrosis typically is managed nonoperatively at first. However, symptoms frequently persist and operative treatment, usually with arthroplasty, commonly is needed.

PVNS and synovial chondromatosis typically are not amenable to nonsurgical treatment. The natural history of PVNS, especially the diffuse form, is progressive joint erosions and arthropathy. As with hemophiliac arthropathy, there is some interest in using radioactive synovectomy in these patients. Although synovial chondromatosis typically is considered to be less aggressive and self-limiting, the loose bodies of this condition often cause pain, loss of function, and eventually secondary joint degeneration.

Surgical Indications and Outcomes

Patients with hemophilic arthropathy were traditionally managed with open synovectomies. Current trends favor the use of arthroscopic treatment. These procedures require less clotting factor support and are less morbid than open surgical approaches.

Management of end-stage hemophilic arthropathy depends on several issues, including the amount of pain and desired level of function and activity. These patients can have compromised bone stock, distorted osseous architecture, and severe soft tissue contractures from superimposed arthrofibrosis. In spite of these potential difficulties, outcomes of knee replacements in this population may be favorable, but are associated with a higher rate of infection.

Arthroscopic or open synovectomy is the treatment of choice for synovial chondromatosis. When possible, arthroscopic procedures allow the surgeon to remove synovium and loose bodies while avoiding the morbidity of an open approach. Occasionally, extensive disease and difficult location require open synovectomy and debridement. Because patients with these conditions often begin with decreased range of motion, an early and closely supervised physical therapy program is essential postoperatively.

The outcome of treatment of synovial chondromatosis usually is favorable. Some patients develop recurrent disease, but the natural history commonly involves regression of disease. Patients may develop secondary arthritis from loose bodies and may require joint replacement.

Treatment of osteonecrosis ranges from symptomatic, nonoperative care to osteotomies, condylar allografts, and joint replacement. Core decompression and arthroscopic debridement also have been recommended with varying rates of success. The main determinants of treatment choice include the location of the lesion, the amount of joint involvement, the extent of secondary degenerative changes, overall limb alignment, and patient age. Historically, outcomes of knee replacement in osteonecrosis have not been as successful as in other conditions. More recent reports have been more encouraging, however.

Although synovial chondromatosis usually follows a self-limiting course over time, diffuse PVNS is locally aggressive. Inadequate removal of involved synovium can lead to recurrent disease; local recurrence rates are reported as high as 50% in the literature. Localized nodular forms of PVNS may be amenable to arthroscopic removal, but diffuse PVNS should be treated with an open total synovectomy. For patients with advanced degenerative changes, treatment options are nonoperative management versus total joint replacement. Knee fusion has fallen out of favor and should be considered a salvage procedure.

Treatment of crystalline arthropathies is symptomatic. In patients with long-standing disease and extensive surface damage, total knee arthroplasty may be indicated with an expectation of success equal to that for osteoarthritis.

Patients with gout should continue their preoperative medical regimen to prevent flares in other joints.

Postoperative Management

Management of patients with these conditions includes the principles of postoperative care outlined in previous chapters. Coordinated multispecialty input often is in the patient's best interest. Patients with long-standing adrenal suppression from oral corticosteroids may need perioperative stress dosing. Hemophiliacs obviously must have appropriately titrated clotting factor levels and perioperative input from a hematology service. These patients need clotting factor support for several weeks following the procedure as they embark on a therapy program. Again, close collaboration with colleagues in internal medicine is essential for appropriate perioperative care.

Especially for those patients undergoing open synovectomies, early institution of a physical therapy program is critical. Patients with synovial chondromatosis and PVNS can be affected by a vicious cycle of decreased motion that is further compromised by open and extensive surgery around the involved joint. These patients should receive particularly close attention from therapists and begin working on range of motion as soon as the periarticular soft tissues allow. Hemophiliacs often have considerable preoperative flexion contractures and they, also, should have especially close follow-up with therapy.

CONCLUSION

Although less common than other knee disorders, the diagnoses discussed above can be treated with reasonable expectations of success if one is aware of the potential difficulties in diagnosis and treatment. Multispecialty care is important and can minimize morbidity and perioperative complications.

SUGGESTED READINGS

Flandry FC, Jacobsen KE, Hughston JC, et al. Surgical treatment of diffuse pigmented villonodular synovitis of the knee. *Clin Orthop.* 1994;300:183–192.

Luck JV, Silva M, Rodriguez-Merchan EC, et al. Hemophilic arthropathy. *J Am Acad Ortho Surg.* 2004;12:234–245.

Mont MA, Rifai A, Baumgarten KM, et al. Total knee arthroplasty in osteonecrosis. *J Bone Joint Surg Am.* 2002;84:599–603.

Siegel HJ, Luck JV, Siegel ME. Advances in radionuclide therapeutics in orthopaedics. J Am Acad Ortho Surg. 2004;12:55–64.

Wold LE, Adler CP, Sim FH, et al. *Atlas of Orthopedic Pathology.* Philadelphia: WB Saunders; 2003.

ARTHROSCOPY

JUSTIN STRICKLAND
DIANE L. DAHM

Knee arthroscopy is the most common operative orthopaedic procedure performed in the United States. It is usually performed as an outpatient procedure and is associated with low morbidity and quick recovery. In addition, multiple types of pathology can be addressed at a single operation. Though the natural history of osteoarthritis is unchanged by arthroscopy, symptomatic relief can be achieved with this modality depending on the pathology found at the time of surgery. Recently, the efficacy of arthroscopy in the treatment of osteoarthritis has been questioned. Patient education and surgical indications are important in the discussion regarding the expectations following arthroscopy in the setting of osteoarthritis.

PREOPERATIVE EVALUATION

Indications

The preoperative evaluation of patients with osteoarthritis is paramount in determining the outcome and expectations following arthroscopy. The following factors suggest higher likelihood of favorable response to arthroscopy:

- Acute onset of pain
- Mechanical symptoms
- Normal or near normal alignment
- Mild to moderate radiographic degenerative changes
- Failure of appropriate nonoperative management program
- Reasonable patient expectations

Clinical Evaluation

When obtaining a history of knee pain from a patient, it is important to note the onset of symptoms and any recent change in symptoms. These patients frequently have a history of chronic knee pain; however, an acute exacerbation or change in the nature of the symptoms may indicate new pathology that may be amenable to arthroscopic treatment. If mechanical symptoms such as catching and locking are present, this may represent meniscal pathology, loose body formation, or an unstable articular cartilage fragment. Localization of pain is also an important factor. Isolated medial or lateral tenderness may indicate a focal articular lesion or symptomatic meniscal pathology. On physical exam, one should note any excessive varus or valgus malalignment or flexion/extension lags. A patient with malalignment in the coronal plane may be a candidate for osteotomy. Finally, patients should be given a trial of nonoperative measures before any operative procedure is undertaken. This might include shoe/heel wedges, use of braces, nonsteroidal anti-inflammatory drugs (NSAIDs) or other medications, injections (steroid and viscosupplementation) and physical therapy. Low-impact exercise and weight loss are also often effective for symptomatic relief in patients with osteoarthritis of the knee.

Radiographic Evaluation

Standing anteroposterior (AP), lateral, posteroanterior (PA) flexion, and sunrise views of the knee should be obtained. One may consider standing full-length hip to ankle films to evaluate alignment. *Severe degenerative disease on plain films is a contraindication for arthroscopic treatment of osteoarthritis.* Magnetic resonance imaging can be helpful to evaluate for focal cartilage defects. New techniques are now available that may differentiate articular cartilage from synovial fluid and subchondral bone, which makes it easier to identify these sometimes discrete lesions. One should interpret MRI findings in patients older than 65 years of age with osteoarthritis cautiously because a very high percentage of these patients will have a degenerative meniscus tear. As always, the radiographic findings should be correlated with the history and physical examination.

Diagnostic Workup Algorithm

An algorithm for evaluation of knee pain for arthroscopic intervention is presented in Figure 22-1.

TREATMENT

Options

The following options are available when performing arthroscopy in the setting of osteoarthritis:

- Lavage and debridement
- Marrow stimulating techniques

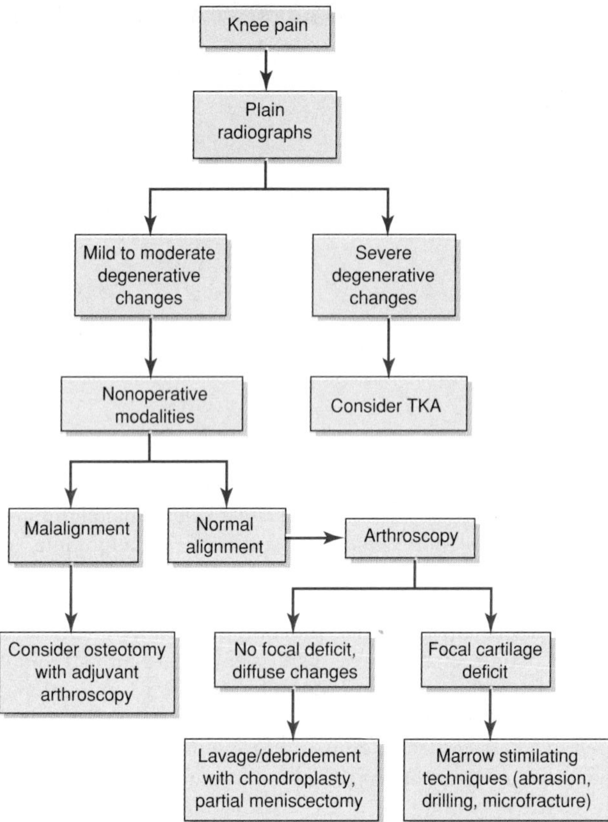

Figure 22-1 Algorithm for treatment of knee osteoarthritis. TKA, total knee arthroplasty.

- Abrasion arthroplasty
- Microfracture/drilling
- Thermal chondroplasty

Multiple goals may be met when a patient with osteoarthritis undergoes an arthroscopic debridement. The degenerative knee has many potential mechanical irritants that may exacerbate a patient's symptoms. These include meniscal tears, unstable flaps of cartilage, and loose bodies. All pathology should be addressed at the time of surgery. It is recommended that chondroplasty and synovectomy be limited to areas that are symptomatic or have the potential to become problematic. Lavage of the joint may be beneficial as this will dilute the degradative enzymes present in the arthritic knee. Osteophytes may also be removed if found to be causing obvious impingement. The advantages of this approach include low morbidity, quick recovery, and the ability to perform a direct assessment of the articular cartilage. It is important to document the findings at the time of arthroscopy as this may influence future reconstructive options such as unicompartmental versus total knee arthroplasty. Even though arthroscopy is a relatively low morbidity, outpatient procedure, the surgeon and patient must remember that no surgical procedure is without risk. Complications such as infection, hematoma, and postoperative stiffness can rarely occur, and patients should be counseled about this possibility before the procedure.

Marrow stimulating techniques such as abrasion arthroplasty, microfracture, and drilling are options typically used for focal cartilage defects. These are more frequently used in younger, active patients with otherwise absent or mild degenerative changes on x-ray views. The goal of these procedures is to penetrate the subchondral bone overlying the defect to stimulate bleeding and the release of marrow contents. This will allow pluripotential mesenchymal cells to invade the defect and begin the process of fibrous metaplasia. Varying amounts of fibrocartilage will eventually fill the defect. Small amounts of hyaline cartilage may be present. Abrasion arthroplasty uses an arthroscopic burr to perform the technique. Simple drilling can also be performed; however, because of its ease of use and lack of heat generation, the so-called microfracture technique has become more widely used. Microfracture is a relatively simple technique using a specialized awl to penetrate the subchondral bone (Fig. 22-2). A depth of 2 to 4 mm is recommended. A bridge of at least 4 mm should be maintained between holes to sustain the integrity of the subchondral bone. Thermal necrosis is not an issue with microfracture as it may be with

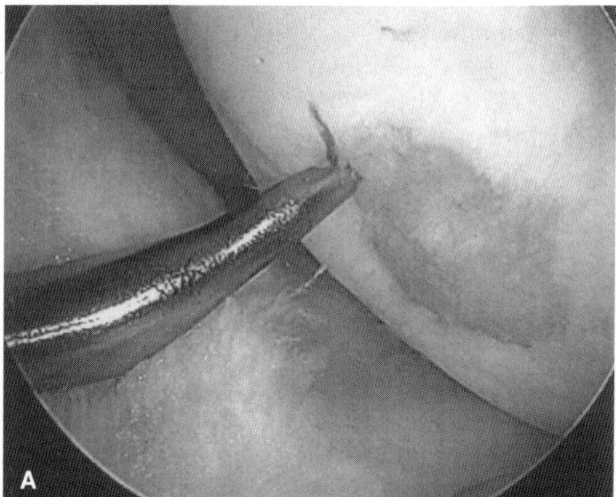

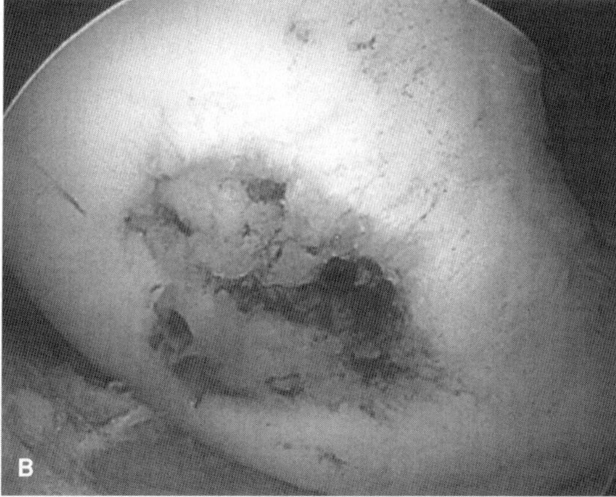

Figure 22-2 **A:** Arthroscopic technique of microfracture for a focal articular cartilage defect. **B:** Confirmation of bleeding subchondral bone in lesion bed.

abrasion arthroplasty, standard drilling, or thermal chondroplasty.

Thermal chondroplasty is a technique that uses a radiofrequency probe to generate heat to denature collagen. This is effective in smoothing and stabilizing articular cartilage defects. However, it has not been proven that this method prevents the propagation of these lesions or that there is a benefit over mechanical chondroplasty. In addition, significant chondrocyte death has been reported with both bipolar and monopolar systems in in vitro studies. This is concerning as it can be difficult to control the temperature of the probe at the cartilage surface. Irreversible damage to articular cartilage occurs at >55°C. Because of these uncertainties, we recommend using this modality with extreme caution and suggest that further studies are needed to justify its routine use to treat cartilage defects.

Results

The clinical results obtained following arthroscopy for osteoarthritis are difficult to interpret. Most published reports are retrospective with variable inclusion criteria, definition of procedures, and outcome measures. These studies have found that arthroscopic debridement yields satisfactory results in 60% to 70% of patients at 2- to 4-year follow-up. There appears to be no clear advantage to subchondral drilling or abrasion arthroplasty in these patients. One prospective study comparing arthroscopic debridement versus placebo surgery found no difference in clinical outcome at 2-year follow-up. In this study, however, patients were not stratified with respect to presence or absence of meniscal pathology, mechanical symptoms/signs, or malalignment. In another prospective outcome study, 44% of patients were found to have improvement in pain at 2-year follow-up. Variables associated with improvement included medial joint line tenderness, a positive Steinman test, and the presence of an unstable meniscus tear at arthroscopy. Older patients (>70 years of age) were more likely to be treated with early total knee arthroplasty following arthroscopic debridement compared with patients younger than 60 years of age. This is consistent with the fact that arthroscopic debridement does not change the natural history of osteoarthritis.

With respect to marrow stimulating techniques, the available data support the use of microfracture for focal cartilage defects. Significant improvements in outcome can be expected in 70% to 80% of patients. Improved results are found in those patients with lower body mass index (<30 kg/m^2), relatively short duration of preoperative symptoms, and higher fill grade as measured by postoperative MRI. In addition, microfracture combined with medial opening wedge osteotomy has been shown in one study to decrease pain and improve function in those patients with chondral defects and varus malalignment at a minimum follow-up of 2 years.

In summary, the role of arthroscopy for osteoarthritis of the knee remains controversial. Symptomatic relief can be expected when patients are carefully selected and properly counseled. The best outcomes are found in patients with a short duration of symptoms of which mechanical symptoms are a significant component, those with unstable meniscal tears and mild to moderate changes on x-ray films, and those who are in the early stages of the disease process without significant malalignment (Table 22-1). Despite these findings, one study showed surgeons were only 60% accurate in predicting which patients would have a successful outcome following arthroscopy.

TABLE 22-1 RESULTS

Stage	Excellent/Good %	Fair %	Poor %
I	100	0	0
II	91	0	9
III	49	28	23
IV	12	52	36

Modified from Jackson RW, Dieterichs C. The results of arthroscopic lavage and debridement of osteoarthritic knees based on the severity of degeneration. *Arthroscopy*. 2003;19:13–20, with permission.

Postoperative Management

Patients may weight-bear as tolerated following simple arthroscopic debridement and lavage for osteoarthritis of the knee. Pain control measures may include intraoperative subcutaneous anesthetic injection, intra-articular anesthetic, corticosteroid or narcotic injection, intra-articular pumps for postoperative local anesthetic delivery, oral pain medications, and edema control. Based on data from experimental and clinical studies, the use of continuous passive motion and protected weight bearing is widely used for 6 weeks following marrow stimulating procedures. There is some evidence to suggest that dynamic compression may facilitate a better-quality repair tissue, which in theory would contain a higher percentage of hyaline cartilage. It is unknown if this protocol affects long-term clinical outcomes following microfracture.

A gradual return to primarily low-impact activities is suggested when pain and swelling have decreased and strength has returned. Return to higher-level impact activities and sports has not been well studied in this population, and recommendations should be individualized based on the patient's goals and clinical outcome.

SUGGESTED READINGS

Bert JM, Maschka K. The arthroscopic treatment of unicompartmental gonarthrosis. A five year follow-up study of abrasion arthroplasty plus arthroscopic debridement and arthroscopic debridement alone. *Arthroscopy*. 1989;5:25–32.

Dervin GF, Stiell IG, Rody K, et al. Effect of arthroscopic debridement for osteoarthritis of the knee on health-related quality of life. *J Bone Joint Surg Am*. 2003;85:10–19.

Harwin SF. Arthroscopic debridement for osteoarthritis of the knee: Predictors of patient satisfaction. *Arthroscopy*. 1999;15(2):142–146.

Hsieh YS, Yang SF, Chu SC, et al. Expression changes in gelatinases in human osteoarthritic knees and arthroscopic debridement. *Arthroscopy*. 2004;20(5):482–488.

Lu Y, Edwards RB, Colby J, et al. Thermal chondroplasty with radiofrequency energy. An in vitro comparison of bipolar and monopolar radiofrequency devices. *Am J Sports Med*. 2001;29:42–49.

Marder RA, Hopkins G Jr, Timmerman LA. Arthroscopic microfracture of chondral defects of the knee: a comparison of two postoperative treatments. *Arthroscopy*. 2005;21(2):152–158.

Mithoefer K, Williams RJ III, Warren RF, et al. The microfracture technique for the treatment of articular cartilage lesions in the knee. A prospective cohort study. *J Bone Joint Surg Am*. 2005;87:1911–1920.

Mosley JD, O'Malley K, Peterson NJ, et al. *New Eng J Med*. 2002;347:81–88.

Rand JA. Role of arthroscopy in osteoarthritis of the knee. *Arthroscopy*. 1991;7:358–363.

Rodrigo JJ, Stedman JR, Stillman JS, et al. Improvement of full thickness chondral defect healing in the human knee after debridement and microfracture using submersion. *Am J Knee Surg*. 1994;7:109–116.

Sterett WI, Steadman JR. Chondral resurfacing and high tibial osteotomy in the varus knee. *Am J Sports Med*. 2004; 32: 1243–1249.

Wai EK, Kreder HJ, Williams JI. Arthroscopic debridement of the knee for osteoarthritis in patients 50 years of age or older: Utilization and outcomes in the province of Ontario. *J Bone Joint Surg Am*. 2002;84-A:17–22.

KNEE OSTEOTOMY

ROBERT T. TROUSDALE

An osteotomy about the knee is a reliable treatment for unicompartmental arthrosis of the knee. Alignment correction procedures about the knee have been used since their introduction by Langenbeck in the 19th century and were popularized by Jackson, Coventry, and Maquet. Paramount to success is understanding the biomechanics and pathophysiology, as well as proper patient selection and surgical execution. In this chapter the pathogenesis, diagnosis, surgical indications, surgical technique, results, and potential complications will be discussed.

PATHOGENESIS AND DIAGNOSIS

Osteoarthritis of the knee has many causative factors including genetic factors, major trauma or trauma from overload secondary to obesity, and/or mechanical malalignment. A concentration of force greater than that which the articular cartilage and subchondral bone can tolerate is a common theme leading to secondary knee osteoarthritis. Malalignment of the limb in excessive varus or valgus will overload the medial or lateral compartments, respectively, and is an important factor in the development of unicompartmental arthritis of the knee. The rationale for realignment osteotomy is to correct the malalignment at the knee by decreasing the excessive load across the affected compartment.

Clinical features of this disease include activity-related knee pain, which is typically located in the affected compartment. Examination should focus on knee range of motion, ligamentous stability, and excluding extra-articular causes of pain (hip, back, vascular, and soft tissue problems). Proper imaging includes radiographs of the knee in three planes and a flexed posterior-anterior weight-bearing view. A long-leg weight-bearing radiograph is essential for preoperative planning. In selected situations, MRI or bone scan may be used to study the status of the noninvolved compartment and meniscus and to look for associated chondral lesions. In most cases prior to considering surgery, patients should have pain sufficient to justify an operation and have failed a structured nonoperative treatment program including appropriate activity modification, weight reduction, use of nonsteroidal anti-inflammatory agents, bracing, and shoe wedges.

TREATMENT

Proper patient selection is critical. The classic indication for osteotomy is unicompartmental osteoarthritis with a secondary varus or valgus malalignment. Osteotomy also has been used for patients with localized avascular necrosis, cartilage defects, and concurrently with osteochondral allografts although little is known about the long-term results of the procedure in these conditions. Ligamentous stability is necessary, although cruciate instability is not an absolute contraindication as ligament reconstruction can be done at the same time or staged with the osteotomy. A reasonable range of motion is necessary with at least 110 degrees of flexion and no more than 10 degrees loss of extension. Age over 60 to 65 years is a relative contraindication, but physiologic age and activity are more important considerations. Inflammatory arthritis, diffuse osteoarthritis, and marked femoral-tibial subluxation are absolute contraindications. Obesity, osteoporosis, chondrocalcinosis, and marked malalignment (>20 degrees) are not strict contraindications, but the success rate and prognosis are compromised.

In general, patients with varus malalignment are best corrected on the tibial side of the joint and those with valgus malalignment are best dealt with on the femoral side to minimize postoperative joint line obliquity. Patients with severe malalignment occasionally should be corrected on both sides of the joint to minimize joint line obliquity. This chapter will focus on the correction of the more commonly seen varus-malaligned limb.

Once indications for high tibial osteotomy are obtained, the decision of whether to do a closing wedge versus an opening wedge needs to be made. Both have advantages and disadvantages (Table 23-1).

Proper Preoperative Planning

Preoperative planning is essential to achieve a proper postoperative mechanical axis. There are multiple ways to plan for an osteotomy, and below is one such technique.

TABLE 23-1 ADVANTAGES AND DISADVANTAGES OF A CLOSING WEDGE VERSUS AN OPENING WEDGE

	Opening High Tibial Osteotomy	Closing High Tibial Osteotomy
Advantages	Technically easy High precision	No bone graft necessary Quicker union time
Disadvantages	Bone graft occasionally necessary Longer union time Potential tibial nerve injury Potential to increase posterior slope	Technically slightly harder to perform Potential peroneal nerve injury Less precise
Relative Indications	Patella alta, loose MCL, moderate OA	Patella baja
Relative Contraindications	Patella baja with patellofemoral symptoms Severe OA (as opening wedge will increase pressure on the medial compartment)	

MCL, medial collateral ligament; OA, osteoarthritis.

Step 1

Using a full-length radiograph, use transparent paper to draw the contours of the whole limb. One should take into account instability of the lateral collateral ligament to avoid overcorrection with the osteotomy. If there is marked lateral collateral ligament instability, stress views can facilitate how much deformity is corrected by the instability versus bony deformity and help determine the proper correction. Depending on the severity of the medial cartilage loss, the new axis is planned to be located 10% to 40% into the lateral compartment. With increasing severity of medial compartment arthritis, the amount of correction is increased.

Step 2

Draw the malaligned mechanical axis from the center of the hip joint to the center of the ankle (Fig. 23-1).

Step 3

Draw the new planed mechanical axis from the femoral head through the desired point in the lateral compartment (10% to 40%) to the ankle (Fig. 23-2).

Step 4

The hinge of the osteotomy is defined and connected distally to the new and old center of the ankle. This gives the angle of desired correction (Fig. 23-3).

Surgical Technique

Closing Wedge

A lateral or midline incision can be used. The anterolateral tibia is exposed to the fibula head. If a major correction is planned (>10 to 12 degrees) resection of the tibia-fibular joint can be performed with an osteotome and/or rongeur. Osteotomy of the tibia is then performed under fluoroscopic control. A K-wire is placed parallel to the joint line, approximately 2.5 cm distal to the joint line. A second K-wire is placed distally, creating a closing wedge at an angle that equals the desired amount of correction. Fluoroscopy can confirm correct size angle of the wedge. The osteotomies are then performed, protecting the posterior structures and patellar tendon. It is important to maintain the integrity of the medial cortex as this serves as a tension band when the osteotomy is closed. The bony wedge is removed, and the osteotomy is closed and fixed with staples or a small laterally based L-plate (Fig. 23-4). Prior to fixation, with the osteotomy closed, it is important to check for overall

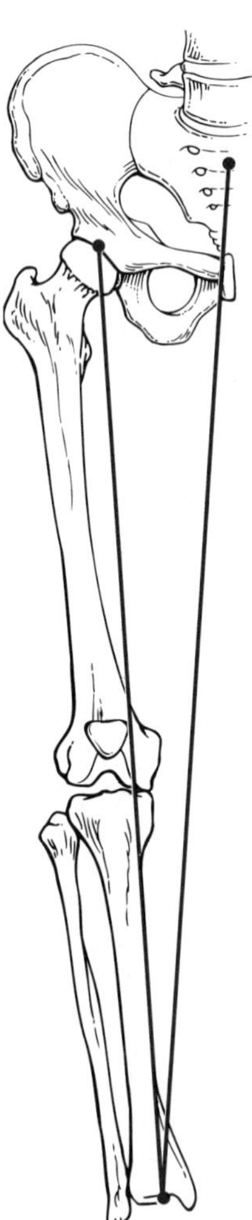

Figure 23-1 Drawing with present mechanical axis placed from center of femoral head to center of ankle.

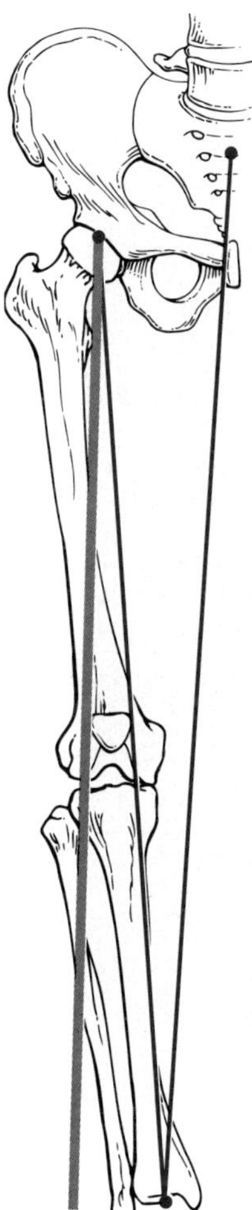

Figure 23-2 Drawing with planned mechanical axis from center of head through lateral compartment.

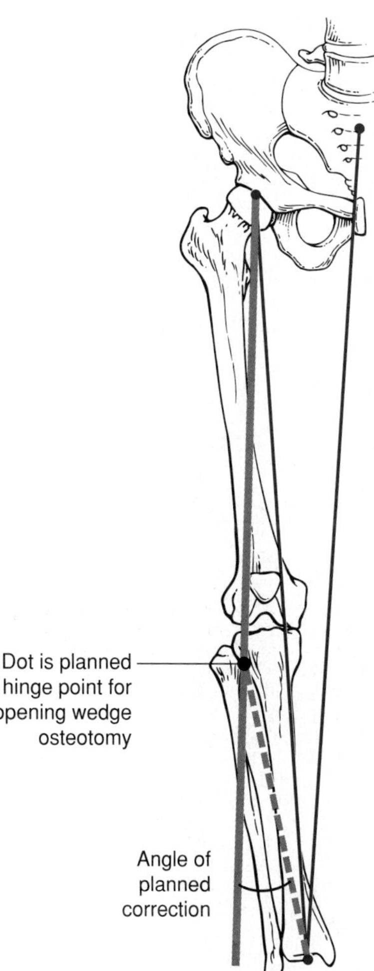

Figure 23-3 Hinge point identified and planned correction angle generated from hinge point to old and new ankle center.

alignment using fluoroscopy. An electrocautery cord or a long metal rod may be superimposed over the center of the hip and center of the ankle to ensure correct placement of the restored mechanical axis into the lateral compartment.

Opening Wedge

The knee is exposed by a longitudinal anterior or anterior-medial incision. A 2-mm K-wire is drilled parallel to the joint line, 3.5 to 4.5 cm distal to the joint line, engaging the opposite cortex. Proper position is confirmed with fluoroscopy. The osteotomy is performed distal to the K-wire to prevent intra-articular fracture into the lateral compartment. The osteotomy is performed proximal to the tibial tuberosity. The posterior structures are protected, and the osteotomy is performed leaving the lateral cortex intact, provided that no sagittal correction is needed. The posterior soft tissues are released to avoid increasing the posterior slope when the osteotomy is opened. The osteotomy is opened slowly using stacked osteotomes or a manufactured wedge to the desired correction. Proper correction is confirmed using intraoperative fluoroscopy with a long rod or a electrocautery cord. Fixation can be obtained with a T-plate or various opening wedge plates designed for this procedure (Fig. 23-5). Small corrections (<10 degrees) can be left alone, but most surgeons favor using allograft bone or bone graft substitute to fill the defect. The plate is placed distally under the pes anserine tendons. Closure is routine over drains.

Complications

Complications after upper tibial osteotomy can occur after closing or opening wedge procedures. Neurovascular problems can be avoided by proper technique and careful retraction. Fracture into the joint is probably more common with the open wedge technique and can be avoided by making sure one has osteotomized at least 90% to 95% across the proximal tibia and gradual opening of the osteotomy. Fracture of the lateral cortex or medial cortex may occur, especially in young patients with hard bone. If this occurs, making sure one obtains stable fixation will minimize the risk of this becoming problematic. Poor correction can be avoided by careful technique and the use of intraoperative fluoroscopy, but this is a relatively crude technique. Inadvertent changing of the tibial slope is more difficult to monitor. Making sure that the osteotomy is done properly in the sagittal plane and that distraction or closure of the wedge is done properly can minimize this problem. One may want

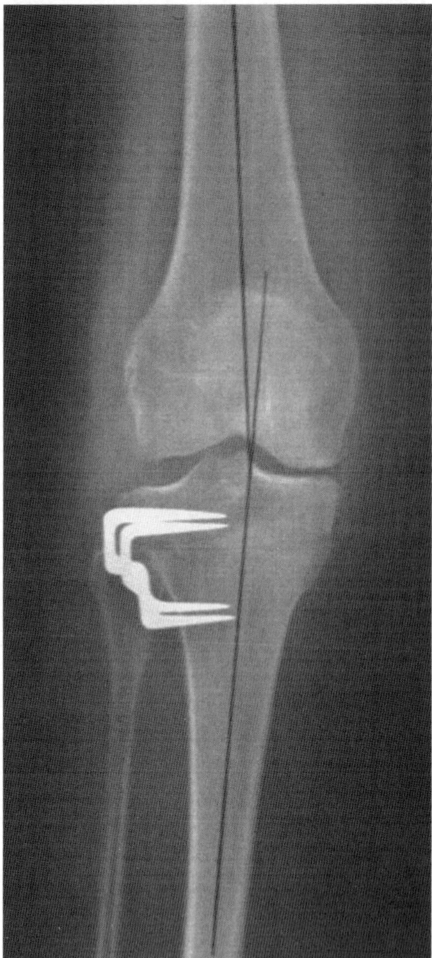

Figure 23-4 Ten-year postoperative radiograph after closing wedge osteotomy fixed with two staples.

to alter the slope intentionally in three situations: (i) In patients with extension lags, decreasing the posterior tibial slope will improve extension; (ii) in patients with hyperextension, increasing the posterior tibial slope will help limit overextension; (iii) in patients with posterior knee instability, increasing the slope will improve stability in extension as the femur slides posteriorly and the tibia anteriorly in this position. Delayed or nonunions can be avoided by maximizing bony apposition and obtaining proper stability. DVT, infection, hematoma, and compartment syndrome have been described.

Postoperative Management

Antibiotics are administered for 24 hours. Drains are removed on the second postoperative day. Mobilization and partial weight bearing (approximately 15 to 20 kg) are begun immediately. With closing wedge osteotomy and good fixation, range of motion is begun at 4 or 5 days with or without a removable splint. Patients with closing wedge osteotomy fixed with staples may be immobilized in a cast for 4 to 6 weeks. If at 6 weeks radiographs show consolidation, progressive weight bearing is allowed. Opening wedge osteotomy patients can begin range of motion immediately and weight bearing after 6 to 8 weeks.

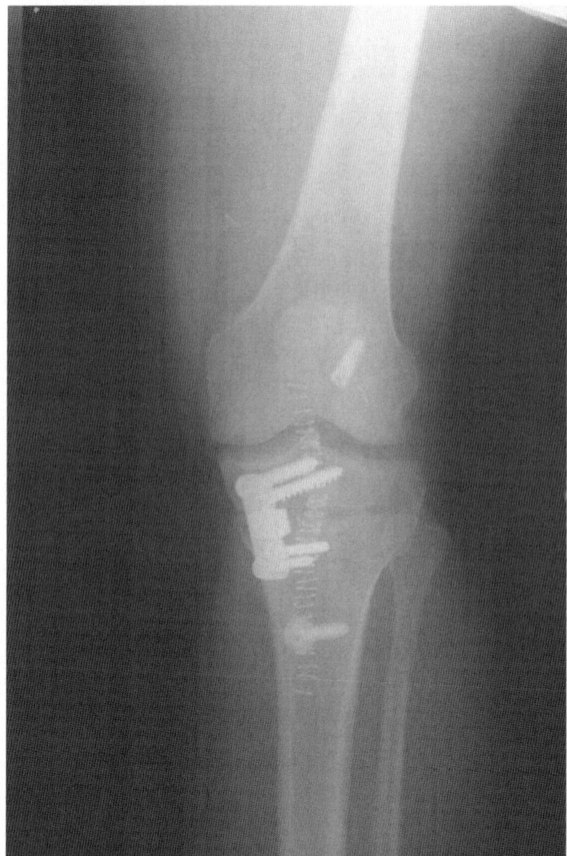

Figure 23-5 Postoperative radiograph after opening wedge osteotomy with simultaneous ligament reconstruction.

Results

Most studies with long-term results have been performed in patients treated with a closing wedge technique. Multiple authors have shown that clinical results deteriorate with time. Insall showed that at 2-year follow-up, 97% of patients had a good or excellent result. The outcome deteriorates to 85% at 5 years and 59% at 9 years. Multiple authors have also reported successful outcome, although with shorter follow-up, with an opening wedge technique. Hernigou has reported on 93 knees treated with opening wedge technique with 90% having a good result at 5 years. Success depends on multiple factors including proper correction, preoperative condition of the noninvolved compartment meniscus, and severity of obesity.

Conclusion

Realignment osteotomy for the young active patient with osteoarthritis secondary to limb malalignment is a reliable and somewhat durable procedure. Proper patient selection and surgical execution will help optimize outcome.

SUGGESTED READINGS

Aglietti P, Rinonapoli E, Stringa G, et al. Tibial osteotomy for the varus osteoarthritic knee. *Clin Orthop*.1983;176:239–251.

Coventry MB. Osteotomy of the upper portion of the tibia for degenerative arthritis of the knee. A preliminary report. *J Bone Joint Surg*. 1965;47A:984.

Fowler PJ, Tan JL, Brown GA. Medial opening wedge high tibial osteotomy: how I do it. *Op Tech Sports Med*. 2000;1:32–38.

Hernigou P. Open wedge tibial osteotomy: combined coronal and sagittal correction. *Knee*. 2002;9:15–20.

Hernigou P, Medevielle D, Debeyre J, et al. Proximal tibial osteotomy for osteoarthritis with varus deformity. A ten to thirteen-year follow-up study. J Bone Joint Surg 1987;69A:332–354.

Insall JN, Joseph DM, Msika C. High tibial osteotomy for varus gonarthrosis. *J Bone Joint Surg*. 1984;66A:1040–1048.

Jackson JP. Osteotomy for osteoarthritis of the knee. Proceedings of the Sheffield Regional Orthopaedic Club. *J Bone Joint Surg*. 1958;40B:826.

Jacobi M, Jakob RP. Open wedge osteotomy in the treatment of medial osteoarthritis of the knee. *Tech Knee Surg*. 2005;4:70–78.

Langenbeck B. Die subkutane Osteotomie. *Dtsch Klin*. 1854;6:327.

Maquet P. Valgus osteotomy for osteoarthritis of the knee. *Clin Orthop*. 1976;120:143–148.

Puddu G, Fowler PJ, Amendola A. *Opening Wedge Osteotomy System by Arthrex: Surgical Technique*. Naples, FL: Arthrex; 1998.

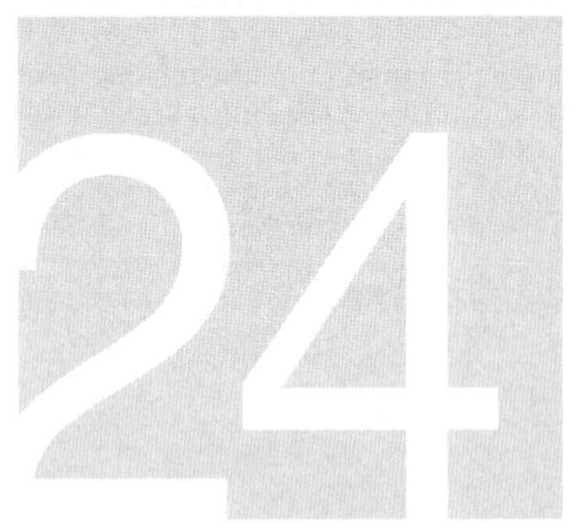

UNICOMPARTMENTAL KNEE ARTHROPLASTY

MARK W. PAGNANO
ROBERT S. RICE

Unicompartmental knee arthroplasty (UKA) has experienced a resurgence of interest in the past decade. For a selected subgroup of patients with isolated advanced degenerative arthritis involving primarily the medial or lateral compartment of the knee, UKA may be the best surgical treatment option. Comparisons of the early outcomes of UKA with those of total knee arthroplasty (TKA) typically reveal faster recovery after UKA. In addition, often there is greater patient satisfaction with UKA because the knee feels more like a normal knee, possibly because of the preservation of both cruciate ligaments after UKA (Table 24-1). Comparisons of the early outcomes of UKA to those of osteotomy typically reveal faster recovery, more predictable pain relief, and fewer surgical complications after UKA. Progression of degenerative arthritis in the unresurfaced portions of the joint after UKA remains a mode of failure that is not faced after TKA. Controversy exists about the ability to predict, through physical exam or radiographs, those patients at risk for developing arthritis in other compartments after UKA. For that reason some surgeons remain reluctant to use UKA and instead rely on TKA for those patients who progress to require a knee arthroplasty. In large cohorts of patients, however, it is fair to conclude that the survivorship of modern UKA and modern TKA are essentially equivalent over the first decade after implantation.

PATHOGENESIS

Isolated advanced degenerative arthritis of the medial compartment of the knee is the most common indication for unicompartmental knee arthroplasty. The pathogenesis of isolated medial compartment disease is well recognized. Progressive loss of articular cartilage leads to varus malalignment of the limb, which then further overloads the articular cartilage and causes additional loss of articular cartilage over time. In most patients with an intact anterior cruciate ligament (ACL), the area of maximal articular cartilage loss is the anteromedial portion of the tibia. When the ACL is intact, most patients will have preservation of full-thickness articular cartilage on the posteromedial portion of the tibia. On the femoral side, almost all of the articular cartilage loss is from the distal femur, with the posterior femoral cartilage relatively well preserved. In patients without an ACL, the knee kinematics are altered substantially and the pattern of arthritis is markedly less predictable. In many, but not all, ACL-deficient patients, sufficient lateral compartment disease or patellofemoral compartment disease will be present such that a UKA is not appropriate.

Isolated advanced degenerative arthritis of the lateral compartment of the knee is decidedly less common than medial-sided disease. Most TKA studies suggest a 10-to-1 predominance of medial over lateral compartment disease, and most UKA studies suggest closer to 20-to-1 predominance of medial UKA versus lateral UKA. In many surgeons' experience, the patient with valgus deformity and lateral compartment disease often presents with concomitant anterior knee pain or patellofemoral radiographic findings that make UKA less appealing. Even in those patients with isolated lateral compartment disease, the pattern of degenerative change is less predictable than in patients with isolated medial disease. This likely reflects the more complex kinematics of the lateral compartment of the knee, which includes greater amounts of gliding and rolling than the medial side.

DIAGNOSIS

Physical Examination and History

The ideal candidate for UKA is able to clearly pinpoint the medial (or lateral) joint line as the source of pain that prevents him or her from carrying out activities of daily living (Fig. 24-1). Those patients who have diffuse knee pain or who clearly identify anterior knee pain as substantially limiting likely will be served better with TKA. Specific anterior knee pain symptoms when squatting or standing from a seated position also would suggest TKA rather than UKA. As with any knee problem, care should be taken to exclude

TABLE 24-1 ADVANTAGES AND DISADVANTAGES OF UNICOMPARTMENTAL KNEE ARTHROPLASTY VERSUS TOTAL KNEE ARTHROPLASTY

Advantages	Disadvantages
1. Preserves bone stock	1. Technically more demanding
2. Preserves both cruciate ligaments	2. Strict patient selection
3. Increased range of motion	3. Potential for disease progression in unresurfaced compartments of knee
4. More normal kinematics	
5. More normal proprioception	

hip disease or a neurologic cause for the pain. Patients with inflammatory arthritis are better suited to TKA than UKA. Considerable debate exists on how to factor age and body weight into the decision to proceed with UKA. Interestingly, at this time the available evidence suggests that weight does not affect early outcome or survivorship through the first decade. This may be because many obese patients are relatively sedentary. In distinction there is evidence from the Swedish Joint Registry that younger age is adversely correlated with survivorship; however, that applies to not just UKA but also TKA.

On physical exam the knee should flex >90 degrees and have no more than a 10- to 15-degree flexion contracture. More substantial flexion contractures typically can be corrected only partially with UKA. Varus or valgus deformity of >10 degrees is typically accompanied by degenerative changes in the other compartments of the knee that make UKA less predictable. Furthermore, varus/valgus deformity of >10 to 15 degrees often requires collateral ligament release at the time of surgery, which most authors have advised against during UKA. The stability of the ACL must be assessed preoperatively. A deficient ACL is a contraindication to the use of a mobile-bearing UKA design because the risk of bearing dislocation is substantial. Some authors suggest that a deficient ACL in a low-demand patient who has not experienced giving way episodes is not a contraindication to a fixed-bearing UKA. When UKA is selected for those low-demand ACL deficient patients, care should be taken not to increase the posterior slope of the tibial component. For active, high-demand patients and for those who have experienced symptomatic giving way episodes, an isolated UKA is contraindicated in the face of ACL deficiency. Some authors have described concomitant or sequential ACL reconstruction and UKA, but the data on that combination is limited.

Radiographic Features

A full-length standing radiograph including the hip-knee-ankle on a 3-foot film is useful. With that film the mechanical axis and anatomic axis can be calculated and the presence or absence of extra-articular bone deformity can be confirmed. On a standing anteroposterior (AP) view of the knee, the contralateral tibiofemoral compartment is examined for evidence of joint space narrowing or osteophyte formation. Some surgeons, particularly those in Europe, routinely obtain stress views of the knee in varus and valgus as part of the evaluation for UKA. These stress views can confirm the integrity of the opposite compartment and determine if adequate correction of the varus-valgus alignment can be obtained without collateral ligament release. On the lateral radiograph, superior and inferior pole patellar osteophytes can be observed. Axial views of the patella are used to grossly assess the patellofemoral articulation for evidence of subluxation or loss of articular cartilage. In the absence of symptoms, some surgeons will ignore the status of the patellofemoral joint; however most surgeons would regard the presence of bone-on-bone changes at the patellofemoral joint as a contraindication to UKA. The presence of diffuse chondrocalcinosis on x-ray films (particularly when accompanied by history or physical findings of recurrent effusion) is a contraindication to UKA.

Typically, plain radiographs and a targeted history and physical exam are sufficient to allow a definitive decision about whether UKA is appropriate. In rare circumstances MRI might be helpful in determining the status of the contralateral compartment or the ACL. MRI, however is helpful in patients with avascular necrosis for whom UKA is contemplated. Some surgeons make a distinction between patients with so-called spontaneous avascular necrosis (AVN) and patients with AVN secondary to corticosteroid use. Patients with spontaneous osteonecrosis typically have small areas of necrotic bone confined to the subchondral region, and those patients are often good candidates for UKA. Some patients with AVN secondary to steroid use have large, geographic avascular bone lesions that could compromise the fixation of the femoral or tibial component after UKA. MRI can be helpful in determining the depth and extent of that necrotic change. If it appears that after the predicted bone cuts a substantial portion of the UKA implant will rest on necrotic bone, then TKA may be a better choice (Fig. 24-2).

TREATMENT

Surgical Goals

Surgeons continue to debate what the appropriate postoperative limb alignment should be after UKA. Most, but not all, surgeons currently recommend that the limb remain slightly undercorrected after UKA. For the typical varus knee undergoing medial compartment UKA, this means leaving the limb with a mechanical axis that passes through the medial compartment just medial to the tibial spines. For most patients the postoperative anatomic femorotibial axis would thus measure 2 to 4 degrees of valgus as opposed to the normal 6 degrees of valgus. The rationale for slightly undercorrecting the mechanical axis is to avoid overloading the articular cartilage in the opposite compartment. Markedly undercorrecting the knee, however, is also inappropriate as

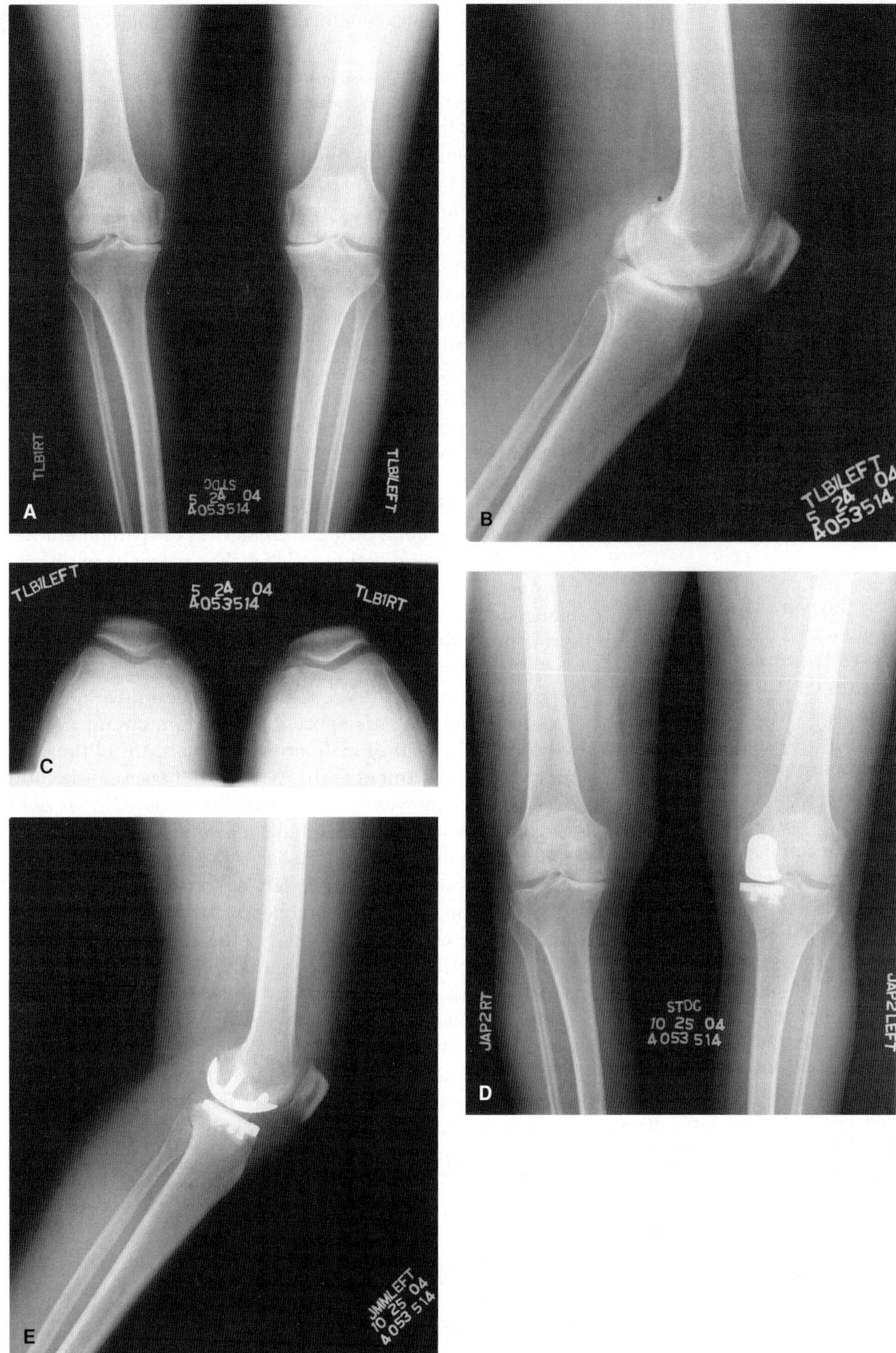

Figure 24-1 A 53-year-old female with advanced medial compartment degenerative arthritis. The symptoms are confined to the medial joint line with no anterior or lateral pain with activities or at rest. The anterior cruciate ligament is intact. **A:** The anteroposterior weight-bearing x-ray film reveals bone-on-bone changes in the medial compartment. The lateral compartment is well preserved. There is no translation of the femur on the tibia and no evidence of tibial spine impingement. **B:** The lateral x-ray film reveals mild degenerative spurs at the superior and inferior poles of the patella. **C:** The axial view of the patella shows a well-preserved patellofemoral joint space with some minimal degenerative changes involving the medial facet of the patella. **D:** The postoperative anteroposterior weight-bearing x-ray film shows a unicompartmental knee in good position. The overall limb alignment has been deliberately left slightly undercorrected, there has been a minimal resection of tibial bone, the femoral and tibial components are parallel in extension, and the femur is well centered over the tibial component. **E:** The postoperative lateral x-ray film reveals that the femoral component is well sized without anterior extension that would impinge on the patella, the tibial component fills the space from anterior to posterior without any overhang, and the posterior slope is not excessive.

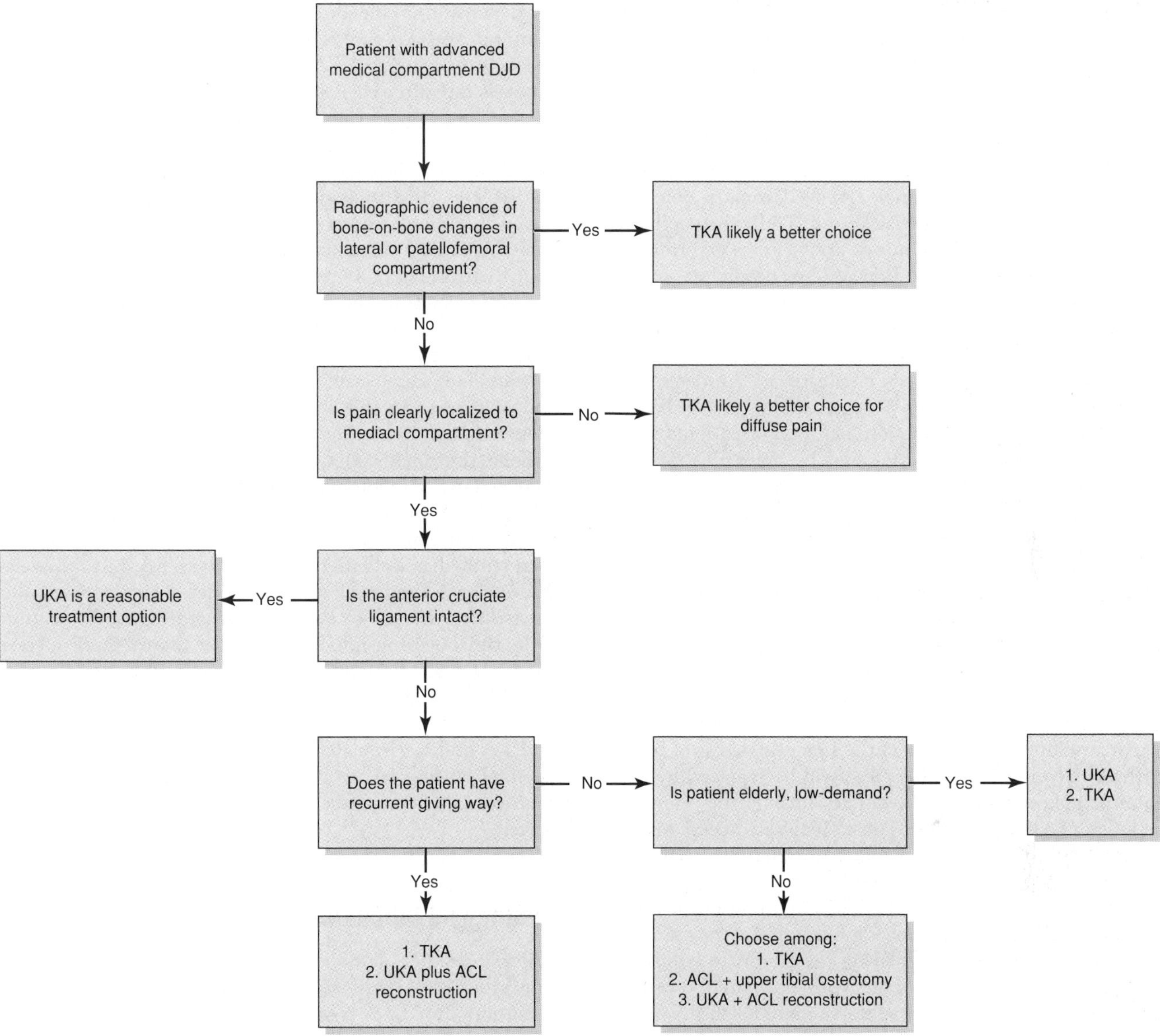

Figure 24-2 A treatment algorithm for the management of advanced medial compartment degenerative arthritis. ACL, anterior cruciate ligament; DJD, degenerative joint disease; TKA, total knee arthroplasty; UKA, unicompartmental knee arthroplasty.

that will place excessive load on the UKA bearing and lead to failure owing to polyethylene wear. In both full extension and at 90 degrees of flexion, the femoral and tibial components should be parallel such that edge loading of the polyethylene does not occur. The knee should be balanced to incorporate 2 mm of laxity in both flexion and extension. The tibial component must not overhang medially where it can irritate the medial collateral ligament. The femoral component must not extend anteriorly beyond the edge of subchondral bone or it can impinge against the patella.

Techniques

Various techniques exist to implant contemporary UKA designs. Those techniques include noninstrumented, freehand preparation through intramedullary, extramedullary, and computer-assisted instrumentation systems. Surgeons must understand the rationale for a given instrumentation system before using the system clinically. Contemporary UKA is often done through a so-called minimally invasive surgical approach (MIS). The MIS technique typically involves an 8- to 12-cm skin incision and a short medial arthrotomy that stops at the superior pole of the patella. A short split into the vastus medialis muscle can be made (mini midvastus approach) or alternatively the subvastus interval can be exploited if more exposure is needed. The patella does not need to be dislocated for UKA, and leaving the patella reduced in the trochlea helps the surgeon avoid some component orientation errors. When UKA is done using a traditional TKA approach with the patella everted and the knee flexed, the tibia tends to externally rotate and the medial flexion space tends to gap open, and that can lead to component orientation problems. MIS techniques continue to be debated in the realm of TKA, but in UKA contemporary instruments are well suited to this approach. A portion of the retropatellar fat pad and the anterior horn of the medial meniscus can be excised for visualization early in the case. In midflexion the status of the ACL, the lateral compartment, and the patellofemoral joint are noted. Any intercondylar osteophytes can be removed from the notch to prevent impingement on the ACL, and patellar osteophytes can be debrided. The sequence of bone cuts is determined by the particular instrumentation system chosen by the surgeon. Typically, on the tibial side the emphasis is on minimal bone resection with at most 2 mm of bone removed from the most worn portion of the tibia. This cut is generally made perpendicular to the long axis of the tibia. The degree of posterior slope is most often 5 degrees but can vary based on patient and implant selection factors. For patients with ACL-deficient knees, less slope may be preferable. When an implant is used that has substantial sagittal plane conformity, then matching the posterior slope to the patient's anatomy is appropriate.

Most tibial instrumentation systems use a vertical freehand cut from anterior to posterior, and this should be done as close to the medial tibial spine as possible without damaging the ACL. The surgeon should reference the tibial tubercle to avoid the tendency to internally rotate that sagittal plane cut. Typically, the largest tibial component that does not overhang should be selected. On the femoral side, most instrumentation systems resect the same thickness of bone (both distally and posteriorly) that will be replaced by the femoral implant. If an intramedullary cutting guide is used, the knee is brought to midflexion to facilitate access to the intramedullary canal. Care is taken to protect the patellar ligament and skin during this part of the procedure. The femoral component is sized from anterior to posterior such that 1 mm of subchondral bone is left exposed at the anterior edge of the component. That sizing will eliminate impingement of the femoral component with the patella even if the patient goes on to develop patellofemoral arthritis years later. In the medial-lateral direction, the femur should be centered over the tibial component without impingement into the notch and without overhang medially. The femoral component should be rotated at 90 degrees of flexion such that the femur and tibia are parallel, thus ensuring that edge loading of the femoral component will not occur. With a trial insert in place, the knee should be balanced with symmetric flexion and extension gaps of 2 mm. The overall mechanical alignment of the leg should be assessed with a cautery cord or long drop rod. If questions exist about component position or limb alignment, an intraoperative x-ray film or fluoroscopy can be used.

Complications

Complications after UKA can involve the entire spectrum of problems encountered with total knee arthroplasty including infection, bleeding, nerve injury, prosthetic loosening, wear, continued pain, thromboembolic disease, and bearing dislocation. The prevalence of infection after UKA has historically been equal to or slightly less than that after TKA. Substantial bleeding after contemporary UKA is uncommon, and it is rare for a patient to require blood transfusion after a single UKA. Injury to the peroneal or tibial nerves is rare after UKA and is substantially lower than that reported after upper tibial osteotomy. Prosthetic loosening, wear, or failure that requires revision surgery can be estimated to occur at a rate of 1% to 1.5% per year over the first decade. Slightly higher rates of failure have been observed in patients younger than 65 years of age compared with those older than 65 years according to the Swedish Joint Registry data and from the group in Oxford, England. Continued pain in the early period after UKA typically is the result of improper patient selection, although infection, early implant loosening, or tibial plateau fracture should be excluded. Late onset of pain can occur from progression of disease in the unresurfaced compartments of the knee, implant loosening, or from polyethylene wear with associated synovitis. Between 10 and 15 years after UKA, symptomatic patellofemoral arthritis has been reported in ≤10% of UKA patients in some series. The prevalence of deep venous thrombosis and pulmonary embolus has not been studied as well after UKA as after TKA, but the available evidence suggests lower prevalence of thromboembolic disease after UKA. For mobile-bearing designs, dislocation of the tibial bearing can occur, and the reported prevalence is 0.5% to 1.5%. Patients with a deficient ACL are at particular risk for bearing dislocation after mobile-bearing UKA. Fracture of the medial tibial plateau has been reported after UKA and is associated with the use of multiple pins to fix tibial cutting jigs to the proximal medial tibia. Similar fractures can occur after excessively deep tibial resections as well.

Results and Outcomes

Multiple studies demonstrate faster recovery after UKA than after TKA. Most studies reveal that the mean range of motion after UKA is substantially better than that after TKA even when accounting for differences in preoperative motion. One prospective randomized trial of UKA versus TKA demonstrated more excellent results after UKA, and those superior results were maintained at 5 years follow-up. Early series of UKA reported survivorship of 85% to 88% at 10 years. More recent series suggest 90% to 98% survivorship at 10 years, which may be attributable to the combination of more appropriate patient selection and improved instrumentation and technique. Most of these studies, however, have been done on elderly patients with a predominance of females over males, and that makes extrapolation of these data to the younger active middle-aged patient difficult. Several recent studies in younger, more active patients have been encouraging with 10 year survivorship of 90% to 92%. Those UKAs that require revision typically are divided equally between patients who fail because of disease progression in the unresurfaced compartments and those who fail because of loosening or wear of the UKA components. Early reports of conversion of the failed UKA to TKA suggested that substantial bone loss was encountered commonly and that these were difficult reoperations. In contrast, many authors now suggest that conversion of the failed contemporary UKA to TKA is relatively straightforward. There are data to suggest that revision of a UKA to TKA is more reliable than revision of UKA to another UKA. Surgeons continue to disagree on whether conversion of a failed UKA to TKA is more or less difficult than conversion of a failed upper tibial osteotomy to TKA.

Postoperative Management

Postoperative pain can be improved by the injection of local anesthetic into the capsule and subcutaneous tissues prior to closing the wound. Patients can typically begin weight bearing as tolerated early after surgery and progress with activities as tolerated. Although some surgeons will perform UKA as an outpatient procedure, most patients are hospitalized for 1 to 3 days. Most surgeons now use some form of rapid rehabilitation protocol such that patients use ambulatory aids for a short period of time after surgery. Just as in TKA, these patients should work diligently early after surgery to regain maximal knee extension and flexion.

PATELLOFEMORAL ARTHROPLASTY

The decidedly poor results with early patellofemoral arthroplasty designs has had a lasting influence on surgeons and has resulted in the continued limited use of patellofemoral arthroplasty. Nonetheless, there likely is a small subgroup of patients for whom contemporary patellofemoral arthroplasty is a good treatment option. For older patients with advanced patellofemoral arthritis, TKA has proved to be a reliable, reproducible, and durable procedure. For patients younger than 55 years of age who have substantial primary or posttraumatic patellofemoral degenerative arthritis without patellar malalignment, patellofemoral arthroplasty may be considered. Furthermore, patellofemoral arthroplasty can be considered in patients with arthritis secondary to trochlea dysplasia. Because a patellofemoral arthroplasty allows retention of both cruciate ligaments, the knee kinematics are better preserved as compared with TKA, and thus patients may perceive the knee to feel more normal. Although contemporary implant designs do offer improvements over historical designs, patellofemoral arthroplasty remains a technically demanding operation. Implant malposition can result in prosthetic impingement, pain, and extensor mechanism instability problems. Implant loosening with contemporary cemented patellofemoral arthroplasty has not proved to be common. With longer-term follow-up, however, a substantial number of patients (25% at 15 years) will go on to develop symptomatic degenerative arthritis in the tibiofemoral articulation. Conversion of patellofemoral arthroplasty to TKA typically is not particularly difficult.

SUGGESTED READINGS

Argenson JN, Komistek RD, Aubaniac JM, et al. In vivo determination of knee kinematics for subjects implanted with a unicompartmental arthroplasty. *J Arthroplasty*. 2002;17:1049–1053.

Cartier P, Sanouiller JL, Khefacha A. Long-term results with the first patellofemoral prosthesis. *Clin Orthop Relat Res.* 2005;436:47–54.

Langdown AJ, Pandit H, Price AJ, et al. Oxford medial unicompartmental arthroplasty for focal spontaneous osteonecrosis of the knee. *Acta Orthop*. 2005;76:688–692.

Lonner JH. Patellofemoral arthroplasty: pros, cons, and design considerations. *Clin Orthop Relat Res.* 2004;428:158–165.

Newman JH, Ackroyd CE, Shah NA. Unicompartmental or total knee replacement? Five year results of a prospective randomized trial of 102 osteoarthritic knees with unicompartmental arthritis. *J Bone Joint Surg Br*. 1998;80:862–865.

Pandit H, Beard DJ, Jenkins C, et al. Combined anterior cruciate reconstruction and Oxford unicompartmental knee arthroplasty. *J Bone Joint Surg Br*. 2006;88:887–892.

Pennington DW, Swienckowski JJ, Lutes WB, et al. Unicompartmental knee arthroplasty in patients sixty years of age or younger. *J Bone Joint Surg Am*. 2003;85:1968–1973.

Price AJ, Dodd CA, Svard UG, et al. Oxford medial unicompartmental knee arthroplasty in patients younger and older than 60 years of age. *J Bone Joint Surg Br*. 2005;87:1488–1492.

Springer BD, Scott RD, Thornhill TS. Conversion of failed unicompartmental knee arthroplasty to TKA. *Clin Orthop Relat Res.* 2006;446:214–220.

Walton NP, Jahroni I, Lewis PL, et al. Patient-perceived outcomes and return to sport and work: TKA versus mini-incision unicompartmental knee arthroplasty. *J Knee Surg*. 2006;19:112–116.

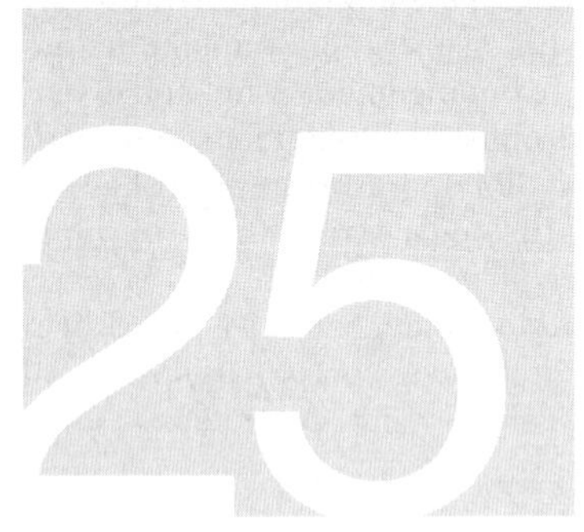

TOTAL KNEE ARTHROPLASTY

HENRY D. CLARKE

Total knee replacement is an excellent treatment option for relieving arthritic knee pain and for improving function. However, it is a technically demanding procedure and the long-term success is dependent on the way the prosthesis is implanted. In this chapter important variables that are associated with achieving optimal results are presented. These include factors related to patient selection, preoperative planning, surgical technique and postoperative management.

PATHOGENESIS

Etiology

The primary indication for knee replacement is for relief of chronic disabling knee pain owing to arthritis that has failed to respond to nonsurgical treatment regimens. In the United States >90% of the patients who undergo total knee arthroplasty (TKA) have osteoarthritis (OA), with the other main causes including rheumatoid arthritis and posttraumatic arthritis. Risk factors for the development of OA include age, body weight, gender, family history of disease, and prior injuries including meniscectomy and cruciate ligament tears. The increased risk in each of these groups is likely multifactorial with both mechanical and chemically mediated components. The composition of both hyaline cartilage and synovial fluid changes with age in both men and women, but women have higher rates of knee OA and therefore, the role of gonadal hormone levels has been debated. A genetic component has also been implicated, although it is likely that many genes contribute to this risk. Genetic differences in cartilage and subchondral bone constituents appear to be involved in this process, and research is ongoing to identify important markers. Patients with a high body mass index are also at increased risk for the development of OA, and this risk may be owing to factors beyond the simple mechanical trauma produced by the elevated joint forces. Clearly some or all of these risk factors may be identified in any individual, and therefore the relative contribution of each is hard to determine.

Epidemiology

Population studies from Western societies have estimated that approximately 10% to 20% of adult patients older than 35 years of age experience chronic knee pain. Among this group of patients, the prevalence of radiographically identifiable OA has been reported to be between 1% and 70%, depending on the age subgroup, but most studies have suggested a rate of between 1% and 15%. In the United States Medicare population, between 30 and 70 people per 10,000, depending on gender and age subgroup, underwent primary TKA in 2000, with the highest rate of 67.9 per 10,000 noted in women between the ages of 75 and 79 years. During this time period, >350,000 primary TKAs were performed annually in the United States.

DIAGNOSIS

Clinical Features

History

Patients with arthritic knees complain of pain that is exacerbated by weight-bearing activity and relieved by rest. Pain may be isolated to one area of the knee in unicompartmental arthritis or diffuse when multiple compartments are involved. Anterior knee pain that is aggravated by stairs or arising from a sitting position is suggestive of patellofemoral involvement. Secondary symptoms include varying degrees of swelling, buckling or giving way, catching, grinding, and stiffness. In some cases, pain may be referred from other areas of the body to the knee. Other causes should always be considered, especially in cases where the pain is not clearly activity related; radiates to the hip, back, or foot; or is inconsistent with the associated physical exam or radiographic studies. In these circumstances, arthritis of the hip, lumbar radiculopathy, and inflammatory diseases without joint destruction should be considered. It is also important to elicit a history of failed nonoperative and operative treatments including steroid or hyaluronic acid injections, oral anti-inflammatory medication, physical therapy, bracing, arthroscopic debridement, ligament reconstruction, and osteotomy.

In addition to reliving arthritic pain, a secondary goal for total knee arthroplasty is to improve patient function. Evaluating the degree of disability experienced by a patient can be difficult but is crucially important. Patient expectations and goals must be clearly understood to optimize satisfaction postoperatively. Some patients may simply be hoping to be able to perform activities of daily living without pain, whereas others may be expecting to be able to participate in vigorous sports such as marathon training or basketball. In patients with high expectations, a frank discussion of the goals of knee replacement and the types of activities that can be realistically pursued postoperatively is necessary.

Relative contraindications to total knee replacement include a history of prior infection in the involved knee or active infection in any other location, neuromuscular conditions such as Charcot arthropathy, prior fusion of the involved knee, and a nonfunctional extensor mechanism. Absolute contraindications include active infection in the involved knee or periarticular region, severe peripheral vascular disease, and lack of adequate soft tissue coverage.

It is also important to elicit a history of any systemic conditions that the patient has experienced. Obesity, diabetes, coronary or pulmonary disease, peripheral vascular disease, and immune compromise owing to cancer or HIV all increase the risks associated with joint replacement. Comprehensive consultation with appropriate specialists is critical to optimize results but rarely precludes joint replacement as long as the patient understands the potential risks.

Physical Examination

Preoperative evaluation should determine the presence of prior skin incisions about the knee, the overall clinical alignment of the leg, joint line and peripatellar tenderness, crepitus, whether the collateral ligaments are competent, and whether the varus or valgus deformity is passively correctable to neutral. In cases where the ligaments may be incompetent, a prosthesis with increased femoral-tibial constraint should be available for use. In addition, the passive range of motion, fixed flexion contractures, and extension lags should be noted. Distal pulses, strength and sensation in the extremity should also be evaluated. Finally, as previously noted, absence of significant hip pain with passive motion and adequate hip range of motion should also be verified.

Radiologic Features

Radiographs of the affected knee are adequate for preoperative counseling in most cases. Standard views include a weight-bearing anterior-posterior (AP) view in full extension, a lateral view, and a Merchant view of the patellofemoral joint. In some cases a posterior-anterior (PA) view in 45 degrees of flexion is helpful for demonstrating significant joint space narrowing when the AP standing view shows only minimal changes. The PA flexion view provides a superior view of the contact between the distal-posterior femoral condyles and the tibia, which is an area where significant cartilage wear can occur. In cases where joint space narrowing is unremarkable or where pain is out of proportion to the radiographic evidence, MRI of the knee may identify meniscal pathology or other periarticular pathology such as avascular necrosis, stress fractures, and bone lesions that require alternative treatment. If lumbar or hip pathology is suspected after physical exam, then adequate radiographs of these areas should also be obtained.

Prior to knee replacement a full length, three-joint view of the lower extremity helps with preoperative planning. However, this is probably only mandatory in cases where there is a history of prior fractures or surgery of the ipsilateral extremity, or physical exam suggests unusual extra-articular deformities.

TREATMENT

Surgical Technique

The key components of the surgical technique for total knee replacement include selecting placement of the skin incision, gaining adequate exposure to the joint, restoring axial alignment of the limb by accurately resecting bone from the femur and tibia, and creation of symmetric flexion and extension gaps with balanced medial and lateral soft tissue tension by releasing the contracted structures. Subtle differences exist depending on whether a posterior cruciate retaining, substituting, or sacrificing prosthesis is implanted, but the broad principles are the same and these are presented in the subsequent sections.

Skin Incision

An anterior midline, vertically oriented skin incision that deviates slightly to the medial side of the tibial tubercle distally is the most utilitarian approach to the knee. Traditionally, incision length was between 15 and 20 cm depending on the size of the patient and surgeon preference. However, with increased emphasis in recent years on reducing incision length and soft tissue dissection in so-called minimally invasive techniques, the incision length has declined and various authors have described the ability to perform TKA through shorter skin incisions.

Prior incisions must be treated with caution as the blood supply to the knee is limited. The vascular supply to the overlying skin is medially biased, and this should be considered in the decision about incision placement when prior incisions exist. In particular, wide scars, lateral incisions, and skin with posttraumatic or postradiation scarring or thinning should be treated with special concern. In general, a single pre-existing transverse incision may be crossed at a right angle with little concern. If a prior anterior incision is present, it should be used unless it lies too far medial or lateral. In circumstances where a prior vertical incision is significantly displaced from the midline, especially with short, well-matured scars, a second vertical midline incision can be made if an adequate skin bridge of about 5 cm can be maintained. However, if multiple vertical or mixed anterior incisions are present, alternative techniques such as tissue expanders or even prophylactic muscle flaps may be required to reduce the risk of postoperative wound-healing problems.

Exposure

The exposure is largely independent of the skin incision that has been used, although with recent minimally invasive techniques, placement of the short incision over the area where the arthrotomy will be performed is optimal. The most utilitarian approach to the knee joint is via a medial parapatellar arthrotomy that begins 5 to 8 cm proximal to the superior pole of the patella, about 5 mm lateral to the medial border of the quadriceps tendon. The arthrotomy extends distally either around the medial border of the patella or directly over the medial edge of the patellar and then extends along the medial edge of the patellar tendon about 5 to 8 cm distal to the joint line. Next, the anterior horn of the medial meniscus is transected and the medial capsule and periosteum is elevated from the proximal 3 to 4 cm of the medial tibia. The infrapatellar fat pad is resected, and the lateral patellofemoral ligament is divided. If at this stage the patella cannot be subluxated laterally, or everted from the field of view, a quadriceps snip can be performed. Beginning at the apex of the arthrotomy in the quadriceps tendon, the arthrotomy is extended laterally and superiorly at an angle of 45 degrees into the vastus lateralis muscle. In the rare case where this maneuver does not relieve tension on the extensor mechanism and the exposure is still inadequate, a tubercle osteotomy can then be performed and will provide adequate exposure.

The recent trend to minimally invasive surgery has prompted renewed interest in alternative approaches to the anterior knee that include subvastus, mini midvastus, and medial and lateral capsular incisions. Although all of these alternatives are believed to cause less damage to the extensor mechanism and allow quicker functional recovery, few controlled studies exist. Furthermore, the visualization of the knee with any of these exposures is limited, and therefore, they are not suitable for every patient in all surgeons' hands. In particular, patients with heavily muscled thighs, obese patients, and patients with patellar baja or large deformities pose special challenges and may not be amenable to these limited approaches.

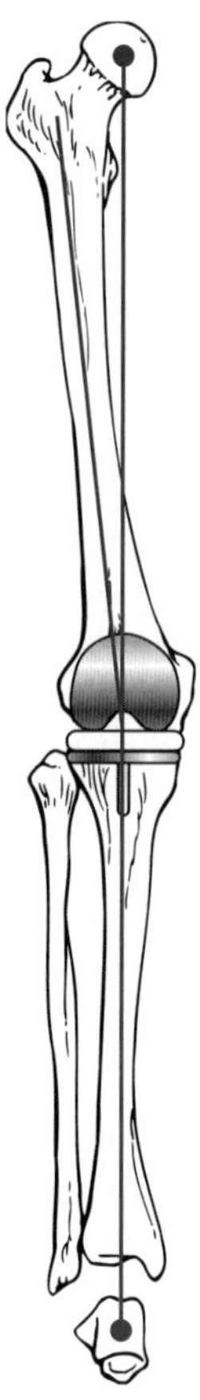

Figure 25-1 The mechanical axis of the knee should pass through the center of the hip, knee, and talus once the prosthesis has been implanted. Both the femoral and tibial components are oriented perpendicular to the mechanical axis. The femoral component is in approximately 5 to 7 degrees of valgus relative to the anatomic axis of the femoral shaft.

Bone Resection

Restoration of axial mechanical alignment of the operated leg within a narrow range of ±3 degrees has been demonstrated to be an important determinant for long-term success following TKA. Therefore, bone resection must be performed in an accurate and reproducible way. Orientation of the femoral and tibial components parallel to the mechanical axis of the leg is the goal of the bone resection in TKA (Fig. 25-1). Many instruments have been designed to help the surgeon optimize the bone resection of the distal and posterior femur and proximal tibia. These include both intramedullary and extramedually alignment guides and cutting blocks that are affixed to the bones. Recently computer navigated systems that use either optical or electromagnetic sensors have been developed to aid in this task and have demonstrated more reproducible results than mechanical guides. The specific order of femoral and tibial cuts is irrelevant as these steps are independent in the classic method of bone resection that is favored by many surgeons. It must be recognized that some surgeons favor the use of tensor systems that rely on a tibial cut made perpendicular to the mechanical axis of the tibia to determine the femoral cuts. In this technique, the tibial cut must be made first.

In a knee with varus deformity, the distal femur usually should be cut in 5 to 7 degrees of valgus relative to the femoral shaft or anatomic axis. However, to avoid persistent excessive valgus alignment in a valgus knee, a distal femoral cut of 4 to 5 degrees of valgus relative to the anatomic axis is suggested in these cases. A three-joint view of the limb can facilitate selection of the optimal distal femoral resection by allowing the angle between the anatomic and mechanical axes of the femur to be measured for the specific individual. Other variables such as the placement of the starting hole and fit of the intramedullary alignment guide in the femoral canal can affect the accuracy of the cut and probably have more of an influence on the ultimate resection angle than surgeon choice of 5 or 6 degrees.

The next important step is to accurately size the femur and set the femoral component rotation (Fig. 25-2). This step will determine the anterior femoral and posterior femoral condylar resections. The epicondylar axis has been shown to be the most reliable landmark for determining accurate rotation and is easily identified intraoperatively. If the femoral component is not set parallel to this axis, it

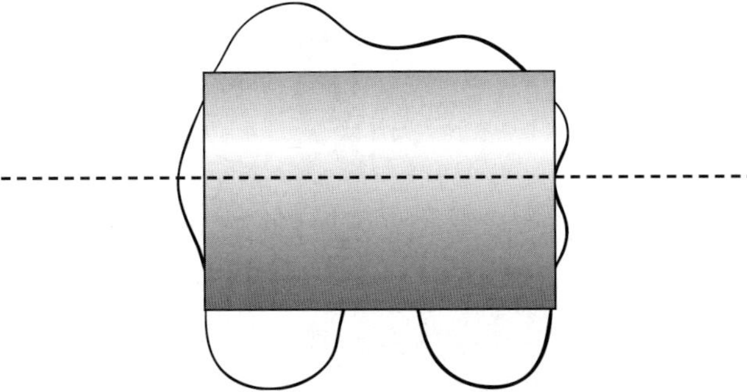

Figure 25-2 The femoral component is aligned parallel to the transepicondylar axis, which passes through the center of the prominence of the lateral epicondyle and the center of the sulcus of the medial epicondyle.

is difficult to produce a symmetric flexion space. The AP axis, or so-called Whiteside line, is a good secondary reference point that links the center of the intercondylar notch and the center of the femoral trochlea. This axis is usually perpendicular to the epicondylar axis. With the femoral cutting block oriented relative to these landmarks, in most circumstances, more bone will be resected from the posterior medial condyle than the lateral condyle because the epicondylar axis is externally rotated relative to the posterior condylar line. In a varus knee the epicondylar axis is generally externally rotated by about 3 degrees relative to the posterior condylar line, whereas in the valgus knee the epicondylar axis tends to be externally rotated by about 5 degrees.

Next, the tibial resection guide is set to produce a bone cut perpendicular to the mechanical axis. Approximately 9 to 10 mm of bone typically will be resected from the unaffected compartment, i.e., from the lateral side in a varus knee. Once the distal and posterior femoral cuts and tibial cut have been made, a spacer block with an extramedullary guide rod is inserted to evaluate whether the optimal limb alignment has been achieved. If the bone cuts fail to achieve the desired limb alignment, then soft tissue balancing of the medial and lateral structures may be difficult to achieve. Furthermore, as previously noted, detrimental mechanical stresses associated with chronic malalignment can lead to progressive laxity and instability. If overall alignment is acceptable, then the next step is creating balanced and symmetric flexion and extension gaps.

Flexion and Extension Gap Balancing

Soft Tissue Releases. Evaluation of the soft tissue tension about the knee begins with an examination of the extremity under anesthesia to evaluate the integrity of the collateral soft tissue restraints. If the deformity can be corrected to neutral, a less aggressive soft tissue release should be anticipated than in a knee with a fixed deformity. Once the bone cuts have been performed as noted previously, re-evaluation of the medial and lateral soft tissue tension is performed with a spacer block as previously noted. In addition to bone and cartilage erosion, the development of deformity associated with degenerative arthritis involves the development of contractures of the soft tissue structures on the concave side of the deformity, and eventually, stretching of the structures on the convex side. For example, in the valgus knee, the lateral structures shorten and the medial soft tissues may become attenuated. The goal of soft tissue balancing is to release or lengthen the tight structures to create symmetric, rectangular flexion and extension spaces (Fig. 25-3). Although mild degrees of soft tissue imbalance may be clinically insignificant, it seems prudent to strive for optimal balance. The techniques described below for soft tissue balancing are based on the principles described by Insall.

In the varus knee, the contracted medial structures include the pes anserine tendons, superficial medial collateral ligament (MCL), posteromedial corner including the semimembranosus insertion, and deep MCL. After the standard arthrotomy and exposure has been performed and the bony cuts on the femur and tibia have been completed, the remnants of the cruciate ligaments and menisci should be excised. This is best performed with the knee in flexion, with a lamina spreader providing gentle joint distraction. It is important to remember that the fibers of the deep MCL attach to the peripheral margin of the midbody of the medial meniscus and must not be damaged during meniscal resection. This is most safely accomplished by leaving a thin rim of 1 to 2 mm of peripheral meniscus. At this stage, posterior condylar osteophytes should be removed with an osteotome.

Next, the largest spacer block that will fit in the flexion gap is inserted and stability is assessed. The knee is then extended and the limb alignment is evaluated. If alignment is acceptable, then the medial-lateral balance is assessed. If the medial structures are still tight, as is frequently found in the varus knee, an incremental release of the medial structures is performed to correct the asymmetry of the medial and lateral soft tissue tension. A 3/4-inch straight osteotome

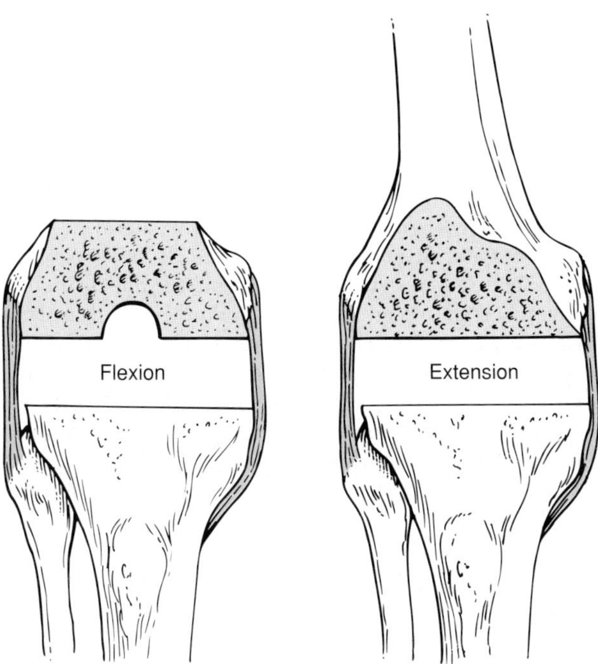

Figure 25-3 Equal and symmetric flexion and extension gaps are created by bone resection and soft tissue releases.

is used to extend the subperiosteal elevation of the distal superficial MCL insertion and deep fascia along the posteromedial border of the tibia. This release may be extended to approximately the level of the middle third of the tibia. In addition, the pes tendons may be released. In some cases, the popliteus tendon may impinge on the posterolateral aspect of the prosthesis, and in these cases of varus deformity it may be released.

Next, the spacer is reinserted and the efficacy of the release is evaluated. In many cases, once the extension space symmetry has been restored by the release, the next thicker spacer block is required. If an imbalance persists, then further subperiosteal elevation of any palpable tight medial bands should be performed distally. In addition, the tibia should be subluxated and externally rotated out from underneath the femur, and in this position a subperiosteal elevation of the semimembranous and posterior capsule from the posteromedial tibia should be completed if not already done.

In the valgus knee, the contracted anatomic structures include the iliotibial band (ITB), lateral collateral ligament (LCL), popliteus tendon, and arcuate ligament/posterolateral capsular complex. If alignment is acceptable when the knee is brought into extension with the spacer block, but the lateral side is tight, then the spacer is removed and laminar spreaders are inserted and gently opened. The lateral soft tissue structures are then released in a graduated fashion using an inside-out technique with the popliteus tendon as a landmark. The arcuate and posterolateral capsular complex are incised horizontally with a number 15 blade at the level of the tibial bone cut. Next, multiple "pie crusting" puncture incisions are made through the ITB and capsule, both at the level of the extension gap and proximal to the joint. Although no specific attempt is made to divide the LCL, it is likely at least partially cut. Once the extension gap appears rectangular, the spacer block is reinserted and the balance re-evaluated. If at this stage the lateral side is still tight, then further pie crusting is performed. In certain cases, the ITB may need to be released entirely from Gerdy's tubercle.

In the valgus knee, the popliteus tendon is preserved, if possible, to act as a lateral stabilizer in flexion and to help prevent rotatory instability. However, in severe valgus knees, typically greater than about 20 degrees, the lateral side may be tight despite the above-noted releases. In these cases, it may be necessary to strip the lateral femoral condyle including the insertion of the popliteus tendon, either sharply or by elevating a wafer of bone from the lateral epicondyle. In these situations, a constrained prosthesis may be required to provide medial and lateral stability. In elderly patients with large valgus deformities, use of a constrained condylar type of prosthesis has been associated with good long-term results despite the theoretical concerns regarding loosening.

Once balanced flexion and extension spaces have been created in either the varus or valgus knee, the knee is assessed to ensure that the size of the overall gaps is equal. The spacer block that allows full extension to be achieved without any tendency to hyperextension is selected, and finally the flexion space must be re-evaluated to ensure that it is symmetric with the extension gap. In cases where the flexion and extension gaps are not equal, further adjustments to the bone resection may be required.

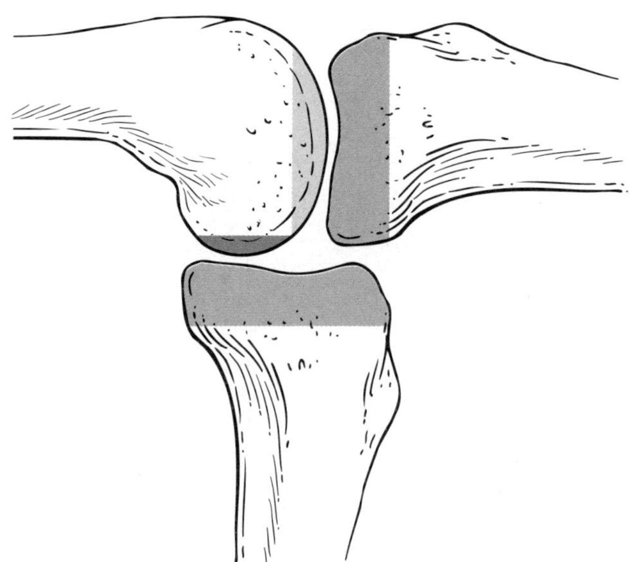

Figure 25-4 The tibial resection influences both the flexion and extension gaps, whereas the distal femoral cut affects only the extension gap and the posterior femoral resection influences only the flexion gap.

To ensure that symmetry is achieved in the size of the flexion and extension gaps, a comprehensive understanding of the impact of the three basic bony cuts in total knee arthroplasty is required. The proximal tibial cut affects both the flexion and extension gap equally, whereas the distal femoral cut selectively determines the extension gap and the posterior femoral resection affects only the flexion gap (Fig. 25-4). These basic principles provide excellent guidance if asymmetric size gaps are encountered.

If the knee is balanced in flexion but tight in extension, with a persistent flexion contracture, an additional 2 mm of femur must be removed as femoral resection selectively changes only the extension gap. In some cases, elevation of the posterior capsule from the femur can correct a slight tendency to residual flexion contractures, especially in the setting of significant preoperative contractures, but bony resection generally provides a more satisfactory result. If the knee is too tight in both flexion and extension to allow insertion of the smallest 10-mm spacer, then additional tibia must be cut as tibial resection changes both the flexion and extension gaps. In the primary setting, with a posterior cruciate retaining implant, it is uncommon to find the knee balanced in extension and too loose in flexion. This may be encountered in a posterior stabilized (PS) knee where release of the PCL may increase the flexion gap more than the extension space. In this setting, resection of additional distal femur and use of a larger polyethylene insert will be the solution. In rare circumstances with either a cruciate-retaining (CR) or PS knee, overresection of the posterior femoral condyles owing to the use of an anterior referencing femoral cutting guide or undersizing of the femoral component may be responsible. In these cases where a CR prosthesis has been used, restoring the posterior condylar offset by upsizing the femoral component and using posterior augments can be considered. With a PS knee, additional distal femur can be resected and a larger polyethylene used. This may move the joint line more proximally, but 5 to 8 mm of elevation is well tolerated with a PS knee. In distinction, joint line elevation with a CR knee is less desirable. Finding that the extension gap is balanced but the flexion gap is tight is more likely to occur in a CR knee where the PCL is too tight. In these cases, graduated release of the PCL or increasing the slope of the tibial cut should be used to solve the gap imbalance.

Component Positioning. Once appropriate extension and flexion gap symmetry has been obtained, the bone surfaces can be prepared for final component positioning. On the femoral side, chamfer cuts must be made as well as a box cut if a PS prosthesis is used. The femoral component should be lateralized on the distal femur, without creating overhang, to optimize patellar tracking. Next, tibial rotation is oriented relative to the junction of the medial and middle thirds of the tibial tubercle. Internal rotation may result in lateral patellar subluxation. Finally, the patellar component is positioned slightly medially and superiorly on the prepared surface, which helps prevent patellar maltracking. The overall composite thickness of the resurfaced patella should restore, or when possible, slightly reduce (1 to 2 mm) the thickness of the native patella. Once these steps have been completed, a reduction using trial components is performed to ensure that appropriate soft tissue balance has been achieved without flexion contracture or hyperextension. If imperfections exist, adjustments are made. Lastly, a "no thumbs" technique is used to evaluate patellar tracking. If the femoral and tibial rotations have been set correctly, the thickness of the patellar has been reproduced, and the other techniques for optimizing patellar tracking have been used, patellar subluxation is uncommon in the varus knee. However, if no technical errors can be identified and maltracking is present, a lateral patellar release should be performed. Once the result with the trial components is acceptable, the surfaces are cleaned and dried and the real components are cemented in place. Once the cement is hard, I routinely release the tourniquet and cauterize any significant bleeding vessels. The joint is irrigated and a deep drain is placed prior to arthrotomy closure, which is performed in extension. After skin closure, a light sterile dressing is used.

POSTOPERATIVE MANAGEMENT AND REHABILITATION

A multimodal approach is used for perioperative pain control. Both nonsteroidal anti-inflammatory medications and narcotic analgesics are given preoperatively in the holding area. Regional blocks including femoral and sciatic nerve blocks are performed preoperatively and are continued postoperatively for 24 to 48 hours. In conjunction with the regional blocks, intravenous narcotics are administered via a patient-controlled analgesia device for breakthrough pain during the first 24 hours. Patients are then switched to oral narcotics for pain control. Passive and active ranges of motion are begun on postoperative day 1 and are advanced as tolerated; the importance of active extension is emphasized to the patient. Ambulation with weight bearing as tolerated is also begun on postoperative day 1, without limitation. Early goals include independent transfers, walking as tolerated, and active motion from full extension to 90 degrees of flexion. Other important perioperative interventions include the use of prophylactic antibiotics given within an hour of the incision and continued for 24 hours postoperatively, and deep vein thrombosis prophylaxis. A multimodal approach to DVT prophylaxis is also used, including the use of thigh-high compression stockings, mechanical sequential compression devices, and low-molecular-weight heparin or adjusted dose Coumadin. The use of continuous passive motion machines is controversial, and there are studies that both support and refute its efficacy.

RESULTS

During the past two decades, the results of total knee replacement have been proven both consistent and durable. Indeed, long-term survivorship has been reported from independent centers to be >90% to 95% at 10 years or greater. In these studies, various prosthesis designs have demonstrated excellent results in both young and old adults. Despite these highly reproducible outcomes, failures do occur. Infection, mechanical failure, periprosthetic fracture, aseptic loosening, polyethylene wear, and instability are the most common modes of failure. Although some of these problems may be unavoidable, long-term success has clearly been noted to be related to patient characteristics and the accuracy with which the prosthesis is implanted. Therefore, both careful preoperative evaluation and optimal surgical technique should be used and remain within the control of the orthopaedic surgeon.

SUGGESTED READINGS

Berger RA, Rubash HE, Seel MJ, et al. Determining the rotational alignment of the femoral component in total knee arthroplasty using the epicondylar axis. *Clin Orthop*. 1993;286:40–47.

Clarke HD, Scuderi GR. Correction of valgus deformity in total knee arthroplasty with the pie-crust technique of lateral soft-tissue releases. J Knee Surg. 2004;17(3):157–166.

Clarke HD, Scuderi, GR. Revision total knee arthroplasty: planning, management, controversies, and surgical approaches. *Instr Course Lect*. 2001;50:359–365.

Insall JN, Easley ME. Surgical techniques and instrumentation in total knee arthroplasty. In: Insall JN, Scott WN, eds. *Surgery of The Knee*. Vol 2. 3rd ed. Philadelphia: Churchill Livingstone; 2001:1553–1628.

Keating EM, Meding JB, Faris PM, et al. Long-term followup of nonmodular total knee replacements. *Clin Orthop Relat Res*. 2002;404:34–39.

Kelly MA, Clarke HD. Long-term results of posterior cruciate-substituting total knee arthroplasty. *Clin Orthop*. 2002;404:51–57.

Lonner JH, Siliski JM, Scott RD. Prodromes of failure in total knee arthroplasty. *J Arthroplasty*. 1999;14:488–492.

Mahomed NN, Barrett J, Katz JN, et al. Epidemiology of total knee replacement in the United States Medicare population. *J Bone Joint Surg Am*. 2005;87:1222–1228.

Malkani AL, Rand JA, Bryan RS, et al. Total knee arthroplasty with the kinematic condylar prosthesis. A ten-year follow-up study. *J Bone Joint Surg Am*. 1995;77:423–431.

Ritter MA, Faris PM, Keating EM, et al. Postoperative alignment of total knee replacement. Its effect on survival. *Clin Orthop*. 1994;299:153–156.

Scott RD, Thornhill TS. Posterior cruciate supplementing total knee replacement using conforming inserts and cruciate recession. Effect on range of motion and radiolucent lines. *Clin Orthop*. 1994;309:146–149

Sowers, MF. Epidemiology of risk factors for osteoarthritis: systemic factors. *Curr Op Rheumatol*. 2001,13:447–451.

COMPLICATIONS AFTER TOTAL KNEE ARTHROPLASTY

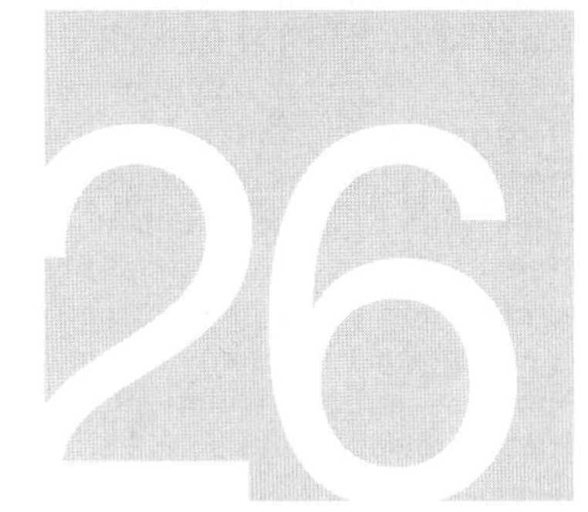

JEFFREY S. ZARIN
ANDREW R. NOBLE
WOLFGANG FITZ

In the United States, over 300,000 total knee arthroplasties are performed each year. Total knee arthroplasty (TKA) is one of the most successful procedures in orthopaedic surgery, and there are excellent reported long-term results with survivorship rates of >90% at 15 years.[1,2,3] In recent years surgical techniques have been changed and new technologies have been introduced for TKA. Patients are now more informed and are requesting newer technologies, better implants, less pain, less blood loss, and quicker recovery from a joint replacement. The introduction of minimally invasive techniques, preemptive analgesia, progressive rehabilitation, computer-assisted surgery, and new materials not only have changed the daily practice for orthopaedic surgeons but also have added new challenges. Beyond the scope of these advances, surgeons must keep in mind that TKA is a major surgery with associated morbidity. This chapter will focus on the postoperative complications including traumatic periprosthetic injuries, the pitfalls of minimally invasive surgery, wound healing problems, nerve injury, and postoperative infection. Also, issues associated with stiffness, tissue balancing, and instability will be addressed.

MORBIDITY AND MORTALITY OF TKA

The overall estimated mortality for total knee arthroplasty during the first 90 days is 0.2% to 0.7%. Increased risk is associated with advanced age, comorbidities, and revision procedures. In a study of >3,000 consecutive TKAs performed by one surgeon, the overall mortality rate was 0.46% during the first 90 days in patients with an average age of 70 years.[4] Gill et al.[4] reported a risk of mortality 16 times higher in patients with cardiac comorbidities such as previous myocardial infarction, ischemic heart disease, and cardiac failure compared with those with no comorbidity. Patients older than 85 years of age had a 14-times increase in the chance of death when compared with patients younger than 85 years of age, with a reported rate of 4.65%. The mortality rate in the Medicare population undergoing primary TKA is reported as 0.6% to 0.7% during the first 90 days in two studies.[5,6] The overall morbidity rates in >80,000 patients during the first 90 days after primary TKA identified in a Medicare population were the following: acute myocardial infarction, 0.8%; pulmonary embolism, 0.8%; pneumonia requiring hospitalization, 1.4%; and infection requiring irrigation and debridement, 0.4%.[5,6]

Surgeon and Hospital Volume

The relationship of surgeon volume to patient outcomes has become a topic of increasing interest. Two recent studies have reported lower mortality and morbidity rates associated with surgeons and hospitals performing a larger volume of TKAs. Katz et al.[5] identified a 30% reduction in mortality rate for patients receiving a TKA in hospitals that perform >25 of these procedures per year. Surgeons performing >50 procedures per year had a 40% lower risk for deep wound infection compared with surgeons performing <12 per year. A steady decline of deep infection was independently related to hospital volume as well, with a reported 40% reduction for hospitals performing >200 cases per year versus those doing <25 per year. The risk of pneumonia also diminished independently for surgeons and hospitals performing >12 and 25 cases, respectively.

Periprosthetic Fractures

Periprosthetic fractures of the femur, tibia, or patella are rare after total knee replacement. The reported prevalence for distal femoral fractures ranges from 0.3% to 2.8%[7] and for tibial fractures from 0.4% to 1.7%.[8] Patellar fractures occurred in 0.05% when unresurfaced[9] and ≤21% with resurfacing.[10]

Distal Femoral Fractures

Supracondylar femur fractures are most frequently traumatic, with a higher incidence seen in patients with osteopenia. Femoral notching may increase the incidence of periprosthetic fractures of the distal femur when both medial and lateral cortices are notched. Nondisplaced fractures with well-fixed implants can be treated by nonoperative intervention with a high success rate. Surgical intervention is required in the setting of displaced supracondylar fractures, and the method of fixation is determined by implant stability. Supracondylar fractures associated with well-fixed femoral components can be treated by several techniques including retrograde nails, blade plates, condylar screw plates, condylar buttress plates, and locked condylar plates.

Retrograde nailing and more recently less-invasive condylar locking plates have become standard treatment methods owing to the preservation of fracture hematoma and minimal soft tissue dissection. Whether the fracture is suitable for a retrograde nail is determined by the length of the distal bone fragment from the fracture to the intercondylar notch. Adequate bone length of the distal fragment is needed for placement of the two distal locking screws. If the most distal aspect of the nail protrudes into the notch, some surgeons have successfully removed this portion after inserting the interlocking screws.[11] The design of the femoral component must also be considered because posterior stabilized systems may preclude insertion of the retrograde nails through a solid cam and post mechanism. Locked plates inserted with minimal soft tissue disruption offer many advantages over retrograde nailing, including rigid fixation with locked screws, ability to combine with posterior stabilized systems, and potentially better fixation in osteopenic patients.[12]

Loose femoral components in combination with supracondylar fractures require a different treatment approach. In certain cases, the periprosthetic fracture can be addressed first and allowed to heal prior to revision of the loose femoral implant. Postponing component revision until fracture healing offers several advantages including less bone loss, ease of revision TKA, reduced need for cortical strut allograft, and less need for augments, wedges, stems, and constrained or hinged prostheses.[8] Combined fixation of the fracture with revision knee arthroplasty is a technically demanding procedure that may require extensive allografts and a hinged prosthesis or oncologic distal femoral replacement prosthesis. Principles include restoration of the joint line, preservation of fixed components, and proper femoral rotation based on a rectangular flexion gap with the tibial component. Bulk allograft may be necessary to restore condylar bone loss. The use of extensive bone cement at the fracture site is discouraged because of risk of nonunion.

Tibial Fractures

Undisplaced or reducible tibial fractures that remain in a stable anatomic position are amenable to nonoperative treatment. Displaced and unstable fracture patterns associated with well-fixed total knee components usually are treated with open reduction and internal fixation with buttress plates or locking plates. Revision total knee replacement is indicated when the fracture involves the tibial component or when the implant is loose. Long-stemmed tibial components should be used to bypass the fracture site and are often secured with a hybrid cement technique. Additional plating or use of bulk allograft may be required based on the fracture pattern and bone loss.

Patellar Fractures

Many factors predispose to patella fractures in TKA. The risk for fracture in nonresurfaced patellae is minimal. Extensive resection with a patella thickness of <15 mm can predispose to fracture.[13] A three-peg design has reduced patellar strain and has a decreased likelihood of fracture compared with a larger single peg. Several other risk factors for patellar fracture have been identified and include overstuffing of the femoropatellar joint, use of oversized femoral components, component malrotation, and placement of the femoral component in too much flexion.[14]

Disruption of the patellar blood supply is another important factor leading to avascular necrosis (AVN) and eventual patellar fracture after total knee replacement. The patellar blood supply may be compromised when a median parapatellar approach is combined with a lateral release. Scuderi et al.[15] demonstrated a 56.4% incidence of reduced blood flow to the patella when a lateral release was performed following a parapatellar approach. However, when a medial subvastus approach is used, there is less risk for AVN when combined with a lateral release because the superior geniculate artery is preserved. No data are available to show that the decreased exposure and reduced soft tissue violation of minimally invasive surgery has an effect on patellar blood supply and associated fractures.

Ortiguera and Berry[10] classified patellar fractures based on fixation of the patellar component, integrity of the extensor mechanism, and quality of the residual patellar bone stock. The fractures are classified as type I with a stable implant and an intact extensor mechanism, type II with disruption of the extensor mechanism, and type III with a loose patellar component and reasonable bone stock (>10 mm thickness, IIIA) or poor bone stock (<10 mm thickness or comminution prohibiting fixation or resurfacing, IIIB). In this study comprising 78 patella fractures, about half were classified as type I and were treated successfully with observation or immobilization.

Disruption of the extensor mechanism typically is treated with surgical intervention. However, type II fractures were associated with a high complication rate of 50% and a reoperation rate of 42%. Open reduction internal fixation was rarely successful owing to a very thin and small piece of bone. Other surgical options included partial or total patellectomy with repair and advancement of the extensor mechanism. Figure 26-1 shows an open reduction internal fixation of a type II fracture with complete rupture of the extensor mechanism. Intraoperatively, it was felt that the remaining distal pole of the patella was large enough for fixation; it ultimately healed without an extension lag or quadriceps weakness (Figs. 26-2–26-4).

Failure of extensor mechanism repair typically is salvaged with an allograft reconstruction consisting of tibial tubercle, patellar tendon, patella, and quadriceps tendon that was first described by Emerson et al.[16] Nazarian and Booth[17] modified this technique by tightly tensioning the

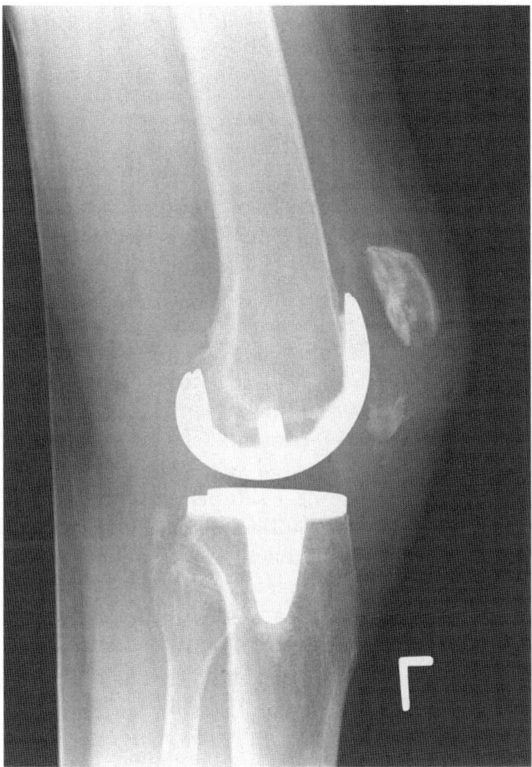

Figure 26-1 Fracture of the inferior patella pole with complete extensor mechanism disruption.

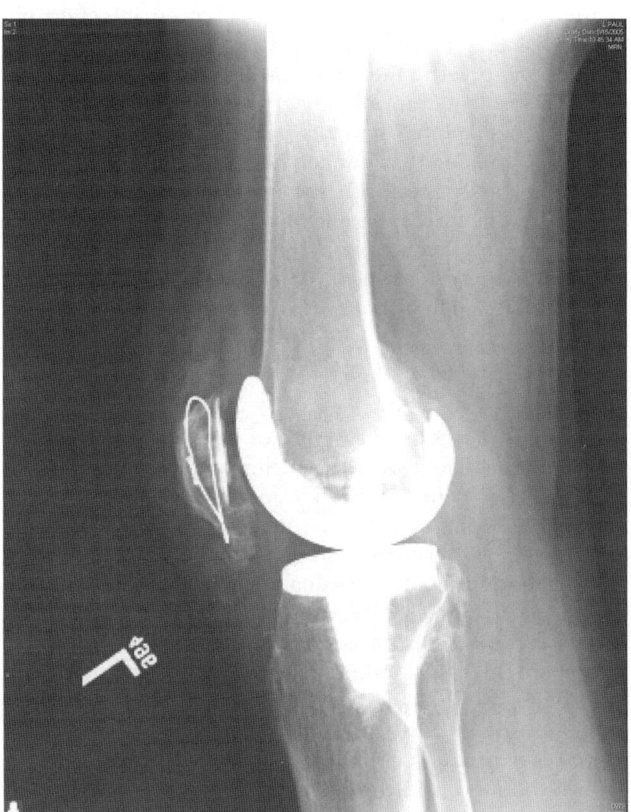

Figure 26-2 Lateral view of left knee with healed repair of patella fracture and extensor mechanism without functional deficit.

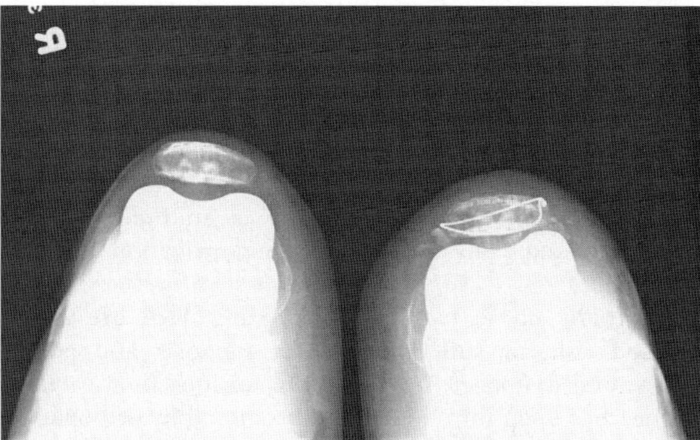

Figure 26-3 Skyline view of repaired and healed patella pole fracture and ruptured extensor mechanism.

repair in full extension and reported improved early results. Burnett et al.[18] reported a series of 20 consecutive reconstructions with one group having minimal tension in extension whereas the second group was tightly tensioned intraoperatively. Loosely tensioned allografts resulted in persistent extensor lag and clinical failure. The tightly tensioned reconstructions were all clinically successful with an average postoperative extensor lag of 4.3 degrees.

Wound Healing Problems

Early wound healing problems after total knee arthroplasty occur infrequently but should be suspected in higher-risk patients who are immunosuppressed, malnourished, taking steroids, or have diabetes or rheumatoid arthritis, as well as those with a history of multiple surgeries or prior infection in the operative knee.

Small amounts of wound drainage that lightly stain dressings may commonly be seen in the first 3 to 4 days after

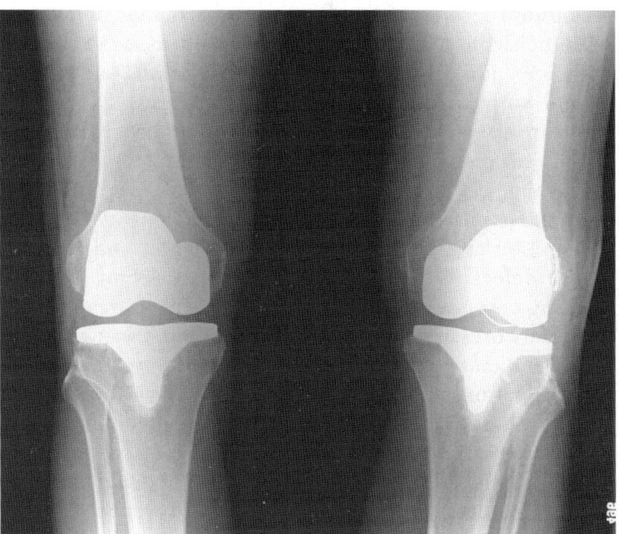

Figure 26-4 Anteroposterior view of bilateral total knee arthroplasties and healed left patella fracture.

surgery. The treatment of postoperative drainage is not clearly presented in the orthopaedic literature but is based on sound clinical judgment. Drainage should be more concerning to the surgeon when it continues after 5 days and if it is associated with diffuse erythema, purulence, or profuse volume. Persistent drainage, particularly of serosanguineous character, usually is an indication for aspiration and consideration of open irrigation and debridement.

Morbidly obese patients undergoing TKA are at increased risk for subcutaneous fat necrosis and potential wound drainage. Application of an incisional vacuum sponge has been introduced and promoted by orthopaedic trauma surgeons to potentially reduce early drainage and wound breakdown in the morbidly obese. After skin closure, an incisional vac with a $^1/_2$-inch-wide strip of sponge is directly applied to a nonadhesive dressing over the closed incision. After 2 to 3 days, the vac dressing and sponge are removed and replaced with a dry dressing (MB Harris, personal communication, 2005).

A suture abscess may present as an infection but is more often a granulomatous reaction to the suture material. The perplexing diagnosis of suture granuloma is more commonly discussed in the general surgery literature, with only a handful of orthopaedic cases being reported. Three cases of culture-negative granulomatous reactions to Vicryl suture were reported within 9 weeks after total hip arthroplasty by Sayegh et al.[19] All cases were successfully treated with excision of the affected tissue, debridement of the joint capsule, and extensive wound lavage. The implants were left in place and the patients were treated with antibiotics pending the negative culture reports, at which time the antibiotics were discontinued. Regarding suture abscesses in total knee replacement, we recommend removal of visible sutures associated with superficial reactions and more formal debridement and antibiotic coverage for deeper cases.

Early postoperative bleeding into a drain is expected but should be more closely observed if profuse and continuous. Temporary immobilization of the knee and avoidance of early motion can often result in spontaneous resolution. However, significant intra-articular hematoma with incisional leakage and excessive soft tissue expansion with impending skin necrosis are indications for prompt formal surgical evacuation with hemostasis. Evacuating the hematoma by squeezing the wound or probing are strongly discouraged because of the potential for retrograde contamination.[20]

Successful treatment of skin necrosis depends on early recognition and is based on the size, depth, and location of the defect. Superficial skin necrosis <4 cm^2 with remaining coverage of bone and tendon may be treated with wet to dry dressing changes or a wound vac. Close observation is imperative to avoid deeper penetration and possible contamination of the prosthesis. An early plastic surgical consult is strongly recommended. For deeper and larger defects of >4 cm^2, a plastic surgeon should plan for local flap coverage. Ries[23] described the use of a medial gastrocnemius flap or latissimus free flap for defects over the patellar tendon and tibial tubercle. Five of the six patients who underwent flap coverage required two-stage revision total knee replacement. Additional adjunctive treatment measures include immobilization as well as appropriate antibiotic therapy with infectious disease consultation.

Deep Infection

Incidence and Risk Factors

All operative procedures are susceptible to bacterial contamination, and the presence of biomaterials places patients undergoing joint replacement at increased risk for the development of deep infection. The incidence of deep infection has been reported to range from 1% to 2.5% in primary TKA and approaches 5.6% in revision TKA. Factors leading to deep infection must be considered with respect to the microbiologic characteristics of the infecting organism, the host, wound, and operative technique.[24]

Biomaterials have an increased susceptibility to bacterial contamination because of a self-perpetuating enlarging immunoincompetent fibroinflammatory zone that develops around the implants.[25] Bacteria may adhere to the implant based on the surface characteristics and the intrinsic properties of the bacteria. Once adherent, bacteria can encase themselves in a hydrated biofilm matrix of polysaccharide and protein. Sessile, biofilm-encased bacteria are less susceptible to antibiotics than free-floating bacteria.[25] This quality of deep bacterial infection of TKA underlies its difficulty in eradication without complete hardware removal.

Patient-specific factors contribute to elevated risk for deep infection as well. Patients with decreased immunity, prior history of deep infection, and higher contamination loads have incidence rates of deep infection between 3% and 10%.[25] Patients with decreased immunity include those with rheumatoid arthritis, diabetes mellitus, organ transplantation, obesity, HIV, poor nutritional status, and hemophilia. Patients with increased contamination loads include those undergoing revision total joint replacement and those with surgical duration >2.5 hours. There is evidence that preoperative nasal screening, topical treatment, and specific perioperative antibiotic prophylaxis in combination with vancomycin reduces the incidence of MRSA infection in orthopaedic operated patients to almost zero.[27,28]

Diagnosis

The key to successful treatment of deep infection is early and accurate diagnosis. Classic clinical presentation of an infected TKA is characterized by increasing persistent pain, warmth, effusion, and less frequently, erythema. Patients with prolonged postoperative pain should be suspected to be infected and should be evaluated for infection. Aspiration of a suspected infected TKA should be performed early and before the first administration of antibiotics.

Repetition of aspiration may increase sensitivity and specificity, as well as increase the chance of identification of the infectious organism with susceptibilities.[30] In a two-stage reconstruction of an infected TKA after hardware removal, followed by a 6-week period of intravenous antibiotic therapy, antibiotic therapy should be discontinued for a $\geq$10 ten days prior to aspiration. Aspiration has been shown to have a 74% positive predictive value and 94% negative predictive value, although rates have been identified in studies of ≤100% sensitivity and specificity.[24] Newer techniques of polymerase chain reaction (PCR) may increase the utility of aspiration in sensitivity but may be associated with an increased false-positive rate. One recent study evaluated the differential gene expression by white blood cells, using a commercially available gene chip. They identified expression of genes from neutrophils present at the site of infection that was different than that expressed at a site of aseptic inflammation. These findings may lead to potential future simple lab tests that can distinguish the causes of inflammation in total joint arthroplasty.[29]

Blood tests should include erythrocyte sedimentation rate (ESR) and C-reactive protein (CRP) level. However, the sensitivity and specificity of ESR has been reported as low as 60% in one series.[24] Therefore, blood tests may be useful for screening but should not be used for the definitive diagnosis of deep infection. Radionucleotide studies, such as indium-labeled leukocyte scans, have been used. Sensitivity and specificity have been reported between 80% and 94%. Increased scan activity can be present in ≤90% of tibial and 65% of femoral components ≥1 year after implantation.[24,30]

Classification and Treatment

The timing of onset from the index procedure defines the classification system of deep infection and can help guide appropriate management. Deep infections have been classified as those with positive intraoperative cultures, early postoperative infection, acute hematogenous infection, and late chronic infection.

Positive intraoperative cultures may occur in the setting of revision TKA for presumed aseptic loosening. Culture results must be interpreted in conjunction with preoperative examination findings and the overall clinical scenario. Multiple intraoperative cultures can help resolve the dilemma of whether a positive intraoperative culture represents contamination or infection. Greater than two of five positive intraoperative cultures can indicate true infection. If felt to be a true-positive, treatment with a 6-week course of suppressive antibiotics can be curative in 90% of patients.[30] This approach is similar to direct-exchange arthroplasty for low-grade infections.

Early postoperative infection occurs within 1 month after implantation. Acute hematogenous infection occurs with seeding of the joint from another primary site of infection, such as urinary tract infection or pneumonia. Invasive procedures leading to transient bacteremia, such as colonoscopy and dental procedures, may contribute to deep joint infection. Presentation is with local inflammation of acute onset and systemic toxicity. Prompt surgical intervention is mandatory, as delays of >2 weeks are associated with decreased rates of implant salvage. A success rate of 60% to 80% has been found with treatment with retention of the implants and multiple debridements. In a study of 24 patients with infected TKA presenting within 30 days of the index procedure or with <30 days of symptoms (acute hematogenous group), Mont et al.[31] reported that the implants were successfully retained in 83% of patients after one to three procedures. On the other hand, Deirmengian et al.[32] reported on a series of 31 TKA patients with disappointing results of infections with *Staphylococcus aureus*. Only one was treated successfully with early debridement, liner exchange, and retention of the implants.

Late chronic infection occurs >1 month after the index TKA and involves extension of the infection through the capsule, with or without sinus formation. Onset is more gradual, with slow deterioration of function and increase in pain. The treatment of late chronic infections has received much attention in the literature of the past 30 years. Single-stage revision in the presence of low-grade organisms has been reported. However, most reports favor a two-stage approach with placement of a temporary antibiotic-impregnated cement spacer after a thorough debridement of the knee joint.[33] The current recommended dosage is ≥3.6 grams of antibiotics per 40 g of acrylic cement for effective elution kinetics and sustained therapeutic levels of antibiotics.[34] We currently use 2 g of vancomycin and 3.6 grams of tobramycin per 40 g of acrylic cement. Premixed antibiotic cements with 1 gram of gentamicin are not recommended for the treatment of deep infection, and an inadequate dosage of antibiotics within bone cement has been described as a cause of treatment failure.[35] Intravenous antibiotics appropriate for the infecting organism are administered for 6 weeks, followed by a second-stage implantation of a permanent prosthesis using low dose antibiotic-impregnated bone cement. Success rates have been identified for two-stage replantation of 80% to 93% when using an antibiotic cement spacer.[36,37,38,39,40,41]

Antibiotic spacer blocks used during the first stage of the two-stage treatment algorithm lead to knee stiffness and may compromise bone stock. Multiple studies have examined the use of an articulated spacer technique. A comparison of static with articulating spacers identified improved preservation of bone stock, increased ease of exposure during replantation, and no apparent increase in reinfection when using articulated spacers.[38] One recent study showed the average range of motion with the articulated spacer was 110 degrees, which was not significantly different than the motion after replantation.[33] Success rates for eradication of infection with the PROSTALAC spacer were found to be 91%.[45] Multiple articulating designs have been described, including all-antibiotic–laden cement, cement and metal composites, and replacement of the original components after autoclave sterilization and loose antibiotic cement technique.[33,36,37,43,39,40] Many variations of spacer design have been described as well, ranging from ball-and-socket type molding, commercially available PROSTALAC designs, and metal-polyethylene-cement composites.[45,44] Most involve the intraoperative production of separate femoral and tibial casted or sculpted cement spacers that mimic the design of the metal implants and allow for motion at the cement/cement interface.[38,43,39,40] All designs show success rates ≥90% for infection eradication and improved patient function with the articulating spacer.

Stiffness

Definition and Incidence

A severely stiff knee after TKA is an uncommon but disappointing and disabling occurrence. Gait studies have suggested increased difficulty of walking occurs with increasing flexion contracture and that flexion of 67 degrees is required for normal gait.[46] Stair climbing requires 83 degrees of flexion, rising from a seated position requires 93 degrees, and tying shoelaces requires 106 degrees.[47]

The overall incidence varies based on the definition criteria used. Severe postoperative stiffness has been defined in the literature as flexion <75 degrees and/or the presence of a knee flexion contracture ≥15 degrees.[46,48] However, others have also suggested that an arc of motion <70 degrees or a flexion contracture >20 degrees with a total range of motion <45 degrees constitutes postoperative stiffness. Prior studies have indicated an incidence of stiffness as high as 12%. Two institutions recently found the incidence of stiffness after TKA to be from 1.3% to 3.7%, based on large consecutive series of >1,000 primary TKAs in both studies.[46,4]

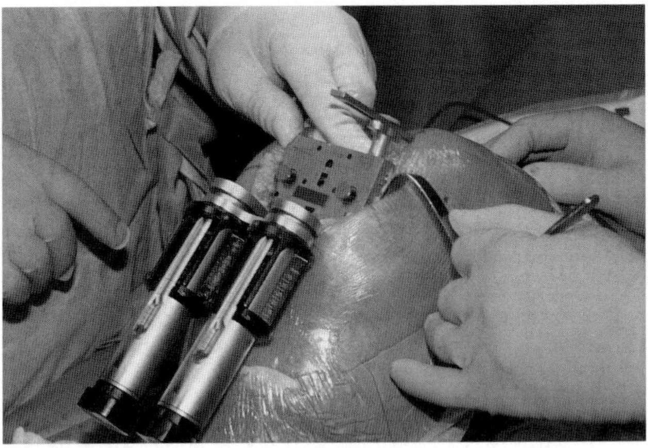

Figure 26-5 Balancing gap technique: Medial and lateral soft tissues are tensioned equally and the femoral size determined (anterior referencing). This creates an equal flexion and extension gap without the use of anatomic landmarks.

Etiologic Factors

Preoperative, intraoperative, and postoperative events can all contribute to a stiff knee after TKA. The range of motion before the index arthroplasty is the most common preoperative predictor of decreased motion after TKA.[46,47] This preoperative stiffness can occur from extensor mechanism or capsular contractures. Although these structures may be released during the index procedure, their elasticity may be restricted owing to chronic fibrosis.[49] Body habitus may also decrease postoperative motion. Obese patients with short stature have earlier impingement of posterior soft tissues, decreasing total flexion.[51] Other patient factors such as posttraumatic arthritis, juvenile rheumatoid arthritis, ankylosing spondylitis, and keloid formation may increase the risk for stiffness.[49,51] Patient noncompliance with postoperative rehabilitation protocols often results in suboptimal knee motion.[51] Whether minimally invasive techniques and preemptive analgesia reduce the incidence of stiffness remains unclear at this time.

Technical aspects of the index TKA may be intrinsic to postoperative stiffness. These may include overstuffing of the patellofemoral articulation by oversizing the femoral component or increasing patellar thickness. A recent study found that on average, passive knee flexion decreased 3 degrees for every 2-mm increment of patellar thickness.[50] Patella height should be restored and not altered.[51,52] Appropriate balancing of the flexion and extension gaps is essential. Gap balancing techniques with spacer blocks or tensiometers help to assess and match intraoperatively composite implant thickness. Femoral or tibial malrotation can be avoided by using the gap balancing technique, in minimally invasive TKA, because anatomic landmarks are not very reliable (Fig. 26-5). Postoperatively, the patellar axis should be parallel to the transepicondylar axis and the tibial axis. Skyline views in 50 to 70 degrees can demonstrate appropriate alignment (Fig. 26-6). An excessively tight flexion and/or extension gap, a tight posterior cruciate ligament (PCL), and femoral and/or tibial malrotation with limited bearing excursion are associated with highly conforming prosthetic designs.[52]

A tight flexion gap is a common error resulting in decreased flexion[51] and can be avoided with the use of spacer blocks. If the posterior femoral condylar bone resection is less than the thickness of the posterior condyles of the femoral component, the flexion gap will be decreased.[52] In this scenario, the extension gap will be larger than the flexion gap. Erroneous selection of an increased tibial polyethylene thickness to balance the extension gap will further limit flexion. Also, positioning the femoral component too posteriorly, in excessive malrotation in the coronal plane, or placing a component with a larger anteroposterior dimension than the patient's anatomy will result in a tight flexion gap.[51] Failure to remove posterior osteophytes sufficiently can block the full sagittal excursion of the tibial polyethylene and prevent full flexion. These osteophytes can also tense the posterior capsule in extension, causing a paradoxic block to full extension as well.[46] Decreased extension may result if the distal femoral resection is too distal, particularly in the setting of a pre-existing flexion contracture. A recent study showed that an average value of 9 degrees of femoral contracture is corrected for every 2 mm of distal femoral resection.[54]

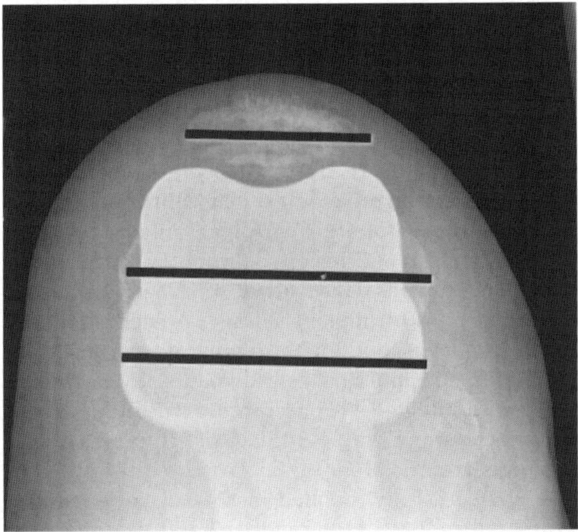

Figure 26-6 Skyline view demonstrating patellar axis, transepicondylar axis, and tibial long axis being parallel.

Femoral and tibial component malposition in the sagittal plane can lead to stiffness postoperatively.[53] The femoral component should optimally be at right angles to the anatomic axis of the femur in the sagittal plane. A hyperflexed component can lead to early cam-post impingement and loss of extension in implants. Figure 26-7 shows a lateral knee radiograph of a PCL-retaining TKA, the femoral component in about 15 degrees of flexion and the tibial component with a slope of 15 degrees. This can be tolerated with a PCL-retaining design, but a PS design would lead to peg impingement.

A hyperextended component can limit flexion and increase the risks associated with anterior femoral cortical notching. It has been suggested that tibial slope in the sagittal plane should equal the patient's bony anatomy preoperatively. An up-sloped tibial cut (i.e., higher posterior than anterior) will lead to a decreased posterior joint space and decreased flexion. Increased down-slope will increase flexion but my lead to anterior tibial translation and early posterior polyethylene wear. Sagittal plane tibial component balance is more critical in PCL-retaining knees, whereas a flat tibial slope is more appropriate in PCL-substituting knees that depend on the cam and post mechanism for sagittal plane behavior of the prosthesis.

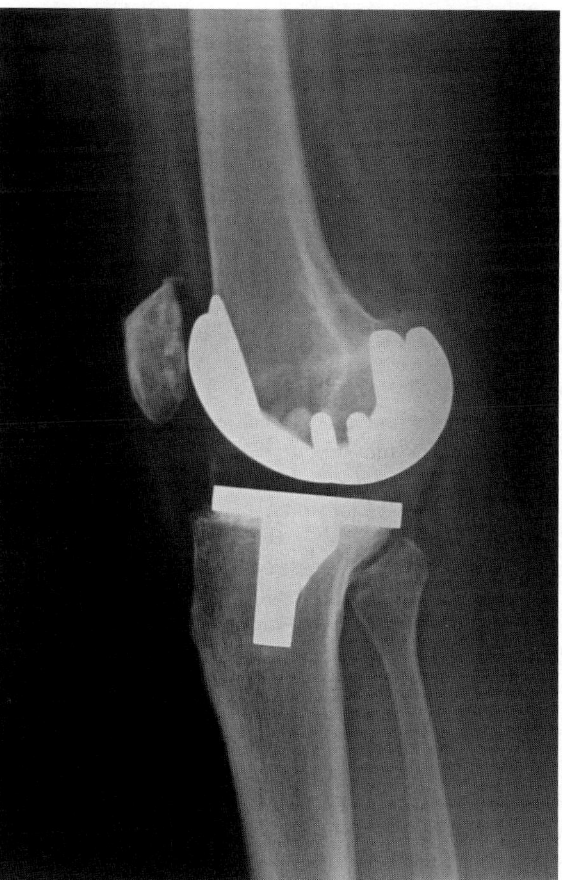

Figure 26-7 Lateral view of a total knee replacement showing a PCL-retaining TKA with about 15 degrees of femoral component flexion and a slope of approximately 15 degrees. In a posterior substituting (PS) design, peg impingement is model specific, but may occur as soon as the combined added angle totals 10 degrees.

Limited knee flexion may result from imbalance of the posterior cruciate ligament in PCL-retaining knee designs. The PCL may result in overtightening in flexion, and imbalance of the flexion and extension gaps will lead to stiffness. Paradoxically, a lax PCL leading to flexion instability may also lead to stiffness, as anterior femoral translation occurs with increasing knee flexion. This can induce earlier posterior impingement and extensor mechanism tightening, decreasing ultimate flexion.[51] Excessive elevation of the joint line with a cruciate retaining implant may lead to patella infera, which has been associated with patellar pain and limited motion.[47,49] Joint line elevation of 3 to 10 mm can substantially increase PCL tension and limit flexion.

Treatment and Outcomes

Postoperative stiffness is best managed by prevention. Preoperative patient education, appropriate postoperative analgesia, and aggressive postoperative rehabilitation help to maximize postoperative motion and function. Continuous passive motion (CPM) machines have been useful adjuncts in the immediate postoperative period, but several studies indicate no significant benefit at 1 year after TKA.[51,49]

The timing of surgical intervention in the setting of a stiff knee replacement remains controversial. Closed manipulation under anesthesia has been shown to be effective when performed within 6 to 12 weeks after primary TKA. Surgical options after 3 months include arthroscopic arthrolysis for focal adhesions, open arthrolysis for general arthrofibrosis, and only if necessary, component revision.[49] Reports of series with arthroscopic arthrolysis and PCL release with a manipulation showed an improvement in only 43% of knees, whereas another group showed an average increase of motion by 30.6 degrees.[49,55] Open arthrolysis with radical scar excision and ligamentous rebalancing has shown some promise. A "pie crust" quadricepsplasty followed by a gradual manipulation has been recommended.[51] Others suggest a quadriceps snip at the time of exposure with similar benefits.[49] A recent study combining aggressive arthrolysis with a customized rehabilitation protocol showed a mean increase in range of motion from 63 degrees to 94 degrees in 94% of knees. However, a flexion contracture averaging 9 degrees remained in 39% of the patients. Sixty-seven percent of the patients had Knee Society scores of good or excellent, with improvement from 34 to 77 points.[46]

Revision total knee replacement is indicated for situations in which an identifiable, intrinsic problem is associated with stiffness. These include situations as discussed above, such as component malposition, incorrect sizing, joint line displacement, inadequate bone resection, and improper soft tissue balancing. One recent study evaluating patients with revision of femoral and tibial components in the setting of stiffness showed Knee Society scores improved from 38 to 87 and arc of motion improved from 55 degrees to 82 degrees in 93% of knees.[48] Another report suggested less promising results, with only 10 of 15 patients satisfied with outcomes, Knee Society scores from 28 to 65, and an increase of arc of motion from 40 degrees to 73 degrees.[56] Successful revision of a stiff knee involves identification of extrinsic sources of stiffness that are uncorrectable, such as ipsilateral hip arthrodesis, neurologic disorders, longstanding extrinsic muscle tightness, and systemic inflammatory conditions. Identification of the cause of failure preoperatively or intraoperatively and assessing correction of the problem after placement of the new prosthesis is associated with the best results.[52]

Instability

Incidence and Risk Factors

Instability after total knee arthroplasty is one of the most common causes of aseptic failure. Although reported incidence rates range from 1% to 2% in all primary total knee replacements, symptomatic instability may account for ≤10% to 20% of patients undergoing revision surgery. Instability may present as medial-lateral instability or flexion instability.

Certain situations increase the risk of an unstable total knee replacement. Greater preoperative deformity requiring large surgical correction and aggressive ligament releases may lead to difficulties with obtaining stability.[58] One study of patients with preoperative valgus deformity averaging >10 degrees noted that 17% of patients had instability postoperatively. In addition, the patients with postoperative knee instability had significantly higher postoperative knee pain than those with stable knees.[2]

Increased strain on the ligaments of the knee may occur with conditions that alter the mechanics of the knee during gait. Neuromuscular pathology such as quadriceps weakness or hip abductor weakness may lead to increased medial forces at the knee, leading to ligamentous laxity and instability. Valgus forces at the knee may be increased by mechanical instability at the ankle with posterior tibialis tendon rupture or at the hip with a valgus alignment of an ipsilateral hip arthroplasty.[58]

Obese patients have increased risk of iatrogenic collateral ligament damage owing to difficult surgical exposure. The use of minimally invasive instrumentation may ease implantation in these patients. Assessment of component position and appreciation of ligament balance can be more difficult with the increased soft tissues and weight of a large limb. Increased thigh circumference will cause a wide-based gait, which increases stresses on the medial collateral ligament. Any or all of these factors may contribute to postoperative instability in obese patients undergoing TKA.

Axial Instability

Varus-valgus instability is the most common and classic type of instability pattern. This type of instability may result from collateral ligament imbalance or failure, incomplete correction of preoperative deformity, and component malalignment and/or failure.

Inadequate or overrelease of contracted collateral ligaments when balancing soft tissues for a fixed axial deformity causes an asymmetric extension gap, leading to medial-lateral instability. Inadvertent damage to the medial collateral ligament (MCL) also leads to instability in extension. Care must always be taken to protect the MCL when performing the medial proximal tibial cut as well as the medial posterior femoral condylar cut. In this setting, medial collateral ligament advancement or reconstruction alone with postoperative bracing has been recommended. However, more predictable stability can be attained by combined repair of the MCL and use of a constrained implant.

Incomplete correction of varus or valgus deformities may lead to axial instability because of imbalance between medial and lateral ligaments and soft tissues. For example, an uncorrected varus deformity will produce a lax lateral sleeve and tight medial sleeve, causing a varus thrust during ambulation. Patients with medial-lateral laxity may compensate by walking with a stiff-legged gait to avoid the pain associated with a thrust or sensation of buckling of the knee.[59] Reconstruction in this situation should be directed toward re-establishing the joint line and appropriate tension in the soft tissue envelope. Asymmetric instability resulting from improper bone cuts or bone loss often requires the use of modular augments or structural bone grafts.

Symmetric varus-valgus instability may be the result of overresection of the distal femur, component loosening, and soft tissue laxity of the medial and lateral collateral ligaments. An overresected distal femur will lead to a larger extension gap than flexion gap. Choosing a thin polyethylene component that fills only the flexion space will lead to a loose extension gap and associated medial-lateral instability as well as genu recurvatum during gait. Loosening of the femoral or tibial component will present as apparent instability on exam. The loose component will tilt with stress, giving the appearance of an unstable opening joint.[59] Global soft tissue laxity may occur in patients with connective tissue disorders such as rheumatoid arthritis or Ehlers-Danlos syndrome. This can result in persistent laxity and instability if not recognized at the time of primary TKA.

Flexion Instability

Mismatch of the flexion and extension gap can lead to flexion instability. This may occur with overresection of the posterior femoral condyles, undersizing the femoral component, and excessive tibial slope.[59] All of these causes lead to a flexion gap that is larger than the extension gap. If a thin polyethylene insert is chosen that fills only the extension gap, flexion instability will result. Patients present with recurrent effusions and a sense of instability without buckling. They will often mistrust the stability of their knee when descending stairs, and there is often associated start-up pain. Posterior translation of the tibia in flexion leads to areas of soft tissue tenderness anteriorly and can be exacerbated by weakness of the extensor complex.[59,60] This could be prevented by using the gap balancing technique: First the extension gap is balanced and the correct insert thickness selected using a spacer block or a tensiometer. Second, femoral rotation is not based on anatomic landmarks since it is sometimes impossible in mini-invasive techniques. A tensiometer is inserted and medial and lateral soft tissues are tensioned. Blocks are used to determine femoral component size, and the anterior cut is completed. Figure 26-4 shows the positioning of a tensiometer in combination with a cutting block to demonstrate how an equal flexion gap could be created using this technique.

Appropriate posterior cruciate ligament (PCL) balancing is critical to prevent stiffness as well as instability in PCL-retaining implants. As mentioned previously, a tight PCL will limit flexion and may contribute to postoperative stiffness and increased polyethylene wear. Typically, lift-off or rollback is observed. A PCL release using a "pie crust" technique of tight fibers, a superior release of the origin, or posterior release of the insertion easily balances the flexion gap. An overreleased PCL may lead to an incompetent ligament, with paradoxic roll-forward of the femur and flexion instability. Flexion instability after cruciate-retaining TKA has been reproducibly treated with revision to a posterior stabilized TKA with careful balancing of the flexion and extension gaps.[60]

Flexion instability in the setting of posterior stabilized TKA has been classically identified as dislocation of the cam and post mechanism. However, with contemporary implant designs, the jump distance has been significantly increased and the prevalence of frank dislocation is approximately only 0.15%.[60] Excessive posterior slope or overresection of the posterior femoral condyles in a PCL-sacrificing TKA can lead to flexion instability because of the associated increased flexion space. This can allow the tibia to subluxate and produce instability with or without dislocation. There have been reports of tibial post fracture, requiring revision. Post failure may be related to increased stresses on the tibial post in the setting of a loose flexion space.[61] Reconstitution of the flexion space in revision TKA for flexion instability is accomplished with the use of posterior femoral augmentation combined with a larger femoral component. Alternatively, more distal femoral bone resection can be made if the bone stock allows, creating symmetric flexion and extension gaps that can be filled with a larger polyethylene insert.[60]

Patellofemoral Instability

The most common causes of pain and the most commonly cited reasons for revision TKA are complications involving the extensor mechanism and patellofemoral joint. Historically, patellofemoral instability after TKA ranged from 10% to 35%. Recent improvements in prosthetic design and surgical technique have lowered these rates to 1% to 12%.[67] Complications include patellar subluxation or dislocation, patellar component wear, and loosening.

Malrotation of the femoral and tibial components is one of the most frequent causes of patellofemoral complications. Limb alignment, preparation of the patella, prosthetic design, and soft tissue balance all contribute to the stability of the patellofemoral joint. Nonsurgical treatments such as bracing and physical therapy are rarely effective in correcting structural abnormalities that lead to patellofemoral maltracking.[67] Treatment should be directed by the cause. Computed tomography (CT) scan is the most accurate and reliable way to assess component positioning and its impact on stability. One study using CT to analyze component rotational alignment found that the combined amount of internal rotation of femoral and tibial components correlated directly with the severity of patellofemoral instability.[64] If malposition is present, revision of one or both components may be indicated. Lateral retinacular release, with or without vastus medialis advancement may also help align the extensor mechanism axis.

Nerve Injury

Neurologic injury after TKA is an uncommon but potentially devastating complication. Multiple retrospective studies examining large consecutive series (>1,000) identify an incidence of 0.3% to 1.3%.[65,68] Subclinical palsy may occur in higher numbers but may be diagnosed only by electrodiagnostic testing.

Predisposing Factors

The cause of peroneal nerve palsy is multifactorial, and no definitive causal relationships have been documented. Conditions associated with peroneal nerve injury include severe flexion and valgus deformity correction, preoperative neuropathy, postoperative epidural analgesia, external leg compression, tourniquet time, and rheumatoid arthritis (RA).

Early studies support the finding that correction of severe valgus and flexion contractures is associated with increased postoperative peroneal nerve palsy. The average preoperative valgus in the patients who developed peroneal palsy ranged from 18 degrees to 23.3 degrees, and average flexion contracture ranged from 15.5 degrees to 22 degrees.[65] The incidence ranges from 3% to 10% for correction of knees with severe valgus and flexion deformity. The mechanism of nerve injury has been suggested to relate to narrowing of the extraneural and intraneural microvasculature associated with stretching of the nerve within its surrounding soft tissue.[55] An anatomic study examining the risk of direct injury to the nerve during releases to allow for correction of valgus deformity measured a mean bone to nerve distance of 1.49 cm at the level of the standard tibial resection. Those authors concluded that the nerve is adequately protected at the posterolateral corner of the knee, but that care should be taken when performing a "pie crust" release.[55]

Epidural analgesia postoperatively may be a risk factor. The sensory block may allow the patient to position the leg in a way that directly compresses the nerve. Also, the patients may tolerate excessive motion in extension or overly constrictive dressings leading to nerve palsy. The epidural may mask a peroneal nerve palsy occurring at the time of surgery and delay diagnosis and initiation of treatment.

Prior neuropathy, both central and peripheral, has been associated with development of peroneal palsy. It is theorized that nerves with prior compromise are more susceptible to a second insult, often termed the "double-crush" phenomenon.[65] No studies have associated diabetic neuropathy with increased risk for peroneal nerve palsy.

Several studies have identified increased rates of peroneal palsy in patients with rheumatoid arthritis.[65,68] In a study by Schinsky et al.,[68] 53% of patients who developed peroneal palsy had a diagnosis of RA, which was significantly higher than the prevalence of RA in their cohort of 1,476 patients. Their patients did not have higher amounts of preoperative valgus or flexion contracture, suggesting that peroneal palsy in RA patients may be via a mechanism unrelated to the deformity of the knee.

Elevated tourniquet times have been associated with electromyogram (EMG) changes in the peroneal and tibial nerves, but the clinical significance of these changes is unclear. The mechanism is thought to be related to both ischemia and mechanical deformation, but most changes have been identified directly beneath the cuff. One study identified tourniquet time of >120 minutes as an independent risk factor for peroneal palsy.[65] Tourniquet release, allowing a reperfusion interval of 10 to 30 minutes, followed by reinflation has been recommended to extend the duration of tourniquet time if needed.[69] One recent study reviewed a consecutive series of >1,000 patients undergoing TKA with a tourniquet time of >120 minutes. The overall incidence of neurologic complications was 7.7% in this population. Complete neurologic recovery occurred in 89% of patients with peroneal nerve palsy.[69]

The peroneal nerve is vulnerable to direct compression, given its superficial anatomic location as it winds around the fibular head. Direct compression on the peroneal nerve by constrictive dressings has been suggested to play a role in the development of palsy. In addition, the development of postoperative hematoma has been identified as a rare source of compression on the nerve leading to palsy.

Treatment and Prognosis

Standard nonoperative management of peroneal nerve palsy includes immediate removal of any constrictive dressings and flexion of the hip and knee to approximately 20 degrees and 45 degrees, respectively. This can be accomplished by elevation of the extremity on several pillows. Initial short-term treatment should be observation and an ankle/foot orthotic (AFO) device for foot drop. Surgical exploration has been indicated if no functional recovery is noted after 3 months from onset, particularly if the AFO is not tolerated. The routine use of surgical decompression remains controversial, despite several reports of full recovery following open exploration.

The potential for recovery after peroneal nerve palsy following TKA ranges from 50% to 89%.[65,69] The less severe the initial palsy, the more likely it is to completely resolve. Despite varying percentages of complete peroneal nerve recovery, most patients have demonstrated good functional capacity after TKA.

REFERENCES

1. Diduch DR, Insall JN, Scott WN, et al. Total knee replacement in young, active patients. Long-term follow-up and functional outcome. *J Bone Joint Surg Am.* 1997;79:575–582.
2. Miyasaka KC, Ranawat CS, Mullaji A. 10- to 20-year followup of total knee arthroplasty for valgus deformities. *Clin Orthop Relat Res.* 1997;345:29–37.
3. Stern SH, Insall JN. Posterior stabilized prosthesis. Results after follow-up of nine to twelve years. *J Bone Joint Surg Am.* 1992;74:980–986.
4. Gill GS, Mills D, Joshi AB. Mortality following primary total knee arthroplasty. *J Bone Joint Surg Am.* 2003;85-A:432–435.
5. Katz JN, Barrett J, Mahomed NN, et al. Association between hospital and surgeon procedure volume and the outcomes of total knee replacement. *J Bone Joint Surg Am.* 2004;86-A:1909–1916.
6. Mahomed NN, Barrett J, Katz JN, et al. Epidemiology of total knee replacement in the United States Medicare population. *J Bone Joint Surg Am.* 2005;87:1222–1228.
7. Healy W. Femoral fractures above total knee arthroplasty. In: Siliski JM, ed. <*Title of Book.*>, New York: Springer-Verlag; 1994:409–415.
8. Engh GA, Ammeen DJ. Periprosthetic fractures adjacent to total knee implants: treatment and clinical results. *Instr Course Lect.* 1998;47:437–448.
9. Grace JN, Sim FH. Fracture of the patella after total knee arthroplasty. *Clin Orthop Relat Res.* 1988;230:168–175.
10. Ortiguera CJ, Berry DJ. Patellar fracture after total knee arthroplasty. *J Bone Joint Surg Am.* 2002;84-A:532–540.
11. Maniar RN, Umlas ME, Rodriguez JA, et al. Supracondylar femoral fracture above a PFC posterior cruciate-substituting total knee arthroplasty treated with supracondylar nailing. A unique technical problem. *J Arthroplasty.* 1996;11:637–639.
12. Kregor PJ, Hughes JL, Cole PA. Fixation of distal femoral fractures above total knee arthroplasty utilizing the Less Invasive Stabilization System (L.I.S.S.). *Injury.* 2001;32(suppl 3):SC64–75.
13. Josechak RG, Finlay JB, Bourne RB, et al. Cancellous bone support for patellar resurfacing. *Clin Orthop Relat Res.* 1987;220:192–199.
14. Windsor RE, Scuderi GR, Insall JN. Patellar fractures in total knee arthroplasty. *J Arthroplasty.* 1989;4(suppl):S63–67.
15. Scuderi GR, Scharf SC, Meltzer LP, et al. The relationship of lateral releases to patella viability in total knee arthroplasty. *J Arthroplasty.* 1987;2:209–214.
16. Emerson RH Jr, Head WC, Malinin TI. Reconstruction of patellar tendon rupture after total knee arthroplasty with an extensor mechanism allograft. *Clin Orthop Relat Res.* 1990;260:154–161.
17. Nazarian DG, Booth RE Jr. Extensor mechanism allografts in total knee arthroplasty. *Clin Orthop Relat Res.* 1999;367:123–129.
18. Burnett RS, Berger RA, Paprosky WG, et al. Extensor mechanism allograft reconstruction after total knee arthroplasty. A comparison of two techniques. *J Bone Joint Surg Am.* 2004;86-A:2694–2699.
19. Sayegh S, Bernard L, Stern R, et al. Suture granuloma mimicking infection following total hip arthroplasty. A report of three cases. *J Bone Joint Surg Am.* 2003;85-A:2006–2009.
20. Insall JN, Scott WN. *Surgery of the Knee.* New York: Churchill Livingstone; 2001.
21. Kindsfater K, Scott R. Recurrent hemarthrosis after total knee arthroplasty. *J Arthroplasty.* 1995;10(suppl):S52–55.
22. Katsimihas M, Robinson D, Thornton M, et al. Therapeutic embolization of the genicular arteries for recurrent hemarthrosis after total knee arthroplasty. *J Arthroplasty.* 2001;16:935–937.
23. Ries MD. Skin necrosis after total knee arthroplasty. *J Arthroplasty.* 2002;17(suppl 1):74–77.
24. Hanssen AD, Rand JA. Evaluation and treatment of infection at the site of a total hip or knee arthroplasty. *J Bone Joint Surg Am.* 1998;80-A:910–921.
25. Jiranek WA, Hanssen AD, Greenwald AS. Antibiotic-loaded bone cement for infection prophylaxis in total joint replacement. *J Bone Joint Surg Am.* 2006;88-A:2487–2500.
26. Pritsch T, Pritsch M, Halperin N. Therapeutic embolization for late hemarthrosis after total knee arthroplasty. A case report. *J Bone Joint Surg Am.* 2003;2003;85-A:1802–1804.
27. Anwar R, Botchu R, Viegas M, et al. Preoperative methicillin-resistant *Staphylococcus aureus* (MRSA) screening: An effective method to control MRSA infections on elective orthopaedics wards. *Surg Pract.* 2006;10(4):135–137.
28. Soriano A, Popescu D, García S, et al. Usefulness of teicoplanin for preventing methicillin-resistant *Staphylococcus aureus* infections in orthopedic surgery. *Eur J Clin Microbiol Infect Dis.* 2006;25(1):35–38.
29. Diermengian C, Lonner JH, Booth RE Jr. The Mark Coventry Award: white blood cell gene expression: a new approach toward the study and diagnosis of infection. *Clin Orthop Relat Res.* 2005;440:38–44.
30. Tsukayama DT, Goldberg VM, Kyle R. Diagnosis and management of infection after total knee arthroplasty. *J Bone Joint Surg Am.* 2003;85-A(suppl 1):75–80.
31. Mont MA, Waldman B, Banerjee C, et al. Multiple irrigation, debridement, and retention of components in infected total knee arthroplasty. *J Arthroplasty.* 1997;12:426–433.

32. Deirmengian C, Greenbaum J, Lotke PA, et al. Limited success with open debridement and retention of components in the treatment of acute *Staphylococcus aureus* infections after total knee arthroplasty. *J Arthroplasty.* 2003;18(suppl 1):22–26.
33. Cuckler JM. The infected total knee. *J Arthroplasty.* 2005;20(suppl 2):33–36.
34. Penner MJ, Duncan CP, Masri BA. The in vitro elution characteristics of antibiotic-loaded CMW and Palacos-R bone cements. *J Arthroplasty.*1999;14:209.
35. Buchholz HW, Elson RA, Engelbrecht E, et al. Management of deep infections of total hip replacement. *J Bone Joint Surg Br.* 1981;63:342.
36. Durbhakula SM, Czajka J, Fuchs MD, et al. Antibiotic-loaded articulating cement spacer in the 2-stage exchange of infected total knee arthroplasty. *J Arthroplasty.* 2004;19:768–774.
37. Emerson RH, Muncie M, Tarbox TR, et al. Comparison of a static with a mobile spacer in total knee infection. *Clin Orthop Relat Res.* 2002;404:132–138.
38. Fehring TK, Odum S, Calton TF, et al. Articulating versus static spacers in revision total knee arthroplasty for sepsis. *Clin Orthop Relat Res.* 2000;380:9–16.
39. Hofmann AA, Goldberg T, Tanner AM, et al. Treatment of infected total knee arthroplasty using an articulating spacer: 2- to 12-year experience. *Clin Orthop Relat Res.* 2005;430:125–131.
40. Pietsch M, Hofmann S, Wenisch C. Treatment of deep infection of total knee arthroplasty using a two-stage procedure. *Oper Orthop Traumatol.* 2006;18(1):66–87.
41. Wilde AH, Ruth JT. Two-stage reimplantation in infected total knee arthroplasty. *Clin Orthop Relat Res.* 1988;236:23–35.
42. Green GV, Berend KR, Berend ME, et al. The effects of varus tibial alignment on proximal tibial surface strain in total knee arthroplasty: the posteromedial hot spot. *J Arthroplasty.* 2002;17:1033–1039.
43. Goldstein WM, Kopplin M, Wall R, et al. Temporary articulating methylmethacrylate antibiotic spacer (TAMMAS). *J Bone Joint Surg Am.* 2001;83-A(suppl 2, pt 2):92–96.
44. Macavoy MC, Ries MD. The ball and socket articulating spacer for infected total knee arthroplasty. *J Arthroplasty.* 2005;20:757–762.
45. Haddad FS, Masri BA, Campbell D, et al. The PROSTALAC functional spacer in two-stage revision for infected knee replacements. *J Bone Joint Surg Br.* 2000;82-B:807–812.
46. Mont MA, Seyler TM, Marulanda GA, et al. Surgical treatment and customized rehabilitation for stiff knee arthroplasties. *Clin Orthop Relat Res.* 2006;446:193–200.
47. Gandhi R, de Beer J, Leone J, et al. Predictive risk factors for stiff knees in total knee arthroplasty. *J Arthroplasty.* 2006;21:46–52.
48. Kim J, Nelson CL, Lotke PA. Stiffness after total knee arthroplasty. *J Bone Joint Surg Am.* 2004;86-A:1479–1484.
49. Scuderi GR. The stiff total knee arthroplasty. *J Arthroplasty.* 2005;20(suppl 2):23–26.
50. Bengs BC, Scott RD. The effect of patellar thickness on intraoperative knee flexion and patellar tracking in total knee arthroplasty. *J Arthroplasty.* 2006;21:650–655.
51. Dennis DA. The stiff total knee arthroplasty: causes and cures. *Orthopedics.* 2001;25:901–902.
52. Nelson CL, Kim J, Lotke PA. Stiffness after total knee arthroplasty, surgical technique. *J Bone Joint Surg Am.* 2005;87-A(supp 1, pt 2):264–270.
53. Laskin RS, Beksac B. Stiffness after total knee arthroplasty. *J Arthroplasty.* 2004;19 (suppl):S41–46.
54. Bengs BC, Scott RD. The effect of distal femoral resection on passive knee extension in posterior cruciate ligament-retaining total knee arthroplasty. *J Arthroplasty.* 2006;21:161–166.
55. Clarke HD, Schwartz JB, Math KR, et al. Anatomic risk of peroneal nerve injury with the "pie crust" technique for valgus release in total knee arthroplasty. *J Arthroplasty.* 2004;19:40–44.
56. Haidukewych GJ, Jacofsky DJ, Pagnano MW, et al. Functional results after revision of well-fixed components for stiffness after primary total knee arthroplasty. *J Arthroplasty.* 2005;20:133–138.
57. Mihalko WM, Krackow KA. Flexion and extension gap balancing in revision total knee arthroplasty. *Clin Orthop Relat Res.* 2006;446:121–126.
58. Vince KG, Abdeen A, Sugimori T. The unstable total knee arthroplasty. *J Arthroplasty.* 2006;21(suppl 1):44–49.
59. Gonzalez MH, Mekhail AO. The failed total knee arthroplasty: evaluation and etiology. *J Am Acad Orthop Surg.* 2004;12(6):436–446.
60. Schwab JH, Haidukewych GJ, Hanssen AD, et al. Flexion instability without dislocation after posterior stabilized total knees. *Clin Orthop Relat Res.* 2005;440:96–100.
61. Boesen MP, Jensen TT, Husted H. Secondary knee instability caused by fracture of the stabilizing insert in a dual-articular total knee arthroplasty. *J Arthroplasty.* 2004;19:941–942.
62. Poilvache PL, Insall JN, Scuderi GR, et al. Rotational landmarks and sizing of the distal femur in total knee arthroplasty. *Clin Orthop Relat Res.* 1996;331:35–46.
63. Bonutti PM, Mont MA, McMahon M, et al. Minimally invasive total knee arthroplasty. *J Bone Joint Surg Am.* 2004;86-A(suppl 2):26–32.
64. Berger RA, Crossett LS, Jacobs, JJ, et al. Malrotation causing patellofemoral complication after total knee arthroplasty. *Clin Orthop Relat Res.* 1998;356:144–153.
65. Nercessian OA, Ugwonali OFC, Park S. Peroneal nerve palsy after total knee arthroplasty. *J Arthroplasty.* 2005;20:1068–1073.
66. Barrack, RL, Schrader T, Bertot AJ, et al. Component rotation and anterior knee pain after total knee arthroplasty. *Clin Orthop Relat Res.* 2001;392:46–55.
67. Eisenhuth SA, Saleh KJ, Cui Q, et al. Patellofemoral instability after total knee arthroplasty. *Clin Orthop Relat Res.* 2006;446:149–160.
68. Schinsky MF, Macaulay W, Parks ML, et al. Nerve injury after primary total knee arthroplasty. *J Arthroplasty.* 2001;16(8):1048–1054.
69. Horlocker TT, Hebl JR, Gali B, et al. Anesthetic, patient, and surgical risk factors for neurologic complications after prolonged total tourniquet time during total knee arthroplasty. *Anesth Analg.* 2006;102:950–955.
70. Olcott CW, Scott RD. The Ranawat Award. Femoral component rotation during total knee arthroplasty. *Clin Orthop Relat Res.* 1999;367:39–42.

SUGGESTED READINGS

Chauhan SK, Scott RG, Breidahl W, et al. Computer-assisted knee arthroplasty versus a conventional jig-based technique. A randomised, prospective trial. *J Bone Joint Surg Br.* 2004;86: 372–377.

Haas SB, Cook S, Beksac B. Minimally invasive total knee replacement through a mini midvastus approach: a comparative study. *Clin Orthop Relat Res.* 2004;428:68–73.

Laskin RS, Beksac B, Phongjunakorn A, et al. Minimally invasive total knee replacement through a mini-midvastus incision: an outcome study. *Clin Orthop Relat Res.* 2004;428:74–81.

Sparmann M, Wolke B, Czupalla H, et al. Positioning of total knee arthroplasty with and without navigation support. A prospective, randomised study. *J Bone Joint Surg Br.* 2003;85:830–835.

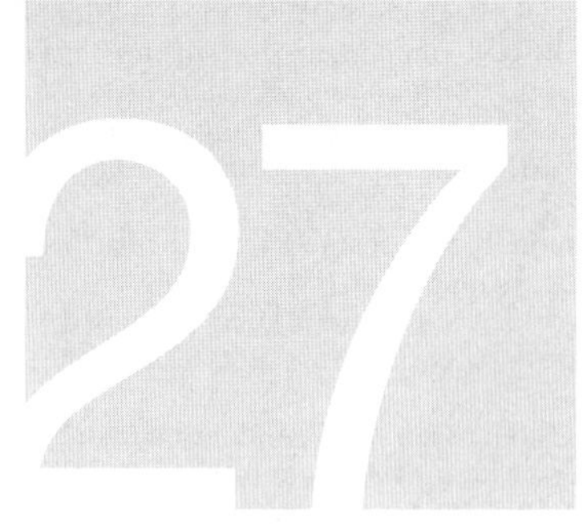

THE PAINFUL TOTAL KNEE ARTHROPLASTY

SATHAPPAN S. SATHAPPAN
JAMES RYAN
DAN GINAT
PAUL E. DI CESARE

Following total knee arthroplasty (TKA), there is normally a progressive decrease in pain and a reciprocal increase in function. Persistent and/or progressive pain is disconcerting to both the patient and surgeon. The causes of pain following TKA are often related to patient anatomy, implant design, and/or surgical technique.

EPIDEMIOLOGY

The occurrence of occasional knee pain after TKA can be as high as 47%; however, only 5% to 7% of patients experience persistent pain. The most common causes of pain are soft tissue tenosynovitis, patella-related complications, malalignment, infection, component loosening, instability, synovitis, and complex regional pain syndrome (CRPS). Less common causes include scarring and retained cement/osteophytes. Patients with preoperative functional limitations, severe pain, low mental health score, or multiple medical comorbidities are more likely to have a painful TKA and a poorer overall outcome.

DIAGNOSIS

When evaluating knee pain in a post-TKA patient, a careful history and clinical examination are prerequisite in making the definitive diagnosis. Diabetic patients may have a higher propensity to infection and neuropathic pain. Establishing the time interval between TKA and development of pain can help with the diagnosis. For example, presence of pain persisting since surgery suggests infection, instability, prosthetic malalignment, or nonarticular causes. When prosthetic infection is suspected, one should inquire about fever, chills, and recent history of invasive procedure (e.g., dental treatment, urologic procedures).

Initial clinical evaluation requires determination of the site of pain. Localized pain is associated with specific causes (Fig. 27-1), and global tenderness is often due to either infection or prosthetic loosening. Constant pain is typically associated with infection, whereas pain associated with mechanical activity is often due to either inflammatory causes or mechanical derangement. Pain that is experienced with weight bearing, but improves with rest, often is caused by prosthetic loosening.

Clinical examination consists of localizing the tenderness and assessing for range of motion (ROM) and stability. Although effusion can be seen in synovitis, erythema and warmth are more often related to joint sepsis. Presence of crepitus is often indicative of either soft tissue impingement or severe polyethylene liner failure leading to metal-on-metal articulation. In addition to a thorough musculoskeletal evaluation, neurologic and vascular assessments are important.

PATHOGENESIS

The causes of a painful TKA are listed in Figure 27-2. Synopses of the most common causes follow.

Soft Tissue Disorders

Pes Anserinus Bursitis

The pes anserinus (Latin for goose's foot) is a bursa that lies deep to the tendons of the sartorius, gracilis, and semitendinosus. Pes anserinus bursitis is an underdiagnosed condition in which patients (often obese females) complain of a tender anteromedial knee mass (2 inches inferior to the medial joint line). Pain is exacerbated with stair climbing. Although nocturnal symptoms predominate, patients may complain of knee stiffness with limited flexion lasting ≤1 hour during daily activities. Most symptoms are secondary to overuse. Infrequently, symptoms can be caused by anteromedial overhang of the tibial component, varus coronal malalignment of the TKA components, or irritation of the pes anserinus bursa by polyethylene debris. First-line treatment consists of rest, nonsteroidal anti-inflammatory drugs (NSAIDs), and injection of steroid and local anesthetics (e.g., lidocaine).

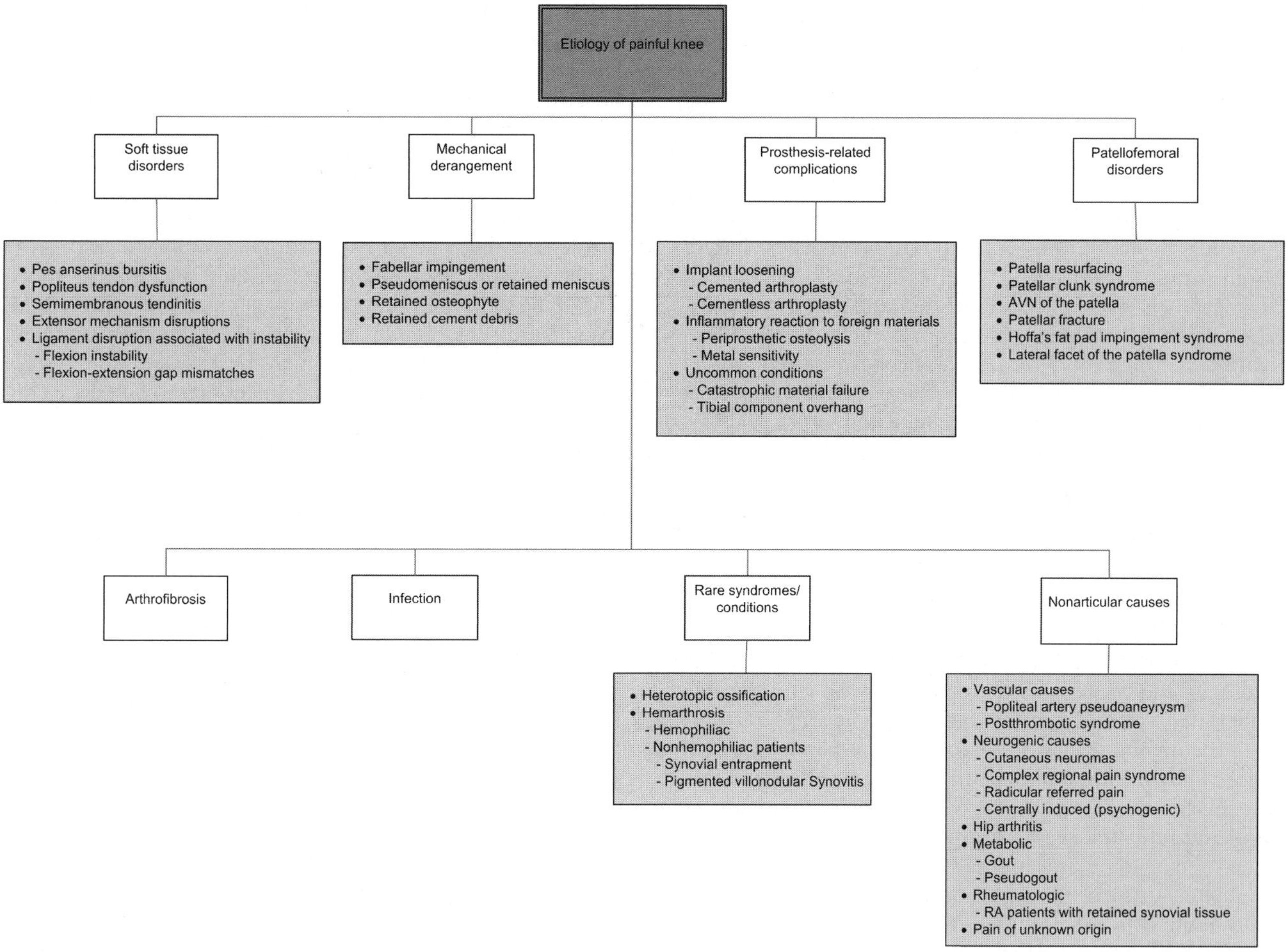

Etiology of painful knee

- Soft tissue disorders
  - Pes anserinus bursitis
  - Popliteus tendon dysfunction
  - Semimembranous tendinitis
  - Extensor mechanism disruptions
  - Ligament disruption associated with instability
    - Flexion instability
    - Flexion-extension gap mismatches
- Mechanical derangement
  - Fabellar impingement
  - Pseudomeniscus or retained meniscus
  - Retained osteophyte
  - Retained cement debris
- Prosthesis-related complications
  - Implant loosening
    - Cemented arthroplasty
    - Cementless arthroplasty
  - Inflammatory reaction to foreign materials
    - Periprosthetic osteolysis
    - Metal sensitivity
  - Uncommon conditions
    - Catastrophic material failure
    - Tibial component overhang
- Patellofemoral disorders
  - Patella resurfacing
  - Patellar clunk syndrome
  - AVN of the patella
  - Patellar fracture
  - Hoffa's fat pad impingement syndrome
  - Lateral facet of the patella syndrome
- Arthrofibrosis
- Infection
- Rare syndromes/ conditions
  - Heterotopic ossification
  - Hemarthrosis
    - Hemophiliac
    - Nonhemophiliac patients
      - Synovial entrapment
      - Pigmented villonodular Synovitis
- Nonarticular causes
  - Vascular causes
    - Popliteal artery pseudoaneyrysm
    - Postthrombotic syndrome
  - Neurogenic causes
    - Cutaneous neuromas
    - Complex regional pain syndrome
    - Radicular referred pain
    - Centrally induced (psychogenic)
  - Hip arthritis
  - Metabolic
    - Gout
    - Pseudogout
  - Rheumatologic
    - RA patients with retained synovial tissue
  - Pain of unknown origin

Figure 27-1 Etiology of the painful knee following total knee arthroplasty (TKA).

Popliteus Tendon Dysfunction

Inflammation of the popliteus tendon (tenosynovitis) can be caused by chronic subluxation of the popliteus tendon over a retained lateral femoral condylar osteophyte or prominent overhang of the posterolateral condyle of the femoral prosthesis. This condition has been reported in about 0.2% of TKA patients. Patients present with lateral knee pain often associated with either a catching sensation or an audible snap at the posterolateral knee. Occasionally recurrent knee effusions mimic symptoms of a septic joint. Women

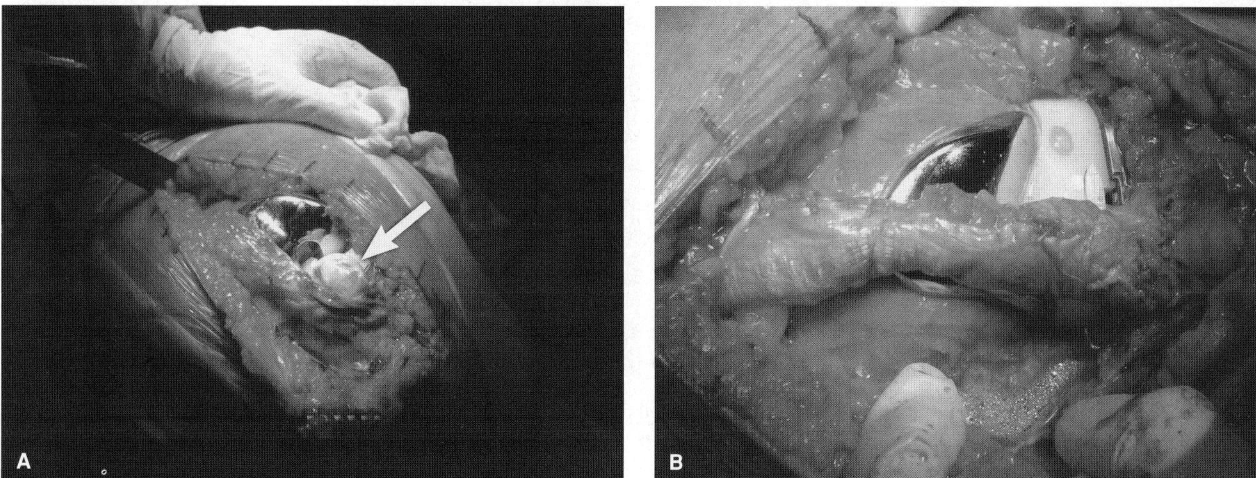

Figure 27-2 Pain pathogenesis in total knee arthroplasty (TKA).

are more likely to have this condition because their relatively smaller femoral geometry may lead to oversizing of the prosthetic component in the medial-lateral plane. Intraoperatively, retained osteophytes, if present, should be excised. In addition, following capsular closure of the knee, the surgeon should perform flexion-extension maneuvers; diagnosis of popliteus tendon dysfunction is suggested by an audible popping sound. If no obvious source of the entrapment is apparent, the popliteus tendon may be released from its femoral insertion.

Diagnosis is made based on history and physical examination; diagnostic arthroscopy may also be required. Conservative treatment options are usually ineffective. Patients may be treated with arthroscopic release of the popliteus tendon from its femoral insertion site, which often provides complete symptom resolution.

Semimembranosus Tendonitis

Semimembranosus tendonitis or tenosynovitis occurs in about 1% of TKA patients. Symptoms include posteromedial knee pain that develops several months following surgery. The pain intensifies with activity, especially during standing from a seated position. Patients with considerable preoperative varus deformity are at risk because restoration of the mechanical axis is associated with an increase in tension on the semimembranosus tendon. Another possible cause of semimembranosus tendonitis is frictional irritation of the reflected segment of the tendon inferior to the posteromedial joint line, particularly in conjunction with osteophytes at the semimembranosus groove.

Although transient pain relief may be achieved with steroid and local anesthetic injections, surgical detachment and excision of the reflected portion of the tendon may be considered. Some authors recommend release of the tendon at the semimembranous groove with lengthening of the tendon to preserve dynamic knee stability.

Extensor Mechanism Disruptions

Extensor mechanism disruptions (quadriceps and patellar tendon ruptures), both of which are uncommon, can be either indirect or direct. Indirect injuries are further subclassified as high-velocity injuries (e.g., motor vehicle accidents) and low-velocity injuries (e.g., slip during daily activities). Hyperflexion with excessive loading causes indirect disruptions. Direct disruptions result from extensor mechanism laceration. Patients typically present with anterior knee pain, weakness, and difficulty negotiating stairs. The patellar tendon ruptures at a force 17.5 times body weight, but detachment of a damaged tendon may occur with less force. Risk factors for these soft tissue disruptions include previous cortisone injections and medical conditions that compromise connective tissue integrity, such as rheumatoid arthritis, chronic renal failure, and diabetes mellitus. Acute disruptions are associated with inflammation and significant pain and can be managed with direct repair; however, rerupture rates are high, and hence one should consider augmentation with autogenous grafts. Neglected ruptures of the patellar or quadriceps tendon typically require direct repair with additional augmentation with either autogenous (e.g., semitendinosus or extended medial gastrocnemius–Achilles tendon) or allograft tissues (quadriceps-patella–achilias tendon–tibial tubercle or achilias tendon–calcaneal bone block) (Fig. 27-3).

Instability

Flexion Instability

Patients may present months to years following index TKA with symptoms of instability and pain with deep-flexion activities (e.g., stair descent or chair transfer). In posterior-cruciate–retaining designs, this has been classically described as flexion instability due to rupture of the posterior cruciate ligament. In posterior-stabilized knees, flexion instability may be secondary to fracture of the polyethylene

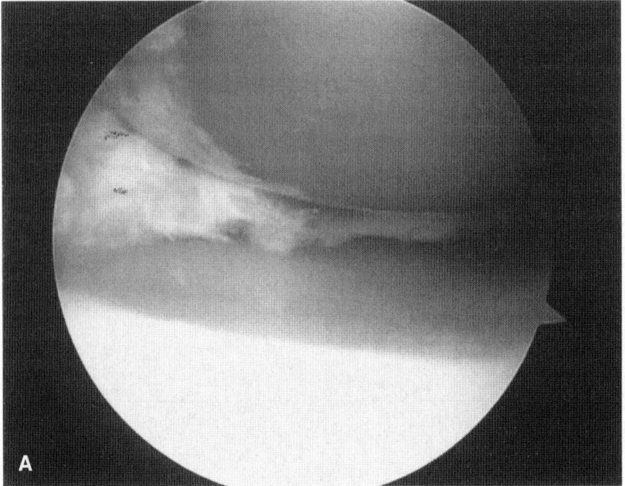

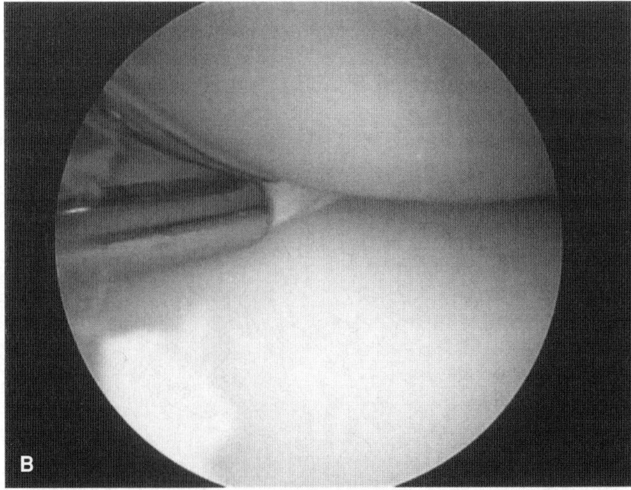

Figure 27-3 Intraoperative photographs of a 60-year-old woman who fell on her knee, suffering a painful extensor mechanism disruption. **A:** The small avascular patella was attached to the quadriceps tendon by thin fibrotic tissue. **B:** The extensor mechanism disruption was addressed using a tendo-Achilles allograft. A Krackow stitch repair of the soft tissue ends was performed with the knee in extension. (Courtesy of Patrick Meere, MD.)

stabilizing cam or an excessively large flexion gap created at the time of index TKA. Additional clinical features include intra-articular effusion, posterior tibial subluxation (sag), and pain. Tenderness is often present over the extensor mechanism, pes anserinus tendon complex, and/or distal iliotibial band. In highly symptomatic cases, revision arthroplasty may be considered (Chapter 28).

Flexion/Extension Gap Mismatches

Inequality between flexion/extension gaps can have consequences on knee stability and kinematics. Unsatisfactory coronal alignment can result in unequal loading of the knee and lead to collateral ligament strain. For example, excessive valgus is associated with medial collateral ligament strain and tenderness. Revision arthroplasty is often required and is discussed in the next chapter.

Mechanical Derangement

Fabella Impingement

The fabella (Latin for little bean) is a sesamoid bone located within the origin of the lateral gastrocnemius tendon and is present in 12% of adults. When the fabella is >2 cm in diameter (mean diameter, 1 cm), there is a risk of fabella impingement following TKA. Symptoms can develop days to months after TKA and are due to the fabella catching on either the posterior femoral, tibial, or polyethylene component. Patients complain of pain at the posterolateral knee (especially with flexion), effusion, palpable popliteal mass, and a sensation of catching. This sensation may be accompanied by a snapping sound. Recurrent impingement leads to articular erosion and notching of the fabella. The adjacent synovial tissue may be laden with birefringent polyethylene particles. In patients with a large fabella identified on preoperative radiographs, intraoperative assessment for possible impingement is accomplished by ranging the knee and listening for an audible snap. If present, the fabella may be excised with electrocautery. Patients presenting with symptoms occasionally get relief with local anesthetic injections. Excision of the fabella via a small posterolateral incision may be required if symptoms are refractory to conservative measures.

Pseudomeniscus or Retained Meniscus

Retained meniscal tissue or pseudomeniscus following TKA can catch and impinge in the tibiofemoral compartment. The suggested pathogenesis includes the production of fibrocartilage from metaplastic transformation of retained meniscal remnants or redundant intra-articular synovium subject to repetitive joint compressive forces. Patients with this condition present with persistent joint line tenderness (posterolateral or posteromedial) about 3 to 6 months following an initially uneventful postoperative course. Patients complain of pain aggravated with stair descent, sometimes accompanied by a catching sensation with knee flexion. Conservative treatment modalities such as physical therapy, bracing, and local anesthetic injections may provide modest relief. Arthroscopic excision of the meniscal tissue typically provides immediate and long-lasting remission of symptoms (Fig. 27-4).

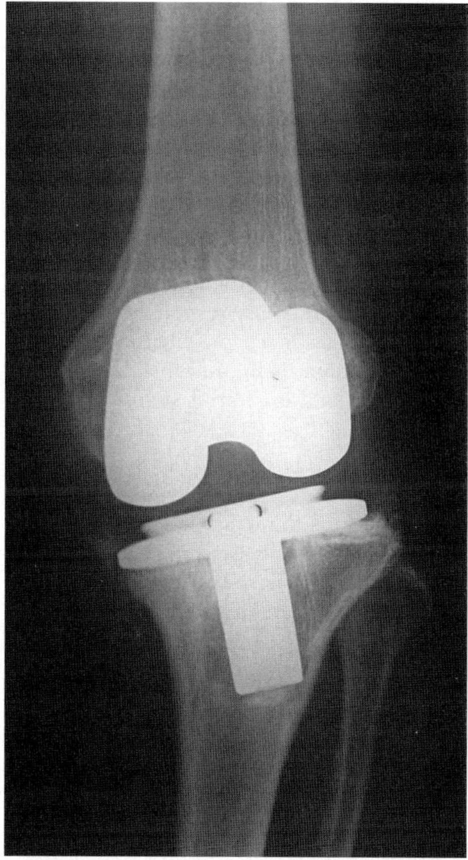

Figure 27-4 Arthroscopic views of medial pseudomeniscus in a 58-year-old man who presented with recurrent posteromedial pain and an associated snapping sensation. **A:** Before treatment. **B:** Arthroscopic shaver being used to debride the impinging pseudomeniscus.

Retained Osteophyte

Meticulous removal of osteophytes is a routine step in all TKAs. However, if large osteophytes remain at the distal femur or proximal tibia, problems can arise. Patients usually present with persistent pain, crepitus, and a knee effusion. Routine radiographs are often negative. Surgical management consists of arthroscopy or open arthrotomy with excision of these osteophytes. Debridement of an associated synovitis may also improve symptoms.

Retained Cement Debris

Uncommonly, cement debris is retained following a primary TKA. The posterior aspect of the knee is the most common site and can lead to pain at this location. With the increasing number of surgeons using smaller incisions for TKA, limited surgical exposure may result in poor visualization of the posterior compartments with subsequent retention of fragments. Patients can present as late as several months after TKA with severe, sharp pain associated with a popping sensation, effusion, and decreased range of motion. Radiopaque cement debris usually can be seen on radiographs. Arthroscopic techniques can be used to remove cement fragments, resulting in symptom resolution.

Periprosthetic Osteolysis

Osteolysis surrounding the femoral, tibial, and patellar components can develop secondary to polyethylene, metal, and/or cement debris. If the debris particles are <15 μm in diameter, they can be ingested by macrophages, which then release numerous inflammatory mediators, including prostaglandin E2, tumor necrosis factor α, and interleukins-2 and -6. The resulting inflammatory response with subsequent activation of osteoclasts is responsible for osteolysis. Patients present with effusion, pain, and instability. Revision TKA is often the only solution to this significant problem.

Metal Sensitivity

Cutaneous contact dermatitis to metal, which can be confirmed on epicutaneous testing, is associated with nickel (Ni), chromium (Cr), cobalt (Co), and CrCoNi alloys and occurs in 8% to 15% of the general population. Metal sensitivity, an allergic reaction of the periprosthetic tissues to metals, has been correlated to contact dermatitis with possible symptom exacerbation following use of conventional prostheses. Clinical features may include eczematid dermatitis, generalized allergic vasculitis, aseptic loosening, and bone necrosis resulting in pain. Pathologic evaluation of tissues can reveal either a cell-mediated immune response or a preponderance of immunoglobulin E antibodies. The frequency of clinically relevant allergic responses to knee implants is unknown, but probably very low. In at-risk patients, titanium-containing or ceramic prostheses may be considered owing to their decreased immunogenic potential.

Catastrophic Material Failure

Most polyethylene wear occurs at the interface between the femoral component and the polyethylene tibial tray. High-molecular-weight polyethylene that has been sterilized by gamma irradiation in air is at the highest risk for catastrophic failure. Modular tibial inserts with suboptimal locking mechanisms can develop wear at the backside of the polyethylene tray. Polyethylene material failure is often associated with a painful chronic effusion and usually occurs many years following TKA. In cases with a metal-backed patella, the thin polyethylene segment can dissociate or wear through, leading to metal-on-metal articulation. Patients present with a grinding or squeaking noise and metallosis. Revision of the patella and sometimes the femoral component usually is required.

Tibial Component Overhang

Tibial component overhang results from malpositioning or oversizing the tibial component with respect to the underlying bony surface. This technical error can result in painful incursion and subsequent inflammation of the collateral ligaments. The medial collateral ligament is more frequently involved than the lateral collateral ligament. Patients who fail medical management, including NSAIDs and/or local anesthetic injection, may be considered for revision surgery.

Patellofemoral Disorders

Patella Resurfacing

Indications for patella resurfacing are still a subject of controversy. Approximately 10% of patients with a nonresurfaced TKA have some persistent anterior knee pain. This may develop several years following the index TKA. If all other diagnoses for anterior knee pain have been excluded, the patella may be resurfaced, especially if the clinical features are suggestive of either inflammatory arthropathy or patellofemoral arthrosis.

Patella Maltracking

Patella maltracking can occur in knees with or without patella resurfacing; it is often due to a tight lateral retinaculum, weak vastus medialis, or more commonly an internally rotated femoral and/or tibial component. If conservative treatment options are unsuccessful, either an extensor mechanism realignment procedure or revision arthroplasty may be required.

Patellar Clunk Syndrome

Patellar clunk is a complication previously described in association with first-generation posterior-stabilized knee designs and is infrequently encountered today. These first-generation implants had a sharp transition between the anterior flange and the intercondylar notch of the femoral component. The condition is characterized by chronic irritation of the quadriceps tendon at the superior aspect of the patella, where the tendon can abut the femoral housing. An inflammatory nodule may form at the junction of the quadriceps tendon and the proximal pole of the patella. When extending the knee from a fully flexed position, at approximately 30 to 40 degrees, patients experience crepitation and catching, frequently accompanied by pain. Treatment consists of arthroscopic or open debridement of the nodule, which is usually successful.

Patellar Fractures

Infrequently (in approximately 1%), TKA can be complicated by patellar fracture in the postoperative period. The incidence is increased with use of a patellar implant with a large central peg or by cutting the patella too thin. Bony resection should match the new prosthetic implant thickness. The minimum postresection thickness is approximately 11 mm. Fracture also may be associated with osteonecrosis of the patella.

Hoffa Fat Pad Impingement Syndrome

Impingement of the Hoffa fat pad has been described following use of mobile bearing TKAs. Compression of the well-innervated fat pad by the anterior border of the polyethylene insert results in anterior knee pain and can be associated with limited ROM. Imaging modalities such as ultrasound and positron emission tomography (PET) scan can aid in confirming the diagnosis. Intraoperative findings suggestive of fat pad impingement include tissue necrosis and sometimes an imprint of the components. If revision surgery is undertaken, it is recommended that the fat pad be removed.

Lateral Facet of the Patella Syndrome

The use of a small inset patella with limited coverage of the lateral patellar facet can lead to painful irritation of the exposed arthritic patellar surface. Patients may complain of anterior knee pain and can have increased radionucleotide uptake over the patella on bone scans. Sunrise view of the patella may indicate abutment of the lateral facet of the patella against the lateral flange of the femoral component. Patella revision may be required for persistent symptoms.

Arthrofibrosis

Patients with arthrofibrosis (stiffness) following TKA typically have a flexion contracture of >15 degrees and/or cannot bend the knee >75 degrees. The incidence of painful postoperative stiffness has been reported to be as high as 10%. Factors associated with knee stiffness include limited preoperative knee ROM, multiple previous knee surgeries, biologic predisposition, history of diabetes, postoperative hemarthrosis, poor patient motivation, inadequate postoperative rehabilitation, improper/insufficient bone cuts, component malposition, tight flexion or extension gap, "overstuffing" of the tibiofemoral or patellofemoral joint, posterior femoral/tibial osteophytes, incorrect component size, a tight posterior cruciate ligament, and heterotopic ossification. Histologic analysis of arthrofibrotic tissue reveals a large population of ovoid and spindle-shaped cells in a dense collagen matrix. Macroscopic variants include simple fibrous bands, exuberant parasynovial fibrous hypertrophy (often in the intercondylar notch), and extensive panarticular scar formation. With diminished ROM, quadriceps work is increased with walking (67 degrees is required for normal gait). Patients may encounter difficulty negotiating stairs and rising from a chair, as these tasks require 85 and 95 degrees of flexion, respectively. Surgical intervention can be early or late. For patients with stiffness within 6 to 12 weeks following TKA, manipulation under anesthesia can be performed. Patients with chronic stiffness may be treated with an arthroscopic or open lysis of adhesions. Revision arthroplasty may be necessary if implant-related causes have been diagnosed.

Infection

The rate of infection following primary TKA is reported to be 1% to 2%. Susceptibility factors include a compromised immune system, obesity, smoking, peripheral vascular disease, venous insufficiency, history of skin ulcers, use of oral steroids, multiple previous surgeries, rheumatoid arthritis, history of knee infection, and recurrent urinary tract infection. Infections following TKA can be categorized as superficial or deep. The deep infections can be further subdivided into direct and hematogenous (seeding from distant infection site). The most common organisms are *Staphylococcus aureus* (coagulase-positive) and *Staphylococcus epidermis* (coagulase-negative). Patients may present with pain, swelling, febrile episodes, erythema, decreased ROM, and sometimes wound drainage (Fig. 27-5).

Treatment options depend on the time of diagnosis. If infections are identified early (<6 weeks) with well-fixed components, an attempt can be made to perform an open, radical debridement with exchange of the tibial insert. Polyethylene exchange is important because the glycocalyx "slime" layer that deposits on the polyethylene bearing can promote recurrence. In cases diagnosed beyond 6 weeks, the following options are considered: primary exchange, two-stage (delayed) exchange, resection arthroplasty, arthrodesis, or amputation. If reimplantation (primary or two-stage) is considered, organism-specific antibiotic-impregnated cement should be used. The most predictable results are achieved with the two-stage exchange

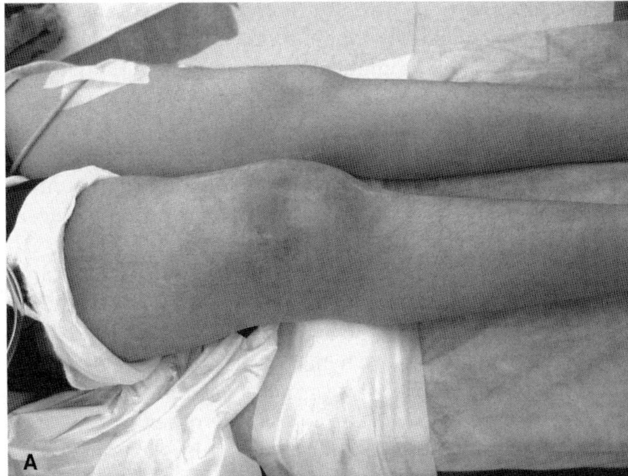

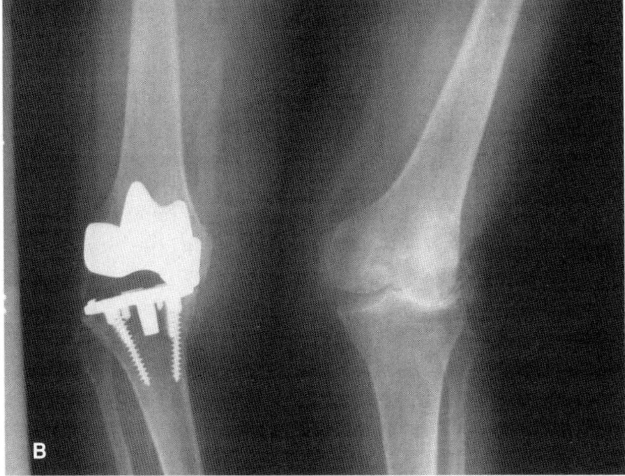

Figure 27-5 A 39-year-old woman with a history of rheumatoid arthritis who had an uneventful cementless total knee arthroplasty. **A:** Four years following the index procedure, she presented with a red and inflamed knee joint; sepsis was confirmed by aspiration and cultures. **B:** Anteroposterior radiograph indicating component loosening secondary to joint infection.

method. Antibiotic suppression can be used in patients with stable implants who are not suitable candidates for surgical intervention and who are infected with a low-virulence organism.

Rare Syndromes/Conditions

Heterotopic Ossification

Heterotopic ossification (HO) tends to occur within the first three postoperative months. It occurs in 5% to 15% of TKA patients, although it is symptomatic in <1% of patients. Presentation is variable and may consist of vague discomfort, stiffness, and, in very rare cases, persistent pain and snapping. New bone formation is evident on radiographs within 3 months following surgery and usually does not change after the first year.

Preoperatively, or within the first 48 hours following surgery, high-risk patients may be given prophylaxis using either a course of indomethacin or radiation. In the occasional patient who experiences symptoms that fail to respond to conservative therapy, surgical excision of the HO may be necessary.

Hemarthrosis

Hemarthrosis may occur from months to several years (mean 2 years) following TKA. The incidence is approximately 5%, and the underlying cause is frequently unknown. In some cases, the pathogenesis is characterized by synovial proliferation secondary to polyethylene, metal, or cement debris, which can frequently bleed owing to entrapment or microtrauma. Tissue histology reveals focal synovial hyperplasia containing histiocytes and hemosiderin deposits. Other possible causes include clotting disorders such as hemophilia, chronic use of anticoagulants, remnant posterior cruciate ligament stump trauma, intercondylar notch fibrosis, pigmented villonodular synovitis, juxta-articular arteriovenous malformation, tumor, component loosening, and knee instability (including flexion instability).

Patients present with a tense, painful effusion with decreased range of motion. Coagulation studies are often normal. In the acute setting, knee aspiration is diagnostic and typically reveals bright red blood. In rare cases angiography may aid in identifying the source of bleeding. Initial management consists of short-term rest, application of ice, limb elevation, splinting, and discontinuation of anticoagulant medication. In patients who fail conservative treatment or who have recurrent hemarthrosis, arthroscopic synovectomy can be considered. In refractory cases, implant revision may provide a satisfactory long-term outcome.

Nonarticular Causes

Vascular Causes

Popliteal Artery Pseudoaneurysm. Vascular injuries constitute a small portion of TKA complications (0.03% to 1.2%). Pseudoaneurysm of the popliteal artery is a rare and painful vascular complication that, if untreated, can result in loss of the operated limb. About 40% of cases are diagnosed within 1 month of disease onset. Symptoms include a painful and pulsatile mass that produces bruits and/or thrills and is usually associated with ecchymosis overlying the popliteal region. In addition, distal pulses may be weak. Magnetic resonance imaging (MRI) can be used to confirm the diagnosis of popliteal artery pseudoaneurysm.

Postthrombotic Syndrome. Following TKA there is a risk of developing deep venous thrombosis (DVT) secondary to stasis, endothelial damage, and increased blood viscosity (the Virchow triad). DVT may precipitate chronic venous insufficiency, and patients may present with a painful, swollen lower limb, sometimes associated with ulceration. Clinical findings can be confirmed with venous Doppler studies. Patients should be treated with compression stockings and referred to a vascular specialist.

Neurogenic Causes

Cutaneous Neuromas. Uncommonly, patients present with a painful TKA secondary to a cutaneous neuroma. A neuroma may develop when the infrapatellar branch of the saphenous nerve, medial femoral cutaneous nerve of the thigh, or medial/lateral retinacular nerves are divided at the index procedure. Conservative measures for neuropathic pain include topical steroids, iontophoresis, transcutaneous electrical stimulation, and medications. If symptoms last >6 months, nerve blocks and selective denervation procedures may be considered.

Complex Regional Pain Syndrome. Complex regional pain syndrome (CRPS), formerly known as reflex sympathetic dystrophy (RSD) or Sudeck atrophy, is a diagnosis of exclusion and arises from autonomic dysfunction. It is a complex interplay of four factors: a local trigger (e.g., surgical trauma), psychologic factors, systemic factors associated with pain exacerbation (e.g., peripheral neuropathy), and sympathetically maintained pain. It is thought to occur in about 0.5% of TKA patients. There is a wide variation in disease presentation. Symptoms may include intense burning or prolonged pain in nonanatomic distributions, sensory abnormalities such as allodynia or hyperalgesia that are out of proportion to the physical examination findings, edema, sudomotor disruptions such as sweating, trophic changes such as smooth, shiny skin, cold intolerance, vasomotor disturbances such as hyperhidrosis and coolness to the touch, stiffness, and weakness. Patients with anxiety and severe pain preoperatively are more likely to develop CRPS. Although there may be a psychologic overlay in CRPS, it is unclear whether the psychologic factors predispose patients to this condition or are a result of this syndrome. Although diffuse pain and hypersensitivity suggest the presence of CRPS, the extensive variability of clinical symptoms warrants a thorough workup to exclude other causes (e.g., mechanical, prosthetic, or soft tissue causes).

In TKA patients with CRPS, osteopenia of the patella may be appreciated on plain radiographs. Technetium-99m bone scans may reveal increased uptake in affected regions. Sympathetic block is useful, both as a diagnostic and therapeutic modality.

Initial treatment consists of NSAIDs, neuromodulating medications, and physical therapy. Narcotics and benzodiazepines are contraindicated in these patients. Instead, anesthetic sympathetic blockade can provide long-term pain relief. Lumbar sympathectomy can be attempted for recalcitrant symptoms.

Pain of Unknown Origin

The diagnosis "pain of unknown origin" is made when all causes are considered (e.g., all causes listed in Fig. 27-1) and none is applicable. The incidence of severe pain without identifiable cause following TKA is about 6%. Associated clinical factors may include history of multiple procedures, fibromyalgia, unreasonable patient expectations, injuries with workers' compensation issues, and patients who had minimal joint disease as determined radiographically prior to TKA.

LABORATORY TESTS

Management of painful knee arthroplasty begins with basic laboratory tests to rule out infection. The usual tests consist of the following:

Erythrocyte sedimentation rate (ESR)

- Returns to normal 3 to 6 months following TKA. Thus, interpretation of this test in the context of the early and intermediate painful TKA may be difficult.
- ESR of >30 has a sensitivity of 80% and a specificity of 63% in predicting infection.

C-reactive protein (CRP)

- An acute-phase protein that returns to normal within 3 weeks following TKA.
- The most useful laboratory test to rule out infection.

Complete blood count (CBC)

- Often normal but can be useful when reviewed with ESR and CRP.
- Lymphocyte count of <1,500 cells/mm^2 is associated with a more than threefold risk of wound complications.

Knee aspiration

- All aspirated fluid should be sent for microscopy and cultures (aerobic and anaerobic bacteria, fungi, and tubercle bacilli). Gram stain has limited sensitivity (10%).
- For diagnosis of infection, knee aspiration has a positive-predictive value of 89.5% and a negative-predictive value of 84.5%.
- Use of antibiotics increases the false-negative rate. Ideally antibiotics should be stopped at least 2 weeks prior to aspiration when chronic infection is suspected.

Synovial biopsy

Synovial biopsy can be performed either arthroscopically or open. The following conclusions can be made based on high-power view:

- A count of ≥10 polymorphonuclear leucocytes (PMNs) per high-power field (HPF) is predictive of infection.
- A count of 5 to 9 PMNs per HPF is not always consistent with infection.
- A count of <5 PMNs per HPF reliably excludes infection.

RADIOLOGIC FEATURES

Radiographic workup depends on the suspected diagnoses. An overview is given below.

Conventional radiographs

- Anteroposterior (AP), lateral, and sunrise views to assess for malposition, patella tilt, periprosthetic fractures, and radiolucent lines.
- Checking for radiographic signs of loosening:
  - Tibial component bone/cement interface is broken down into five to seven zones, depending on whether or not a stem is present (as seen on AP view).
  - Femoral component bone/cement interface is broken down into five to seven zones, depending on whether or not a stem is present (as seen on lateral view).
  - Patellar component bone/cement interface is broken down into three to five zones, depending on number of fixation lugs (as seen on sunrise view).
  - The width of radiolucent lines for each zone is measured in millimeters. The total widths are added for each zone for all three components.
  - For each component, if the cumulative total widths are ≤4 and these lines have been nonprogressive on subsequent radiographs, the component is not significant for implant loosening; cumulative total widths of 5 to 9 should be followed closely, as loosening is likely; cumulative total widths of ≥10 signify failure or impending failure.
- Special films may occasionally be required:
  - Full-length radiograph: To assess overall limb alignment.
  - Oblique films: To evaluate for periprosthetic osteolysis.
  - Dynamic fluoroscopy: To confirm mechanical derangement (e.g., fabella impingement), component loosening, and instability.
  - Fluoroscopically positioned radiographs: May be obtained to gain perfectly tangential views of uncemented implant bone/prosthesis interfaces. These radiographs are useful in evaluation of uncemented knee component loosening.

Arthrography

- An invasive nonspecific test that may help diagnose component loosening (especially tibial).
- Current use is limited and superseded by other tests described below.

Ultrasound

- Permits dynamic, real-time evaluation of moving structures such as muscles and tendons.
- Often unavailable.

Sinography

- Can be used to determine whether a draining sinus communicates with the knee joint.

Technetium-99m bone scintigraphy

- Although a negative scan rules out significant knee pathology, a positive scan is nonspecific. Positive scans are seen most commonly in infection, component loosening, stress fracture, and bone remodeling.

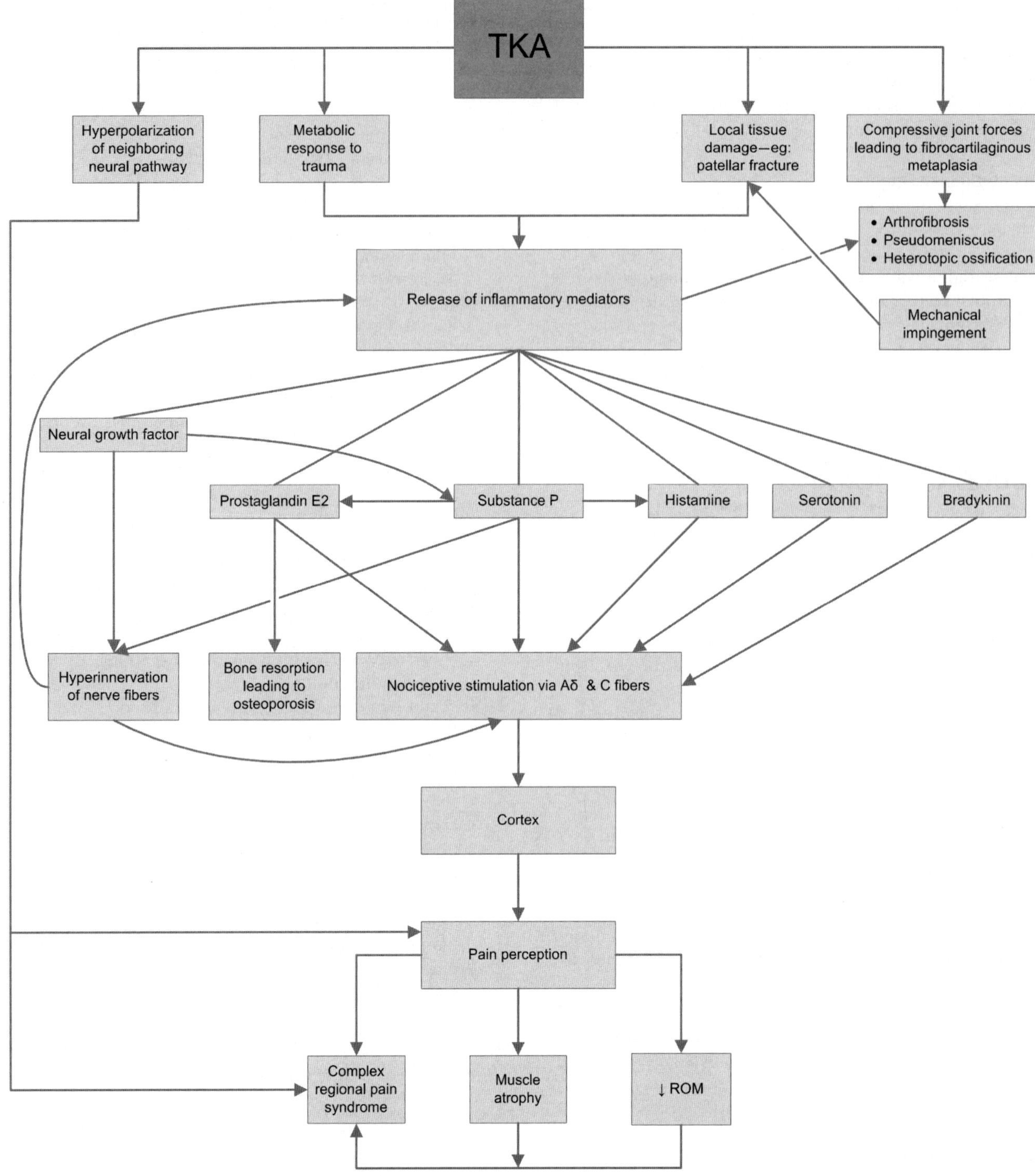

Figure 27-6 Diagnostic evaluation and management of pain following TKA.

Computed tomography scan

- Significant metal artifact can arise.
- Newer reformatting software allows for artifact suppression and improved imaging of bone/cement and cement/implant interfaces and allows for better quantification of osseous defects.

Magnetic resonance imaging

- Conventional MRI sequences have extensive metallic susceptibility artifact.
- Newer metal subtraction software programs aid in diagnosis of various soft tissue and bone-related causes of painful TKA, e.g., collateral ligament disruptions, bursitis, synovitis, fat pad scarring, intramuscular hematoma, pigmented villonodular synovitis, and osteolysis.

Diagnostic Workup and Management Algorithm

A flowchart outlining clinical history, physical examination, diagnostic procedures, and possible treatment options of painful TKA is presented in Figure 27-6.

SUMMARY

Clinical evaluation and subsequent management of patients presenting with pain following TKA can be a diagnostic challenge even for the experienced surgeon. A systematic approach is essential to elucidating the cause of a painful TKA. Patients with definable causes of knee pain following TKA such as loosening, malalignment, oversized components, or heterotopic ossification improve most predictably from surgical intervention. Revision TKA performed prior to defining a specific cause for the patient symptoms can lead to inferior functional results and persistent or worsened symptoms.

SUGGESTED READINGS

Bong MR, Di Cesare PE. Stiffness after total knee arthroplasty. *J Am Acad Orthop Surg*. 2004;12(3):164–171.

Dennis DA. Evaluation of painful total knee arthroplasty. *J Arthroplasty*. 2004;19(4 suppl 1):35–40.

Gonzalez MH, Mekhail AO. The failed total knee arthroplasty: evaluation and etiology. *J Am Acad Orthop Surg*. 2004;12(6):436–446.

Greipp ME, Thomas AF. Reflex sympathetic dystrophy syndrome: pain that doesn't stop. *J Neurosci Nurs*. 1986;18(1):23–25.

Lindenfeld TN, Bach BR Jr, Wojtys EM. Reflex sympathetic dystrophy and pain dysfunction in the lower extremity. *Instr Course Lect*. 1997;46:261–268.

Mont MA, Serna FK, Krackow KA, et al. Exploration of radiographically normal total knee replacements for unexplained pain. *Clin Orthop Relat Res*. 1996:331:216–220.

Sharkey PF, Hozack WJ, Rothman RH, et al. Insall Award paper. Why are total knee arthroplasties failing today? *Clin Orthop Relat Res*. 2002;404:7–13.

Sofka CM, Potter HG, Figgie M, et al. Magnetic resonance imaging of total knee arthroplasty. *Clin Orthop Relat Res*. 2003;406:129–135.

REVISION TOTAL KNEE ARTHROPLASTY

GAVIN PITTMAN
THOMAS K. FEHRING
J. BOHANNON MASON

GENERAL PRINCIPLES

Total knee arthroplasty (TKA) has become one of the most successful orthopedic procedures with at least 95% good or excellent results reported after 10 years of follow-up. Despite this success, a painless, well-functioning prosthetic knee joint cannot be uniformly guaranteed. Approximately 32,000 revision total knee replacements were performed in 2002 in the United States alone, and that number continues to rise annually.

Although there are various reasons for TKA revision surgery, the most prevalent causes of failure can be grouped into early and late mechanisms of failure based on the length of time from the index operation. Early failures most commonly result from postoperative infections, joint instability, aseptic component loosening, and patellofemoral issues. Some of these failures are attributed to poor surgical judgment or surgical technique during the initial arthroplasty. Common causes of late failures include infections from a hematogenous source or the sequelae of polyethylene wear. Late failures appear to be more closely related to host factors and material limitations.

As discussed in previous chapters regarding the assessment of the painful TKA, a systematic approach using the patient history, physical exam, laboratory analysis, and radiographic images is required to determine the mechanism of failure. Surgical exploration of a painful total knee without clearly defined treatable mechanism of failure is rarely successful. A firm understanding of the underlying pathology and methods of addressing it is mandatory before intervening. The purpose of this chapter is to help the surgeon establish a sound preoperative plan and to execute this plan in an efficient manner to provide the patient with a durable, successful revision total knee replacement.

Preoperative Planning

Accomplishing a successful revision total knee arthroplasty can be a challenging task even for the most seasoned surgeon. Despite the added difficulties of addressing infection, malalignment, bone loss, and instability, the primary goals of revision surgery should remain the same as those in primary knee arthroplasty. These goals include establishing proper alignment, balancing the extension space in the coronal plane, and creating a flexion space that equals the extension space. Preoperative planning allows the surgeon to visualize these goals prior to entering the operating room and provides the opportunity to determine what additional tools and devices will be necessary to facilitate the revision.

Although nuclear studies, MRI, and CT scanning may be beneficial during the assessment of the painful total knee, conventional radiographs continue to be the most useful references for planning a revision. Weight-bearing anteroposterior (AP), lateral, and Merchant views offer an informative and quick method for evaluating the prosthetic components and the surrounding bone. Previously obtained radiographs may be available for comparison to assess progressive changes in bone quality or component stability. Oblique flexion views of the distal femur improve the ability to detect and estimate the size of osteolytic lesions that may exist adjacent to the femoral prosthesis. Fluoroscopy may also be helpful in eliminating small degrees of obliquity seen in conventional radiographs that may obscure radiolucent lines at component interfaces. This is particularly useful in evaluating whether or not a cementless implant is bone ingrown.

The hip-knee-ankle radiograph allows assessment of lower extremity alignment and is used to determine the proper femoral and tibial mechanical axes. The distal femoral cut is made based on the femoral mechanical axis. A line is drawn from the middle of the femoral head to the middle of the knee. A perpendicular from this line at the level of the distal femur denotes a proper distal femoral resection. The tibial mechanical axis is defined in a similar fashion, drawing a line from the middle of the talus to the middle of the knee. A line perpendicular to this line at the level of the proximal tibia denotes a proper proximal tibial resection. Deformities of the femur and tibia, such as bowing or fracture that may compromise the position of intramedullary alignment guides or stem insertion are detected with this radiograph. This information allows templating of the revision distal femoral and tibial resections to recreate a neutral lower extremity alignment and alerts the surgeon to potential pitfalls if intramedullary alignment guides are used.

Exposure of the Revision Knee

A thoughtfully designed surgical approach is necessary to avoid potentially devastating healing problems and to obtain adequate access to the knee. These issues should be addressed during the initial history and exam of the patient. Inquiries regarding delayed wound healing, wound drainage, stiffness, or any other complications after primary knee surgery should be made. The examination should clearly document the location of previous skin incisions, presence of sinus tracts, mobility of the soft tissues and patella, active and passive range of motion, and whether an extensor lag is present. Investigating these issues preoperatively may prevent unexpected difficulties in the operating room.

The surgical incision must be of adequate length to fully expose the knee joint safely without applying excessive tension on the skin edges. It has been shown that a midline incision is less disruptive to the anterior arterial network of the knee. However, when multiple prior incisions are present, the most lateral skin incision should be used. Since the blood supply to the skin over the knee comes from medial to lateral, a medial incision in the presence of a previous lateral incision compromises the blood flow to the skin between the incisions. When a medial and lateral incision is encountered, the lateral incision usually should be used and extended in both directions. A flap is created, which must be done in the subfascial plane to preserve the dermal plexus' contribution to vascularity of the flap. Frequently it is necessary to incorporate or cross a previous incision. Any scar that must be intersected should be done in a perpendicular fashion. Similarly, the incorporation of a previous incision must avoid acute angles to minimize the risk of skin necrosis and a resultant narrow bridge of skin tissue. Adherent skin must be mobilized in the subfascial plane to identify the proper location of the capsular incision and allow retraction of the underlying tissues.

The capsular incision is performed along the medial border of the quadriceps tendon, the patella, and the patellar tendon with the knee in flexion. Less invasive approaches, such as the midvastus or subvastus incisions, generally do not provide sufficient exposure for revision surgery. Adhesions, synovium, and scars beneath the quadriceps tendon and throughout the medial and lateral synovial recesses are removed with the knee extended. Care must be taken while releasing scar over the epicondyles to prevent damage to the collateral ligaments. The medial joint capsule is released from the underlying tibial metaphysis, maintaining an intact sleeve around the medial border of the proximal tibia to the posterior midline. The tibia is externally rotated while flexing the knee until anterior subluxation of the proximal tibia ensues. With this patellar inversion technique, no attempt to evert the patella is made until the femoral and tibial components have been removed. Attempts to evert the patella early risks avulsion of the patellar tendon and should be discouraged in revision surgery.

When revision surgery is performed on a stiff knee, more extensile exposures may on occasion be necessary. The quadriceps snip is the most commonly used method to relax the extensor mechanism. It is accomplished by completely incising the quadriceps tendon at a 45-degree angle from distal medial to proximal lateral in line with the fibers of the vastus lateralis 4 to 6 cm above the patella. The quadriceps V-Y turndown is typically reserved for the near ankylosed knee. This technique divides the quadriceps tendon at its junction with the rectus muscle, at a 45-degree angle, in a distal and lateral direction. Although effective for exposure, this approach is frequently accompanied by extensor lag postoperatively. A tibial tubercle osteotomy provides excellent exposure and is preferable to the V-Y turndown in extremely stiff knees. However, persistent anterior knee pain and nonunion have been described with this technique. The routine use of extensile exposure is unnecessary and should be discouraged. More than 90% of revisions can be performed with the patellar inversion technique previously described.

Component Removal

Depending on the stability and type of fixation, the removal of total knee components can be a time-consuming and frustrating process. However, the benefits of a safe and orderly extraction must be considered. Avoidance of condylar bone loss or fracture can greatly facilitate a successful reconstruction. Familiarity with implant removal instruments and their proper use assists in making this step more efficient and less complex.

The order in which the implants are removed decreases the risk of complications and enhances the ability to remove the next component. The tibial polyethylene insert is removed first. Knowledge of implant-specific removal instruments for modular inserts is necessary. Most modular inserts can be removed with an osteotome that will disengage the plastic from the underlying tibial tray. Initial removal of the tibial insert will increase space in the knee that is needed to remove the other components.

The femoral component is generally removed second. The implant/cement interface for cemented implants is disrupted with thin osteotomes or ultrasonic devices. Working at this interface from both the medial and lateral sides limits bone loss. The implant/bone interface for cementless implants is most easily divided with thin osteotomes, power saws, or thin high-speed cutting burrs. The anterior condylar, distal, and chamfer interfaces are usually readily accessible. The posterior condylar interface is more difficult to reach and may require angled osteotomes or a Gigli saw for disruption if this portion of the component is well fixed. Once loosened, the femoral implant can be removed by gently tapping the anterior flange with a metal punch and mallet in a distal direction. Vigorous disimpaction should be discouraged as this indicates that the fixation has not been sufficiently disrupted to proceed with removal.

Removal of the femoral component provides access to the tibial tray. The same instruments used to disrupt the femoral interfaces are also used here. However, cemented implants with a roughened surface may require a saw or ultrasonic device to separate the cement from the implant. After the component is loosened, the knee is hyperflexed and the tibia is anteriorly translated. Osteotomes can then be stacked under the tray to elevate it out of the proximal tibia.

Uncemented stems without biologic fixation typically are removed with their respective implant during the extraction process outlined above. However, well-fixed cemented stems and roughened stems secured biologically to bone can be very difficult to remove. If the stems cannot be disimpacted with the attached implant, the condylar portion should be disengaged or cut away from the stem. This provides direct access to the stem. Cemented stems can then be removed by breaking the cement/stem interface with a high-speed burr or ultrasonic device. Biologically fixed stems can be removed with trephines designed to remove cementless total hip arthroplasty femoral stems or a narrow high-speed burr. Rarely a femoral window or tibial tubercle osteotomy is required for the removal of well-fixed cemented or cementless stems.

Extraction of failed components is an often overlooked step of the revision. Use of proper tools and patience is warranted to avoid making the surgery more complex by removing excessive bone or initiating fractures.

Joint Alignment and Ligament Balance

With the failed components removed, adequate space should be available within the joint to observe bone quality and deficiency and begin preparing the femur and tibia for reimplantation. The hip-knee-ankle radiograph may be reassessed to determine whether an intramedullary guide may be used and to review the resection level and angle for the distal femoral and proximal tibial resections.

In most cases, the revision distal femoral cut may be referenced from an intramedullary rod that is secured within the diaphyseal cortex. If the femoral canal is not amenable to an intramedullary guide, an extramedullary guide or computer assistance may be used. The former is less accurate than intramedullary guidance, and the latter adds complexity to the case. Regardless, a flat cut is made with an oscillating saw through the cutting guide at an angle perpendicular to the mechanical axis. The amount of bone removed should be minimal to prevent elevating the joint line excessively. Exceptions to this include a significant preoperative flexion contracture from an inadequate primary distal femoral resection or if nonsupportive bone is encountered that will eventually require augmentation. The estimated level of the joint line is 2 to 2.5 cm distal to the epicondyles, 1 cm distal to the inferior pole of the patella with the knee in extension or more simply when the patella rests in the proper position in the trochlear groove in full extension.

The proximal tibial resection provides the foundation on which the revision is built. Therefore, the importance of creating an accurate cut that is perpendicular to the mechanical axis cannot be overstated. This resection can be referenced from intramedullary or extramedullary alignment guides. Intramedullary guides may be influenced by bowing within the proximal tibia or by the presence of sclerotic bone within the intramedullary canal.

Although several techniques exist, we prefer using the classic method of balancing the knee if the collateral ligaments are not attenuated. After the components are provisionally sized, a coronally symmetric extension gap is created with the appropriate medial and lateral releases. The height of this gap is measured with the knee in extension. The knee is then flexed and the flexion gap is measured and then tensioned. The appropriate AP cut guide is placed on the distal femur and is rotated until parallel with the tibial cut. A stylus is used anteriorly to prevent notching the distal femur. The size of the AP cutting block can then be manipulated to match the height of the flexion gap with the previously measured extension gap. Other methods used to establish rotation of the femoral component, such as the posterior condylar axis or trochlear axis, are difficult to reference in the revision situation because of previous bony resections and bone loss. While we prefer to use the classic method described above to set femoral rotation and balance the flexion gap, the epicondylar axis can be used to assess femoral rotation when collateral ligaments are severely attenuated.

After the flexion and extension gaps are balanced, the femoral box and chamfer cuts are made. If the use of augments has been calculated into the gap balancing, augments should be added to the femoral cutting blocks to avoid unnecessary bone resection. The necessity of stems, augments, and degree of articular constraint can now be determined.

Managing Bone Loss: Augments, Allograft, and Custom Implants

Some degree of bone loss is to be expected when performing a revision total knee replacement. Significant deficiencies may be seen when aseptically loosened components have been neglected or the primary total knee failed owing to osteolysis or infection. Although bone deficiencies cannot be comprehensively evaluated before the failed components have been removed, assessment of the preoperative radiographs should alert the surgeon to existing defects and allow preparation of a surgical strategy to manage these defects. Bone loss can be categorized into cavitary defects, which have an intact surrounding cortical rim, or segmental defects, with no surrounding cortex. Depending on the severity of the bone loss, cement, cement and screws, bone graft, modular metallic augments, and custom implants can be used to fill the deficiencies and recreate the joint line.

Cement is frequently used to fill small contained defects of both the femur and the tibia. When cement is used to fill more significant defects, screws partially embedded in host bone can be added to strengthen the cement construct. This technique can be extremely effective in moderate-sized deficiencies, especially in older patients.

Bone graft has been used to address a wide variety of osseous deficiencies around the knee from small cavitary lesions to extensive segmental defects. Because autograft is usually in short supply, allograft bone is generally used in revision total knee arthroplasty. Although a thorough discussion of bone graft basic science is beyond the scope of this chapter, familiarity with the types of allograft, sterilization methods, storage process, disease transmission, and incorporation with the host is required before its use.

Particulate allograft is typically used to fill contained cavitary defects when sufficient host bone is present to provide structural support for the revision components. If healthy host bone is encountered at the base of the lesion, vascularization of the allograft and replenishment of bone stock can be expected.

Structural allografts are most commonly used to manage segmental defects that are too large to be managed with metallic augments. This scenario is commonly seen in cases of advanced osteolysis or infection. Femoral head allografts have been used successfully to fill large cavitary defects of both the distal femur and proximal tibia in these situations and provide a structurally sound surface on which stemmed cemented revision components are used.

Segmental defects that extend proximal to the collateral insertions on the femoral epicondyles impair ligamentous stability as well as component stability. This situation may be encountered with a comminuted supracondylar periprosthetic fracture or severe cases of osteolysis. Partial or full distal femoral allografts (depending on the bone defect location), may be cemented to stemmed revision components using a back table technique. The allograft-prosthetic composite is then secured to the host femur using a diaphyseal engaging stem. Another alternative in this situation is a salvage system or tumor prosthesis which uses a rotating hinge device. This is particularly useful in the elderly, limited-demand population.

Concerns regarding structural allograft resorption, nonunion, fracture, and disease transmission have encouraged the use of metallic devices to fill segmental osseous defects. Modular metallic augments use the predictable properties of metal to manage segmental deficiencies adjacent to both tibial and femoral revision prostheses. These devices allow the surgeon to re-establish the joint line, assist in component alignment, and adjust soft tissue balance to improve knee kinematics. The augments are available in various sizes and shapes, with corresponding trials, creating a versatile system that has greatly reduced the necessity for structural bone grafts and custom implants.

Tibial augmentation devices are available in full wedge, hemiwedge, and block geometries, depending on the manufacturer. They usually are applied to fill segmental medial, lateral, or combined defects of 5 to 20 mm in depth. The location and size of the defect determines which type of augment is appropriate to preserve supportive host bone. Although joint line elevation may be accomplished with the use of a thicker insert, this has the disadvantage of placing increasing stress on the locking mechanism of the tibial insert to the baseplate. Combined medial and lateral block augments will elevate the joint line without applying undue stress on the locking mechanism. A longer stem should be considered in this situation, as the augments will effectively shorten stem penetration into host tibia.

Femoral modular augments are available in the block geometry in various thicknesses and may be applied to the medial and/or lateral condyles distally and posteriorly. Distal augments fill segmental defects below the epicondyles or depress the joint line to its anatomic location. As in the tibia, a longer stem may be required to effectively engage the host femur when distal augmentation is employed. Posterior augments are beneficial in decreasing the flexion gap, which is usually greater than the extension gap in the revision situation. Laterally placed posterior augmentation assists patellar tracking by externally rotating the femoral component when posterolateral bone is deficient.

Significant bony anatomic deficiencies occasionally require tumor prostheses or custom implants. Modern tumor prostheses may have cemented or press-fit intramedullary fixation to the host bone and are equipped with modular diaphyseal segments. These features provide a versatile implant that has intraoperative flexibility. However, most tumor prostheses use a rotating hinge articulation that increases stresses placed on the bone/implant interface and may not be ideal for more active patients.

Use of Stemmed Components

As previously discussed, some degree of bone loss is to be expected when performing a revision total knee replacement. The use of stems on revision components is designed to transfer stress away from the damaged periarticular bone to the shaft. Contemporary revision total knee systems are equipped with numerous stem options: variable length stems designed to engage the metaphyseal or diaphyseal bone, cemented or press-fit interfaces, and straight or offset stems. Although the use of stems in revision total knee arthroplasty is routine, the appropriate use of the stem options available remains controversial.

Several biomechanical studies comparing cemented versus noncemented stems in cadaveric tibias reveal significantly less tibial tray micromotion in the cemented group. Similarly, retrospective clinical studies consistently show higher rates of radiolucent lines adjacent to noncemented stems at 18 months to five years postop. The only retrospective comparison revealed significantly greater radiographic stability when cemented stems were used.

Uncemented diaphyseal engaging stems have become popular because they are simple to use and help guarantee acceptable implant alignment in most circumstances. However, in some cases, diaphyseal stem engagement may compromise tibial component position owing to the limitations of a canal-filling stem. An unrecognized valgus tibial bow will malalign the tibial component into valgus when a canal-filling diaphyseal engaging stem is used. Also, the frequent anteromedial location of the shaft in reference to the plateau will cause the baseplate to overhang medially when a canal-filling stem is used. Although an offset tibial stem may decrease such malposition, a relatively narrow metaphyseal engaging cemented straight or offset stem may be adjusted within the cement mantle to fully accommodate these anatomic variants.

Canal-filling stems can have a similar negative effect on the alignment of the femoral prosthesis. Because of the anterior femoral bow, a diaphyseal engaging stem may contact the anterior endosteal surface of the canal, causing flexion of the component. Alternatively, if the canal-filling stem slides past the anterior endosteal surface, the femoral component may translate anteriorly, both overstuffing the patellofemoral joint and increasing the flexion gap. As in the tibia, a narrow metaphyseal engaging cemented stem may be positioned more posteriorly within the cement mantle of the distal femur to decrease the flexion gap without being biased by the femoral bow.

The judicious use of offset stems may limit component malposition when canal-filling stems are used. However, the intraoperative flexibility, as well as biomechanical and radiographic comparisons, prompts some surgeons to continue to use cemented metaphyseal engaging stems in most cases.

Articular Constraint

Articular constraint refers to the degree of stability afforded to the knee joint by prosthetic design. Additional constraint must be supplied by the implants if the soft tissues around the knee are insufficient to maintain joint stability. In the revision situation, the choices of constraint include posterior stabilized articulations, nonlinked constrained prostheses, and rotating hinge constrained designs. Because increased levels of constraint generate larger stresses on the implant/bone interface, the least amount of constraint that provides a stable joint should be selected. Although a thorough preoperative examination may alert the surgeon to potential instability issues, a final decision regarding the degree of articular constraint often cannot be made until bone defects are addressed and ligament balancing has been accomplished.

Most revision total knee replacements can be accomplished with posterior stabilized implants. These prostheses provide minimal constraint through a congruent tibiofemoral articular surface and a spine and cam mechanism that promotes femoral rollback and prevents posterior displacement of the tibia in flexion. This design requires functional collateral ligament support for varus and valgus stability in flexion and extension. Equalizing the flexion and extension gaps is necessary to prevent the spine from dislocating posterior to the cam if an excessive flexion space exists.

Nonlinked constrained implants are used when one or both collateral ligaments are insufficient, creating varus or valgus laxity or an excessive flexion gap that cannot be balanced with the extension gap. This design is equipped with a taller and thicker polyethylene spine or post that may be reinforced with an underlying metal pin. The post closely approximates the intercondylar box providing rotational, translational, and varus/valgus support to the knee joint. Stems should be used to dissipate forces transmitted to the implant/bone interface.

Rotating hinge constrained components are generally reserved for cases of severe bone loss or global instability where the flexion gap is so excessive that the condylar post of a nonlinked constrained device will be unable to prevent posterior displacement of the tibia under the femur. Because rotating hinge devices do not constrain rotation, less stress may be placed on the implant/bone interface than with nonlinked constrained devices. Generally, the use of rotating hinge constrained components is discouraged except in elderly patients with global instability, severe bone loss, and low functional demands because the large osseous resection necessary for implantation limits salvage options (including arthrodesis).

SPECIAL CONSIDERATIONS

Infection in Total Knee Arthroplasty

Infection is the cause of failure in approximately 1% to 2% of total knee replacements. Therefore a high index of suspicion for infection is warranted during the evaluation of all failed total knees. Prompt diagnosis not only may decrease the risk of morbidity and mortality but also increases the available treatment options.

An investigation for infection should occur during the evaluation of every patient with a painful total knee. Unfortunately, the presentation varies considerably depending on the length of time since surgery, the duration of the infection, the virulence of the offending organism, the host status, and use of antibiotics. Nevertheless, a history of continuous knee pain, swelling, warmth, problems with postoperative wound healing, drainage, or an active infection in another area of the body prompts further scrutiny. Radiographs are valuable for assessing the components and periarticular bone quality but rarely distinguish infectious from aseptic failures.

Because of inaccuracies of diagnostic tests, none can be used in isolation to reliably predict the presence of infection, but when used in concert, they allow detection of approximately 90% of infections. Serologic tests including white cell count, sedimentation rate, and C-reactive protein are sensitive but relatively nonspecific screening tests. Routine use of various radioisotope scans appears impractical owing to their low sensitivity. Aspiration of the knee may provide the most useful preoperative information if there is clinical suspicion for infection and the patient has not received antibiotics within 2 weeks. Although the sensitivity of culture results after aspiration is limited, analysis of the synovial fluid revealing >2,500 white blood count (WBC)/mm and >90% polymorphonuclear (PMN; leucocytes) is highly sensitive and specific for infection in the prosthetic knee joint. If an infectious cause for total knee failure remains questionable intraoperatively, frozen histologic analysis by an experienced pathologist should be performed with tissue taken from multiple sites in search of evidence of acute inflammation. Despite clinical scenarios, such as the presence of inflammatory arthropathies or indolent organisms, that continue to impair our ability to distinguish septic from aseptic failures, the judicious use of diagnostic tests improves the ability to identify infected total knee replacements.

The treatment of an infected total knee depends on the timing and duration of the infection, the virulence of the organism, and the patient's overall health. Fluid and tissue cultures must be obtained to guide antibiotic therapy. Acute infections, whether in the early postoperative period or hematogenous in origin, are typically managed with attempted prosthetic retention. Open surgical debridement, radical synovectomy, and tibial insert exchange followed by a short period of intravenous (IV) antibiotics and chronic suppression are recommended in the proper situations. Required criteria include the following: no evidence of osteomyelitis, component loosening, or sinus tract formation; an organism of low virulence that is susceptible to antibiotics; and symptoms that have been present for a short period of time (i.e., <4 weeks postop or within 48 hours of a hematogenous infection). The presence of resistant organisms or an immunocompromised host appear to provide less favorable results with prosthetic retention.

Exchange arthroplasty is the preferred treatment for infections that have been present for >4 weeks or involve more virulent organisms. This process involves resection of the infected components, a thorough joint debridement, and prosthetic reimplantation.

Delayed exchange arthroplasty has been preferred by most surgeons in North America. Eradication of infection consistently approaches 90% in the literature with a two-stage approach. During the first stage, after component removal and debridement, a cement spacer that is impregnated with heat-stable antibiotics is used to discourage soft tissue contracture while delivering high local doses of antibiotics to the infected knee. Some surgeons currently fashion an articulating spacer to minimize bone loss and knee stiffness while improving patient function between stages. This technique also facilitates exposure at reimplantation without any apparent increase in reinfection rates. Systemic antibiotics usually are discontinued about 6 weeks after the spacer is placed. An aspiration prior to reimplantation may be performed and serologic tests for inflammation (erythrocyte sedimentation rate [ESR], C-reactive protein [CRP]) are followed for a gradual return to normalcy prior to reimplantation. Reimplantation usually is performed 2 to 3 months after the first stage. If serologic tests do not normalize, or if frozen section analysis at the time of reimplantation suggests continued active infection, a repeat debridement with articulating spacer exchange is performed and reimplantation is delayed.

Functional results after revision TKA for infection have improved with more rapid diagnosis and the availability of modern revision systems. However, results have been tempered by increasing rates of bacterial antibiotic resistance as well as more immunocompromised hosts. Failure to eradicate total knee infections after repeated attempts at reimplantation leaves the surgeon with few options. Resection arthroplasty is reserved for patients with poor baseline functional requirements. Arthrodesis remains a viable option in patients with irreparable extensor mechanism disruption, multiple recurrent infections, or an inadequate soft tissue envelope provided the contralateral limb and ipsilateral ankle and hip are functional. Above-knee amputation is generally reserved for situations where other reconstructive or salvage efforts are deemed futile.

Periprosthetic Fractures

Based on the Mayo Clinic Joint Registry, the prevalence of periprosthetic fractures adjacent to primary TKAs is 2.3% and rises to 6.3% after revision TKAs. The number of patients with this problem appears to be increasing as the volume of total knees being implanted climbs and patients live longer and more active lives. Distal femur fractures are seen more frequently than patellar or proximal tibia fractures. Issues relevant to the treatment of these periprosthetic fractures include the anatomic location, bone quality, functional requirements of the patient, and whether the fracture occurred intraoperatively or postoperatively.

Intraoperative distal femur fractures typically involve the condyles and occur during removal of failed components or during the insertion of a posterior stabilized implant into an incompletely prepared intercondylar box. Although screws may provide sufficient fixation for a nondisplaced fracture, transferring stress away from the condyle to the shaft through the use of a stemmed component is warranted when fractures are unstable.

Most postoperative fractures of the distal femur are traumatic in origin. Previous notching of the distal femur may contribute to torsional failure. Treatment is based on fracture displacement and component stability. Nonoperative treatment using a cast or brace should be considered for nondisplaced fractures when the femoral component remains stable, especially while treating a patient with low functional demands. Close radiographic follow-up is required to ensure that the fracture remains well aligned.

Displaced fractures with stable implants are treated with rigid internal fixation or intramedullary nails. Although several types of plates have adequate reported results, fixed-angle devices with proximal and distal locking screws are an attractive option. Fixation in the osteopenic bone that is frequently encountered is improved significantly when locking screws are used. The precontoured distal femoral plate may also assist with indirect reduction of the fracture and can be placed through a smaller incision to produce minimal disturbance to the fracture hematoma. Modern retrograde intramedullary nails also provide rigid fixation. However, distal fixation can be a problem in some fracture patterns. The ability of a specific posterior stabilized femoral component to accept a retrograde nail must be investigated preoperatively. Occasionally bone grafting or cement augmentation is required to enhance distal fixation when extensive comminution or osteopenia is present.

Distal femur fractures with loose femoral components require component revision in addition to fracture fixation. A stemmed component with adjuvant fixation is used. However, if comminution is severe, a rotating hinge tumor prosthesis can be used to reconstruct the knee.

Periprosthetic fractures of the tibia plateau that occur intraoperatively may be secured with cancellous screws or a low-profile plate. A longer tibial stem is recommended to protect the fractured plateau. Metaphyseal fractures that occur adjacent to the stem are usually nondisplaced and vertical in orientation. They often occur during removal of a failed tibial component. When recognized, they should also be treated with a longer stem to bypass the defect. Nondisplaced intraoperative fractures that are distal to the stem have been successfully treated with a brace or cast and limited weight bearing. However, displaced fractures distal to the stem require internal fixation for stability.

Postoperative periprosthetic fractures of the tibia plateau commonly lead to tibial implant failure. Prosthetic malalignment, osteopenia, osteolysis, and osseous necrosis have been implicated as predisposing factors. Revision of the tibial component with a stemmed implant and managing the bone loss with modular augments or bone graft are recommended.

Postoperative fractures adjacent to the stem of a stable tibial prosthesis are generally caused by a traumatic mechanism. These fractures are often nondisplaced and may be treated in a long-leg cast. Displaced fractures are best managed with a plate and screw construct. Metaphyseal fractures with an unstable prosthesis require revision to a longer stemmed prosthesis. Stable tibial components with a postoperative fracture distal to the stem often can be treated nonoperatively in a long-leg cast with protected weight bearing. If the tibial prosthesis is loose, revision surgery is indicated. However, delayed reconstruction after the fracture has healed in a cast may simplify the surgery.

Tibial tubercle fractures that occur in the postoperative setting may be the result of trauma or owing to the nonunion of a tubercle osteotomy. Nondisplaced fractures are amenable to casting in extension. Displaced fractures require reduction and internal fixation with screws or wires.

Intraoperative periprosthetic patella fractures usually occur during the removal of a failed patellar implant with deficient underlying bone. Postoperative fractures generally are the consequence of direct impact onto the knee or the result of indirect trauma from a forceful quadriceps contraction. Increased vulnerability to patella fractures occurs after excessive bone resection, overstuffing of the patellofemoral joint, or eccentric position of the component. The method of periprosthetic patella fracture management is controversial and depends on the location, extensor mechanism function, stability of the implant, and medical status of the patient.

Patella fractures with a stable implant and a functional extensor mechanism generally are treated nonoperatively with a brace or cast keeping the knee in extension while allowing full weight bearing. Occasionally a nonunited marginal fracture fragment may require excision for continued pain. Surgical repair is recommended for fractures associated with a significant extensor lag. When fractures with an intact extensor mechanism are accompanied by a loose implant, the decision to simply remove the component versus attempted revision should be based on the remaining patellar bone stock.

Stiffness Following Total Knee Replacement

Difficulties with obtaining adequate knee motion after TKA can be a frustrating experience for the patient as well as the surgeon. Although the normal knee range of motion is approximately 0 to 140 degrees, most functional activities can be accomplished with 95 to 100 degrees of flexion. Less excursion of the knee makes walking, stair use, and sitting problematic.

Arthrofibrosis is the most commonly identified cause of limited motion after a technically sound total knee replacement has been performed. Dense adhesions develop within the joint, resulting in limited flexion and extension. Aggressive range of motion protocols have been instituted at most hospitals to prevent prolonged immobilization, which can exacerbate this condition. However, it is difficult to predict which patients will require further intervention to maintain motion. A careful manipulation under general or regional anesthesia may restore knee motion to near its observed intraoperative level if performed prior to the maturation of adhesions in the first 6 weeks postoperatively. Once scar has matured, arthroscopic lysis of adhesions has been used effectively to disrupt fibrous bands around the fat pad and superior pole of the patella. Arthroscopic release of the posterior cruciate ligament also has provided significant improvements in motion when a cruciate-retaining prosthesis presents with a stiff knee.

Physical examination and radiographs of the knee may reveal technical problems with the primary surgery that may impede motion. Retained osteophytes, implant malalignment, improper component sizing, and imbalance of flexion and extension gaps can mechanically limit motion. Unlike arthrofibrosis, diminished motion was most likely present at the completion of the primary surgery in these situations. Manipulation and arthroscopic releases are rarely helpful under these circumstances. Revision surgery is necessary to improve these motion limitations. Since significant complications may accompany revision TKA, careful consideration must be taken before embarking on this effort to re-establish motion.

Retained osteophytes located on the posterior femoral condyles can impair both flexion and extension. A mechanical block caused by impingement of the osteophyte on the posterior tibia may limit flexion. Extension is impaired by the mass of the osteophyte, tenting the posterior capsule. Removal of the tibial insert is required to access the posterior knee prior to the cautious removal of the osteophytes with an osteotome.

Component malalignment can also limit motion, particularly concerning the slope of the tibia baseplate in the sagittal plane. Excessive posterior slope may limit full extension and cause flexion instability. Anterior slope of the baseplate may cause hyperextension of the knee and limit flexion. Knowledge of the required slope for the specific implant in question is needed prior to its revision.

Improper femoral component sizing and the mismatch of flexion and extension gaps are closely related. A common error is underresection of the distal femur. This produces a tight extension gap and a resultant flexion contracture. Similarly, an insufficient posterior femoral resection will lead to oversizing the femoral component and create a tight flexion space. Flexion of the knee may also be impaired if insufficient patellar bone is resected, creating an "overstuffed" patellofemoral joint.

Surgical management of a stiff total knee should be undertaken cautiously because several mechanisms are not amenable to operative repair. A thorough evaluation is necessary to determine the appropriate treatment. Although surgical intervention has provided statistically significant improvements in motion, functional improvements are not consistently realized.

Polyethylene Wear and Osteolysis

Modern ultra–high-molecular-weight polyethylene provides a low-friction surface intended to articulate with a polished femoral component. However, even with a highly congruent articulation, small polyethylene particles are released from the tibial insert owing to the complex shearing and rotational motions of the knee joint, even during the normal gait cycle. Furthermore, tibial locking mechanisms in modular components allow some degree of insert micromotion, producing backside polyethylene wear. Several additional variables have been implicated in accelerating particle release: abrasive wear, method of polyethylene sterilization and shelf life, coronal alignment of implants, congruency of prosthetic articulations, patient size, and activity levels. Polyethylene wear produces various total knee problems ranging from aseptic synovitis to osteolytic defects that can impair component fixation and complicate reconstructive efforts. As total knee replacements are now implanted in young, active patients, long-term survivorship may become increasingly impaired by material limitations.

The clinical triad of effusion, pain, and progressive changes in coronal alignment of the knee characterizes accelerated polyethylene wear. The effusion is related to the inflammatory reaction induced by macrophage engulfment of the shed particles creating a boggy synovitis that may be accompanied by pain. The asymmetric wear may produce symptomatic instability. If neglected at this point, progressive osteolysis will ensue. Therefore, it is important to revise the patient presenting with these symptoms promptly.

Management of osteolysis depends on the extent and location of the lesions as well as component stability. Preoperative radiographs, including oblique flexion views, should alert the surgeon to loose components and allow an estimation of bone loss. Revision components with alternate levels of articular constraint, stems, modular augments, and allograft may be necessary to facilitate reconstruction. The damaged tibial insert is removed and a full synovectomy is performed. All components should be stressed to ensure stability. If stable, consideration of filling defects with particulate allograft or cement is warranted. Unstable components are removed and revised as described in the section above.

The continuum of problems associated with polyethylene wear highlights the need for routine postoperative surveillance of total knee patients. It has also led to innovative devices intended to reduce backside wear, which appears to correlate with osteolysis. All-polyethylene, nonmodular metal-backed, and rotating-platform tibial components are currently being investigated to determine their ability to limit osteolysis.

SUGGESTED READINGS

Barrack RL, Smith P, Munn B, et al. Comparison of surgical approaches in total knee arthroplasty. *Clin Orthop*. 1998;356:16–21.

Emerson RH, Head WC, Malinin TI. Reconstruction of patellar tendon rupture after total knee arthroplasty with an extensor mechanism allograft. *Clin Orthop*. 1990;260:154–161.

Fehring TK, Griffin WL. Revision of failed cementless total knee implants with cement. *Clin Orthop*. 1998;356:34–38.

Fehring TK, McAvoy G. Fluoroscopic evaluation of the painful total knee arthroplasty. *Clin Orthop*. 1996;331:226–233.

Fehring TK, Odum S, Griffin WL, et al. Patella inversion method of exposure in revision total knee arthroplasty. *J Arthroplasty*. 2002;17:101–104.

Fehring TK, Odum S, Griffin WL, et al. Early failures in total knee arthroplasty. *Clin Orthop*. 2001;392:315–318.

Felix NA, Stuart MJ, Hanssen AD. Periprosthetic fractures of the tibia associated with total knee arthroplasty. *Clin Orthop*. 1997;345:113–124.

Ritter MA, Keating M, Faris PM. Screw and cement fixation of large defects in total knee arthroplasty. A sequel. *J Arthroplasty*. 1993;8:63–65.

Spangehl MJ, Masri BA, O'Connell JX, et al. Prospective analysis of preoperative and intraoperative investigations for the diagnosis of infection at the sites of two hundred and two revision total hip arthroplasties. *J Bone Joint Surg*. 1999;81-A:672–683.

Springer BD, Hanssen AD, Sim FH, et al. The kinematic rotating hinge prosthesis for complex knee arthroplasty. *Clin Orthop*. 2001;392:283–291.

Whiteside LA, Ohl MD. Tibial tubercle osteotomy for exposure of the difficult total knee arthroplasty. *Clin Orthop*. 1990;260:6–9.

PHYSICAL EVALUATION OF THE SHOULDER

ARASH AMINIAN
JASON KOH

Shoulder pain is one of the most common complaints seen by an orthopaedic surgeon. A careful physical examination can reveal a significant amount of information about the patient's complaint. Shoulder pain can be due to intrinsic diseases of the shoulder joint or pathology originating from the spine, chest, or visceral structures. Assessment of these regions along with a detailed history is important in the complete patient evaluation.

PATIENT HISTORY

History is a critical aspect of the patient evaluation (Table 29-1) and can help narrow the differential diagnosis of a patient presenting with shoulder pain. The history should include general questions about the patient's age, handedness, and activities, and more specific questions about the nature of the complaint. Hand dominance can give insight into mechanism of injury as well as determination of extent of disability and recovery. Activities, both work and recreational, again have important implications for cause of injury and treatment. Overhead workers or competitive athletes will have significantly higher demands on the shoulder compared with sedentary individuals. Age will also provide insight into potential causes of pain, with younger patients associated with instability and secondary impingement, and older patients with arthritis and outlet impingement.

The location and nature of the pain can aid in the diagnosis of shoulder injuries. Lateral arm pain, particularly with overhead activity, is often associated with rotator cuff pathology or impingement. Superior discomfort, especially with cross-arm adduction, can be associated with acromioclavicular (AC) joint pain. Deep shoulder pain or posterior shoulder pain at the glenohumeral (GH) joint is associated with labral pathology.

Anterior shoulder pain is associated with biceps tendonitis. Neck or periscapular pain is relatively nonspecific since many will have this secondary to abnormal compensatory scapulothoracic (ST) movement (shrug sign).

Mechanical symptoms, such as clicking, catching, or popping, may have multiple possible causes. However, it is sometimes possible to distinguish between subacromial crepitus (often owing to bursitis or rotator cuff pathology) and glenohumeral clicks and pops that may be related to labral tears or arthritis. Complaints of a "loose" shoulder or one that "comes apart" suggest instability that is more subtle than a frank dislocation. These may be accompanied by reports of neurologic symptoms such as numbness, tingling, or a "dead arm" feeling. These neurologic complaints in this context are usually nonradicular and may be related to subtle traction on the brachial plexus during an instability episode. Persistent pain associated with paresthesias in a radicular distribution suggests a cervical cause. (Table 29-1)

PHYSICAL EXAMINATION

Observation

The patient must be dressed so that the examiner can observe the normal bony and soft tissue contours of both shoulders, including the scapular border, and determine any asymmetry. When looking at the anterior view, the examiner should look for step-off deformity of the AC joint and any bumps on the clavicle indicative of prior fracture. Flattening of the normally round deltoid contour may indicate an anterior shoulder dislocation or paralysis of the deltoid muscle. A "Popeye" deformity (bulging of the upper arm) from a distally migrated biceps can occur after biceps tendon rupture. From the posterior view, the examiner can appreciate any atrophy of the supraspinatus or infraspinatus muscle indicative of a compressive neuropathy of the suprascapular nerve. Winging of the scapula in which the medial border of the scapula moves posterior to the chest wall is seen with long thoracic nerve injury.

Palpation

As with any assessment, the examiner is comparing one side of the body with the other. Initially palpate the bony landmarks around the shoulder starting at the sternoclavicular (SC) joint, the clavicle, the AC joint, and the coracoid. Tenderness along these anatomic landmarks can be indicative of arthritic changes, joint sprains or separation, and fracture.

TABLE 29-1 HISTORY

Handedness
Activities (work and recreational; overhead, repetitive, golf, tennis)
Age
Acute or chronic injury
Pain (onset, location, duration, intensity, radiation, quality, better/worse)
Mechanical symptoms (clicking, catching, popping)
Instability ("loose" or dislocating shoulder)
Neurologic symptoms (numbness, tingling, "dead arm")
Prior injury/treatment
Medication use
Physical therapy
Prior surgeries
Review of systems
History of joint laxity
Other joint or systemic arthritis
Cervical spine (radiculopathy)
History of malignancy
History of lung disease or smoking (Pancoast tumor)
History of abdominal or chest pain
Family history of joint problems

The biceps tendon can also be palpated in its groove proximally. Simultaneous palpation of bilateral biceps tendons in the groove proximally can reveal relatively increased pain consistent with tenosynovitis; absence would indicate proximal rupture. Tenderness along the anterior GH joint capsule can occur with adhesive capsulitis.

Range of Motion and Strength

Both shoulders are simultaneously examined for active range of motion to help identify side-to-side differences. If there is a loss of active range of motion, passive motion should be evaluated. The pattern of movement, such as an abnormal shrug sign in which scapulothoracic motion attempts to compensate for painful glenohumeral motion, should be noted.

The movements of the shoulder that are tested include the following (Fig. 29-1):

- Forward flexion (normal range 150 to 180 degrees).
- Abduction (normal range 170 to 180 degrees).
- External rotation
  - with the elbow at the side (normal range 30 to 60 degrees)
  - With the arm abducted 90 degrees (normal range 70 to 90 degrees)
- Internal rotation
  - (measured by height reached behind the back with the thumb, normal range thoracic level 4 to 8) (Fig. 29-2)
  - With the arm abducted 90 degrees (normal 30 to 60 degrees)

The combined internal and external arc of motion with the arm abducted 90 degrees should be symmetric. It is common that there is a relative lack of internal rotation of the dominant arm.

A discrepancy between active and passive motion suggests loss or inhibition of muscle activity, most likely owing to impingement or other rotator cuff pathology. Pain with forward flexion and abduction but maintained passive external rotation suggests impingement or rotator cuff pathology. A global loss of motion (forward flexion/abduction plus internal rotation plus external rotation) suggests arthritis or adhesive capsulitis. Loss of external rotation past neutral in the context of recent trauma suggests a posterior dislocation.

Muscle Testing

A full assessment of the cervical roots with motor testing is performed (Table 29-2).

Rotator cuff muscles are tested as follows:

- Supraspinatus is tested with shoulders in 90 degrees of abduction. Both the "empty can" (thumbs down) and "full can" test (thumbs up) activate the supraspinatus; the empty can test may also trigger impingement as the greater tuberosity passes under the coracoacromial arch.
- Teres minor/infraspinatus (external rotators) are tested with shoulders in neutral abduction/adduction and elbow in neutral rotation and flexed to 90 degrees.
- Subscapularis (lift-off test or belly-press test):
  - Belly press test: The patient presses the hand against the stomach with the elbow brought in front of the body and the wrist straight. Inability to maintain the elbow in front demonstrates weakness of the upper portion of the subscapularis. (Fig. 29-3)
  - Lift-off test: With the patient's back of the hand touching his or her lower spine, the hand is lifted off against resistance (Fig. 29-4), testing the lower portion of the subscapularis.

Special Tests

Biceps Pathology

Speed and Yergason tests are performed for biceps pathology. The Speed test is performed by resisting forward elevation from 90 degrees with the arm in neutral abduction/adduction and the forearm in full supination. The Yergason test is performed with the arm at the side and elbow in 90 degrees of flexion and resisting supination. Pain with resisted movements during these tests is indicative of proximal biceps tendon pathology.

Impingement Signs/Rotator Cuff Pathology

Physical examination signs that aid in diagnosing subacromial impingement include the Hawkins-Kennedy and Neer impingement signs, the painful arc sign, cross-body adduction test, and the drop arm sign.

Neer Impingement Sign (Fig. 29-5). The scapula is stabilized and the arm is passively forward flexed by the examiner until the patient reports pain or until full elevation is reached. Pain in the anterior or lateral part of

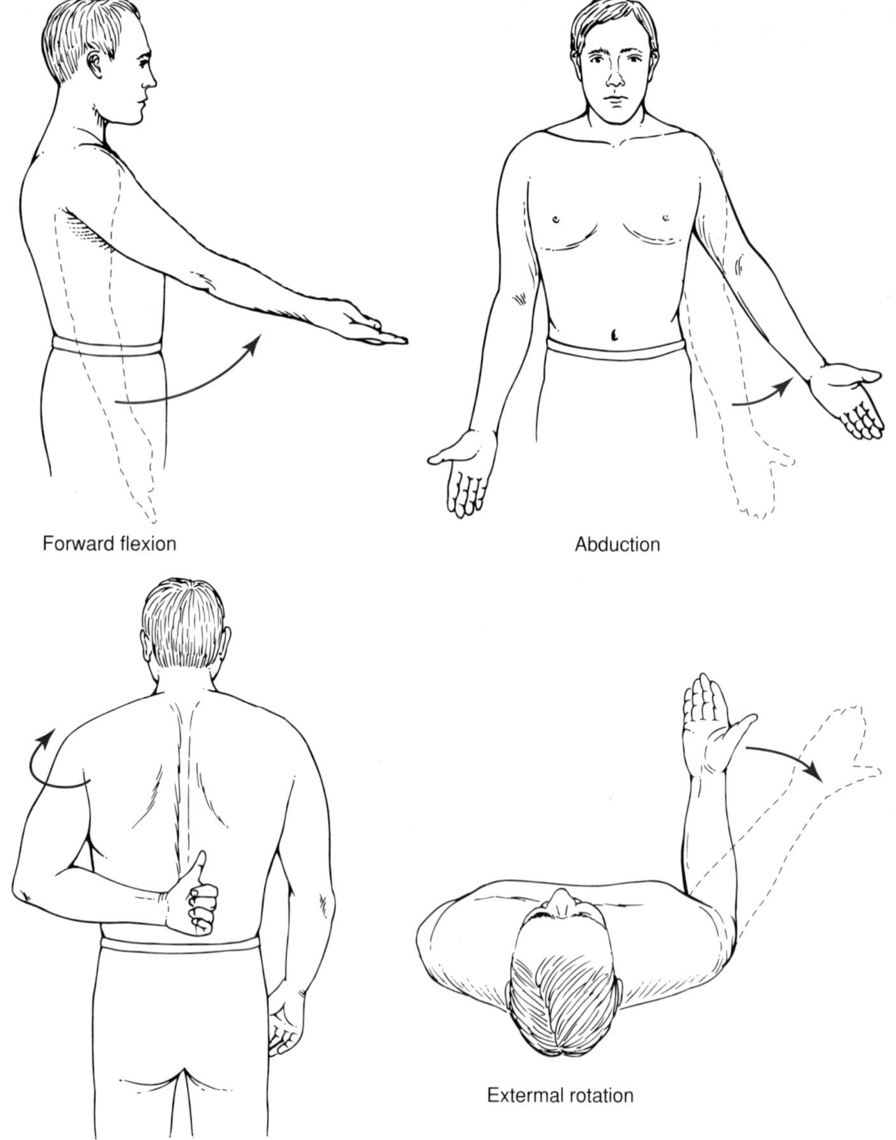

Figure 29-1 Range of motion.

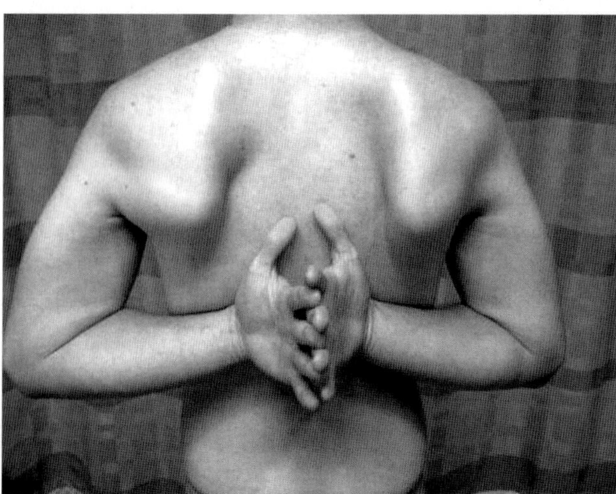

Figure 29-2 Internal rotation.

TABLE 29-2 MUSCLE TESTING—UPPER EXTREMITY

Cervical Root	Muscle Group
C4	Deltoids
C5	Biceps
C6	Wrist extension
C7	Elbow extension
C8	Grip
T1	Finger abduction

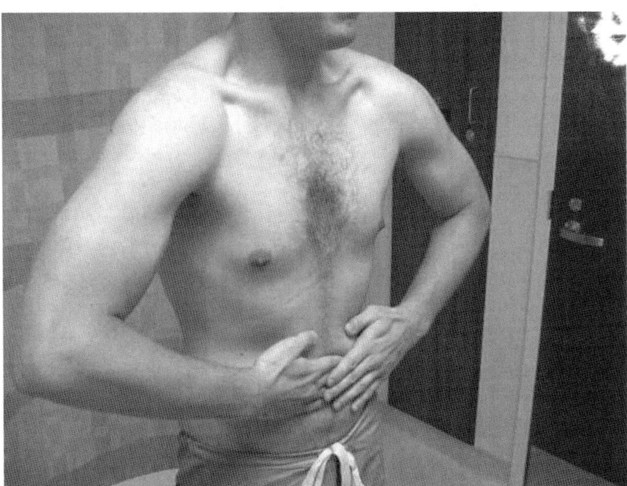

Figure 29-3 Belly press.

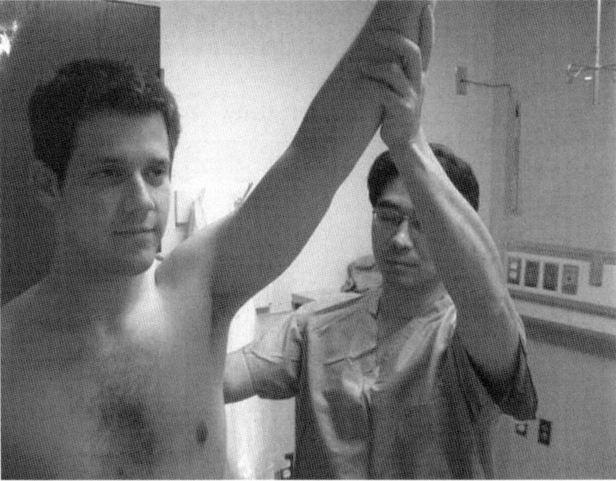

Figure 29-5 Impingement—Neer.

the shoulder in the range of 90 to 140 degrees is considered a positive test

Hawkins-Kennedy Impingement Sign (Fig. 29-6). The arm is placed in 90 degrees of forward flexion and then internally rotated. The end point of rotation is when the patient feels pain or when rotation of the scapula is felt. Pain with internal rotation is a positive sign.

Painful Arc Sign. The patient is asked to elevate the arm in the scapular plane until full elevation is reached, and then the arm is brought down in the same arc. The test is considered positive if the patient has pain between 60 and 120 degrees of elevation.

Cross-Body Adduction Test. The arm is put in 90 degrees of forward flexion and then adducted across the body by the examiner. The test is considered positive with pain produced by adduction.

Drop Arm Test. The patient is asked to elevate the arm fully and then slowly reverse the motion. If the arm is dropped suddenly or the patient has pain, the test is considered positive.

The diagnostic value of these clinical tests for subacromial impingement is summarized in Table 29-3.

Superior Labrum Anterior-Posterior Lesions

The O'Brien test is used to assess superior labral anterior posterior (SLAP) lesions. The goal is to load the biceps tendon and transmit the force to the biceps anchor at the superior labrum. It is performed with the arm in 10 degrees of adduction, 90 degrees of forward flexion, and thumb pointing to the floor. Forward elevation is resisted in this plane and pain is assessed. If the patient has pain that is resolved with supination of the arm, the test is considered positive. Studies in the literature have shown this test to be sensitive but not specific.

The crank test (Fig. 29-7) is used to evaluate for posterior-superior labral tears. The patient is positioned supine, and the arm is abducted to 90 to 120 degrees and externally rotated. This generates internal impingement of the posterior-superior rotator cuff against the

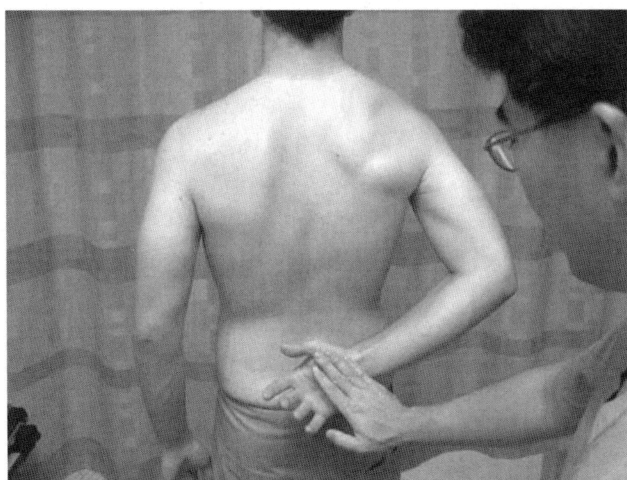

Figure 29-4 Lift off.

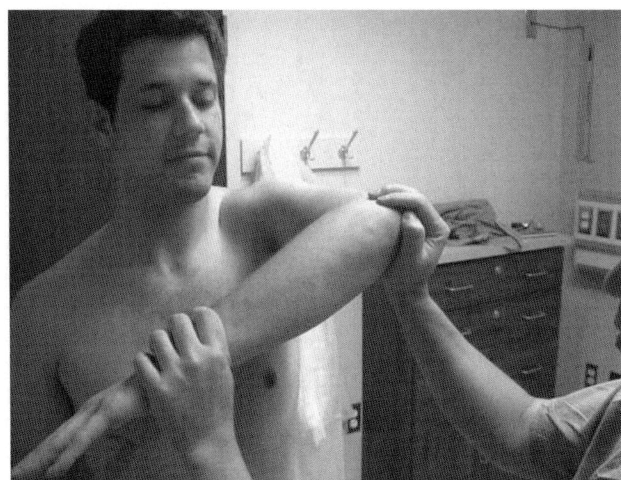

Figure 29-6 Impingement—Hawkins.

TABLE 29-3 DIAGNOSTIC VALUE OF CLINICAL TESTS FOR IMPINGEMENT

	Sensitivity (%)	Specificity (%)	Positive-Predictive Value (%)	Negative-Predictive Value (%)
Neer sign	68	68.7	80.4	53.2
Hawkins-Kennedy sign	71.5	66.3	79.7	55.7
Painful arc sign	73.5	81.1	88.2	61.5
Cross-body adduction test	22.5	82	69.3	36.9
Drop arm test	26.9	88.4	81	39.7

posterior-superior glenoid rim and labrum. Posterior pain at the GH joint line is positive.

Instability

Instability of the shoulder can be in different planes: anterior, posterior, inferior, or multidirectional. The direction of the instability is important to determine because of the treatment implications. When assessing for instability, the examiner should test for generalized joint laxity with thumb to forearm flexibility or forearm recurvatum. Instability is tested by several tests.

In the apprehension sign test (Fig. 29-8), with the shoulder in 90 degrees of abduction and the elbow in 90 degrees of flexion, the shoulder is externally rotated. Patients with anterior instability will have a feeling of possible anterior shoulder dislocation, subluxation, or pain with this maneuver. For posterior instability the arm is adducted, internally rotated, and a posterior force is applied. If pain is elicited, this may signal a posterior labral tear.

The load and shift test for anterior instability (Fig. 29-9). is performed with the shoulder in 90 degrees of abduction and 90 degrees of elbow flexion. The examiner loads the humeral head into the glenoid and translates it anteriorly and posteriorly. This test is graded based on the amount of translation of the humeral head on the glenoid. Translation is 1+, 2+, or 3+ (1+, humeral head to the rim; 2+, humeral head over the rim and reduces by itself; 3+, the humeral head dislocates and does not reduce).

Sulcus sign testing (Fig. 29-10) is performed with the arm to the side, and inferior translation of the humeral head is assessed from the acromion. Typically, inferior translation is maximized with internal rotation of the arm. Translation is graded based on the amount of translation (1+, <1 cm of translation; 2+, 1 to 2 cm of translation; 3+, >2 cm of translation). When patients have a large sulcus sign, the examiner should consider the diagnosis of multidirectional instability. Alternatively, a significant SLAP tear may result in clinically evident inferior translation.

Posterior instability (Fig. 29-11) is assessed by bringing the arm into 90 degrees of forward flexion, internal rotating, and applying a posterior force. This may elicit pain or apprehension, and posterior translation of the humeral head may be appreciated. If there is pain that is relieved by bringing the arm into 90 degrees of abduction, there may be a posterior labral tear (Kim test).

Cervical Spine

A complete examination of the shoulder should always include an assessment of the cervical spine. Cervical radiculopathy can present as shoulder pain and must be evaluated. Range of motion of the cervical spine and a motor

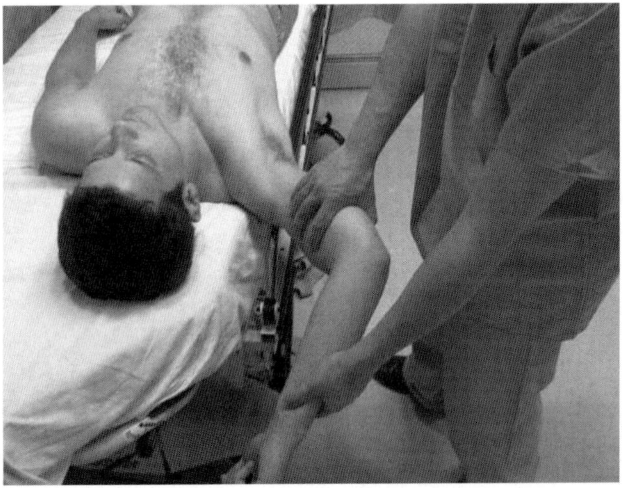

Figure 29-7 Crank.

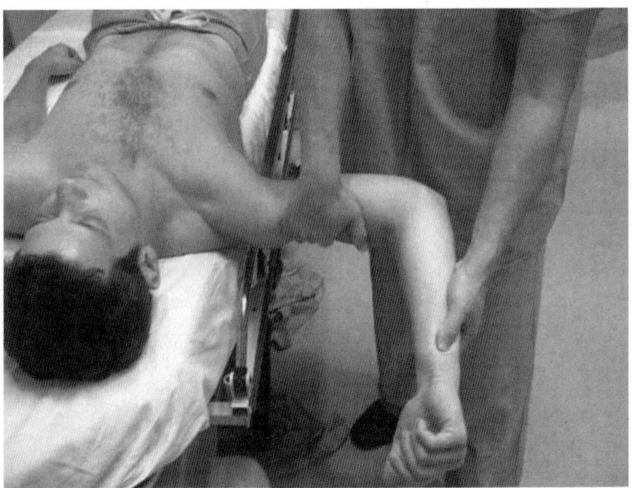

Figure 29-8 Apprehension.

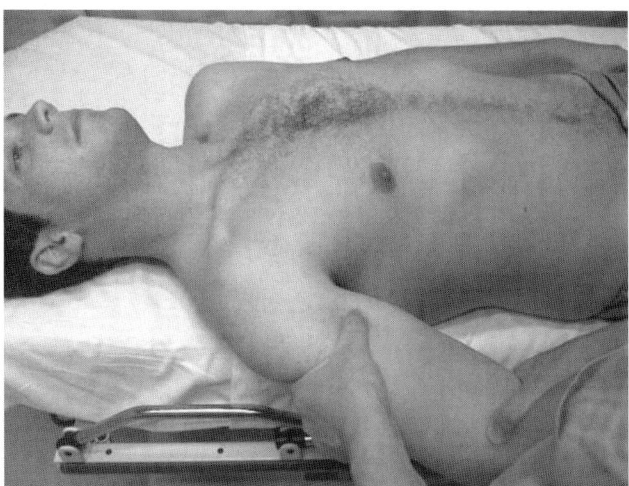

Figure 29-9 Load and shift.

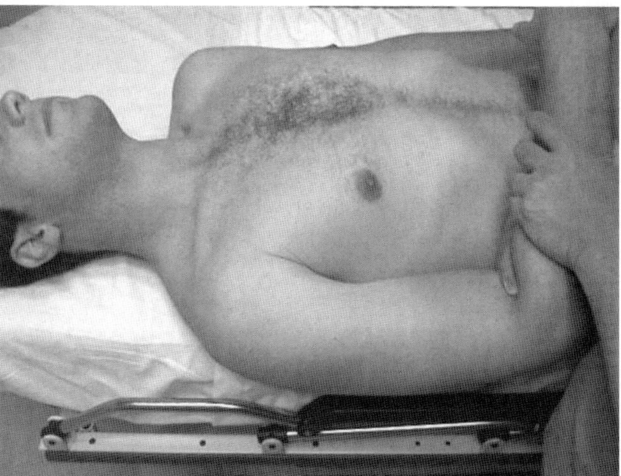

Figure 29-10 Sulcus.

and sensory evaluation of the cervical roots and dermatomes is needed for completeness.

Pain distribution of patients with cervical pathology is mostly over the trapezial region, whereas pain due to primary shoulder pathology is typically located over the deltoid. The Spurling test and Lhermitte test can help delineate nerve root compression. The Spurling test involves extending, laterally flexing, and rotating the neck to the affected side with axial compression. This causes narrowing of the neural foramina and produces nerve root compression. The Lhermitte test involves vertical pressure on the head, which causes a shocklike sensation in the affected extremity.

Authors' Step-by-Step Physical Examination

Have the patient expose both shoulders. Stand in front of the patient. Evaluate the neck (Spurling, Lhermitte) and palpate the shoulders (SC, AC, biceps tendon). Have the patient go through bilateral active forward flexion, abduction, and external rotation. Note range of motion and if there is any dyskinesis (shrug sign, painful arc test). If there is a lack of active motion in a plane, evaluate passive range of motion. Perform Neer and Hawkins impingement tests. Test resisted abduction. Test cross-arm adduction. Test for the O'Brien sign. Test Speed and Yergason. Test active internal and external rotation. Perform belly press test. Have patient turn around and evaluate scapular position and motion with abduction and forward flexion. Evaluate internal rotation. Evaluate lift-off test.

Have the patient lie supine with the shoulder at the edge of the bed. Evaluate passive external rotation, sulcus sign, and load and shift test. Abduct the arm to 90 degrees. Externally rotate the arm, assessing for any apprehension and noting range of motion. If there is apprehension, test relocation. Evaluate crank test. Evaluate internal rotation at 90 degrees. Adduct the arm with the arm flexed 90 degrees and test posterior instability.

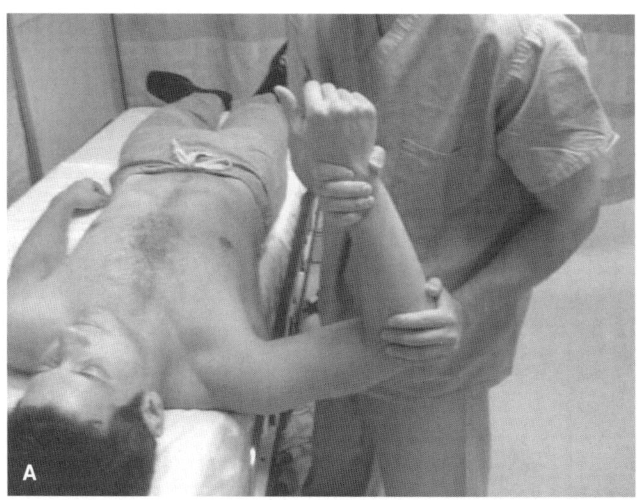

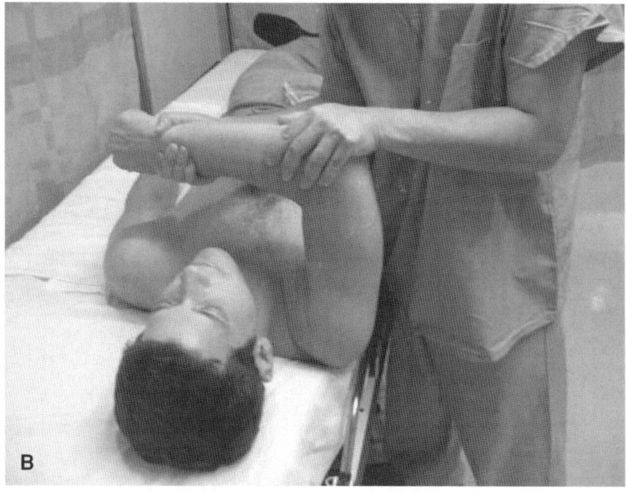

Figure 29-11 A and B: Posterior instability—Kim test.

SUGGESTED READINGS

Cofield RH, Irving JF. Evaluation and classification of shoulder instability. *Clin Orthop Relat Res*. 1987;223:32–43.

Davies GJ, Gould JA, Larson RL. Functional examination of the shoulder girdle. *Phys Sports Med*. 1981;9:82–104.

Gerber C, Ganz R. Clinical assessment of instability of the shoulder. *J Bone Joint Surg*. 1984;66B:551–556.

Hawkins JR, Mohtadi NGH. Clinical evaluation of shoulder instability. *Clin J Sports Med*. 1991;1:59–64.

Hawkins R, Bokor DJ. Clinical evaluation of shoulder problems. In Rockwood CA Jr, Matsen FA III, eds. *The Shoulder*. Philadelphia: WB Saunders; 1990:149–177.

Hoppenfeld S. *Physical Examination of the Spine and Extremities*. Norwalk, CT: Appleton-Century-Crofts; 1976.

Neer CS, Welsh RP. The shoulder in sports. *Ortho Clin North Am*. 1977;8:583–591.

Norwood LA, Terry GC. Shoulder posterior and subluxation. *Am J Sports Med*. 1984;12:25–30.

Park HB, Yokota A, Gill HS, et al. Diagnostic accuracy of clinical tests for the different degrees of subacromial impingement syndrome. *J Bone Joint Surg*. 2005;87A:1446–1455.

Post M, Silver R, Singh M. Rotator cuff tears: diagnosis and treatment. *Clin Orthop Relat. Res*. 1983;173:78.

Tzannes A, Murrell GA. Clinical examination of the unstable shoulder. *Sports Med*. 2002;32(7):447–457.

SURGICAL EXPOSURES OF THE SHOULDER

JOHN-ERIK BELL
SARA L. EDWARDS
THEODORE A. BLAINE

PATIENT POSITIONING

Shoulder surgery is typically performed in either a beach-chair or lateral decubitus position. In the beach-chair position, the head of the bed is elevated approximately 60 degrees. It is lowered if a concealed axillary approach is planned. The patient is shifted to the ipsilateral side of the bed, allowing the arm to be put through a full range of motion without coming into contact with the table. The head and neck are placed in neutral position and secured with tape to the head holder. A short arm board is placed on the table just above the elbow, which can be supplemented after draping by a sterile bolster. A hydraulic arm positioner can also be used as an alternative to the short arm board. For the posterior approaches, the patient is typically placed in a lateral decubitus position.

SKIN INCISIONS

It is very important to take care to make the incision as cosmetically acceptable as possible. Although the most cosmetically acceptable incisions follow the Langer skin tension lines, it is also important to keep in mind sensory dermatomes to avoid neuromas and hypesthetic areas. Supraclavicular nerves supply sensation to the superoanterior shoulder, the axillary nerve supplies skin over the middle deltoid, and the posterior rami of cervicothoracic spinal nerves supply posterior skin from trapezius to scapula. The vascularity of the shoulder area is excellent, so flap viability is high despite extensive undermining in the plane of the deep muscle fascia. Small incisions also afford a great deal of exposure owing to the mobility of the shoulder joint, since seemingly hidden pathology can often be brought into view simply by rotating the arm.

DELTOPECTORAL APPROACH

Standard Deltopectoral Approach

The standard deltopectoral approach is the workhorse for shoulder reconstruction (Fig. 30-1). It exploits the internervous plane between the axillary (deltoid) and medial/lateral pectoral nerves (pectoralis major). The standard incision is made from just inferior to the clavicle, over the coracoid process, extending down the arm to the area of the deltoid insertion in an oblique fashion. Needle-tipped electrocautery is used to create full-thickness flaps medially and laterally. This dissection extends superiorly to the clavicle and inferiorly to the insertion of pectoralis major. Two Gelpi retractors are placed in the superior and inferior aspects of the wound. The deltopectoral interval is then identified. It is typically highlighted by a stripe of fat overlying the cephalic vein, which should be carefully preserved. It is most convenient to retract the vein laterally with the deltoid, because there are fewer venous tributaries from the pectoralis than from the deltoid. Once the vein is freed from the pectoralis and hemostasis is achieved, the subdeltoid space is identified. The easiest way to identify this interval accurately is to begin in the subacromial space and sweep laterally and distally. A Richardson retractor is then placed beneath the deltoid, and the pectoralis tendon is identified.

In shoulders with limited external rotation, the proximal 5 to 10 mm of the pectoralis tendon may require release but should be repaired at the end of the case. Care should be taken when releasing the pectoralis tendon to avoid injury to the long head of biceps tendon running immediately laterally. A second Richardson retractor is then placed deep to the pectoralis muscle, revealing the clavipectoral fascia. This fascia is then incised just lateral to the conjoint tendon, and a medium Richardson retractor is placed to retract the conjoint tendon medially. Whereas both the short head of biceps and coracobrachialis are tendinous proximally, at the

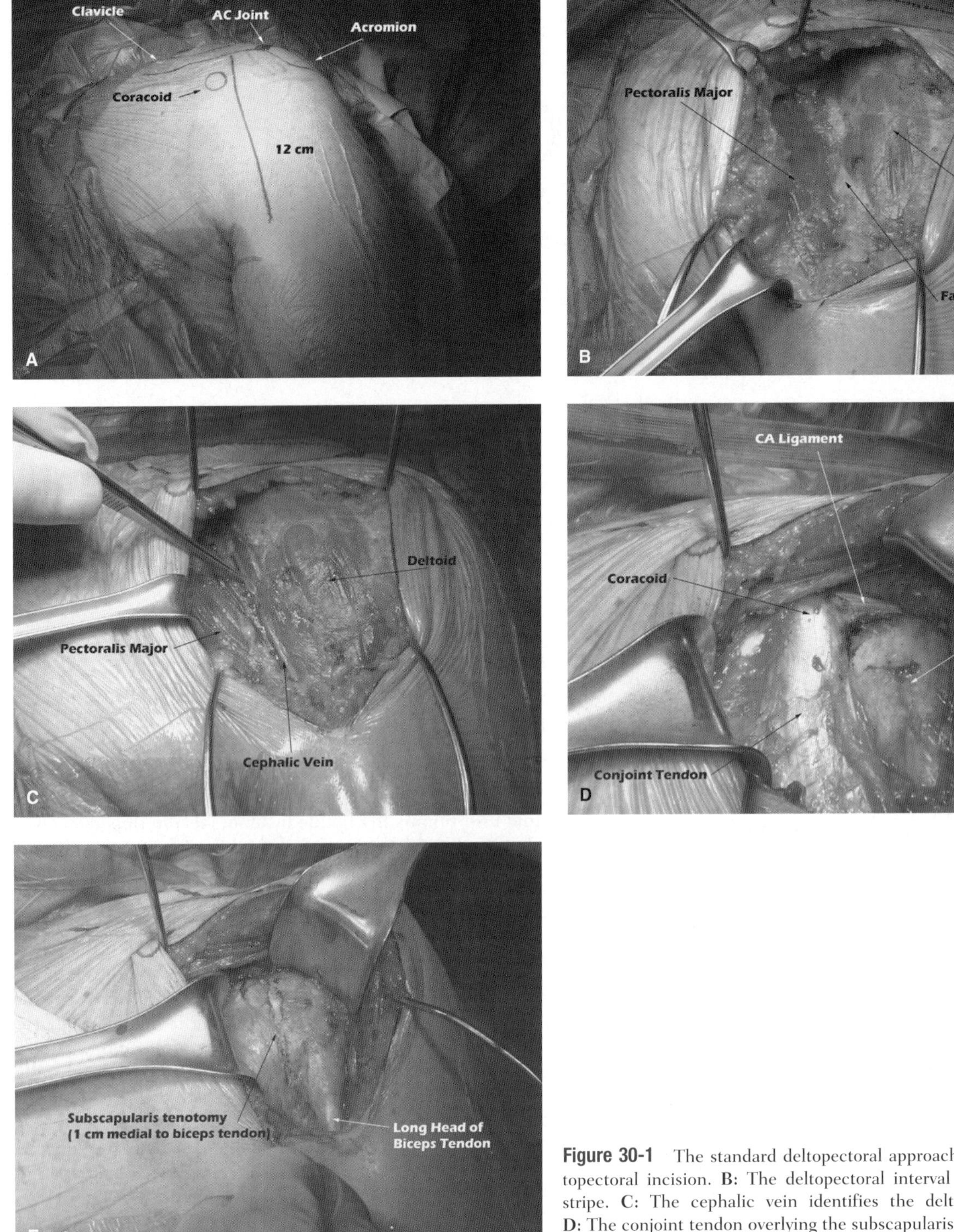

Figure 30-1 The standard deltopectoral approach. **A:** Standard deltopectoral incision. **B:** The deltopectoral interval with overlying fat stripe. **C:** The cephalic vein identifies the deltopectoral interval. **D:** The conjoint tendon overlying the subscapularis. **E:** Incision of the subscapularis tendon.

distal portion of the wound the short head of biceps muscle belly lies medial to the tendon of coracobrachialis, so, as the medium Richardson retractor is placed, care should be taken to avoid placing it in the interval between the short head of biceps muscle belly and coracobrachialis. With the conjoint tendon retracted medially, the coracoid and the coracoacromial ligament are identified. Ideally, the coracoacromial ligament should be preserved because it is an important part of the coracoacromial arch, but occasionally the leading edge must be released to facilitate superior exposure. A Darrach retractor is then placed beneath the deltoid and used to gently lever the humeral head anteriorly. The anterior bursa is completely removed, affording clear visualization of the subscapularis.

The rotator interval is then identified, which demarcates the upper border of the subscapularis, and the lower border is recognized by the adjacent leash of vessels. These vessels are controlled with cautery or ligation. Many options exist regarding treatment of the subscapularis. The subscapularis can be removed from the humerus directly from bone, beginning just medial to the biceps tendon, which is advantageous if there is significant stiffness and loss of external rotation, since the subscapularis can be repaired back to bone more medially. The subscapularis tendon can also be divided 1 cm medial to its insertion, or a thin osteotomy of the lesser tuberosity can be performed, leaving the subscapularis attached to the bony fragment. The arthrotomy is continued superiorly through the rotator interval. Care must be taken to protect the axillary nerve and posterior circumflex humeral artery, which run under the muscular portion of the subscapularis toward the quadrangular space.

Concealed Axillary Incision

A variation on the standard deltopectoral approach is the concealed axillary incision (Fig. 30-2). This can be used for shoulder arthroplasty or for anterior stabilization procedures. Here, the incision strictly follows the Langer lines. Whereas the traditional deltopectoral approach is approximately 15 cm in length, the concealed axillary incision begins 3 to 5 cm inferior to the coracoid and extends only 5 to 7 cm into the axillary crease. Skin flaps are widely elevated, and the deltopectoral interval is identified. The rest of the approach is the same as in the deltopectoral. This approach may not give sufficient exposure of the tuberosities for large rotator cuff tears or for fracture cases.

Mini-Incision Approach

Current shoulder arthroplasty instrumentation usually exits the skin in a 5-cm arc centered just lateral to the coracoid process. In addition, the average diameter of the humeral head at the surgical neck is 49 mm. These facts suggest that the minimum incision length for shoulder arthroplasty is at least 5 cm. A 5-cm incision centered just lateral to the coracoid process can be used in shoulder arthroplasty and allows better access to the tuberosities for fracture cases than the concealed axillary incision. Again, wide subcutaneous flaps are created and the deltopectoral interval is identified. The cephalic vein is retracted laterally with the deltoid muscle. The remainder of the exposure is similar to the standard deltopectoral approach. Since glenoid exposure is often difficult even with traditional incisions, minimally invasive approaches should be reserved for only select patient populations. It is most appropriate for thin patients with good range of motion.

Extensile Deltopectoral Approach

For revision shoulder surgery, the exposure sometimes needs to be more extensile than the standard deltopectoral approach. The deltopectoral approach is extended distally by extending the incision along the lateral border of the biceps. The interval between biceps and brachialis is identified, and the biceps is retracted medially. Because the brachialis has dual innervation, it can be split longitudinally along its midline. The periosteum is then split, and subperiosteal dissection allows safe exposure of the humeral shaft. The radial nerve pierces the intermuscular septum 10 cm proximal to the lateral epicondyle of the humerus.

ANTEROSUPERIOR APPROACH

Standard Anterosuperior Approach

This approach is used for the repair of a massive rotator cuff tear and can also be used for shoulder arthroplasty in the setting of a massive rotator cuff tear. The skin incision is made extending from the anterior lip of the acromion 8 cm distally in line with the deltoid fibers. Dissection is carried through subcutaneous tissue with cautery, and full-thickness flaps are raised anteriorly and posteriorly at the level of the superficial deltoid fascia. There is an avascular raphe separating the anterior and middle thirds of the deltoid, which is identified and incised from its acromial attachment distally to a point approximately 4 cm from the acromion. A stay suture is placed at the distal edge of the deltoid split to prevent propagation of the split beyond 5 cm, where the axillary nerve is known to lie. Richardson retractors are placed to retract the anterior deltoid anteriorly and the middle deltoid posteriorly. A complete bursectomy is then performed, allowing excellent exposure of the rotator cuff tear anatomy or, if the cuff is absent, the glenohumeral joint. Detachment of the deltoid origin from the lateral acromion is considered a last resort for increased exposure because of the postoperative complication of deltoid rupture, which is often not salvageable. If some fibers of deltoid origin are detached, it should be done strictly subperiosteally so that a cuff of stout tissue remains for repair.

Mini-Open Approach for Rotator Cuff Repair

The mini-open rotator cuff repair has been extensively studied and is considered an improvement over larger incisions that detach some of the deltoid origin. The approach consists of a 3- to 4-cm incision, which is often an extension of a previously placed midlateral arthroscopy portal. It is carried to the superficial deltoid fascia, above which full thickness flaps are elevated. The superficial deltoid fascia is then split in line with its fibers, again taking care to avoid propagating the split beyond 5 cm distal to the lateral edge of the acromion. The deltoid is then divided, exposing the subdeltoid/subacromial bursa. A bursectomy is performed, which allows excellent direct visualization of the rotator cuff, the anatomy of the cuff tear, and the cuff footprint on the greater tuberosity.

COMBINED APPROACH

For special cases, the advantages of both the deltopectoral and anterosuperior approaches can be exploited. This allows, in addition to the excellent deltopectoral exposure, visualization of the posterior glenohumeral joint and posterior cuff, especially the infraspinatus. If this approach is planned preoperatively, the standard deltopectoral skin incision is made slightly more laterally; otherwise, the combined

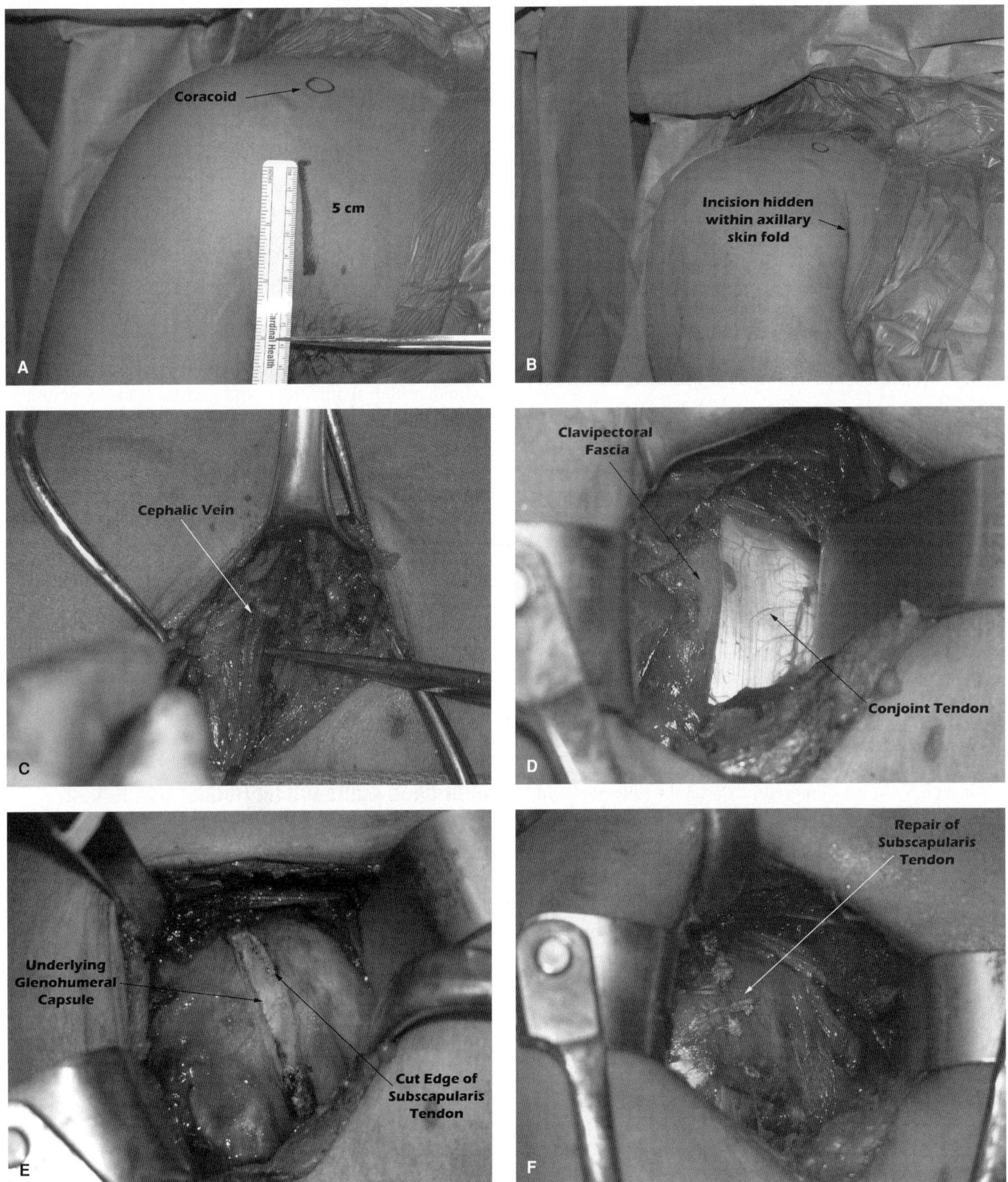

Figure 30-2 The concealed axillary approach. **A:** The concealed axillary incision. **B:** With the arm adducted, the incision is hidden in the axillary fold. **C:** Identification of the cephalic vein by mobilizing full-thickness skin flaps. **D:** Identification of the conjoint tendon. **E:** Incision of the subscapularis tendon. **F:** Repair of the subscapularis tendon.

approach can be done through the standard deltopectoral incision. Again, large full thickness flaps of skin are created and mobilized extensively. The deltopectoral approach is performed as described previously and then a second approach is made between the anterior and middle deltoid as described in the anterosuperior approach, but both approaches are made through the same deltopectoral incision.

POSTERIOR APPROACH

Muscle-Sparing Approach

This approach is used for posterior instability and for fractures of the scapula and glenoid (Fig. 30-3). The patient is positioned in a lateral decubitus position, 60 degrees from

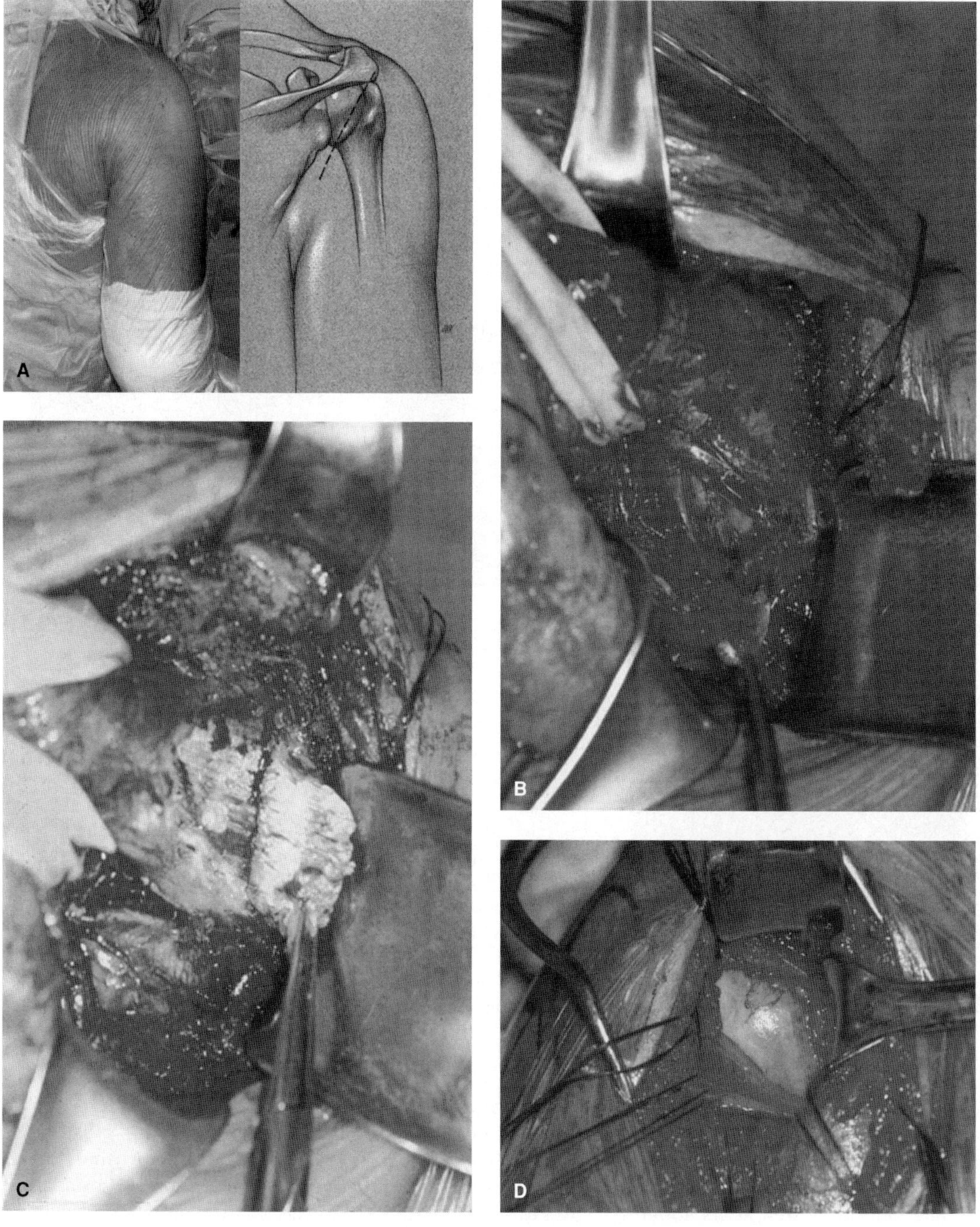

Figure 30-3 The posterior approach. **A:** The skin incision. **B:** Retraction of the deltoid and identification of the interval between infraspinatus and teres minor. **C:** Incision of the infraspinatus and dissection off the posterior capsule. **D:** Capsulotomy exposing the glenohumeral joint.

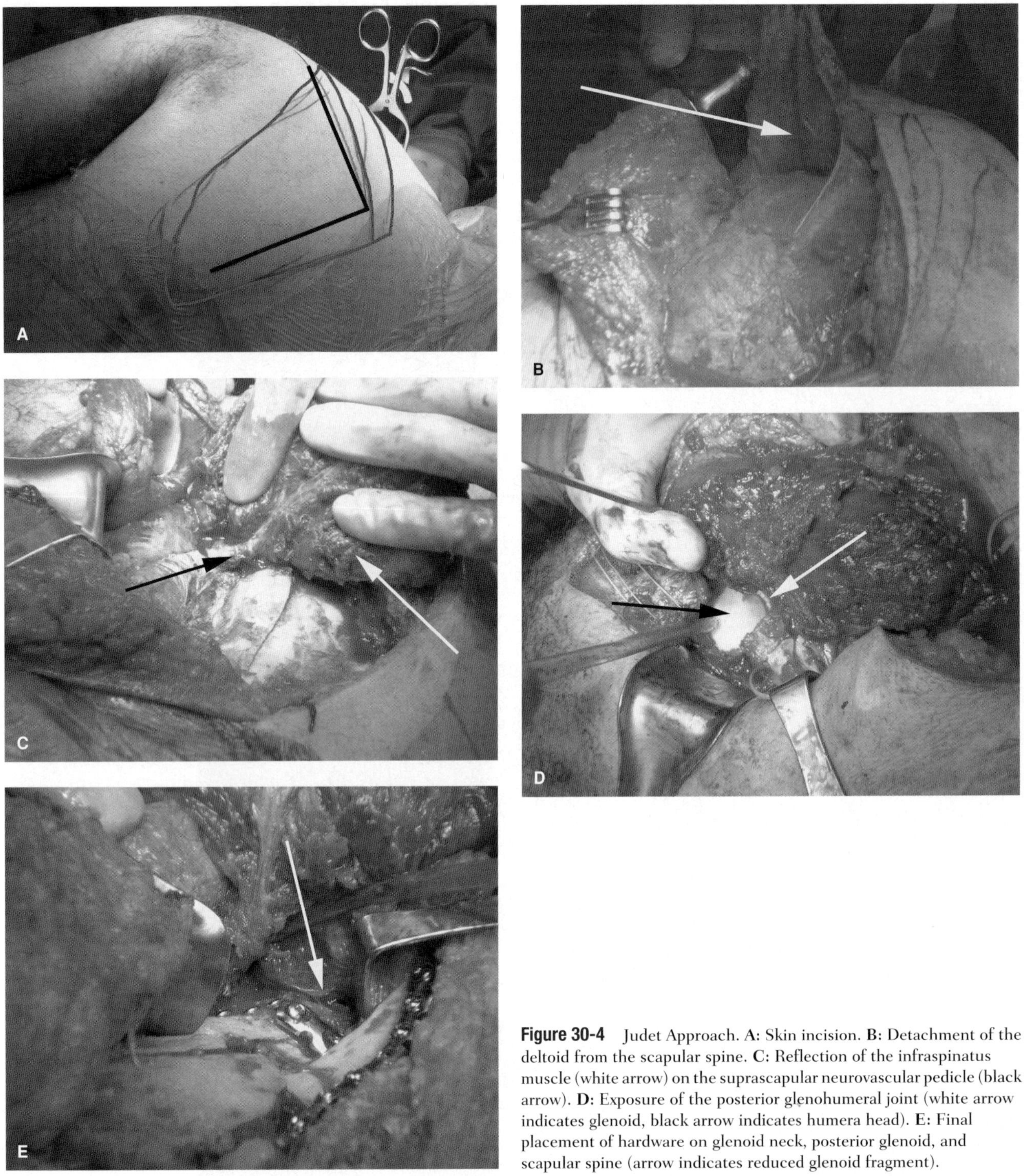

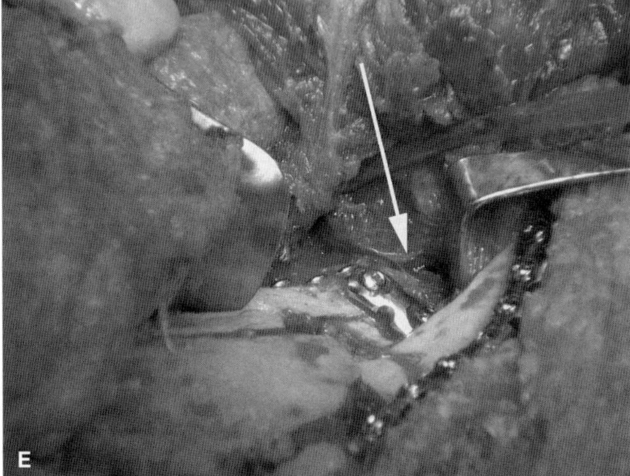

Figure 30-4 Judet Approach. **A:** Skin incision. **B:** Detachment of the deltoid from the scapular spine. **C:** Reflection of the infraspinatus muscle (white arrow) on the suprascapular neurovascular pedicle (black arrow). **D:** Exposure of the posterior glenohumeral joint (white arrow indicates glenoid, black arrow indicates humera head). **E:** Final placement of hardware on glenoid neck, posterior glenoid, and scapular spine (arrow indicates reduced glenoid fragment).

prone. An incision is made vertically following the Langer lines along a line drawn from the posterolateral lip of the acromion to the posterior axillary fold, centered 2 cm beneath the acromion. Full-thickness flaps are raised at the level of the deep fascia. The deltoid as well as its superficial and deep fascia is split in line with its fibers. This deltoid split must not propagate beyond the teres major to avoid injury to the axillary nerve. The internervous plane between infraspinatus (suprascapular nerve) and teres minor (axillary nerve) is used for this approach. It is most easily identified at the medial aspect of the wound proximal to the musculotendinous junction and is often marked by a stripe of fat. It is important, however, that the dissection stays lateral to the glenoid neck to avoid injury to the suprascapular nerve. On entering the interval between infraspinatus and teres minor, the posterior joint capsule is apparent.

Judet Approach

The Judet approach is a posterior approach used for complex posterior fracture patterns of the scapula and glenoid (Figure 30-4). The patient is positioned prone, and the skin incision begins at the posterolateral lip of the acromion, extends along the spine of the scapula, and turns at a right angle inferiorly along the medial border of the scapula. The posterior deltoid is elevated off the spine of the scapula. The underlying infraspinatus is elevated off the medial border of the scapula and retracted laterally on its suprascapular neurovascular pedicle, while care is taken to protect the pedicle.

SUGGESTED READINGS

Bigliani LU. Treatment of two- and three-part fractures of the proximal humerus. *Instr Course Lect*. 1989;39:231–244.

Brodsky JW, Tullos HS, Gartsman GM. Simplified posterior approach to the shoulder joint. A technical note. *J Bone Joint Surg Am*. 1987;69:773–774.

Henry AK. *Extensile Exposure*. 3rd ed. Edinburgh: Churchill-Livingstone; 1995.

Leslie JT, Ryan TJ. An anterior axillary incision to approach the shoulder joint. *J Bone Joint Surg*. 1962;44A:1193.

Neer CS. Anatomy of shoulder reconstruction. In: Neer, CS, ed. *Shoulder Reconstruction*. Philadelphia: WB Saunders: 1990;32–39.

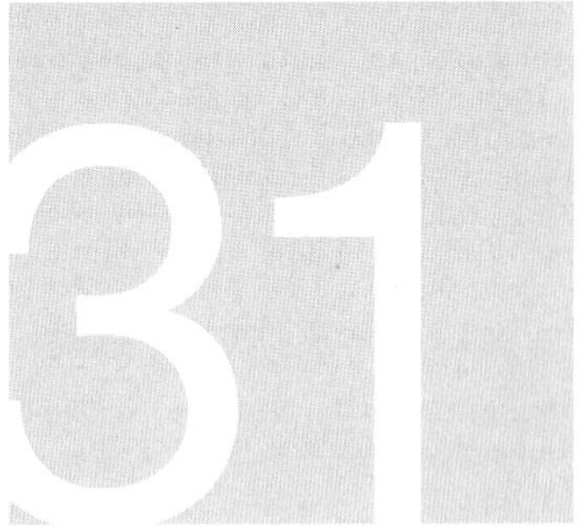

STERNOCLAVICULAR JOINT DISORDERS

GEORGE S. ATHWAL

Disorders of the sternoclavicular joint are uncommon in comparison to other shoulder girdle problems. The sternoclavicular joint may be affected by traumatic conditions, such as dislocation and fracture, or atraumatic conditions such as arthritis and infection. Diseases like sternocostoclavicular hyperostosis, osteitis condensans, Friedrich disease and spontaneous joint instability also affect the sternoclavicular joint but are rare. Posterior joint dislocations, although uncommon, are of particular concern owing to their high risk of serious complications including respiratory compromise, vascular compromise, hoarseness, brachial plexus compression, and death. A thorough understanding of these disorders and the associated clinical and radiograph findings will allow accurate diagnosis and appropriate treatment.

PATHOGENESIS

Etiology

Dislocation of the sternoclavicular (SC) joint requires a remarkable amount of force, which may be applied directly or indirectly. A direct force dislocation occurs when a sufficiently strong posterior directed force is applied to the anterior aspect of the medial clavicle, and as a result the medial clavicle dislocates posteriorly toward the mediastinal structures. An indirect force dislocation, the most common mechanism of injury, may result in anterior or posterior sternoclavicular joint instability. An anterior SC joint dislocation occurs when an anterolateral compressive force is applied to the shoulder creating an external rotatory torque on the clavicle with resultant anterior displacement of the medial clavicle. A posterior dislocation results when the opposite occurs, a posterolateral compressive force results in an internal rotatory torque on the clavicle with associated posterior dislocation of the medial clavicle. The two most frequent causes of SC joint subluxation or dislocation are motor vehicle collisions (40%) and contact sports (27%), such as rugby or football. Other traumatic causes of injury are falls, crush injuries and heavy lifting.

Degenerative arthritis is the most common condition affecting the sternoclavicular joint. Its exact cause is unknown; however, it is thought to be multifactorial in origin (e.g., hereditary, trauma, aging, and joint laxity). Sternoclavicular arthritis has also been associated with spinal accessory nerve palsy secondary to radical neck surgery. The nerve palsy results in shoulder ptosis, which increases stresses transmitted across the SC joint resulting in early degenerative changes. A history of manual labor is also a risk factor for the development of symptomatic osteoarthritis. Rheumatoid arthritis involvement of the SC joint is variably reported in the literature.

Infections of the sternoclavicular joint are usually bacterial and are commonly associated with intravenous drug use and immunocompromised states such as acquired immunodeficiency syndrome (AIDS) or chemotherapy. Other predisposing conditions for SC joint sepsis include rheumatoid arthritis, alcoholism, bacteremia, and chronic diseases.

Epidemiology

Sternoclavicular joint injuries are rare and represent <1% of all joint dislocations. With respect to the shoulder girdle, they represent only 3% of injuries—compared with 85% for glenohumeral dislocations and 12% for acromioclavicular joint injuries. Anterior SC joint dislocations are much more common than posterior dislocations, with an anterior-to-posterior ratio of 20:1.

The incidence of sternoclavicular degenerative arthritis is likely underreported as it is very often misdiagnosed and mistreated. The frequency of SC degenerative arthritis increases with age, and studies have found degenerative changes in 90% to 100% of patients over the age of 70 years. Postmenopausal women are more susceptible than either men or premenopausal women to osteoarthritis; however, the etiology is unknown. Rheumatoid arthritis (RA) involvement of the SC joint has been reported in as many as 30% of patients, and changes were usually present within 1 year of diagnosis.

Septic arthritis of the sternoclavicular joint appears to have a higher incidence in intravenous drug abusers. Common causative organisms are *Staphylococcus aureus* and *Streptococcus* species. Immunocompromised patients

TABLE 31-1 CLASSIFICATION OF STERNOCLAVICULAR JOINT INSTABILITY

Etiology	Traumatic	Anterior sternoclavicular (SC) joint dislocation more common than posterior dislocation (ratio, 20:1)
	Atraumatic	*Congenital*—malformation or hypoplasia of the medial clavicle and/or manubrium with resultant joint instability
		Developmental—instability develops in a previously normal SC joint owing to arthritis, clavicle malunion, scoliosis, or nerve palsy
		Spontaneous—recurrent SC joint instability with arm elevation that spontaneously reduces with arm lowering; unknown etiology, but associated with generalized ligamentous laxity
Direction	Anterior	Medial clavicle dislocates/subluxates anterior to the manubrium
	Posterior	Medial clavicle dislocates/subluxates posterior to the manubrium, toward mediastinal structures
Degree of instability	Subluxation	Translation of the medial clavicle, without dislocation, owing to disruption of the sternoclavicular ligaments
	Dislocation	Dislocation of the sternoclavicular joint owing to disruption of the sternoclavicular and costoclavicular ligaments
Chronicity	Acute	<6 weeks
	Chronic	>6 weeks
	Recurrent	Recurrent episodes of sternoclavicular joint subluxation or dislocation

have other causative organisms, such as *Pseudomonas aeruginosa*, *Neisseria gonorrhoeae*, and *Candida albicans*.

Pathophysiology

The sternoclavicular joint is a diarthrodial, saddle-type joint which is the only true synovial articulation between the upper extremity and the axial skeleton. The epiphysis of the medial clavicle is the last to appear and the last to close at 23 to 25 years of age. The SC joint has limited intrinsic bony stability as less than half of the medial clavicle articulates with the superolateral manubrium; therefore, stability is provided by the robust capsular ligaments and the strong costoclavicular and interclavicular ligaments. An intra-articular disc ligament exists that divides the joint into two separate spaces; it functions to reduce incongruities between the articular surfaces and as a restraint to medial displacement of the clavicle.

Ligament sectioning studies have found increased anterior and posterior joint translation (41% and 106%, respectively) with release of the posterior joint capsule. Anterior capsular release was found to increase only anterior translation, and sectioning of the costoclavicular and the interclavicular ligaments resulted in insignificant joint translation. Therefore, it is thought that the posterior joint capsule is the most important restraint to anterior and posterior sternoclavicular joint translations.

Anatomically, the sternoclavicular joint is located anterior to vital superior mediastinal structures. These structures include the innominate artery and vein, the subclavian artery and vein, the recurrent laryngeal nerve, the phrenic nerve, the vagus nerve, the esophagus, and the trachea. Posterior dislocation of the medial clavicle may compromise any of these structures with potential life-threatening consequences. These vital structures are also placed at risk during operative management of sternoclavicular disorders, such as arthrotomy for infection and open reduction of dislocations.

Classification

Sternoclavicular joint disorders are relatively uncommon and span a wide spectrum of orthopedic diseases (trauma, arthritis and infection). Therefore, a universal classification scheme does not exist.

Sternoclavicular joint instability may be classified according to etiology, chronicity, direction, and degree of instability (Table 31-1). A formal classification system for degenerative arthritis of the sternoclavicular does not exist; therefore, standard principles may be applied. Degenerative changes in the SC joint initiate at the inferior part of the medial clavicular head, which articulates with the manubrium. Mild osteoarthritis has radiographic changes consisting of minimal joint space narrowing and small osteophytes. Moderate osteoarthritis has further joint space narrowing, subchondral sclerosis, and larger peripheral osteophytes while severe arthritis has complete cartilage loss.

DIAGNOSIS

Physical Examination and History

Clinical Features

Instability. Sternoclavicular joint injury is most frequently the result of a motor vehicle collision or a sports-related trauma. A detailed history will allow determination of the mechanism of injury as patients may describe a direct blow to the anterior chest or medial compression to the shoulder girdle with resultant indirect SC joint injury. Patients may complain of pain, tenderness or deformity around the SC joint. Symptoms of hoarseness, shortness of breath, difficultly swallowing, or choking should be elicited as they may indicate posterior dislocation of the medial clavicle with concomitant mediastinal compression.

Patients with acute SC joint dislocation will present with swelling, tenderness, and severe pain that is exacerbated with arm movement. The differentiation between anterior and posterior dislocation can usually be made on physical examination; however, in cases of severe swelling, accurate diagnosis may be difficult. With an anterior dislocation, the medial clavicle is prominent and can be palpated anterior to the manubrium. In patients with a posterior dislocation, the prominent medial clavicle is absent and the manubrium is more easily palpated. Patients with posterior dislocations may also exhibit signs of damage to the pulmonary and vascular systems, such as stridor, venous congestion, or hemodynamic instability.

Sternoclavicular joint subluxation without dislocation may be subtle and consist of only mild pain, tenderness, and swelling. Joint instability may be tested by translating the medial clavicle joint in the anteroposterior direction and comparing with the contralateral side. Patients with atraumatic or spontaneous sternoclavicular joint instability can usually demonstrate with minimal discomfort subluxation or dislocation with arm elevation that spontaneously reduces when the arm is brought down.

Arthritis. Patients with degenerative arthritis report activity-related pain and swelling at the sternoclavicular joint. Symptoms are exacerbated by palpation of the joint and active shoulder elevation. The medial clavicle may be prominent owing to osteophytes and may also be in fixed subluxation. Patients with rheumatoid arthritis usually report similar findings of pain, swelling, and joint crepitus; however, isolated joint involvement of the SC joint in RA is rare.

Joint Sepsis. Septic arthritis of the sternoclavicular joint is uncommon and is usually associated with immunocompromised states (human immunodeficiency virus [HIV]), rheumatoid arthritis, renal dialysis, or intravenous drug abuse. The hallmark features are pain, swelling, tenderness, and erythema over the SC joint. Constitutional symptoms, such as fever, chills, and night sweats, are common.

Radiographic Features

Radiography. Standard radiographic projections are difficult to interpret for sternoclavicular joint injuries because of overlapping anatomic structures. Several special projections have been described to aid in the diagnosis of SC joint pathology, including the serendipity and Hobb views. The serendipity view is performed with the patient supine and the radiography tube angled at 40 degrees cephalad, centered on the manubrium; this image allows a relative axial view of the joint. The Hobb view approximates a 90-degree lateral view of the SC joint and is performed with the patient leaning over the radiography table so that the flexed neck is almost parallel to the table. Radiographs should be assessed for joint congruity (instability), signs of arthritis (OA), and erosions with joint destruction (neoplasm, sepsis).

Computed Tomography. Computed tomography (CT) provides a simple and accurate method of assessing the SC joint and has been reported as being the best imaging modality. It is important to image both sides for comparison of the pathologic to the normal contralateral side. CT scans can also be reformatted into three-dimensional images to allow accurate representation of the SC joint (Fig. 31-11). When interpreting studies with posterior SC joint dislocations, a particular benefit is the ability to assess mediastinal structures and their potential compromise (Fig. 31-2). In patients with such findings, CT with angiography is indicated.

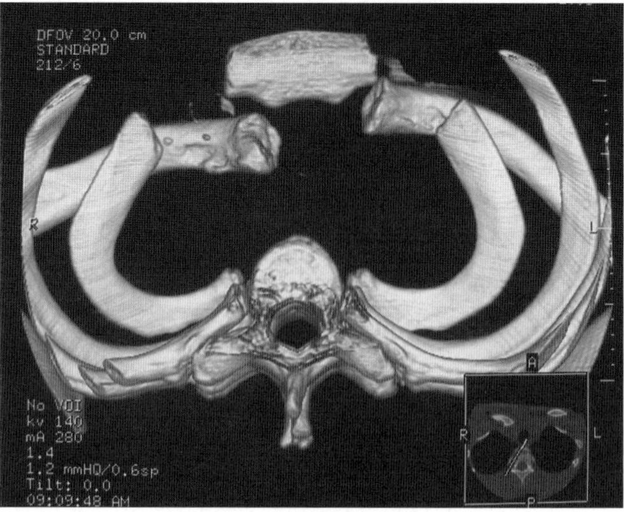

Figure 31-1 Three-dimensional CT reconstruction of a traumatic right posterior sternoclavicular joint dislocation.

Magnetic Resonance Imaging. Magnetic resonance imaging (MRI) provides a more detailed and specific identification of SC joint soft tissues and mediastinal structures. Coronal MRI images are ideal for evaluation of the SC joint

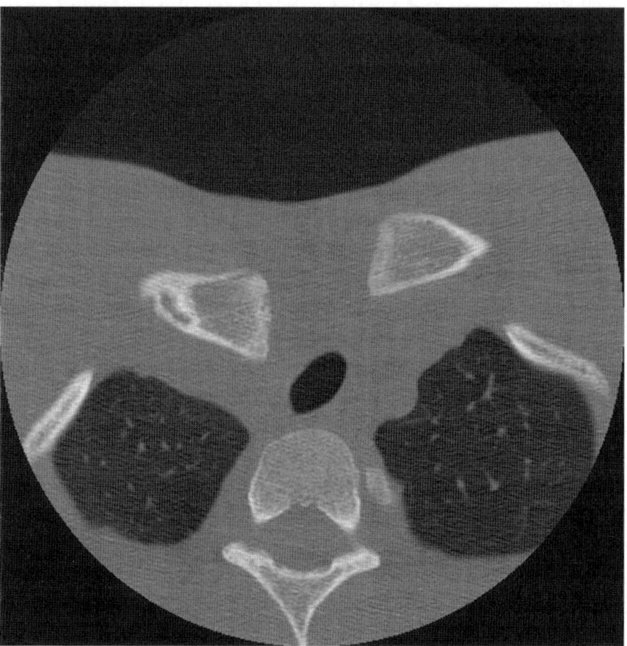

Figure 31-2 Axial CT image of a posterior sternoclavicular joint dislocation with associated compression of the mediastinal structures, notably the trachea.

articular surfaces, the intra-articular disc, and the interclavicular and costoclavicular ligaments. The axial views are useful in assessing the anterior and posterior sternoclavicular ligaments, joint congruity, and the relationship between vital mediastinal structures and the SC joint.

Diagnostic Workup Algorithm

The SC joint is subject to the same disease processes that occur in other joints (instability, osteoarthritis, rheumatoid arthritis, infection, fracture). A detailed history outlining symptom onset, systemic complaints, family history, and social history will lead to a provisional diagnosis. Physical examination with a focus on joint translation, swelling, fluctuance, warmth, and signs of pulmonary-vascular compromise will further hone the diagnosis. Imaging with radiographs and CT will be confirmatory and assist with treatment planning.

TREATMENT

Surgical Indications/Contraindications

Instability

Anterior Sternoclavicular Joint Dislocation. Acute traumatic anterior SC joint dislocations are generally treated with closed reduction under sedation or general anesthesia. Anterior dislocations are generally easily reduced; however, they tend to remain unstable and there is a high redislocation rate. Because of the high complication rate of surgery and the low rate of persistent symptoms or functional deficit with nonoperative treatment, it is recommended that redislocated SC joints be treated conservatively.

The technique of closed reduction involves the patient being supine with a moderate-sized bolster placed between the shoulders. The arm is abducted to 90 degrees with gentle traction followed by a posterior-directed force applied to the medial clavicle. If a stable reduction ensues, the patient may be immobilized in a figure-of-eight bandage, a Velpeau bandage, a clavicle strap harness, or a bulky pressure pad taped over the medial clavicle for 6 weeks. If the SC joint redislocates, the patient may be placed in a shoulder sling for comfort until symptoms subside.

Operative stabilization of traumatic anterior SC joint instability should be considered only in patients who have failed nonoperative treatment. Patients may complain of pain, deformity, and crepitus. Various procedures have been described to stabilize the medial clavicle or reconstruct the SC joint. The author's preferred technique is reconstruction of the anterior and posterior SC joint capsule and sternoclavicular ligaments with tendon graft woven through the manubrium and medial clavicle (Fig. 31-3). The patient is positioned in a 40-degree upright beach-chair position. The surgical approach involves an oblique 6- to 8-cm incision centered over the medial clavicle extending over the manubrium. The platysma muscle is divided, and the medial clavicle and SC joint are exposed. Drill tunnels (3 to 4 mm in diameter) are created in the medial clavicle, and the manubrium followed by passage of the tendon graft.

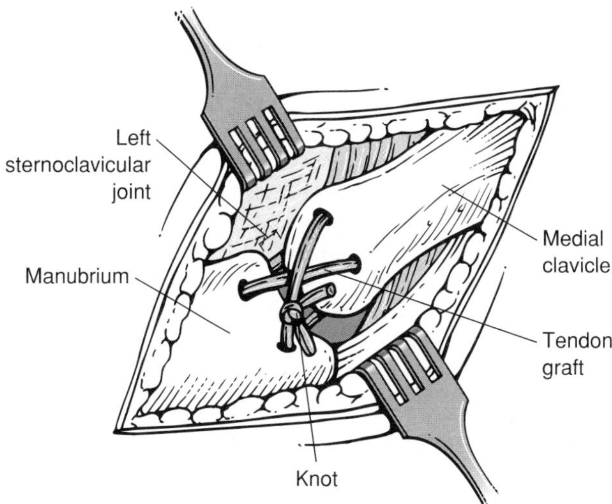

Figure 31-3 Tendon-weave reconstruction of the anterior and posterior sternoclavicular joint capsule and sternoclavicular ligaments. The tendon graft is passed through drill tunnels created in the medial clavicle and manubrium.

The joint is reduced, and the tendon graft is secured. This is followed by suture repair of the costoclavicular ligaments and remaining soft tissues to augment the reconstruction. Other surgical options include the Burrow procedure (subclavius tendon tenodesis to medial clavicle), sternal head of sternocleidomastoid muscle transfer, costoclavicular ligament reconstruction with tendon graft, and distal clavicle resection with soft tissue stabilization.

Posterior Sternoclavicular Joint Dislocation. Patients with a posterior SC joint dislocation should undergo a thorough history and physical examination assessing for associated mediastinal injuries. Mediastinal injuries, if present, should be completely investigated and the appropriate referrals made to vascular, cardiothoracic, or general surgery.

Acute traumatic posterior SC joint injuries that present within 7 to 10 days should be treated with an attempted closed reduction. Once reduced, unlike anterior dislocations, posterior dislocations tend to remain stable. Closed reduction should be conducted in the operating room with appropriate anesthesia and with vascular or thoracic surgery available. The most commonly described reduction maneuver is the abduction-traction technique, in which the patient is positioned supine with a medium-sized bolster placed between the shoulders. The arm is abducted to 90 degrees with traction; as the arm is gently extended, the medial clavicle is levered forward with a reduction occurring usually with an audible snap. If the reduction is unsuccessful, the medial clavicle may be manually manipulated to bring it forward, and if this is also unsuccessful, a sterile towel clip may be used to grasp the clavicle to pull it forward. Resistant posterior SC joint dislocations have also been reduced by another maneuver termed the *adduction-traction technique*. This technique involves gentle traction to the adducted arm with a posterior-directed force applied to both shoulders, which levels the medial clavicle over the first rib and into its normal position.

Indications for surgical treatment of posterior SC joint dislocations include an unsuccessful or unstable closed reduction, chronic posterior instability, or chronic posterior dislocations. Patients with chronic posterior SC joint dislocations without initial symptoms of mediastinal compromise have experienced significant late complications such as vascular compromise, thoracic outlet syndrome, and erosion of the medial clavicle into vital mediastinal structures (arteries and veins). The operative technique of open reduction and stabilization is identical as for anterior SC joint dislocations, and the reader is referred to the previous section.

Arthritis

Patients with symptomatic arthritis of the sternoclavicular joint are best managed with nonoperative treatment, such as anti-inflammatory medications, local steroid injections, and activity modification. Patients with rheumatoid arthritis should also be managed medically in conjunction with a rheumatologist.

Indications for the surgical management of SC joint arthritis include persistent pain and functional limitation despite maximized nonoperative treatment. Operative treatment involves excision of the medial end of the clavicle with preservation of the posterior sternoclavicular and costoclavicular ligaments. On average, 8 to 10 mm of medial clavicle is excised; if too much is excised or if damage to the stabilizing ligaments occurs, clavicular instability may occur.

Infection

Sternoclavicular joint sepsis is managed medically with organism-specific parenteral antibiotics, along with surgical irrigation and debridement. In subacute and chronic cases with delayed diagnosis, abscess formation with bone destruction may necessitate partial SC joint resection and first rib debridement. Untreated or partially treated infections may progress to extrapleural or intrathoracic abscess with potentially life-threatening complications. In severe cases with extensive debridement, patients may require transposition of the ipsilateral pectoralis major muscle to obliterate residual space and to reconstruct the chest wall.

Complications

Complications from anterior SC joint dislocations are usually mild. Patients may complain of a noncosmetic bump at the medial end of the clavicle or symptoms consistent with late degenerative arthritis.

Nonoperative management of posterior SC joint dislocations has been associated with a wide variety of complications owing to the proximity of the joint to the mediastinal structures. Documented complications include pneumothorax, respiratory distress, venous congestions, laceration of the superior vena cava, compression of the subclavian artery, brachial plexopathy, esophageal rupture, tracheoesophageal fistula, and hoarseness. Although the rate of complications has been documented at 25%, the reported fatality rate is low.

Complications from the operative treatment of SC joint disorders vary depending on the type of surgical procedure. Complications of medial clavicle resection usually relate to damage of the stabilizing ligaments leading to instability and pain. Most complications associated with past operative stabilization procedures for traumatic SC joint injuries related to hardware migration. Kirschner wires, Steinmann pins, and Hagie pins used to transfix the SC joint have migrated and punctured vital structures; therefore, alternative means of joint stabilization are recommended such as autograft or allograft tendon reconstruction.

Results and Outcome

Because of the uncommon nature of sternoclavicular joint disorders, there are few good outcomes studies. Studies in the literature are limited by their retrospective design, few patient numbers, and variable clinical follow-up.

In general, the literature on nonoperative management of anterior sternoclavicular joint dislocations states a 70% to 80% satisfaction rate (return to normal activities and no SC joint pain). Posterior SC joint dislocations that are successfully managed with closed reduction appear universally to do well in the literature, with minimal pain and disability, no recurrences, and minimal crepitus.

There is little information in the literature on the outcomes of surgically treated posterior SC joint dislocations. Analysis of the few studies available shows the results are highly variable and may depend on the type of operative procedure. Procedures involving resection of the medial clavicle without stabilization appear to have poor outcomes owing to residual instability. Medial clavicle resection procedures with maintenance or reconstruction of the supporting ligaments have a 70% good to excellent outcome. Outcomes with open reduction and ligament reconstruction are also variable and range from 42% to 90% good to excellent results.

The management of sternoclavicular arthritis with medial clavicle resection with preservation of the stabilizing joint structures provides a 70% to 90% good to excellent outcome at medium- to long-term follow-up. Once again, the studies available are few, retrospective, with low patient numbers, and use variable outcome measures.

Postoperative Management

Instability

The postoperative management of SC joint instability surgery involves protection of the shoulder and SC joint with a shoulder immobilizer and limited motion consisting of pendulum exercises for 6 weeks. Patients may then progress to passive range of motion, active assisted motion, and then to active range of motion. Shoulder-strengthening exercises are initiated at 3 months.

Arthritis

The postoperative management of medial clavicle resection for arthritis is similar to the postoperative management of SC joint instability surgery. The rehabilitation goals are to allow adequate healing of the sternoclavicular soft tissues to prevent late instability while allowing protected shoulder motion.

Infection

Sternoclavicular joint arthrotomy, irrigation, and debridement should be managed in a shoulder immobilizer for comfort. Patients requiring aggressive debridement with medial clavicle excision should be managed similarly to patients with medial clavicle resections for arthritis.

SUGGESTED READINGS

Allman FL Jr. Fractures and ligamentous injuries of the clavicle and its articulation. *J Bone Joint Surg Am*. 1967;49:774–784.

Bicos J, Nicholson GP. Treatment and results of sternoclavicular joint injuries. *Clin Sports Med*. 2003;22(2):359–370.

Ernberg LA, Potter HG. Radiographic evaluation of the acromioclavicular and sternoclavicular joints. *Clin Sports Med*. 2003;22(2):255–275.

Higginbotham TO, Kuhn JE. Atraumatic disorders of the sternoclavicular joint. *J Am Acad Orthop Surg*. 2005;13(2):138–145.

Hiramuro-Shoji F, Wirth MA, Rockwood CA Jr. Atraumatic conditions of the sternoclavicular joint. *J Shoulder Elbow Surg*. 2003;12(1):79–88.

Nettles JL, Linscheid RL. Sternoclavicular dislocations. *J Trauma*. 1968;8(2):158–164.

Pingsmann A, Patsalis T, Michiels I. Resection arthroplasty of the sternoclavicular joint for the treatment of primary degenerative sternoclavicular arthritis. *J Bone Joint Surg Br*. 2002;84:513–517.

Wirth MA, Rockwood CA Jr. Acute and chronic traumatic injuries of the sternoclavicular joint. *J Am Acad Orthop Surg*. 1996;4(5):268–278.

Yeh GL, Williams GR Jr. Conservative management of sternoclavicular injuries. *Orthop Clin North Am*. 2000;31(2):189–203.

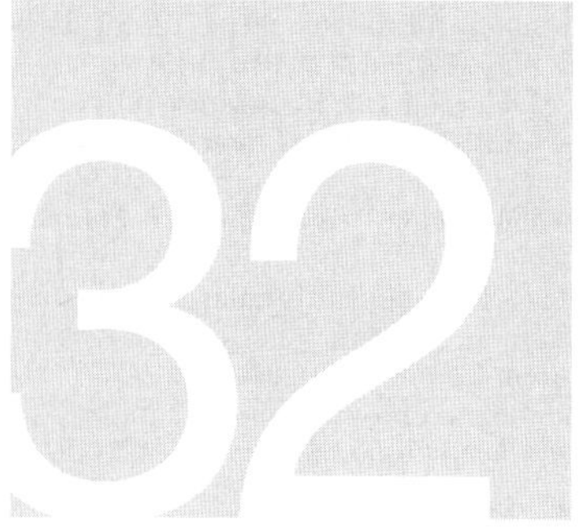

ANTERIOR GLENOHUMERAL INSTABILITY: PATHOANATOMY

JONATHAN B. SHOOK
GUIDO MARRA

OVERVIEW

In 1906 Perthes first described the capsulolabral defect that, >30 years later, Bankart went on to coin the "essential lesion." Since then, a plethora of anatomic and biomechanical studies have helped to clarify the elements that contribute to anterior glenohumeral instability (AGI). We now know that the shoulder joint is the most frequently dislocated joint and that >90% of these dislocations are anterior. The innate bony anatomy of the glenohumeral joint makes it particularly prone to instability. It has been likened to a golf ball on a tee. A small glenoid matched to a large humeral head allows the joint to be very mobile. The joint is thus quite dependent on the surrounding soft tissues for stability. When the bony anatomy is disrupted, or when the soft tissues fail, instability is the result. The specific pathoanatomy related to AGI is discussed below under two general categories: static stabilizers and dynamic stabilizers (Table 32-1).

STATIC STABILIZERS

Capsule and Ligaments

More time and effort has probably been spent trying to elucidate the structures of the capsule and ligaments of the glenohumeral joint than any other aspect of the shoulder. It has been >150 years since investigators first described distinct ligaments that contributed to the shoulder joint's stability. Since then, many others have collaborated in their efforts to arrive at a generally accepted model of the capsuloligamentous complex. We consider three major ligaments when discussing anterior glenohumeral instability: the inferior, middle, and superior (Fig. 32-1). These ligaments act as checkreins and countervail forces on the humeral head at the extremes of range of motion. When they become lax or disrupted, the humeral head translates beyond its normal boundaries of the glenoid.

The inferior glenohumeral ligament complex (IGHLC) is universally accepted as the primary static restraint to AGI. Investigators have conducted cadaveric dissections, histologic analysis, and biomechanical studies to delineate the individual components of the complex. The most popular model describes the complex with an anterior and posterior band with an interposed axillary pouch. It functions as a sling, or hammock, that changes position and undergoes reciprocal tightening and loosening with arm rotation. The anterior band is particularly important at limiting anterior translation when the arm is externally rotated and abducted to 90 degrees. Injury to this band of the complex is one of the most significant factors leading to AGI.

The IGHLC can rupture as the result of a traumatic anterior dislocation. Traumatic failure of the IGHLC most frequently occurs when it is avulsed with the anterior labrum, forming a Bankart lesion. Additionally, it may become stretched out over time by repetitive microtrauma. Overhead athletes are especially prone to this type of injury. With either type of injury, the anterior capsule can undergo plastic deformity as a result of trauma. The capsule becomes more and more voluminous, causing increased glenohumeral translation.

The middle glenohumeral ligament (MGHL) appears to function as the primary restraint to anterior translation when the arm is externally rotated and abducted from 60 to 90 degrees. The MGHL can be absent in ≤30% of individuals, and some feel that this predisposes to AGI. Additionally, the MGHL can be avulsed along with the IGHLC with a Bankart lesion.

The superior glenohumeral ligament (SGHL) has little to do with limiting pure anterior translation. But more recently it has been implicated for its role in the rotator interval laxity. Some believe that a widened rotator interval as a result of a deficient SGHL may be implicated in recurrent AGI. Table 32-2 summarizes each of these ligaments' roles in preventing AGI.

A less common and often overlooked cause of AGI is the humeral avulsion of the glenohumeral ligament (HAGL) lesion. Unlike the more commonly seen avulsion of the ligaments from the glenoid/labrum side, it is possible to detach the ligaments from the humeral side. This may be caused by either an anterior shoulder dislocation or hyperabduction.

TABLE 32-1 STATIC AND DYNAMIC STABILIZERS

- Static
  - Capsule and ligaments
  - Labrum
  - Humeral and glenoid bony anatomy
    - Bony borders
    - Humeral and glenoid version
  - Rotator cuff
  - Negative intra-articular pressure
- Dynamic
  - Rotator cuff and surrounding musculature
  - Scapulothoracic motion
  - Long head of the biceps
  - Proprioception

TABLE 32-2 GLENOHUMERAL LIGAMENTS

- Inferior glenohumeral ligament complex
  - Limits anterior translation of the humeral head when the arm is externally rotated and abducted to 90 degrees
  - Anterior band of complex is the most important structure
- Middle glenohumeral ligament
  - Limits anterior translation of the humeral head when the arm is externally rotated and abducted from 60 to 90 degrees.
  - Absent in ≤30% of individuals
- Superior glenohumeral ligament
  - Little role in limiting pure anterior humeral translation
  - May be implicated in recurrent anterior instability owing to its role in the rotator interval

The HAGL lesion must be identified and anatomically repaired to restore stability to the shoulder.

Glenoid Labrum

Few structures are as important when considering AGI as is the glenoid labrum. It serves as the anterior anchor point for the capsuloligamentous complex, as well as a chock block during anterior translation of the humeral head. Additionally, it deepens the glenoid and increases the surface area contact of the humeral head.

When this structure becomes detached from the glenoid rim and scapular neck, it is called a *Bankart lesion* (Fig. 32-2). Whether this is truly the "essential lesion," as Bankart proposed, remains a topic of debate. Cadaveric studies have shown that simply detaching the labrum is not sufficient to cause AGI. In contrast, multiple authors have observed intraoperatively that detachment of the labrum is quite common after traumatic anterior instability episodes. One study has demonstrated detachment of the labrum in ≤97% of first time anterior dislocators without evidence of associated intracapsular injury. It has also been observed that recurrent anterior subluxers and dislocators have a fraying of the labrum. The severity of the deleterious effect on the labrum appears to be additive based on the number of instability episodes.

Another variety of labral injury, an anterior labral periosteal sleeve avulsion, or ALPSA, can result in AGI. This injury differs from the classic Bankart lesion in that the labrum is incompletely dissociated from the glenoid. A periosteal sleeve remains attached to the labrum that allows it to displace medially and rotate inferiorly. The lesions heal but will lead to recurrent AGI owing to excessive anterior capsular laxity. The sleeve must be detached, creating a full Bankart lesion, and then anatomically reattached to restore the labrum and capsule to proper function.

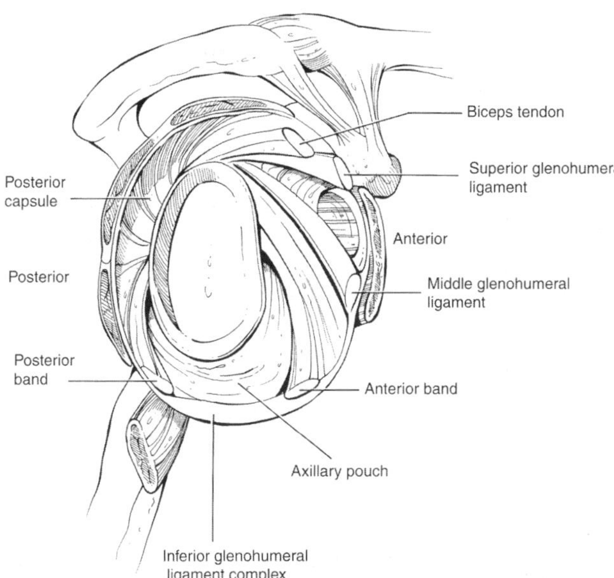

Figure 32-1 Glenohumeral capsuloligamentous complex. (From O'Brien SJ, Neves MC, Amoczky SP, et al. The anatomy and histology of the inferior glenohumeral ligament complex of the shoulder. *Am J Sports Med.* 1990;18:449–456, with permission.)

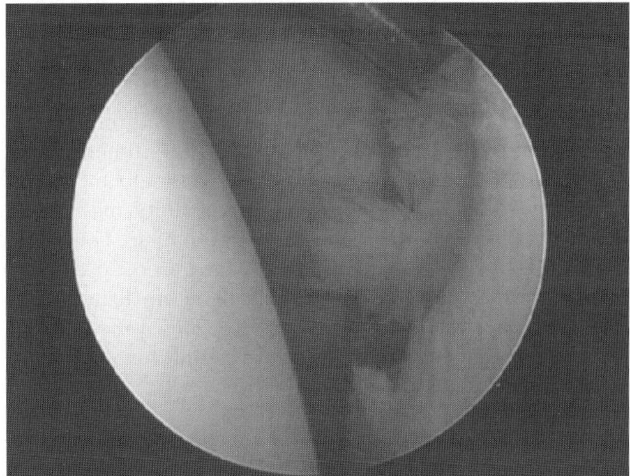

Figure 32-2 Arthroscopic picture of a Bankart injury viewed from the posterior portal (humeral head on the **left** and glenoid on the **right**).

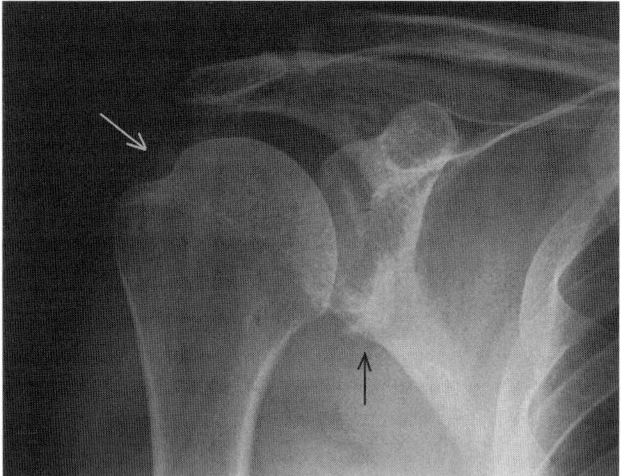

Figure 32-3 Anteroposterior radiograph demonstrating a bony Bankart injury (*black arrow*) and Hill-Sachs lesion (*white arrow*).

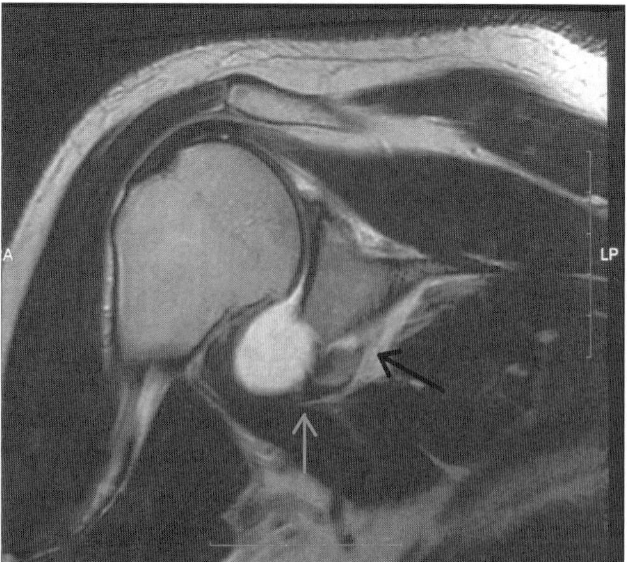

Figure 32-4 Coronal plane MRI demonstrating fracture of the anteroinferior glenoid (*black arrow*) and maintenance of the labral attachment to the glenoid rim (*gray arrow*).

Humeral and Glenoid Bone Loss

When the humeral head dislocates anteriorly, its posterolateral margin comes into contact with the anterior glenoid rim. In the process of dislocating, the portion of the humeral head in contact with the glenoid can sustain an impression fracture. This fracture and bone loss is termed a *Hill-Sachs lesion* (Fig. 32-3). It can occur in ≤80% of anterior dislocations and may be present in an even higher percent of recurrent dislocators. Small lesions usually do not affect stability of the joint, but those >30% of the articular surface deserve attention. These larger lesions can predispose one to recurrent AGI, and they require reconstruction to restore stability to the glenohumeral joint. Despite capsular and labral repairs, large Hill-Sachs lesion can render the joint unstable.

Bone loss can take place on the glenoid side of the joint, and most frequently occurs as a *bony Bankart* (Fig. 32-3). This arises when a portion of the anteroinferior rim of the glenoid is fractured off with the capsulolabral attachments as the humeral head dislocates anteriorly (Fig. 32-4). When the fractured piece contains >20% to 25% of the glenoid surface area, it should be repaired back to the remaining glenoid.

Glenoid bone loss may also occur as a result of chronic wear. Recurrent anterior subluxation of the humeral head can cause gradual deterioration of the glenoid rim. When this defect becomes large enough, instability may result even after capsulolabral repair. As with traumatic bone loss, large defects require bone grafting. Many procedures have been described to augment glenoid bone stock including the transfer of the coracoid process (Bristow procedure or Latarjet procedure) and the use of autograft bone block.

Humeral and Glenoid Version

Although humeral and glenoid version appears to have some influence on posterior glenohumeral instability, it most likely has little or no effect on anterior instability. Clinical studies and sophisticated CT analyses have failed to show any significant relationship between version and AGI. However, one must be sure that apparent changes in glenoid version are not the result of glenoid bone loss.

Rotator Cuff

The rotator cuff is generally viewed as a dynamic rather than static stabilizer, but passive tension within the cuff appears to play some role in preventing AGI. Specifically, the subscapularis has been shown to limit anterior translation of the humeral head at low ranges of shoulder abduction. When the subscapularis becomes injured or ruptured, as such is the case particularly in older individuals who suffer traumatic anterior dislocations, its static block to anterior translation is lost.

Negative Intra-Articular Pressure

Negative intra-articular pressure develops within the shoulder joint because of the relatively higher osmotic pressure in the surrounding interstitial tissue that causes water to be drawn out of the joint. This effect appears to be important when dynamic stabilizers are not functioning properly. A defect in the capsule or labrum, or degenerative changes in the glenohumeral joint, eliminate the effect. The importance of this negative pressure is probably negligible, though, when dynamic stabilizers are functioning properly.

DYNAMIC STABILIZERS

Traditionally, the dynamic stabilizers of the shoulder have received less attention than static stabilizers. Most early stabilization procedures were nonanatomic reconstructions, which resulted in altered biomechanics of the joint. This subsequently led to secondary problems, such as decreased range of motion and glenohumeral arthritis. But with advancements in laboratory and surgical techniques, we have been able to understand better the dynamic factors that affect shoulder stability.

Rotator Cuff and Surrounding Musculature

We are increasingly recognizing the importance of the rotator cuff as a dynamic stabilizer of the shoulder. The coordinated contracture of the rotator cuff causes a force coupling of the muscles and a joint reaction force vector toward the center of the glenoid. The net result is a joint compression force that keeps the humeral head located within the glenoid fossa. Dysfunction of the rotator cuff muscles owing to poor neuromuscular control, injury, atrophy, contracture, or tendon deficiency can result in uncoupling of the muscles and a net force vector directed away from the center of the glenoid. Consequently, excessive translation of the humerus occurs and undue strain is placed on the capsuloligamentous structures and the labrum. The net result of rotator cuff dysfunction is instability.

Scapulothoracic Motion

Motion in the scapulothoracic plane is also a very important factor in glenohumeral joint stability. Dysfunction of the coordinated timing and positioning of the glenoid and humeral head can be caused by dyskinesis of the scapular rotators. Most often, this is caused by fatigue of the serratus anterior and trapezius muscles. Less commonly, dysfunction may be caused by long thoracic nerve palsy.

Long Head of the Biceps

It appears that the long head of the biceps brachii serves an important function in dynamic shoulder stabilization, especially when the rotator cuff or capsuloligamentous structures are overwhelmed. It serves its greatest role in preventing anterior displacement when the arm is in internal rotation at the middle and lower levels of elevation. When there is a Bankart lesion, the function of the biceps in preventing humeral head displacement may be even more important than the rotator cuff muscles. Indeed, in patients with rotator cuff weakness, the biceps tendon may become hypertrophied.

Proprioception

Multiple investigators have found mechanoreceptors in the shoulder capsule and ligaments. These receptors are thought to provide feedback information about the joint position and motion. This enables a coordinated interaction of the dynamic shoulder stabilizers. Individuals with a history of AGI appear to have a higher threshold for detecting passive motion of their shoulder. Whether or not these feedback loops function at speeds fast enough to prevent instability episodes remains a topic of debate.

SUGGESTED READINGS

Arciero RA, Wheeler JH, Ryan JB, et al. Arthroscopic Bankart repair versus nonoperative treatment for acute, initial anterior shoulder dislocation. *Am J Sports Med.* 1994;22:589–594.

Bankart ASB. The pathology and treatment of recurrent dislocation of the shoulder joint. *Br J Surg.* 1938;26:23–29.

Bigliani LU, Kelkar R, Flatow EL, et al. Glenohumeral stability. Biomechanical properties of passive and active stabilizers. *Clin Orthop Relat Res.* 1996;330:13–30.

Iannoti JP, Williams GR, eds. *Disorders of the Shoulder: Diagnosis and Management.* Philadelphia: Lippincott Williams & Wilkins; 1999.

Lippitt S, Matsen F. Mechanisms of glenohumeral joint instability. *Clin Orthop.* 1993;291:20–28.

O'Brien SJ, Neves MC, Arnoczky SP, et al. The anatomy and histology of the inferior glenohumeral ligament complex of the shoulder. *Am J Sports Med.* 1990;18:449–456.

O'Brien SJ, Schwartz RS, Warren RF, et al. Capsular restraints to anterior-posterior motion of the abducted shoulder: a biomechanical study. *J Shoulder Elbow Surg.* 1995;4:298–308.

Taylor DC, Arciero RA. Pathologic changes associated with shoulder dislocations. Arthroscopic and physical examination findings in first-time traumatic anterior dislocations. *Am J Sports Med.* 1997;25:306–311.

Turkel SJ, Ithaca MW, Panio MW, et al. Stabilizing mechanism preventing anterior dislocation of the glenohumeral joint. *J Bone Joint Surg Am.* 1981;63-A:1208–1217.

ANTERIOR GLENOHUMERAL INSTABILITY: TREATMENT OF ACUTE INJURY

MARK LAZARUS
VIP NANAVATI

Anterior dislocation of the glenohumeral joint is among the most common traumatic dislocations in the human body. The soft tissues to the glenohumeral joint must be disrupted for the humeral head to escape the glenoid fossa. The most important factor determining the location of tissue disruption is the age of the patient. In patients older than 40 years of age, the posterior mechanism of dislocation is common. This involves a tear in the rotator cuff with or without labral tissue involvement. In patients younger than 40 years of age, the predominant tissue injury is a tear of the anterior inferior glenoid labrum (Bankart tear). A study delineating the arthroscopic findings after initial traumatic anterior dislocation in patients younger than 24 years of age revealed that 61 of 63 patients (97%) sustained an avulsion of the anterior inferior glenoid labrum. Fourteen of the 63 patients (22%) had an associated osseous lesion of the glenoid rim. The most important risk for recurrence after initial dislocation may be the underlying pathologic tissue disruption. An arthroscopic study of 45 patients who sustained an initial traumatic dislocation showed that most had Bankart tears. Moreover, these patients also were found to have gross instability on examination under anesthesia. Six of the 45 patients who did not have labral pathology were found to be stable on examination under anesthesia.

Multiple studies have addressed the outcomes of patients after first-time traumatic anterior dislocation. The risk of recurrence after initial dislocation has been reported as high as 95% for patients younger than 20 years of age. For patients younger than 25 years of age, the recurrence rate has been reported as high as 50% to 75%. After the age of 25 years, the risk of recurrence has been shown to rapidly decrease. Despite the varying rates of recurrence that have been reported, studies have clearly demonstrated that the risk of recurrence after initial traumatic anterior dislocation is extremely high. This risk is inversely related to the age of the patient at the time of initial dislocation. Therefore, treatment should be based on the age of the patient.

PATIENT PRESENTATION AND EVALUATION

Diagnosis of an anterior glenohumeral dislocation is normally a straightforward process. The patient's history most often presents a mechanism of an eccentrically applied load to the hand while the arm is outstretched. At presentation, the patient typically appears as leaning forward with the humerus in slight abduction, flexion, and internal rotation. Usually, the humeral head is palpable anteriorly with a concomitant hollowing and visible deficiency posteriorly under the acromion. Patients may present after the dislocation has spontaneously reduced, in which case the diagnosis may not be evident. The mechanism of injury, history of a "dead arm" event, and reported information of a pop at the time of injury or pain that was relieved after a pop often represent key clues toward diagnosis.

Initial evaluation must include a thorough neurovascular examination. The more common neurapraxias can be ruled out with resistance testing of the posterior and middle deltoids and biceps. Pulses, warmth, and capillary refill should be compared with the unaffected extremity. Symmetry, however, does not necessarily exclude axillary artery injury. In the case of a spontaneously reduced dislocation, the patient will present with prominent guarding against combined abduction and external rotation.

Preliminary radiographic evaluation, usually consisting of a single oblique view, has often been completed prior to orthopaedic consultation. This view can adequately rule out fractures about the humeral head and neck that may prevent closed reduction. If additional injuries are not present, the surgeon should reduce the shoulder prior to ordering further radiographs. In the event radiographs cannot be taken at the time of presentation, such as in the event of an on-field injury, a gentle attempt at reduction is warranted.

MANAGEMENT

Reduction

Several reduction maneuvers have been described in the literature. These include the hippocratic technique, the Stimson technique, and the Milch technique. The hippocratic technique involves using countertraction either with the surgeon's foot across the axillary folds against the chest wall or with a sheet pulling countertraction from across the patient's body in a cephalad direction by an assistant. Simultaneously, axial traction is applied to the affected shoulder. Internal and external rotation of the humeral head will help reduce the glenohumeral joint. The Stimson technique involves placing the patient prone with approximately 5 pounds of axial traction strapped at the wrist. With the Milch technique, an abduction and external rotation maneuver with concomitant gentle pressure on the humeral head with the thumb enables reduction on the supine patient. Perhaps more important than any particular method of reduction is to ensure that the patient is adequately relaxed and that adequate analgesia has been provided. Intravenous sedatives and anxiolytics are often helpful. Several authors have reported the successful use of intra-articular lidocaine for anesthetic. The glenohumeral joint can be easily penetrated posteriorly with an 18-gauge spinal needle. Aspiration of hemarthrosis verifies joint penetration. Fifteen to 20 mL of 1% lidocaine will provide adequate analgesia for the patient to cooperate with reduction efforts. Regardless of the maneuver used, successful reduction is confirmed with the restoration of normal humeroscapular relationships and smooth glenohumeral rotation. Patients generally experience dramatic pain relief after reduction. A thorough postreduction neurovascular exam must be performed.

Imaging

Having had adequate analgesia and sedation, the postreduction patient can readily tolerate a more thorough radiographic evaluation. Radiographs generally include a true glenohumeral anterior posterior (AP) in internal and external rotation and an axillary lateral. A true shoulder AP view is an x-ray view taken in the plane of the scapula (at approximately 30 to 40 degrees). Internal and external rotation views provide information regarding humeral head and tuberosity injuries. An axillary view confirms reduction of the glenohumeral joint and aids in the diagnosis of tuberosity fractures and Hill-Sachs lesions.

Various axillary views have been described. These include a true axillary view, which involves placing the arm in 70 to 90 degrees of abduction and then directing the x-ray beam superiorly through the axilla. A safer, less traumatic axillary technique involves elevating the arm in the plane of the scapula. This modification tends to prevent the humeral head from being placed into a vulnerable position. Other axillary images include the West Point view. In this technique, the patient is placed prone with the shoulders raised approximately 7 cm off the x-ray table. With the head and neck turned away, the x-ray beam is directed 25 degrees inferior from the horizontal and 25 degrees medial. The Velpeau view places the patient standing and leaning backward over the radiographic cassette. The x-ray beam is then directed vertically downward.

If a glenoid rim osseous defect is suspected, an apical oblique (Garth) view should be obtained. This radiographic technique places the scapula flat against the x-ray cassette similar to a true AP view. The x-ray beam is then directed in a 45-degree caudad direction.

Special radiographic techniques used to view humeral head defects in addition to the internal and external AP views include the tangential view, the Hill-Sachs view, and the Stryker-Notch view. The tangential and Hill-Sachs views involve AP x-rays in increasing degrees of internal rotation. The Stryker-Notch view is taken with the patient in the supine position with the affected hand placed on the head. The x-ray beam is then directed 10 degrees in a cephalad direction.

With any of these radiographic techniques, the surgeon may be required to assist in patient and extremity positioning. Obtaining high-quality postreduction radiographs, however, will provide critical information that will aid the orthopaedic surgeon in formulating the proper treatment algorithm for the patient.

If radiographic assessment demonstrates the possibility of an osseous Bankart lesion that involves >25% to 30% of the glenoid width, further evaluation with CT imaging with three-dimensional reconstructions is required. A recent study quantitatively demonstrated that CT imaging was superior to plain radiographs in assessing the size of a bony defect of the glenoid.

Magnetic resonance imaging (MRI) has a limited but specific use in the evaluation of acute anterior glenohumeral dislocations. An MRI should be obtained when examination in the subacute postdislocation period yields evidence of a rotator cuff tear, particularly a subscapularis rupture (Fig. 33-1). A prospective study analyzing the accuracy of subacute MRI scans to identify labral tears in

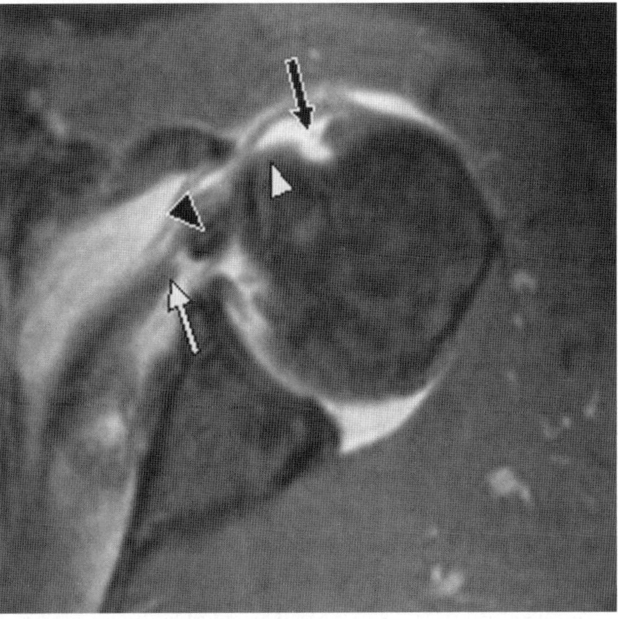

Figure 33-1 MRI of subscapularis tear.

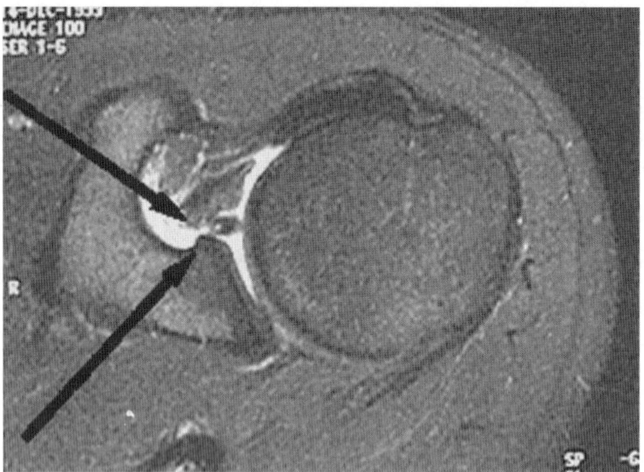

Figure 33-2 MRI of an anterior labral tear.

patients with first-time traumatic dislocations showed only a 70% correlation with arthroscopically confirmed labral tears. Another prospective study examining the accuracy of MRI arthrography to identify labral pathology in patients with traumatic anterior instability showed a specificity of 98% (Fig. 33-2). Diagnostic sensitivity, however, was only 76%.

In the event of persistent deltoid or rotator cuff weakness without other clinical evidence of rotator cuff tear, electromyographic studies are indicated.

POSTREDUCTION TREATMENT

Immobilization

Generally, a simple sling has traditionally been used for postreduction immobilization. A sling with strap padding is often better tolerated than a shoulder immobilizer. Patients are encouraged to wear the sling during sleep to protect the shoulder during this initial period. In addition, patients are encouraged to remove the sling to exercise the elbow, wrist, and digits frequently. The duration of immobilization has typically been continued for $\leq$3 weeks, but absolutely no longer. Investigators have demonstrated that the length of immobilization has had no effect on the rates of recurrent dislocation. Alternatively, recent studies have suggested that the position of immobilization may affect the healing potential of labral lesions, thereby potentially affecting the redislocation rates for first-time dislocators. In a recent study, 19 traumatic anterior dislocations with Bankart tears were evaluated with MRI scans with the shoulders placed in both external and internal rotation. Findings included decreased separation and displacement of the labrum from the glenoid when the arm was in external rotation compared with when it was in internal rotation. A follow-up study of 40 patients with acute traumatic anterior dislocations was recently conducted. The patients were equally randomized to immobilization in sling and swathe in internal rotation or in a prefabricated splint in external rotation for 3 weeks. Results showed that none of the 20 patients immobilized in external rotation had a recurrent anterior dislocation at a mean 15-month follow-up. Whether immobilization in external rotation prevents long-term recurrence rates still remains to be seen.

Assessment

Repeat examination is critical during the subacute phase after dislocation. Re-evaluation should be during the first week of index dislocation. A prospective study of 538 first-time traumatic anterior dislocation patients showed a redislocation rate of 3.2% within the first week after original dislocation. Factors associated with increased risk for redislocation included neurologic deficit, associated large rotator cuff tears, and associated glenoid rim fractures with or without fractures of the greater tuberosity.

During physical examination, range of motion will likely demonstrate appreciable tightening of the shoulder, especially with external rotation in the unelevated position. External rotation that is greater than the unaffected side suggests a possible subscapularis rupture. Rotator cuff function should be assessed, particularly in patients older than 40 years of age as several studies have demonstrated the increased incidence of rotator cuff tears in this age group. Focused attention should be placed on examination of the subscapularis in all age groups. The lumbar lift-off test as described by Gerber has been shown to accurately predict subscapularis integrity and function. This test can usually be performed at the 3-week postdislocation assessment. An examination that reveals evidence of a rotator cuff tear mandates further evaluation with an MRI.

Nonoperative Therapy

The patient is started on a gentle supine self-passive stretching program at 3 weeks postdislocation. Exercises consist of gentle forward elevation and external rotation, with an external rotation limit of 40 degrees. An over-door pulley may be used for assistance in regaining forward elevation. Next, a scapular strengthening and postural program are used. Pendulum exercises are avoided as they promote poor scapular mechanics and increase anteroinferior translation of the humeral head. Formal, supervised therapy is instituted during the sixth week postdislocation. Passive stretching is used to correct any residual contractures. The mainstays of treatment at this stage are rotator cuff and scapular strengthening. Devices that promote normal humeroscapular rhythm are implemented: the body blade, pulleys, and upper body ergometers. Athletes generally can return to their sport midseason. Harnesses and prophylactic taping may provide proprioceptive feedback against extreme abduction and external rotation. At 12 weeks postdislocation, sport-specific exercises are started. Plyometrics for athletes and work hardening for heavy laborers may be necessary.

Early Surgical Intervention

The ability to prevent recurrent dislocation through exercise therapy is controversial. Studies involving cadets at military academies have demonstrated success rates of ≤75% after coordinated therapy programs for first-time dislocators. It is unclear whether such results could be reproduced in a more general population over a longer period of time. One study demonstrated only a 16% decrease in recurrence rates in patients treated with exercise therapy after traumatic subluxation.

The role of early surgical intervention for patients with initial dislocation has become more accepted with the advent of more refined arthroscopic techniques and instrumentation. Theoretically, these generally young patients have more clearly defined pathology and healthier tissue, making them good candidates for arthroscopic repair. In a prospective study comparing nonsurgical management and arthroscopic repair in West Point military cadets with initial dislocations, the recurrence rate was 80% in the nonsurgical group and 14% in the surgical group. In another study comparing randomized patients younger than 30 years of age with initial dislocations, those treated with immobilization and rehabilitation had a recurrence rate of 47% at 33 months compared with 15.9% in the group treated with arthroscopic Bankart repair. Although repair techniques vary among studies, most data suggest that arthroscopic Bankart repair is most advantageous if done after the initial dislocation, before the development of chronic pathologic changes associated with recurrent instability.

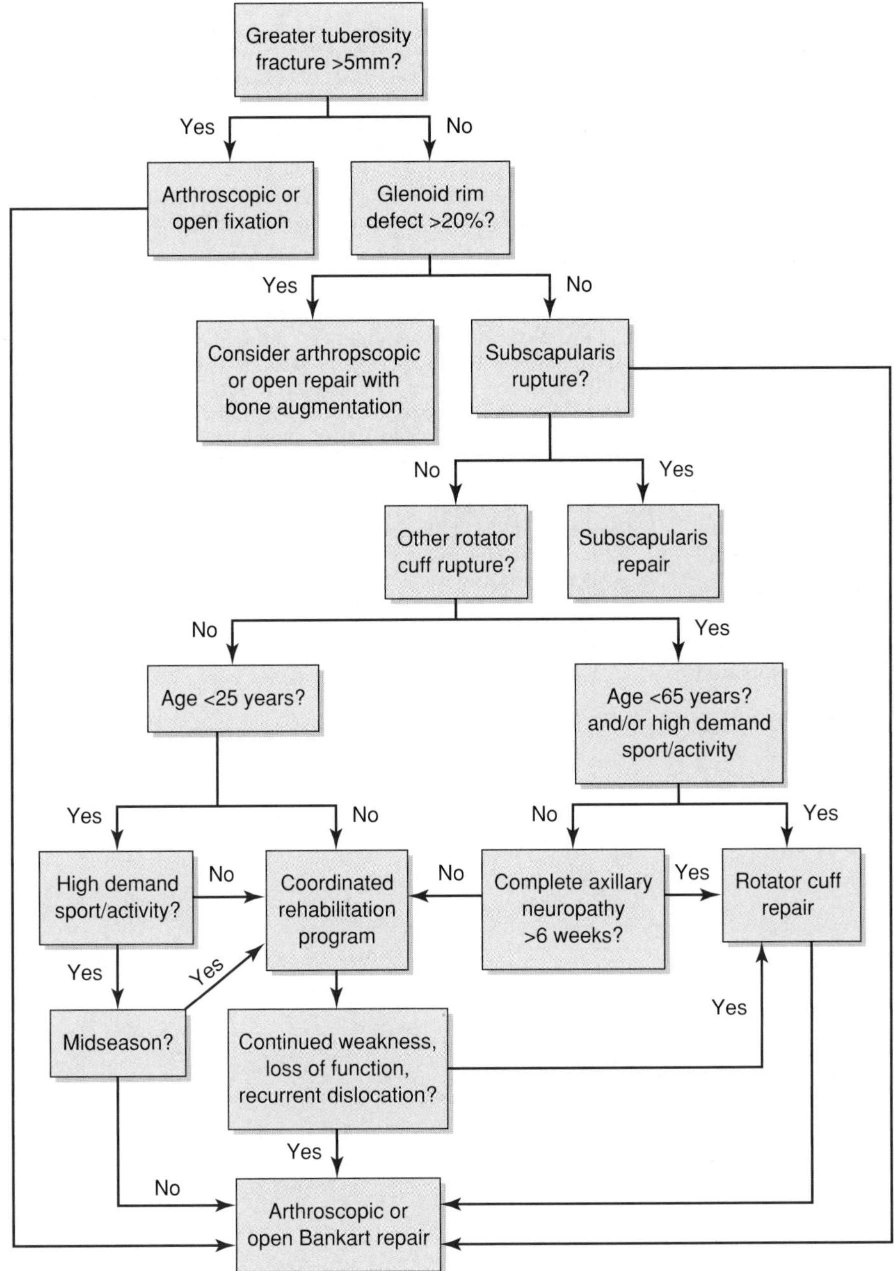

Figure 33-3 Algorithm for the management of first-time traumatic dislocations.

TREATMENT ALGORITHM

The treatment of patients with first-time dislocations should be based on current science. The surgeon's algorithm must take into account the patient's age, activity level, and goals (Fig. 33-3). Several key points must be recognized in formulating a treatment plan. Tuberosity fractures displaced more than 5 mm require reduction and fixation. In young patients, concomitant arthroscopic Bankart repair should be strongly considered. Repair of traumatic subscapularis rupture should be performed as soon as possible to avoid musculotendinous retraction and scarring, regardless of age. Glenoid rim fractures equaling >20% of the intact glenoid width will often require bone augmentation in addition to a Bankart repair. For patients who lead an active lifestyle or are involved in a high-demand occupation and who have sustained a full-thickness rotator cuff tear from a dislocation, surgical treatment should involve both a rotator cuff repair and Bankart repair, if present. For the older patient with a large full-thickness rotator cuff tear and axillary neuropathy, rotator cuff repair should be considered if deltoid function does not return in 6 to 12 weeks postdislocation. For competitive athletes younger than 25 years of age, arthroscopic Bankart repair should be considered in the off season. For any patient younger than 25 years of age with a first-time dislocation, the benefits and risks of early arthroscopic Bankart repair should be discussed and offered as a reasonable option.

Open versus Arthroscopic Repair

Open Bankart repair has traditionally been advocated as the technique of choice for collision and contact athletes. A recent study demonstrated excellent long-term results in American football players treated with open Bankart repair. No patient had recurrent dislocations postoperatively, and only 2 of 58 had recurrent subluxation. In another study involving 194 patients with arthroscopically repaired Bankart lesions, 101 of whom were contact athletes, a recurrence rate of only 6.5% was present in patients without associated bone defects. In contrast, a recurrence rate of 87% was reported for those patients with marked bone loss.

Despite the advances in shoulder arthroscopy, there are a few absolute indications for open surgical repair in first-time dislocators. These include substantial humeral and/or glenoid bone loss, or irreparable rotator cuff deficiency, particularly those of the subscapularis. Relative contraindications to arthroscopic repair include humeral avulsions of the glenohumeral ligaments and capsular ruptures. In general, however, arthroscopic Bankart repair is probably indicated for first-time dislocations as there has never been any significant difference demonstrated in the surgical ease or outcome between early and late open Bankart repair.

SUGGESTED READINGS

Arciero RA, Wheeler JH, Ryan JB, et al. Arthroscopic Bankart repair versus non-operative treatment for acute, initial anterior shoulder dislocations. *Am J Sports Med*. 1994;22:589–594.

Burkhart SS, De Beer JF. Traumatic glenohumeral bone defects and their relationship to failure of arthroscopic Bankart repairs: significance of the inverted-pear glenoid and the humeral engaging Hill-Sachs lesion. *Arthroscopy*. 2000;16:677–694.

Burkhead WZ Jr, Rockwood CA Jr. Treatment of instability of the shoulder with an exercise program. *J Bone Joint Surg Am*. 1992;74;890–896.

Itoi E, Lee S, et al. Quantitative assessment of classic anteroinferior bony Bankart lesions by radiography and computed tomography. *Am J Sports Med*. 2003;31(1):112–118.

Lazarus MD. Acute and chronic dislocation of the shoulder. *Orthopaedic Knowledge Update: Shoulder and Elbow 2*. Rosemont, IL: American Academy of Orthopaedic Surgeons; 2002:71–81.

Levine WN, Rieger K, McCluskey GM. Arthroscopic treatment of anterior shoulder instability. *Instr Course Lect*. 2005;54:87–96.

Millett PJ, Clavert P, Warner JJP. Open operative treatment for anterior shoulder instability: when and why? *J Bone Joint Surg Am*. 2005;87:419–432.

Robinson C, Kelly M, Wakefield AB, et al. Redislocation of the shoulder during the first six weeks after a primary anterior dislocation: Risk factors and results of treatment. *J Bone Joint Surg Am*. 2002; 84:1552– 1559.

Sanders T, Morrison W, Miller MD, et al. Imaging techniques for the evaluation of glenohumeral instability. *Am J Sports Med*. 2000;28:414–434.

ANTERIOR GLENOHUMERAL INSTABILITY: CONSERVATIVE TREATMENT; TRAUMATIC AND MULTIDIRECTIONAL

ADAM M. SMITH

TRAUMATIC DISLOCATION

Acute, traumatic dislocation of the shoulder is a common injury. Anterior dislocation is usually associated with a shoulder that is positioned in abduction and external rotation with an anteriorly directed force on the humeral head.

At the patient's initial presentation, care should be taken to complete a comprehensive examination of the entire upper extremity for any evidence of neurovascular injury, with special care to examine the axillary and musculocutaneous nerve distributions. Shoulder dislocation has been shown to result in clinically apparent neurologic injury in about 10% of patients.[1] Although most of these injuries are clinically insignificant and recovery is complete, appropriate documentation is important. Accurate examination of neurologic function is vital prior to any reduction maneuver. Although neurologic studies are not routinely recommended, patients who present with initial muscular paralysis may be examined with electromyogram (EMG) and nerve conduction studies at least 3 weeks after the injury if clinical recovery does not occur.

Imaging

Initial imaging studies of the glenohumeral joint should include a minimum of three views and must include an adequate axillary view. Patients and staff may be reluctant to perform an axillary radiograph owing to concerns about pain with arm positioning. However, an adequate axillary radiograph can be safely obtained using a Velpeau view (Fig. 34-1).

Hill-Sachs lesions (impaction injury of the humeral head to the glenoid) and fractures of the humeral neck, glenoid, or tuberosities are not uncommon and should be noted prior to reduction to avoid confusion with an iatrogenic injury. Large humeral head impactions (engaging Hill-Sachs lesions) and glenoid bone loss have been identified as poor prognostic predictors of outcome in patients who undergo arthroscopic instability repair.[2]

Pathoanatomy

With an acute anterior-inferior dislocation of the glenohumeral joint, an injury to the anterior soft tissues of the shoulder occurs with detachment of the labrum and the inferior glenohumeral ligament complex from the anteroinferior aspect of the glenoid Bankart lesion.[3] Although multiple intra-articular injuries have been documented with arthroscopy after shoulder dislocation, Bankart lesions have been described as the "essential" lesion of shoulder instability and are seen in more than 90% of acute, traumatic shoulder dislocations.[4] However, labral tearing alone is often not enough to lead to recurrent shoulder instability and is usually associated with capsular stretching. Initial management, both operative and nonoperative, is directed at the management of these labral and capsular injuries.

Reduction

A cooperative, relaxed patient is imperative when attempting reduction of the glenohumeral joint. Although some physicians are able to successfully reduce shoulders without sedation on the playing field or immediately after a dislocation event, muscle spasm and pain occur, with most patients requiring medication to assist with the reduction maneuver. Injection of the glenohumeral joint with intra-articular lidocaine has been found to be a safe and effective method of analgesia to assist with reduction maneuvers.[5] With this

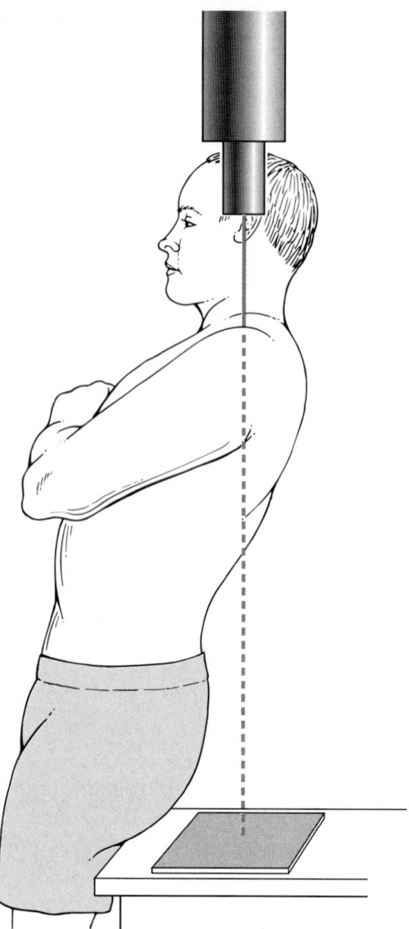

Figure 34-1 Positioning for the Velpeau axillary view is easy to perform.

method, 10 to 15 mL of 1% lidocaine is injected into the glenohumeral joint.

Multiple reduction maneuvers have been discussed in the literature for anterior-inferior dislocations. Postreduction radiographs with at least three views including an axillary are recommended to evaluate the glenohumeral joint for a complete concentric reduction and the presence of any fracture.

One of the most common methods used is the traction-countertraction technique.[6] In this method the patient lies in the supine position with a sheet around the upper thorax. An assistant provides a steady countertraction force to the thorax while the surgeon applies steady gentle traction to the arm in the direction of the dislocation.

The Stimson technique is an excellent technique (Fig. 34-2). The patient is placed prone and the arm allowed to hang off the side of the table perpendicular to the body. A light weight (approximately 5 pounds) is attached to the wrist, and the patient is allowed to relax. Reduction is usually achieved within 10 to 20 minutes as the gentle prolonged traction allows muscle relaxation and reduction of the glenohumeral joint.

The external rotation method can be performed by one person.[7] The reduction is performed with the patient in the supine position, and the affected elbow flexed to 90 degrees with the arm adducted to the level of the chest and the shoulder flexed forward 20 degrees. With the elbow stabilized, the surgeon gently externally rotates the shoulder with minimal force until the shoulder is reduced. Elderly patients or those with subclavicular dislocations should not undergo this technique because of the risk of iatrogenic fracture.

Immobilization

After the initial dislocation has been reduced and the glenohumeral joint is concentric on radiographic examination, a period of immobilization is warranted to maintain reduction, promote healing of the injured soft tissues, and decrease the chance for recurrent dislocations. Recommendations for length of immobilization of acute dislocations are usually 4 to 6 weeks.

Although the most desirable position for immobilization is debated, most authors recommend use of a simple sling with the shoulder in the internally rotated position. Immobilization of the shoulder in external rotation has recently been suggested. With this method, a brace is used to immobilize the shoulder in the externally rotated position. This position has been shown on MRI to reduce anterior joint cavity volume and allow a more anatomic reduction of the Bankart lesion to the glenoid neck and rim owing to increased tension on the anterior soft tissues and subscapularis muscle. This position is not tolerated well by most patients. Further studies examining the role of external rotation bracing in the immediate postinjury period will be required.[8,9]

Therapy

Early therapy with trained personnel is warranted to regain shoulder motion and strength. Motion exercises including active-assisted motion such as pulley and wand therapy are started after the immobilization period. Rotator cuff, periscapular, and body core strengthening and neurore-education are instituted after pain and motion have improved.

Athletes with an injury that occurs in season offer special challenges. In uncomplicated initial cases, return to play or activities is allowed only when range of motion and strength are equal to the uninjured shoulder.[10] Special braces designed to limit overhead motion (abduction and external rotation) have been used with varying degrees of success to prevent instability so that athletes can return to play after in-season dislocation. If the athlete has recurrent instability in season, athletes and their parents should have a thorough understanding of the risks of continued participation with a grossly unstable shoulder.

Results

The results of conservative care of acute shoulder dislocation are mixed and seem to depend on the age of the patient and desire to continue participation in the inciting event. Patients 18 years old or younger and contact athletes

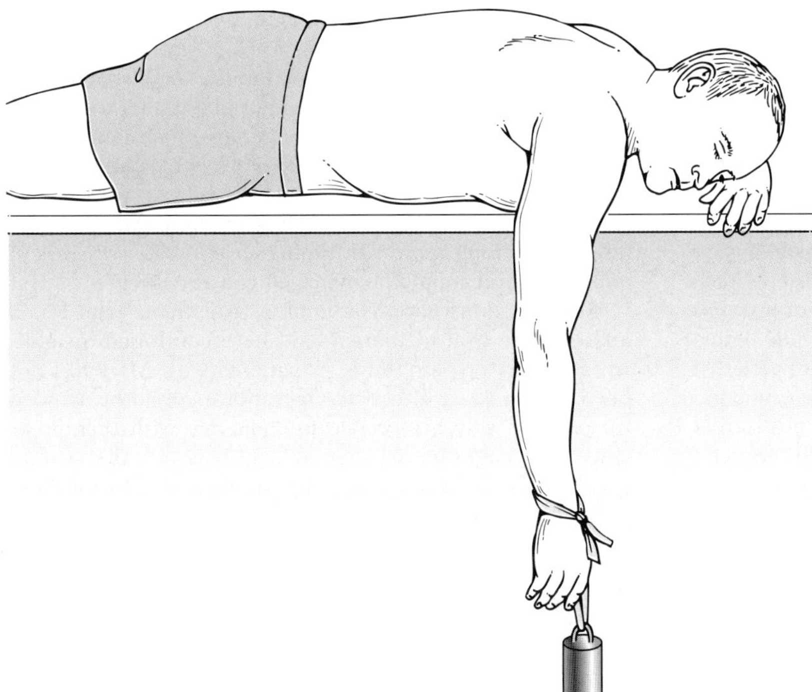

Figure 34-2 Stimson technique for glenohumeral reduction.

have higher rates of recurrent dislocation and have been reported to have recurrent instability in >90% of patients with standard nonoperative regimens (immobilization in internal rotation in a sling, therapy, and return to activities). This high recurrence rate has led some authors to pursue other forms of nonoperative therapy such as initial immobilization in external rotation to minimize the rate of recurrence. Early results from multicenter trials are not yet available.[8,9] Other authors have explored early operative intervention when managing younger patients with arthroscopic Bankart repair with short-term results that have been favorable.[11] Long-term sequelae of recurrent shoulder instability include glenohumeral arthritis and have been identified in approximately 20% of patients with long-term follow-up.[12]

Older patients with less demanding activities usually can be managed with conservative treatment and rehabilitation. Although prolonged weakness of the shoulder may be owing to neurologic injury, rotator cuff tearing is known to occur in patients older than 35 years of age. Patients with continued weakness of the rotator cuff after a few weeks of rehabilitation should be examined closely for cuff tearing and may require appropriate imaging. Patients with tears of the subscapularis are particularly prone to developing recurrent instability and should be aggressively managed with operative treatment.[13,14] Patients with subscapularis tearing may demonstrate increased passive external rotation of the shoulder and inability to perform lift-off, belly-press, or bear-hug tests.[15]

Surgical treatment is generally warranted for patients who fail nonoperative intervention and continue to dislocate despite aggressive rehabilitation. Patients with irreducible dislocations or open injuries warrant urgent surgical intervention. The treatment of young patients (<18 years of age) or contact athletes with acute dislocations is controversial, and recommendations continue to emerge. Although characterization of what constitutes a chronic dislocation is not well-defined in the literature, patients with a shoulder dislocation present for ≥3 weeks are managed much differently than those with acute dislocations and frequently require operative intervention. These patients are generally cognitively impaired or multitrauma patients and should undergo attempts at closed reduction only in a well-controlled setting with adequate sedation and muscle relaxation to avoid iatrogenic fracture or neurovascular injury.

MULTIDIRECTIONAL INSTABILITY

Multidirectional instability (MDI) is difficult to define. Diagnosis of MDI is usually subjective, and agreement on classification has not been achieved.[16] However, it is generally accepted that patients with MDI have instability in more than one direction (anterior, inferior, or posterior). The treatment of MDI was first defined by Neer and Foster.[17] Our understanding continues to evolve and is the subject of several ongoing studies.

Pathoanatomy/Diagnosis

Anatomic changes in patients with MDI include a large, patulous inferior capsule that increases glenohumeral joint volume, thus diminishing the checkrein effect of the glenohumeral ligaments. Rotator interval tissue is usually thinned and less robust than normal. Although the tissue in patients is often less than ideal, neurologic abnormalities also exist and seem to play a key role in the MDI syndrome,[18] A large joint capsule combined with loss of proprioceptive control of the rotator cuff likely leads to loss of concavity compression. Periscapular muscle control for scapular positioning may lead to inappropriate glenoid position, thus leading to instability. This is supported by recently reported data that atypical patterns of muscle activity with resulting dysfunctional neuromuscular control of the rotator cuff and periscapular musculature is a major contributing factor to the pathologic cause of MDI.[19,20]

Although some patients complain of gross instability or frequent complete dislocation of the shoulder, most patients with MDI complain of vague sensations of pain or instability with routine activities of daily living or at the end points of motion. MDI is seen in two broad categories of patients: patients with general ligamentous laxity at baseline, and patients who have long-standing microtrauma with no discreet injury (swimmers, gymnasts, throwers, weight lifters, and patients involved in racquet sports).

Patients with generalized ligamentous laxity are able to demonstrate hyperextendable joints (elbows, knees, wrists, metacarpophalangeal). These patients generally have no tear of the labrum (Bankart lesion), but may have an excessively "loose" shoulder with an enlarged inferior capsular pouch. Patients with recurrent microtrauma also frequently have loose shoulders from acquired activities, such as swimming, that require extreme ranges of motion for maximum performance and result in stretching of the shoulder capsule through repetitive stress. However, in these patients, an acute event occurs causing injury to the already capacious capsule. These patients may have a labral or capsular tear and should be differentiated from patients with generalized ligamentous laxity.

Patients with MDI often present with subtle physical findings. Loose shoulders are common findings in young patients (particularly girls), and reproduction of new or pathologic instability leading to the patient's symptoms should be the focus of the examination. Examination of the asymptomatic shoulder is important and can give insight to abnormalities in the affected shoulder. Identification of a sulcus sign with prominent humeral head depression below the acromion with gentle inferior traction applied to the wrist indicates lax capsular rotator interval tissue. Asymmetric shoulder laxity can be identified by examining for the amount of humeral head translation off of the glenoid rim. Examination under anesthesia is extremely useful and allows the surgeon to examine the shoulder with variable amounts of rotation to identify areas of asymmetrical laxity.[21,22]

Rehabilitation

Patient education is an important first step in rehabilitation. An adequate understanding of the underlying problem seems to facilitate patient compliance. Functional activities should not only include strengthening of the rotator cuff and periscapular muscles, but also should emphasize retraining of the scapula and dynamic stabilizers of the shoulder for appropriate positioning of the glenoid. Patients should be discouraged from any voluntary subluxation. Rehabilitation may take several months, and patients (and physicians) may become frustrated. However, a minimum of 6 months of therapy (some authors recommend a year) is required for maximum benefit.

Although the reported data are limited somewhat by how MDI is defined, long-term outcomes of patients with MDI are generally favorable with nonoperative treatment. Satisfactory results were reported in 29 of 33 (88%) patients with MDI by Burkhead and Rockwood.[23] Children with voluntary dislocation/subluxation of the glenohumeral joint usually do well long term with no increase in osteoarthritis in adulthood and should be managed conservatively.[24]

Surgical intervention is limited to patients who failed an adequate trial of therapy and have continued instability. Surgery for pain alone in patients with MDI has not been shown to be effective. Operations should be avoided for patients who are unable to cooperate with therapy or who have cognitive or mental health issues that would preclude full participation in a postoperative rehabilitation program.

REFERENCES

1. Visser CP, Coene LN, Brand R, Tavy DL. The incidence of nerve injury in anterior dislocation of the shoulder and its influence on functional recovery. A prospective clinical and EMG study. *J Bone Joint Surg Br*. 1999;81:679–685.
2. Burkhart SS, De Beer JF. Traumatic glenohumeral bone defects and their relationship to failure of arthroscopic Bankart repairs: significance of the inverted-pear glenoid and the humeral engaging Hill-Sachs lesion. *Arthroscopy*. 2000;16:677–694.
3. Bankart AS. The pathology and treatment of recurrent dislocation of the shoulder-joint. *Br J Surg*. 1938;26:23–29.
4. Hintermann B, Gachter A. Arthroscopic findings after shoulder dislocation. *Am J Sports Med*. 1995;23:545–51.
5. Matthews DE, Roberts T. Intraarticular lidocaine versus intravenous analgesic for reduction of acute anterior shoulder dislocations. A prospective randomized study. *Am J Sports Med*. 1995;23:54–58.
6. Matsen FA III, Thomas SC, Rockwood CA Jr. Glenohumeral instability. In: Rockwood CA Jr, Matsen FA III, eds. *The Shoulder*. Philadelphia: WB Suanders; 1990:526–622.
7. Eachempati KK, Dua A, Malhotra R, et al. The external rotation method for reduction of acute anterior dislocations and fracture-dislocations of the shoulder. *J Bone Joint Surg Am*. 2004;86:2431–2434.
8. Itoi E, Sashi R, Minagawa H, et al. Position of immobilization after dislocation of the glenohumeral joint: a study with use of magnetic resonance imaging *J Bone Joint Surg Am*. 2001;83:661–667.
9. Itoi E, Hatakeyama Y, Kido T, et al. A new method of immobilization after traumatic anterior dislocation of the shoulder: a preliminary study. *J Shoulder Elbow Surg*. 2003;12:413–415.
10. Buss DD, Lynch GP, Meyer CP, et al. Nonoperative management for in-season athletes with anterior shoulder instability. *Am J Sports Med*. 2004;32:1430–1433.
11. Bottoni CR, Wilckens JH, DeBerardino TM, et al. A prospective, randomized evaluation of arthroscopic stabilization versus nonoperative treatment in patients with acute, traumatic, first-time shoulder dislocations. *Am J Sports Med*. 2002;30:576–580.
12. Hovelius L., Augustini BG, Fredin H, et al. Primary anterior dislocation of the shoulder in young patients. A ten-year prospective study. *J Bone Joint Surg Am*. 1996;78:1677–1684.
13. Neviaser RJ, Neviaser TJ, Neviaser JS. Concurrent rupture of the rotator cuff and anterior dislocation of the shoulder in the older patient. *J Bone Joint Surg*. 1988;70:1308–1311.
14. Hawkins RJ, Bell RH, Hawkins RH, et al. Anterior dislocation of the shoulder in the older patient. *Clin Orthop*. 1986;206:192–195.

15. Barth JRH, Burkhart SS, de Beer JF. The bear-hug test: the most sensitive test for diagnosing a subscapularis tear. *Arthroscopy*. 2006;22:1076–1084.
16. McFarland EG, Kim TK, Park HB, et al. The effect of variation in definition on the diagnosis of multidirectional instability of the shoulder. *J Bone Joint Surg Am*. 2003;85:2138–2144.
17. Neer CS II, Foster CR. Inferior capsular shift for involuntary inferior and multidirectional instability of the shoulder. A preliminary report. *J Bone Joint Surg Am*. 1980;62:897–908.
18. Lephart SM, Warner JJP, Borsa PA, et al. Proprioception of the shoulder joint in healthy, unstable, and surgically repaired shoulders. *J Shoulder Elbow Surg*. 1994;3:371–380.
19. Barden JM, Balyk R, Raso VJ, et al. Atypical shoulder muscle activation in multidirectional instability. *Clin Neurophysiol*. 2005;116:1846–1857.
20. Morris AD, Kemp GJ, Frostick SP. Shoulder electromyography in multidirectional instability. *J Should Elbow Surg*. 2004;13:24–29.
21. Cofield RH, Irving JF. Evaluation and classification of shoulder instability. With special reference to examination under anesthesia. *Clin Orthop Relat Res*. 1987;223:32–43. Review.
22. Oliashirazi A, Mansat P, Cofield RH, et al. Examination under anesthesia for evaluation of anterior shoulder instability. *Am J Sports Med*.;27:464–468.
23. Burkhead WZ, Rockwood CA. Treatment of instability of the shoulder with an exercise program. *J Bone Joint Surg*. 1992;74:890–896.
24. Huber H, Gerber C. Voluntary subluxation of the shoulder in children. A long-term follow-up study of 36 shoulders. *J Bone Joint Surg Br*. 1994;76:118–122.

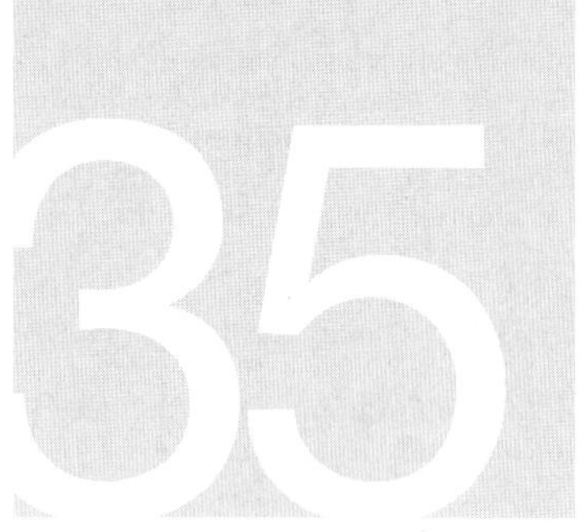

SURGICAL MANAGEMENT OF TRAUMATIC UNIDIRECTIONAL AND ATRAUMATIC MULTIDIRECTIONAL INSTABILITY

XAVIER DURALDE

The indication for surgical management of glenohumeral instability is a failure of conservative treatment modalities. The goal of surgery is to reconstruct glenohumeral anatomy in a balanced fashion avoiding excessive tightening in any one direction, in other words, to obtain a stable yet mobile shoulder without causing stiffness. Pathoanatomy will vary from case to case, so a versatile treatment strategy is necessary allowing adjustment of operative technique based on the pathology encountered. Instability presents in an extremely variable fashion from one patient to another as mentioned in previous chapters and is associated with various pathologic lesions.

The commonly described ends of this spectrum are TUBS (*t*raumatic *u*nidirectional instability due to a *B*ankart lesion that typically requires *s*urgery) and AMBRI (*a*traumatic *m*ultidirectional instability that is often *b*ilateral and treated with *r*ehabilitation or *i*nferior capsular shift when conservative treatment fails).

Significant overlap occurs between these two groups, and surgical planning must take this into account. As arthroscopic techniques improve, a larger percentage of these operations may be performed arthroscopically, but the principles of treatment remain the same whether the surgery is performed open or arthroscopically. The surgeon should strive to identify all pathoanatomy based on history, physical examination, radiographic studies, evaluation under anesthesia, and diagnostic arthroscopy. Surgery can then be performed to repair all damaged structures and re-establish balanced stability of the glenohumeral joint.

Wide variation currently exists in the orthopaedic community regarding the definition of multidirectional instability.[1] This diagnosis is overestimated if it is based on laxity testing alone. Neer and Foster[2] first reported on the results of the inferior capsular shift for multidirectional instability in 1980, describing a group who had uncontrollable, involuntary inferior subluxation or dislocation associated with both anterior and posterior dislocations or subluxations of the shoulder. These patients had both signs and symptoms of instability in all three directions. Unfortunately, many patients with unidirectional or bidirectional instability with associated asymptomatic laxity of the shoulder in another direction have been lumped into this extreme category. The balanced surgical approach described in this chapter can be successfully adapted irregardless of the degree of instability encountered, but in the severely affected group described by Neer and Foster, a modified rehabilitation program may be in order to allow greater time for soft tissue healing.

BENEFITS OF ARTHROSCOPY

As in other areas of shoulder pathology, arthroscopy has greatly increased the surgeon's diagnostic and therapeutic capabilities.[3] A careful diagnostic arthroscopy prior to instability repair allows the surgeon to identify all pathology contributing to the patient's instability.[4] Bankart lesions have been reported in combination with superior labral tears[5] as well as significant stretching of the glenohumeral joint capsule.[6,7] Failure to identify and treat all contributing pathology may lead to failure of the instability repair.[8,9] Some lesions such as superior labral tears are best treated arthroscopically, emphasizing the importance of arthroscopic evaluation even if open instability repair is planned. Other cited advantages of arthroscopic instability techniques include lower morbidity, decreased pain, shorter surgical time, improved cosmesis, and better maintenance of motion postoperatively.[3,10] The degree to which these theoretical advantages apply will vary from surgeon to surgeon depending on his or her own level of experience with arthroscopic surgical technique. Currently arthroscopy does have its limitations, with higher failure rates reported in cases of significant glenoid bone loss (<25% loss of inferior glenoid).[9,11,12] Modern arthroscopic techniques with suture anchors are well suited to manage labral pathology,[13] whereas cases involving humeral avulsions of the glenohumeral ligaments (HAGL lesion), capsular insufficiency following previous surgery,[3] and multidirectional instability due to diffuse capsular laxity may be better suited to open techniques. In cases in which the surgeon cannot achieve stability with arthroscopic techniques, he or she should not hesitate to proceed with an open instability repair.

SURGICAL OPTIONS

Wide variability exists in both the spectrum of pathologic lesions causing shoulder instability and surgical techniques available to address pathology. Patients with traumatic shoulder instability most commonly have a Bankart lesion whereas the hallmarks of atraumatic instability are a redundant capsule and a widened rotator interval.[14] Although traumatic instability is generally unidirectional, atraumatic instability is generally bidirectional or multidirectional and can occur because of congenital laxity, repetitive microtrauma to the shoulder, or traumatic events superimposed on pre-existing laxity.[15] As long as the surgeon understands that significant overlap exists in these patient groups and is ready to treat all encountered pathology, a successful surgery can be planned and expected.

Currently, arthroscopic techniques are ideal for management of labral pathology such as Bankart lesions and can be adapted to treat associated capsular and rotator interval pathology. Recent reports on suture anchor techniques have shown comparable results to open Bankart repairs.[16] The open inferior capsular shift offers a versatile and highly effective approach to diffuse capsular laxity and has significant advantages over other described open techniques. The capsular shift procedure described by Neer can be modified to adjust the tightening of the capsule depending on the amount and location of laxity in a particular shoulder. It can be modified for unidirectional, bidirectional, or multidirectional instability.[14] The inferior capsular shift is designed to reduce capsular volume on all sides including anterior, inferior, and posterior through a single approach. It allows overlapping and therefore reinforcement of tissues in the direction of greatest instability with tightening of the capsule inferiorly and on the opposite side. This procedure also avoids asymmetric tightening, which can lead to abnormal joint mechanics and a fixed subluxation in the opposite direction.[17] The operation is laterally based to allow for greater volume decrease than medially based or centrally based techniques because the glenohumeral joint capsule is a laterally based, truncated cone.[18] This approach also allows treatment of associated labral avulsions anteriorly and rotator interval closure. It does not allow adequate exposure of the superior labrum, and diagnostic arthroscopy is beneficial prior to open surgery to allow visualization of the superior labrum and arthroscopic superior labral repair if needed arthroscopically.

For these reasons, the technique for the open inferior capsular shift will be described for the treatment of atraumatic instability and the arthroscopic Bankart repair using a suture anchor technique will be described for the treatment of traumatic instability. Although these techniques are by no means the only procedures recommended for the treatment of shoulder instability, they are both versatile and effective and afford surgeons the ability to adapt their techniques to all encountered pathology.

OPERATIVE TECHNIQUE

Anesthesia

Instability repair can be performed under interscalene regional anesthesia, general anesthesia, or a combination of both. The interscalene block provides pre-emptive analgesia as well as excellent postoperative analgesia and has been proven to be reliable and safe.[19] Its shortcomings include the fact that the posterior shoulder (posterior arthroscopic portal) and axilla are not adequately covered by the block and require the addition of local or general anesthesia. In addition, the pectoralis major is not completely included, and tension in this muscle may limit exposure during deep dissection in open repairs. For arthroscopic techniques, muscle paralysis is generally not required although it is helpful for open approaches. This author uses a combination of general anesthesia and interscalene block for all instability repairs. A laryngeal mask airway is generally used in arthroscopic cases unless airway issues require the use of an endotracheal tube. In open cases, an endotracheal tube is used so that muscle paralysis can be used to relax the pectoralis major.

Patient Positioning and Setup

Both arthroscopic and open instability repairs can be performed in the beach-chair position. In open cases, the torso is placed at a 30-degree angle to the floor. This position allows easy access to the axilla if an axillary skin incision is to be used and offers excellent access to the inferior pouch. The trunk is placed more vertically in arthroscopic cases to allow easier access to the posterior shoulder. In arthroscopic cases, the beach-chair position allows easy conversion to open surgery if necessary. Distraction of the humeral head away from the glenoid is most easily achieved, however, in the lateral decubitus position with traction on the arm and the weight of the patient's dependent body as countertraction. In the beach-chair position, distraction of the glenohumeral joint for improved arthroscopic visualization runs the risk of displacement of the patient's body off the operating table. In these cases, the patient's torso can be tied to the operating table, using a sheet to prevent displacement. A neurosurgical headrest is helpful with either approach to allow better access to the shoulder.

Examination under Anesthesia

Examination under anesthesia serves to clarify the direction and degree of instability. This rarely contradicts the preoperative diagnosis but may be helpful, especially in muscular patients who guard on examination in the office. It is also helpful in defining the primary area of instability. The surgeon must be careful to relocate the humeral head in the glenoid prior to each maneuver to maintain a frame of reference. Translation of the humeral head over the glenoid rim is abnormal in any direction. With the arm at the side, the sulcus test in neutral will demonstrate laxity in the superior portion of the glenohumeral capsule including the superior glenohumeral ligament as well as the rotator interval. This is also indicative of an enlarged inferior pouch. Failure of the sulcus sign to improve significantly by placing the shoulder in an externally rotated position is indicative of incompetence of the rotator interval tissue as this should normally tension in external rotation. With the arm in 90 degrees of abduction and neutral rotation, the shoulder can be gently forced anteriorly and posteriorly to test the laxity of the inferior glenohumeral ligament and the anterior and posterior capsule. Crepitus on dislocation and relocation is suggestive of labral pathology. If the humeral head locks out of joint, this is suggestive of a Hill-Sachs lesion.

Diagnostic Arthroscopy

The diagnostic arthroscopy is of great benefit in identifying pathologic lesions contributing to the patient's shoulder instability whether an arthroscopic or open technique of repair is planned. A standard posterior portal is established in the soft spot, and a 30-degree arthroscope is used to perform a systematic evaluation of the glenohumeral joint. Placement of the anterior portal must be carefully planned as two anterior portals are required for arthroscopic instability repair. For the diagnostic arthroscopy, an 8-mm cannula can be placed anterosuperiorly through the rotator interval adjacent to the glenoid and labrum. This allows space for later placement of an additional cannula (usually 5 mm) farther inferiorly and laterally, which enters the rotator interval laterally at the triangular convergence of the supraspinatus and subscapularis tendons. Areas of concern include the articular surfaces, the labrum, the capsule, and the rotator cuff and biceps tendons.

The humeral head is carefully inspected for a Hill-Sachs lesion posterosuperiorly. Burkhart and DeBeer[11] have described a method to determine arthroscopically how much anteroinferior glenoid bone is missing in the case of a bony Bankart lesion. Bone loss >25% of the glenoid would be an indication for open bone grafting. Secondary degenerative changes of the articular surfaces owing to chronic instability or large chondral lesions from an acute traumatic dislocation can be documented as these may affect prognosis.

The labrum must be evaluated circumferentially both by visual inspection and tactile examination with a probe. The superior labrum may normally be meniscoid, with the diagnosis of a torn labrum reserved for cases with fraying and granulation. A torn superior labrum can generally be elevated off the glenoid rim by 1 cm. Anteriorly, the labrum may be detached and clearly visible or it may be healed along the anterior glenoid neck (anterior labroligamentous periosteal sleeve avulsion lesion, or ALPSA lesion).[20] In this latter case, the anteroinferior glenoid appears bare with the capsule attaching medially on the glenoid neck. This lesion must be identified so that the labrum can be elevated and reduced back onto the rim of the glenoid.

The capsule is inspected for signs of stretching, midsubstance tearing, or tearing from its humeral insertion (HAGL lesion). The drive through sign describes the ability to easily push the arthroscope between the humeral head and glenoid, passing the scope from the back to the front of the glenohumeral joint. The drive through sign indicates capsular laxity, and if it persists following arthroscopic labral repair, suggests a concomitant capsular stretching, which may require further capsular imbrication or open repair.

Undersurface rotator cuff injuries may be associated with glenohumeral instability, and arthroscopy allows identification and treatment. The biceps anchor may be involved with superior labral tears and is readily identified arthroscopically.

OPEN INFERIOR CAPSULAR SHIFT

The crux of the capsular shift procedure is adequate release of the capsule far enough inferiorly and posteriorly to allow obliteration of the inferior pouch and any associated posterior capsular laxity. Understanding and performing several key maneuvers are critical to success and should help give the surgeon confidence with this operation. Proper takedown of the capsule is critical to avoid bisecting the inferior pouch. The capsular insertion inferiorly on the medial humeral neck is broad and somewhat variable anatomically.[21] Safe techniques with release of both the superior capsular reflexion and the more inferior capsular insertion under direct vision are critical in avoiding potential injury to the axillary nerve. Simple guidelines are available to determine the amount of capsular release and amount of shift needed in each individual case.

For the open inferior capsular shift, a neurosurgical headrest is used to allow the assistant access to the superior shoulder. A short arm board is built up with sheets to maintain arm position anterior to the anterior axillary line (Fig. 35-1). Local anesthesia is infiltrated in the axilla and the posterior portal site as these areas are not adequately covered by the interscalene block. The table back is elevated to position the trunk at a 30-degree angle to the floor, and the table is placed in reverse Trendelenburg during the diagnostic arthroscopy. The table back is then returned to the 30-degree position for the open portion of the case. This maneuver precludes the need to readjust the headrest between the arthroscopic and open portions of the procedure.

The skin incision is made in the deltopectoral interval for muscular men and typically measures 10 cm in line between the coracoid and axillary fold.[22] In thin women, a 5- to 6-cm axillary incision can be made in the skin folds. The axillary skin folds can be marked with a needle scratch prior to draping, which allows the incision to be hidden.

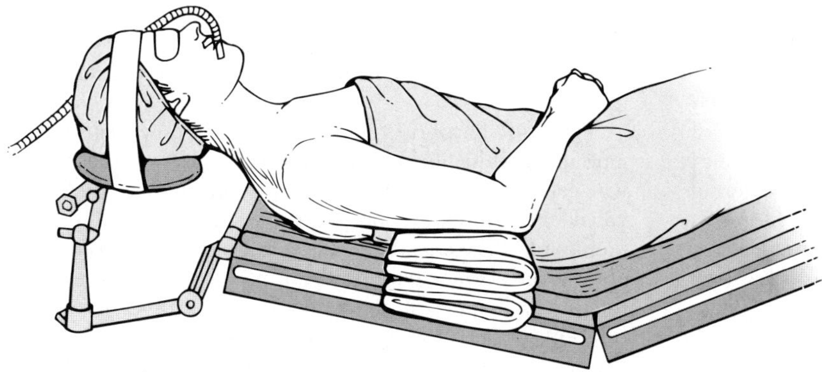

Figure 35-1 In a beach chair position, the front and back of the shoulder are exposed to allow access to both sides. A neurosurgical headrest is helpful in positioning. A built-up arm rest with two sheets allows the arm to rest in the midaxillary line during capsular reconstruction.

Skin flaps are elevated from the inferior rolled border of the pectoralis major to the clavicle with either incision. A needle-point cautery is useful for careful dissection while allowing hemostasis. The deltopectoral interval is then developed using blunt and sharp dissection taking the cephalic vein laterally. The clavipectoral fascia is incised along the lateral border of the conjoined tendon, and this structure is retracted medially. Excessive traction on this structure is avoided to prevent damage to the musculocutaneous nerve. The subacromial and subdeltoid bursal adhesions are released, and the terminal branch of the posterior humeral circumflex vessel is cauterized as it passes between the deltoid and proximal humerus just lateral to the bicipital groove. The anterior humeral circumflex vessels are ligated using no. 0 polyester sutures. This allows access to the inferior portion of the capsule and has not been associated with avascular necrosis. The sutures are placed 1 cm apart so that the vessels can be cauterized in between and released. Care must be taken to not grasp the joint capsule with the medial suture as this will not allow the subscapularis to be separated from the capsule in later dissection.

The inferior veil of the coracoacromial ligament is released sharply to the level of the ligament itself to allow clear visualization of the rotator interval. The deep dissection is begun with an incision of the subscapularis tendon 1 cm medial to the lesser tuberosity. The superficial two-thirds of this tendon are dissected off of the capsule using blunt and sharp dissection. Typically, a pointed Adson clamp is used to spread the subscapularis fibers, and these are cut with a long-handled no. 15 blade. The thickness of the subscapularis can be determined by opening the rotator interval and palpating the thickness of the tendon so that the superficial two-thirds can be reliably peeled off of the underlying capsule while leaving some tendinous tissue attached to the capsule for reinforcement. During the inferior portion of this dissection, the axillary nerve must be palpated and protected. The tug test, as described by Flatow, is useful to localize the nerve.[23] The surgeon passes the index finger of the inside hand along the subscapularis muscle beneath the conjoined tendon. With the outer hand, the surgeon palpates the axillary nerve on the undersurface of the deltoid muscle lateral to the humerus. By gently tugging back and forth with two hands, the surgeon can be sure which medial structure is indeed the axillary nerve. The ability to tug the nerve medially and feel tension on it laterally assures the surgeon of continuity of the nerve through the axilla. The inferior portion of the subscapularis has a very muscular insertion onto the capsule. This can be released using electrocautery, and the plane between the subscapularis and the capsule clearly visualized from this inferior portion of the approach. The needle-point cautery is used to carefully cut through most of the subscapularis thickness inferiorly until just a few muscle fibers are visible overlying the capsule. These last few fibers are released using a blunt elevator (a rounded blunt Cobb-like elevator is preferred). This elevator can then be passed medially gently to define the plane between the capsule and the subscapularis tendon. The tendon dissection off the capsule can then proceed both from a medial-to-lateral and a lateral-to-medial direction. It is important to free all subscapularis fibers off of the capsule so that the capsule is free to be shifted and not tethered by the subscapularis muscle. This also allows a Bankart repair to be performed more easily if this is required. If subscapularis fibers are left attached to the capsule medially at the level of the glenoid, visualization for passage of sutures during the open Bankart repair will be obscured. Suturing the subscapularis to the capsule with the Bankart sutures can potentially tether the subscapularis and limit motion. After release of the subscapularis, the capsule can be clearly visualized.

Capsular release begins at the level of the rotator interval. The capsule is transected 5 mm medial to the stump of subscapularis tendon. This leaves enough capsule laterally to anchor the repair later during capsular reconstruction. Traction sutures are placed in the medial limb of the capsule during this maneuver. At the inferior border of the subscapularis insertion, it is critical to deviate the incision in the capsule in a hockey stick fashion laterally along the neck of the humerus, essentially vertical and parallel to the line of the humerus. This avoids amputation of a portion of the inferior pouch. The axillary pouch is now palpated to determine its size. The pouch does have a variable pattern of insertion on the anatomic neck of the humerus. The periosteum and broad capsular insertion are incised vertically along the anterior humerus just distal to the most inferior aspect of the subscapularis stump. Inferior to subscapularis tendon, the entire capsule can be released from the humerus without leaving a lateral cuff as capsular repair will not require suture placement that far inferiorly. The vertical portion of the capsular and periosteal release is carried to the level of the latissimus dorsi tendon. An elevator can then be used to elevate the capsule off the medial anatomic neck, placing the elevator just inferior to the articular reflection of the capsule. This allows any capsular reflection adjacent to the articular surface (usually superior to the elevator) to be incised under direct vision without risk of damage to the axillary nerve. Flexion and external rotation will bring that portion of the neck of the humerus into the surgical field and allow the capsule to be released from the humerus under direct vision. This arm position also reduces tension on the axillary nerve and allows it to fall away from the inferior pouch. Additional traction sutures are placed into the margin of the capsule as more capsule is liberated from the humerus. The more inferior portion of the capsular insertion (that part inferior to the elevator) is cut under direct vision with scissors just superior to the latissimus dorsi tendon. This dissection can be carried posteriorly to the level of the posterior band of the inferior glenohumeral ligament if needed. The amount of capsular release and amount of shift required will vary from patient to patient. Guidelines for capsular release are the following. The capsule should be released from the anatomic neck of the humerus until traction on the anterior capsule obliterates the inferior pouch and also eliminates posterior subluxation of the glenohumeral joint with the arm in neutral rotation. These two observations at surgery indicate that the inferior and posterior pouches are adequately tightened by anterior tension to allow for a balanced reconstruction of the shoulder joint capsule.

At this point, a humeral head retractor (usually a Fukuda ring retractor) is inserted and the anterior labrum is carefully inspected. If a Bankart lesion is noted, it can be repaired at this time. The labrum is freed from the anterior glenoid neck, and the glenoid neck is debrided down to bleeding bone. This can be done with a curette, osteotome, or burr. This creates a fresh bleeding bed for healing of the labrum. Suture anchors are generally placed on the rim of the glenoid between the equator and most inferior point of the defect depending on the amount of labrum avulsed. The labrum is shifted superiorly with the sutures to afford a medial as well as lateral shift with this procedure. Both suture limbs can be brought underneath the labrum and out of the capsule, tying the knots extra-articularly. If the patient has a hypoplastic labrum and the labral repair does not create an adequate bumper, a no. 2 polyester suture can be placed parallel to the glenoid through the labrum from approximately the 5 o'clock to the 3 o'clock position to create a purse-string type imbrication of the labrum in that location. Palpation of the Bankart repair should demonstrate a firm bumper of the labrum at the location of the repair.

It is critical to understand that a capsular shift cannot be effectively performed if the labrum and capsule are not attached to the glenoid. A Bankart lesion must be repaired prior to performing the capsular shift. Once the labral repair is performed, a T cut can be made in the capsule obliquely along the superior border of the inferior glenohumeral ligament (IGHL). Scissors are generally used to cut the capsule. This T cut can also be performed prior to the Bankart repair to help exposure. The IGHL is usually visible, but in patients with hypoplastic ligaments, the capsular incision should proceed obliquely superiorly to end at the equator of the glenoid. This capsular incision generally passes anterior to the labrum, and the labrum should not be incised.

The shift portion of the procedure is now begun. The amount of shift performed will vary from case to case and will depend on the amount of capsule released, degree of capsular redundancy, and the arm position selected for reattachment of the capsule. Deep retractors are now removed, and for the average patient, the arm is positioned in approximately 30 degrees of abduction and 30 degrees of external rotation for performance of the capsular shift. In overhead throwing athletes, this position can be adjusted even up to 80 degrees of external rotation and abduction to allow for greater mobility in the abducted/externally rotated position. The 30/30 position, however, is the most common recommended position. The first step of capsular repair involves placement of two sutures of no. 0 polyester at the lateral aspect of the rotator interval superiorly. These are placed prior to repair of the inferior pouch to avoid having to position the arm in extension to visualize this area following repair of the inferior portion of the capsule. These sutures will be later passed through the superior margin of the superior limb of the capsule both to close the lateral aspect of the rotator interval and to anchor the superior portion of the capsule as it is pulled over the inferior capsule to complete the capsular reconstruction. With the arm in 30 degrees of abduction and external rotation, the inferior capsule is then pulled superiorly as far as possible and is repaired to the lateral stump of capsule using multiple no. 0 polyester interrupted figure-of-8 sutures (Fig. 35-2). The

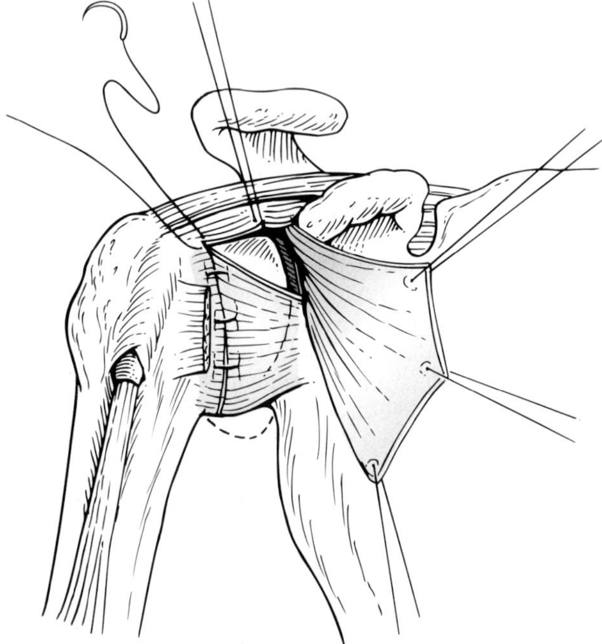

Figure 35-2 The inferior limb of the capsule is pulled superiorly as far as possible with the arm in the 30/30 position and typically can be repaired to the stump of the capsule laterally at the level of the rotator interval. Note the two rotator interval sutures, which will later anchor the superior limb of the capsule prior to overlap.

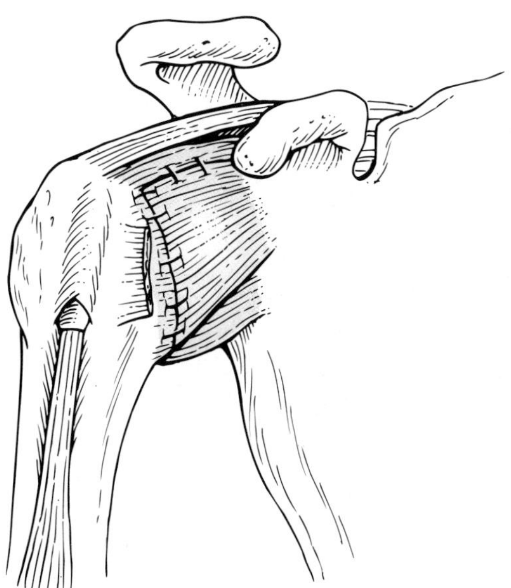

Figure 35-3 The final capsular reconstruction following inferior capsular shift. Notice that the anterior capsule is double thickness whereas the inferior pouch and posterior capsule have both been tightened with this approach.

amount of shift possible will vary from patient to patient, customizing the repair to that particular patient's degree of instability. The superior limb of the capsule is then repaired to the rotator interval using the previously placed polyester sutures. The superior limb of the capsule is then pulled in a vest-over-pants fashion over the inferior limb and is sutured laterally to the stump of capsule using multiple no. 0 polyester interrupted figure-of-8 sutures. The two limbs of the capsule are then sutured together medially (Fig. 35-3). The subscapularis is now repaired anatomically using no. 0 polyester interrupted figure-of-8 sutures back to the stump of subcapularis left laterally. The continuity of the axillary is verified using the tug test. Routine deltopectoral closure and skin closure are then performed. Suction drainage is generally not required.

ARTHROSCOPIC BANKART REPAIR

The pathology and surgery will be described in reference to a right shoulder.

Patient Positioning

This operation can be performed in either the beach-chair or the lateral decubitus position. The lateral decubitus position has the advantage of easier joint distraction without tying up an assistant or running the risk of displacing the patient's torso off the table. If the beach-chair position is used, some type of restraining device to hold the patient's torso firmly to the operating table is recommended to avoid pulling the patient off the table. We generally use a combination of general anesthetic and interscalene block for patient comfort both during and after the procedure, but paralysis is not required for the arthroscopic procedure. Three arthroscopic portals are required for arthroscopic Bankart repair, one posterior and two anterior portals. The posterior portal is made in the soft spot centrally in the posterior aspect of the glenohumeral joint. One anterior portal should be placed to allow an 8-mm cannula to enter the joint along the most medial and superior aspect of the rotator interval into the joint. The second anterior portal is placed laterally and slightly inferior to the first but not so inferior that the cannula is aimed superiorly. This cannula will be used to drill holes and pass suture anchors into the glenoid rim. Inferior orientation of this cannula facilitates placement of the 5 o'clock anchor anteroinferiorly. A 5-mm cannula is placed through this portal, entering the rotator interval at its most lateral apex. A diagnostic arthroscopy is performed to visualize all damaged structures. The Bankart lesion classically presents as an avulsion of the labrum from the 3 o'clock to approximately the 6 o'clock position. The labrum must be carefully inspected circumferentially, however, as superior labral tears are commonly seen in association with an anteroinferior labral avulsion. The status of the biceps and rotator cuff are also carefully inspected. The posterior aspect of the humeral head is carefully evaluated for the presence of the Hills-Sachs lesion. The anterior labrum is often healed along the anterior neck of the glenoid and may not therefore be visualized on initial arthroscopic inspection. Presence of the ALPSA lesion can be confirmed by looking at the anterior glenoid neck through one of the anterior portals. An arthroscopic elevator is placed through the more superior medial portal while the surgeon views from posterior, and the displaced labrum is then elevated sharply off the anterior neck of the glenoid. This will allow the labrum to float laterally and lie adjacent to the rim of the glenoid. A 5.5-mm full-radius resector is then used to debride the anterior glenoid neck down to bleeding bone. This creates a good healing surface for labral repair.

The labrum will be repaired to the rim of the glenoid using 3-mm bioabsorbable suture anchors. Two or three suture anchors are typically used at the 5 o'clock, 4 o'clock, and 3 o'clock positions along the anteroinferior glenoid rim. Metal suture anchors are also acceptable.

It is critical that the labrum be repaired up onto the rim of the glenoid to re-establish the anteroinferior "bumper" and deepen the socket to increase the concavity compression effect of the shoulder.[13] To achieve this, anchors must be placed either on the apex of the glenoid rim or slightly onto the face of the glenoid. Anchor placement on the anterior glenoid neck will not allow the labrum to be repaired to its anatomic position and may result in recurrent instability postoperatively.[9] Just as in the open Bankart repair, a superior shift of the labral tissues is desirable during repair. A traction suture through the labrum will assist in achieving this shift prior to placement of suture anchors. This technique described by Boileau and Ahrens[24] consists of passing a traction suture through the labrum via the superior portal using either a Caspari-type punch or a suture shuttle. This suture is then placed outside the superior medial cannula and is used as a traction suture to pull the labrum superiorly. This allows the suture shuttle to pass sutures from the anchors more inferiorly through the labrum. If significant capsular laxity is noted along with the Bankart lesion, more capsule can be grasped with the suture shuttle to create a shift of tissue medially and superiorly while simultaneously making the labrum more bulky by the addition of capsular tissue. Specific guidelines for the amount of shift of capsular tissues needed during arthroscopic repair are not as well defined as they are for open inferior capsular shift. The surgeon can view inferiorly while tension is applied to the traction suture to determine how much of a shift is needed to obliterate the inferior pouch. There are no reports available to judge the efficacy of this technique. The first anchor is placed at the 5 o'clock position directly onto the rim of the glenoid via the more inferior-lateral cannula. The drill cannula is tapped with the mallet to secure its position on the rim of the glenoid. The drill hole is made to the depth of the drill stop, and the 3-mm bioabsorbable anchor is tapped into place. One suture limb is then grasped and retrieved out the anteromedial cannula. A 90-degree cannulated suture hook is then placed through the more anteromedial cannula and is used to pass a suture shuttle through the labrum inferior to the position of the suture anchor while tension is applied via the traction suture. This shuttle is retrieved using a suture grasper via the more inferior lateral portal and is used to pass the one suture limb in that cannula back through the labrum (Fig. 35-4). One suture limb then passes directly from the anchor out through the superior cannula while the second suture limb passes through the labrum and out through the superior cannula. The labrum can now be secured at this location using a sliding knot. This sliding knot is best tied via the more inferior lateral portal as it is in line with the anchor. The post of the sliding knot is the suture limb passing through the labrum itself as this will more reliably keep the knot off the articular surfaces (Fig. 35-5). Suture anchors are now placed at the 4 o'clock and 3 o'clock positions, and these steps are repeated to create a bumper of labrum along the anteroinferior glenoid rim (Fig. 35-6). The normal sublabral foramen superior to the 3 o'clock position should not be closed as this will not enhance the repair and will lead to a loss of external rotation. The most difficult anchor to place and suture to pass is the first. The next two suture anchors are relatively straightforward.

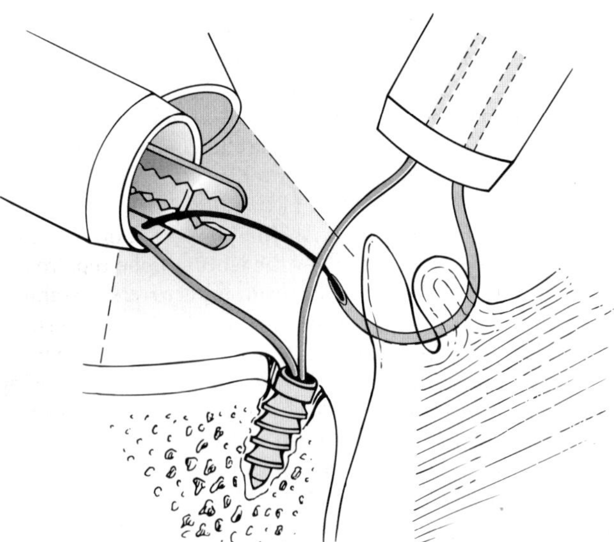

Figure 35-4 A 90-degree curved suture hook is used to pass a shuttle through the labrum and a portion of capsule. The suture limb from the anchor can then be transported through the labrum.

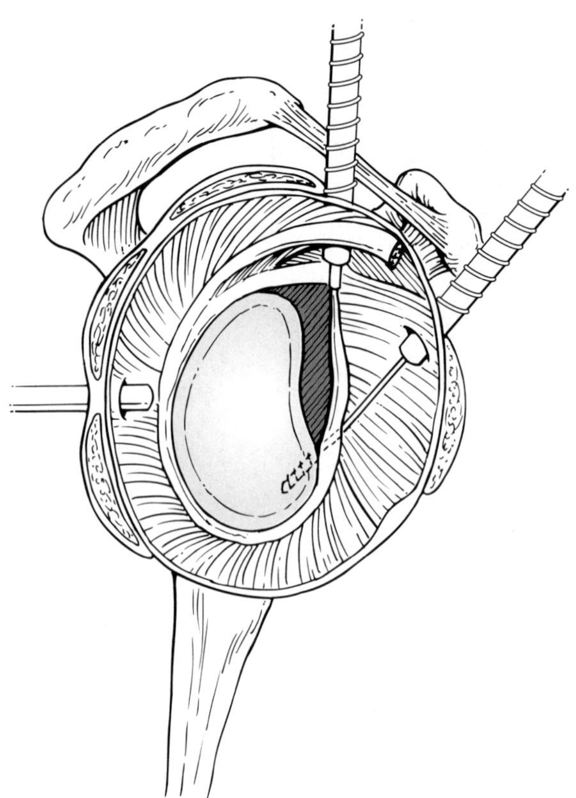

Figure 35-5 The three-portal technique of arthroscopic Bankart repair. The arthroscopic anchor is placed at the 5 o'clock position via the more inferior and lateral of the anterior portals. The suture shuttle is used to pass one limb of suture from the suture anchor through the labrum. Notice the traction suture pulling the labrum superiorly to facilitate a superior shift of the labrum and capsule.

Superior Labral Repair

If a superior labral anterior to posterior (SLAP) tear is noted, an additional anchor can be placed at the 1 o'clock position easily through these two cannulas. The surgeon must be cautious in placing the 1 o'clock anchor because the most superior cannula is relatively medial and the drill must be aimed medially to avoid penetrating the glenoid face. Again, one suture limb can be pulled out the inferior cannula. A bird-beak tissue penetrator can be passed through the superior cannula and through the labrum grasping the suture limb that is passing out the inferior cannula. This suture is then pulled back through the labrum, and a sliding knot is again used for repair. The 11 o'clock suture anchor posterosuperiorly can usually be reached using the aforementioned cannulae. If not, a midlateral portal can be established using a spinal needle as a guide, and a 5-mm working cannula is placed directly through the rotator cuff to allow access to the 11 o'clock position posterosuperiorly. The glenoid neck superiorly in the area of the SLAP lesion is debrided

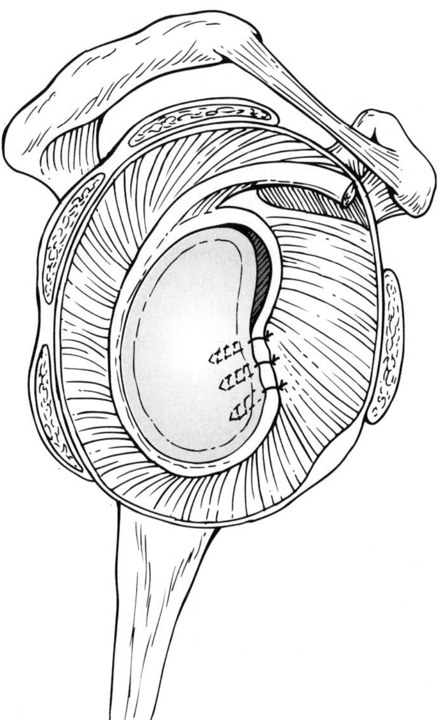

Figure 35-6 The final repair with arthroscopic Bankart repair showing suture anchors at the 3 o'clock, 4 o'clock, and 5 o'clock positions re-establishing a normal attachment for the inferior glenohumeral ligament and recreating an anatomic bumper.

down to bleeding bone. The 3-mm bioanchor is placed in a similar fashion to the previous anchors. One suture limb is grasped out an anterior portal. The 90-degree cannulated suture hook is placed through the anteromedial cannula and is used to pass the suture shuttle through the labrum just posterior to the biceps anchor. This shuttle is retrieved out the midlateral cannula and is used to pass the suture through that cannula through the labrum. Both sutures are retrieved out the midlateral cannula, and a sliding knot (using the suture limb through the labrum as the post) is used to secure the labrum.

POSTOPERATIVE REHABILITATION

The vast majority of patients following open or arthroscopic instability repair can begin an identical postoperative rehabilitation program. The exception to this is the patient with true multidirectional instability who had signs and symptoms of true instability in all three directions preoperatively and who had an extremely patulous capsule of questionable quality at the time of surgery. That particular patient will benefit from a brace postoperatively holding the arm in neutral rotation to protect both the anterior and posterior capsule evenly and supporting the arm to avoid inferior subluxation for the first 6 weeks following surgery. Patients with instability this extreme rarely develop stiffness following capsular reconstruction, and this type of delay will allow for more scar tissue formation in the capsule.

The main difference between arthroscopic and open repairs involves the detachment of the subscapularis tendon and the subsequent need for its protection in the early postoperative period. Protection of the capsular and labral repair in these two patient groups, however, is identical and requires greater restrictions than those typically needed for the protection of the subscapularis alone. Following open repair, patients are cautioned for the first 6 weeks to avoid lifting >5 pounds, avoid excessive external rotation outside the treatment protocol, and avoid using the arm to get up from a seated position. The act of pushing oneself up from a seated position with the arm in the internally rotated position places significant stress on the subscapularis and should be avoided during the first 6 weeks following open surgery. Other than these few restrictions, the therapy protocol is identical for both groups (Table 35-1).

TABLE 35-1 POSTOPERATIVE REHABILITATION FOLLOWING OPEN AND ARTHROSCOPIC INSTABILITY REPAIR

Weeks 0–2	Weeks 2–6	Weeks 6–12	12+ Weeks
Active assisted motion	Goal: Gain 10 degrees per week in FE and ER	Patient should be at ≈130 degrees FE and 40 degrees ER.	Allow patient to run.
Sling outdoors and to sleep for 6 weeks	Light ADL Limit to 5-lb force	Continue stretching. Goal: Gain 10 degrees per week in FE and ER.	Add proprioceptive exercises.
Forward elevation 0–90 degrees	No internal rotation	Add internal rotation as tolerated.	Begin light throwing at 6 months.
External rotation to 0 degrees	No resistive exercises	Add resistive exercises.	Advance to full throwing program at 9 months.
No internal rotation	Isometrics for muscle re-education		May begin contact sports at 9 months.
Elbow, wrist, finger ROM			

FE, forward elevation; ER, external rotation; ADL, activities of daily living.

RESULTS

Neer and Foster first described the inferior capsular shift procedure in 1980[2] and reported uniformly satisfactory results in a series of 40 patients with multidirectional instability. A follow-up series of 100 additional patients in 1990 revealed similar results.[14] Pollock et al.[25] demonstrated the versatility of this procedure with 94% excellent and good results in a series of patients with unidirectional and bidirectional instability. Multiple other authors have subsequently shown the procedure's reliability sometimes with slight modification in technique.[7,25–30] Good and excellent results are noted routinely in approximately 90% of patients with recurrent instability ranging from 4% to 11% postoperatively. Although 70% to 90% of athletes return to play following open inferior capsular shift surgery, elite overhead athletes have only about a 50% chance to return to play at the same level.

Current arthroscopic techniques of Bankart repair using suture anchors have demonstrated results equal to open techniques and are laying to rest the notion that arthroscopic techniques are unreliable for instability surgery.[16] Although older techniques using bioabsorbable tacks and transglenoid techniques were not as reliable as open Bankart repair,[31] newer series reporting on suture anchor techniques routinely demonstrate good and excellent results between 91% and 95%.[4,8,12,32–34] Fabricciani et al.[16] reported no recurrences in a prospective series of 60 patients, half of whom were treated with open Bankart repair while the other half were treated arthroscopically. Better final range of motion was noted in the arthroscopic group, supporting one of the major theoretical advantages of this arthroscopic technique. Recurrent instability has been reported ranging from 0% to 11% with this arthroscopic technique. Return to sports ranges between 74% and 100%,[4,12,32,33] but overhead athletes still have more difficulty in returning to sport at the same level of play, with results between 55% and 68% reported.[4,33] Glenoid bony defects greater than 25% to 30% remain a significant cause of failure[9,11,12] and are an indication for open repair and bone grafting.

SUMMARY

The two extremes in the spectrum of instability include traumatic unidirectional instability, usually associated with labral pathology such as a Bankart lesion, and atraumatic multidirectional instability, usually associated with capsular laxity. Glenohumeral instability is a spectrum with significant overlap in presentation and pathologic lesions contributing to the problem. The surgeon must be able to identify all pathoanatomy contributing to the instability through a careful preoperative and intraoperative evaluation. Surgery is reserved for failure of conservative management, but when performed, should address all pathology contributing to the instability. The capabilities of arthroscopy are expanding continuously, and current arthroscopic techniques have been proven equal to open techniques for Bankart repair, the usual lesion of traumatic instability. Inferior capsular shift enjoys similar success in treating the usual lesions of atraumatic instability, a patulous capsule, and widened rotator interval. Successful management with arthroscopic or open procedures depends on identification of pathology, adequate mobilization and balanced repair of tissues, protection of the axillary nerve, and a safe rehabilitation program that allows adequate healing time for the repaired tissues. Current contraindications for the arthroscopic technique include glenoid bone loss >25% and an inability to repair capsular avulsions or defects. Each surgeon should use techniques with which he or she feels comfortable to achieve the above stated goals for successful management of either traumatic or atraumatic glenohumeral instability.

REFERENCES

1. McFarland EG, Kim TK, Park HB, et al. The effect of variation in definition on the diagnosis of multidirectional instability of the shoulder. *J Bone Joint Surg*. 2003;85A:2138–2144.
2. Neer CS II, Foster CR. Inferior capsular shift for inferior and multidirectional instability of the shoulder: a preliminary report. *J Bone Joint Surg*. 1980;62A:897–908.
3. Cole BJ, Millett PJ, Romeo AA, et al. Arthroscopic treatment of anterior glenohumeral instability: indications and techniques. *Instr Course Lect*. 2004;53:545–548.
4. Gartsman GM, Roddey TS, Hammerman SM. Arthroscopic treatment of anterior-inferior glenohumeral instability. *J Bone Joint Surg*. 2000;82A:991–1003.
5. Maffet MW, Gartsman GM, Moseley B. Superior labrum-biceps tendon complex lesions of the shoulder. *Am J Sports Med*. 1995; 23(1):93–98.
6. Bigliani LU, Pollock RG, Soslowsky LJ, et al. "Tensile properties of the inferior glenohumeral ligament." *J Orthop Res*. 1992;10:187–197.
7. Altchek DW, Warren RF, Skyhar MJ, et al. T-plasty modification of the Bankart procedure for multidirectional instability of the anterior and inferior types. *J Bone Joint Surg*. 1991;73A:105–112
8. Gartsman GM, Roddey TS, Hammerman SM. Arthroscopic treatment of bidirectional glenohumeral instability: two-to five year follow up. *J Shoulder Elbow Surg*. 2001;10(1):28–36.
9. Tauber M, Resch H, Forstner R, et al. Reasons for failure after surgical repair of anterior shoulder instability. *J Shoulder Elbow Surg*. 2004;13(3):279–285.
10. McIntyre LF, Caspari RB, Savoie FH III. The arthroscopic treatment of multidirectional shoulder instability: two-year results of a multiple suture technique. *Arthroscopy*. 1997;13:418–425.
11. Burkhart SS, DeBeer JF. Traumatic glenohumeral bone defects and their relationship to failure of arthroscopic Bankart repairs: significance of the inverted-pear glenoid and the humeral engaging Hill-Sachs lesion. *Arthroscopy*. 2000;16:677–694.
12. Kim SH, Ha KI, Cho YB, et al. Arthroscopic anterior stabilization of the shoulder: two to six-year follow-up. *J Bone Joint Surg Am*. 2003;85A:1511–1518.
13. Okamura K, Takiuchi T, Aoki M, et al. Labral shape after arthroscopic Bankart repair: comparisons between the anchor and Caspari methods. *Arthroscopy*. 2005;21(2):194–199.
14. Neer CS II. *Shoulder Reconstruction*. Philadelphia: WB Saunders, 1990:273–341.
15. Bigliani LU, Flatow EL. History, physical examination, and diagnostic modalities. In: McGinty JB, Caspari RB, Jackson RW, et al., eds. *Operative Arthroscopy*. New York: Raven Press; 1991:453–464.
16. Fabbriciani C, Milano G, Demontis A, et al. Arthroscopic vs. open treatment of Bankart lesion of the shoulder: a prospective randomized study. *J Bone Joint Surg Am*. 2004;86A:2574.
17. Wang VM, Sugalski MT, Levine WN, et al. Comparison of glenohumeral mechanics following a capsular shift and anterior tightening. *J Bone Joint Surg Am*. 2005;87:1312–1322.

18. Miller MD, Larsen KM, Luke T, et al. Anterior capsular shift volume reduction: an in vitro comparison of 3 techniques. *J Shoulder Elbow Surg*. 2003;12:350–354.
19. Bishop JY, Sprague M, Gelber J, et al. Interscalene regional anesthesia for shoulder surgery. *J Bone Joint Surg*. 2005;87A:974–979.
20. Neviaser TJ. The anterior labroligamentous periosteal sleeve avulsion lesion: a cause of anterior instability of the shoulder. *Arthroscopy*. 1993;9:17–21.
21. Sugalski MT, Wiater M, Levine WN, et al. An anatomic study of the humeral insertion of the inferior glenohumeral capsule. *J Shoulder Elbow Surg*. 2005;14:91–95.
22. Leslie JT Jr, Ryan TJ. The anterior axillary incision to approach the shoulder joint. *J Bone Joint Surg*. 1962;44A:1193–1196.
23. Flatow EL, Bigliani LU. Locating and protecting the axillary nerve in shoulder surgery: the tug test. *Orthop Rev*. 1992;21:503–505.
24. Boileau P, Ahrens P. The TOTS: a new technique to allow easy suture placement and improve capsular shift in arthroscopic Bankart repair. *Arthroscopy*. 2003;19:672–677.
25. Pollock RG, Owens JM, Flatow EL, et al. Operative results of the inferior capsular shift procedure for multidirectional instability of the shoulder. *J Bone Joint Surg Am*. 2000;82A:919–928.
26. Choi CH, Ogilvie-Harris DJ. Inferior capsular shift operation for multidirectional instability of the shoulder in players of contact sports. *Br J Sports Med*. 2002;36(4):190–294.
27. Cooper RA, Brems JJ. The inferior capsular-shift procedure for multidirectional instability of the shoulder. *J Bone Joint Surg*. 1992;74A:1516–1521.
28. Bigliani LU, Kurzweil PR, Schwartzbach CC, et al. Inferior capsular shift procedure for anterior inferior shoulder instability in athletes. *Am J Sports Med*. 1994;22:578–284.
29. Bak K, Spring BJ, Henderson JP. Inferior capsular shift procedure in athletes with multidirectional instability based on isolated capsular and ligamentous redundancy. *Am J Sports Med*. 2000;28(4):466–471.
30. Pagnani MJ, Dome DC. Surgical treatment of traumatic anterior shoulder instability in American football players. *J Bone Joint Surg*. 2002;84A:711–715.
31. Freedman KB, Smith AP, Romeo AA, et al. Open Bankart repair vs. arthroscopic repair with transglenoid sutures or bioabsorbable tacks for recurrent anterior instability of the shoulder: a meta-analysis. *Am J Sports Med*. 2004;32:1520–1527.
32. Mazzocca AD, Brown FM Jr, Carreira DS, et al. Arthroscopic anterior shoulder stabilization of collision and contact athletes. *Am J Sports Med*. 2005;33(1):52–60.
33. Ide J, Maeda S, Takagi K. Arthroscopic Bankart repair using suture anchors in athletes: patient selection and postoperative sports activity. *Am J Sports Med*. 2004;32:1899–1905.
34. Potzl W, Witt KA, Hackenberg L, et al. Results of suture anchor repair of anteroinferior shoulder instability: a prospective clinical study of 85 shoulders. *J Shoulder Elbow Surg*. 2003;12:322–326.

POSTERIOR SHOULDER INSTABILITY: DIAGNOSIS AND TREATMENT

WILLIAM N. LEVINE
ERIC M. GORDON

Sir Astley Cooper's 1839 report from Guy's Hospital on the details of a dislocation in an epileptic is considered the classic on posterior glenohumeral instability and contains a description of the characteristic findings of loss of external rotation, an anterior void with posterior fullness, and a detached subscapularis and reverse Hill-Sachs lesion confirming the diagnosis on postmortem exam. Cooper referred to this injury as "an accident which cannot be mistaken." Sixteen years later and still 40 years prior to the advent of x-ray studies, Malgaigne published a report of 37 cases of posterior dislocation, illustrating that with a thorough physical exam one can make a proper diagnosis. Despite these early reports of posterior instability, it remains one of the most commonly misdiagnosed and mistreated disorders in all of orthopaedics.

PATHOGENESIS

Etiology

Posterior instability is complex and multifactorial. It includes both dislocation and subluxation and may result from trauma, repetitive overuse or microtrauma, or without trauma. Traumatic posterior instability may result from direct forces applied to the humeral head or proximal shaft, or indirectly by way of a lever arm and/or muscle imbalances. Repetitive overuse or microtrauma is most often seen in younger athletic patients who participate in contact or overhead sports. Atraumatic instability may result from underlying bony and/or soft tissue abnormalities. Furthermore, it may be unidirectional, bidirectional with a posterior component, or multidirectional with a predominantly posterior component.

The most vulnerable position for traumatic posterior instability occurs with the shoulder in forward flexion, adduction, and internal rotation. This position will also reproduce symptoms in patients with recurrent instability. Axial loading through the humeral shaft acting as a lever arm, as occurs during a motor vehicle accident, drives the humeral head posteriorly. In cases of electrical shock or seizure, violent muscular contraction of the adductors and internal rotators (latissimus dorsi, pectoralis major, subscapularis, and teres major) may overwhelm the opposing external rotators (infraspinatus and teres minor) as well as bony and soft tissue restraints.

Certain anatomic variations predispose patients to atraumatic posterior instability. Bony abnormalities including excessive retroversion of the glenoid and humeral head, and glenoid dysplasia and hypoplasia have been implicated in the development of posterior instability. Ligamentous laxity, posterior or inferior capsular laxity, or labral dysplasia and aplasia further predispose patients to subluxation or frank posterior dislocation. Instability may also occur in the setting of muscular or structural imbalance exacerbated by certain positions. This may be further complicated by the presence of a volitional component of the patient to sublux or dislocate posteriorly.

Epidemiology

Posterior instability has a reported incidence of 2% to 5%. The incidence may in fact be higher owing to undetected and missed cases. Posterior dislocations and subluxations are very commonly missed in the emergency room with a reported incidence as high as 60% to 80%. This is typically owing to inappropriate radiographs—it is critically important to obtain 90-degree orthogonal radiographs to avoid this preventable missed diagnosis.

Approximately 50% of cases occur traumatically, mostly in men between 35 and 55 years old with as many as 15%

of cases bilaterally. Recurrent posterior shoulder instability primarily affects younger men between ages 20 and 30 years who participate in competitive overhead or contact sports with only about half of patients reporting a previous initiating injury.

More than 97% of posterior dislocations are *subacromial* in which the main component is internal rotation and the humeral head is fixed posteriorly. The lesser tuberosity is located in glenoid, and the greater tuberosity is no longer seen lateral to humeral head. Although historically, posterior dislocations were associated with shock or electroconvulsive therapy, this is now rarely the case.

Pathophysiology

Shoulder stability is a function of static and dynamic stabilizers as well as arm position. Contributing factors to static stabilization include bony, labral, ligamentous, and capsular contributing factors. Dynamic stabilizers include the rotator cuff and muscular attachments to the humerus. Variations in the anatomy may predispose patients to developing instability or may be the result of a traumatic event or series of events leading to recurrence of subluxation or dislocation. While a number of specific individual variations have been implicated in the development or recurrence of instability, the cause is multifactorial.

Normal glenoid osseus retroversion is approximately 4 to 7 degrees and varies widely among the population. Although excessive retroversion of the glenoid, as well the humeral head, have been implicated as primary causes of posterior instability, they may be more accurately considered as contributing factors if present. Localized erosion of the posterior glenoid occurring either primarily or as a result of repeated events of instability may further contribute to symptoms of instability. Primary or congenital glenoid dysplasia/hypoplasia is a very rare disorder characterized by incomplete ossification of the lower two thirds of the glenoid and adjacent scapular neck, and may be isolated or associated with other anomalies such as humeral head flattening or hypoplasia (Fig. 36-1). Far more common bony abnormalities include engaging defects of the anterior humeral head and fractures of the posterior rim of the glenoid, which, depending on size, play a critical role in posterior instability and require thorough evaluation to determine effective treatment.

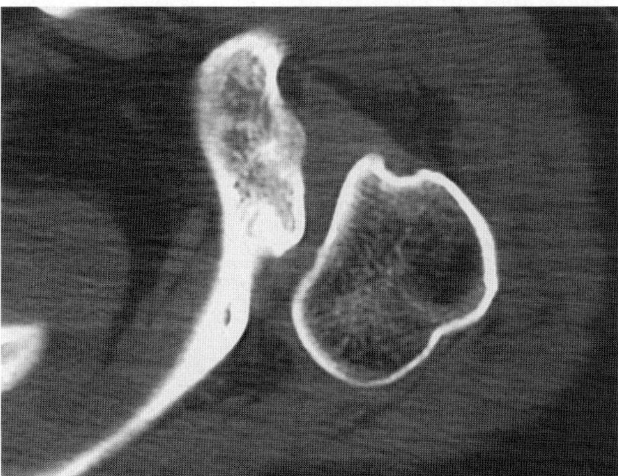

Figure 36-1 Axial computed tomogram of a 28-year-old RHD female with congenital hypoplasia and dislocation of the left shoulder.

Classification

Numerous systems of classification have been described, subdividing various types of posterior instability to assist in proper treatment and outcome determination. To date, however, no single classification system has been agreed on.

Acute: <6 weeks prior to reduction
Chronic: >6 weeks prior to reduction

Posterior dislocation may be unidirectional, bidirectional, or multidirectional with primarily posterior instability.

Heller classified posterior instability with the following system:

I. Traumatic dislocation/subluxation (dislocation: trauma, convulsions, electrocution; subluxation major and minor trauma)
   (a) Primary dislocation/primary subluxation
      i. Acute
      ii. Persistent
   (b) Recurrent dislocation/subluxation
      i. Posttraumatic
      ii. Posttraumatic voluntary
II. Atraumatic dislocation/subluxation
   (a) Primary dislocation/subluxation
      i. Acute
      ii. Persistent
   (b) Recurrent dislocation/subluxation
      i. Atraumatic
      ii. Atraumatic voluntary
      iii. Voluntary

DIAGNOSIS

History and Physical Examination

Diagnosis begins with a thorough history, which may or may not indicate a traumatic event. Patients may complain more about stiffness or functional disability than pain at the time of evaluation—especially if the evaluation is nonacute (past the first several weeks following the instability event). There is often a history of radiographs that have been interpreted as "normal." Patients with missed posterior dislocations often are being treated for "frozen shoulder." Other important components include a history of seizures (a posterior fracture-dislocation occurring without trauma is considered pathognomonic of seizure), diabetes (hypoglycemic seizure), alcohol or drug use, polytrauma, and psychiatric illness. Inquiry should be made regarding diseases or illness associated with ligamentous laxity such as Ehlers-Danlos syndrome. In athletes complaining of shoulder pain, it is important to ascertain details of their activities and which motions or positions elicit or aggravate their symptoms. Activities such as pitching, volleyball, gymnastics, swimming,

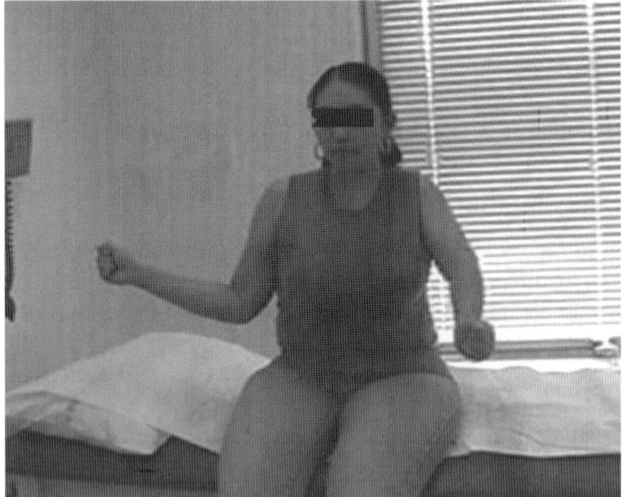

Figure 36-2 Clinical photo of patient from Figure 36-1 attempting maximal external rotation of both upper extremities. Notice the fixed internally rotated position of the left shoulder.

golf, archery, and contact sports place increased physiologic stresses on the glenohumeral joint that may lead to or exacerbate posterior instability. Attempts to reproduce symptoms with specific movements and positions should be made during the exam.

Physical examination begins with inspection, which may demonstrate difficulty with removal of coat or movements such as touching one's head. Attention should be paid to the symmetry and contour of the shoulders, muscle size and tone, and the appearance of bony prominences including the acromion, coracoid, and proximal humerus. Active and passive range of motions should be evaluated with the patient seated and in supine positions. The classic finding in fixed posterior dislocation is the inability to externally rotate on the affected side (Fig. 36-2). All patients should be evaluated for generalized ligamentous laxity, which includes the four standard parameters of index finger metacarpophalangeal (MCP) hyperextension, thumb abduction with palmar-flexed wrist, knee hyperextension, and elbow hyperextension.

Specific tests are useful in patients with recurrent instability who are reduced and/or asymptomatic at the time of exam. A positive posterior apprehension test elicits pain (and apprehension) with flexion, adduction, and internal rotation. The anterior and posterior load and shift test is performed with the patient positioned supine at the edge of the exam table, shoulder in neutral rotation, 45-degree abduction, and forward flexion. After gently loading the humeral head with an axial force directed proximally at the elbow, anteriorly and posteriorly translating forces are applied by directly grasping and moving the humeral head. This test is graded in the following manner:

+1 = Noticeable translation short of the glenolabral rim
+2 = Translation over the glenolabral rim with spontaneous reduction
+3 = Translation with complete dislocation requiring manual reduction

A translation of 2+ in any direction may be normal and therefore requires additional attention to patient responses of pain or apprehension with testing to properly diagnose posterior instability. The sulcus test/sulcus sign is performed by placing downward traction on the neutrally positioned arm and measuring the dimple or sulcus between the lateral acromion and humeral head. Voluntarism should be ascertained during the physical examination as it is a negative prognostic indicator for surgical intervention.

Radiologic Features

The minimum requirement for the proper radiologic evaluation of the shoulder in all cases should include three views: an anteroposterior (AP) (preferably performed perpendicular to the scapular plane), a scapular-Y or outlet view (90 degrees from the true AP), and an axillary view. Because routine AP and lateral x-ray views are often inadequate to establish diagnosis, it is imperative that an axillary view be obtained to confirm diagnosis (Figs. 36-3 to 36-5).

In the case of posterior dislocation, several findings may be present on AP radiographs. The *vacant glenoid* or *posterior rim sign* occurs with the loss of normal humeral overlap on the glenoid. A distance of >6 mm between the anterior glenoid rim and humeral head suggests a posterior dislocation. A *trough line* or compression fracture of the anteromedial humeral head occurs in approximately 75% of posterior dislocations. This *reverse Hill-Sachs lesion*, often occurring at the time of the original injury, may enlarge with subsequent dislocations. The cystic head sign or *light bulb sign* results from the fixed internal rotation of the humerus. On the scapular-Y view with a posterior dislocation, the humeral head may be seen posterior to the glenoid. Up to 50% of traumatic posterior dislocations will have nondisplaced fractures, mostly of the lesser

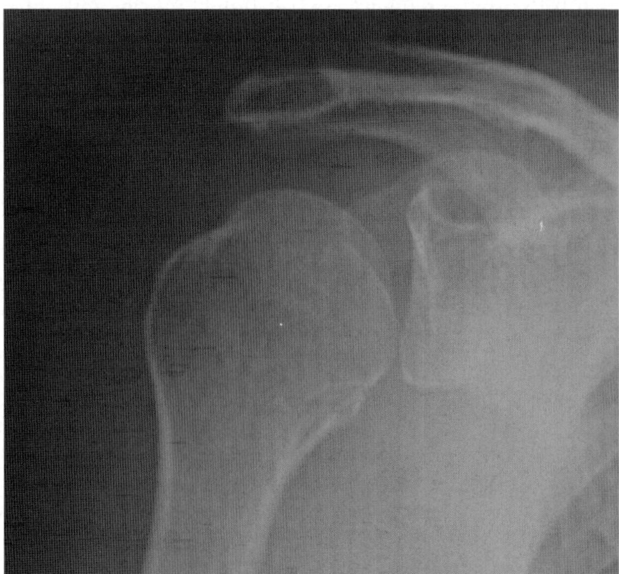

Figure 36-3 A 47-year-old RHD male with a missed posterior dislocation. True anteroposterior (AP) read by radiologist as "normal."

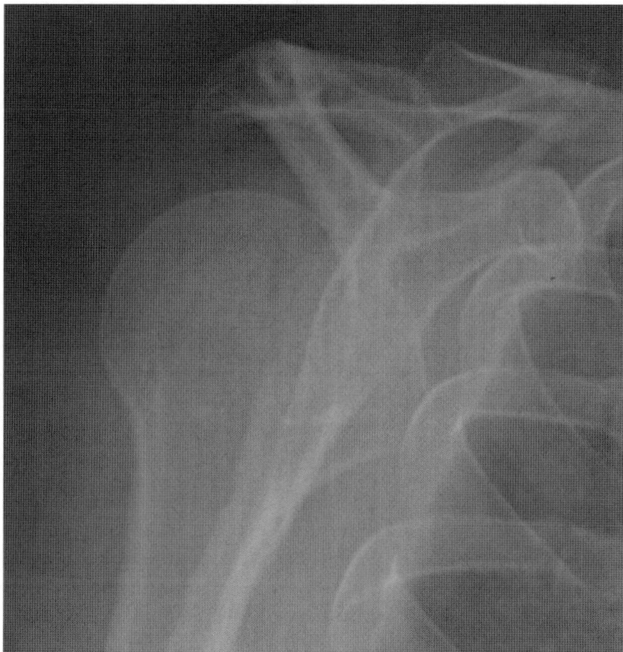

Figure 36-4 Scapular lateral radiograph of patient from Figure 36-3 also read as "normal."

tuberosity, owing to avulsion of the subscapularis, and less often of the posteroglenoid rim (reverse Bankart). Computed tomography is useful for further diagnosis and bony evaluation as well as preoperative planning in the case of bony injury or abnormality requiring surgical reconstruction (Fig. 36-6).

MRI may be necessary in cases that do not have significant bony abnormalities and may show any of the following:

- Reverse Bankart: Avulsion of posterior glenoid labrum
- POLPSA lesion: Posterior labral capsular periosteal sleeve avulsion

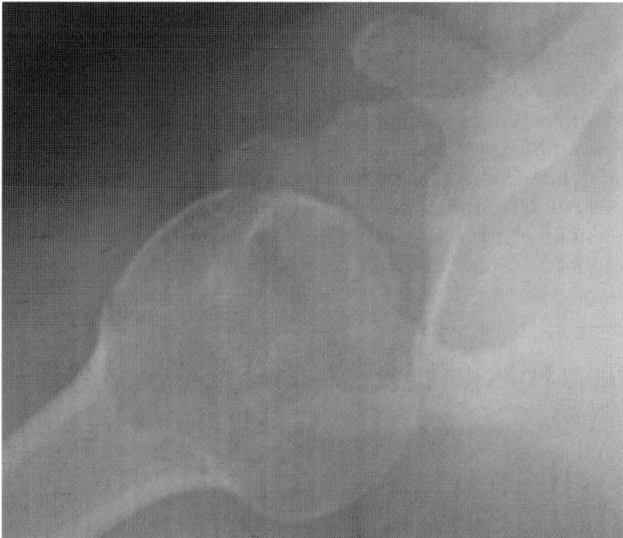

Figure 36-5 Axillary radiograph confirming the posterior dislocation in same patient from Figures 36-3 and 36-4.

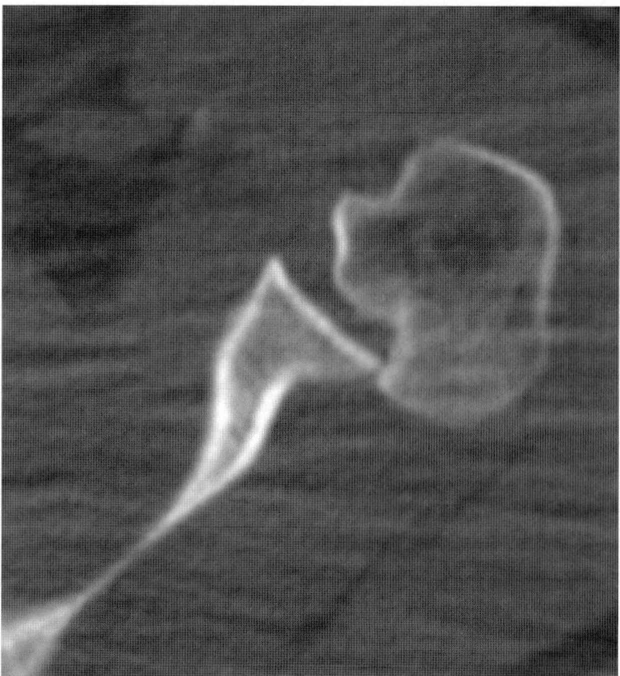

Figure 36-6 Axial computed tomogram in a 37-year-old RHD male following a seizure.

- Reverse HAGL: A posterior humeral avulsion of the inferior glenohumeral ligament
- The Kim lesion: An incomplete and concealed lesion of the posteroinferior labrum

Diagnostic Workup Algorithm

From the history:

- Traumatic, microtraumatic, atraumatic
- Acute or chronic
- Voluntary, involuntary; psych history
- Associated injury, abnormality, illnesses (diabetes mellitus, alcohol abuse, seizure)
- Previous treatment/therapy

From the physical exam:

- Unidirectional, bidirectional, or MDI with posterior instability
- Subluxation or dislocation
- Reduced or fixed
- Is there generalized ligamentous laxity?
- Positional instability

From diagnostic imaging:

- Is there a frank dislocation or subluxation present?
- Associated fractures/bony abnormalities (x-ray views, CT)
  - Bony reverse Bankart or reverse Hill-Sachs (percent/size of defect)
  - Other fractures: tuberosity, proximal humerus
  - Glenoid hypoplasia/dysplasia
  - Excessive glenoid retroversion

- Soft tissue injury or abnormality
  - Reverse Bankart (soft tissue)
  - Posterior HAGL
  - POLPSA
  - Kim Lesion
  - Redundant axillary pouch
  - Widened rotator interval

TREATMENT

Acute Traumatic Posterior Instability

Acute, traumatic posterior dislocations can be managed in much the same way as anterior dislocations, when recognized acutely. Following satisfactory muscular relaxation and pain control, with the patient in the supine position, longitudinal and lateral traction should be applied with gentle internal rotation followed by external rotation to disimpact the head and stretch and then relax the posterior capsule. Another method of disimpaction is to flex the arm to 90 degrees and gently adduct. Pressure is then applied directly to the posterior humeral head anteriorly to complete the reduction.

Care should be taken to perform maneuvers gently and avoid creating fractures if the head is locked. Following reduction, a sling in neutral to external rotation may be used for immobilization; however, if there is concern for recurrent instability, a gunslinger type brace or spica cast should be applied. The recommended position of immobilization to optimize stability and healing of the posterior labrum and capsule is abduction, external rotation, and extension for a period of 4 weeks.

Open reduction is indicated when there is a large impaction defect or the injury is more than 6 weeks old (chronic, "locked"). Other indications for surgery in the acute setting include displaced tuberosity or glenoid fracture requiring reduction, or an open injury. A deltopectoral approach is made and is usually all that is necessary in most patients. A separate posterior incision is rarely required to facilitate reduction.

Following disimpaction, defects smaller than 25% can be repaired using subchondral elevation with bone grafting if the injury is <2 weeks old. Small defects >2 weeks old may be filled using transfer of the subscapularis (McLaughlin) or the lesser tuberosity (Neer); however these are nonanatomic repairs that risk rotator cuff weakness or dysfunction and can complicate future procedures. Larger defects ≤40% to 50% can be filled with structural allograft. Repairs should be assessed intraoperatively for stability, addressing injuries to the labrum, capsule, rotator cuff, or glenoid if necessary. In the case of defects >50% of the humeral head or presence of significant osteoarthritis, a hemiarthroplasty should be performed. Total shoulder arthroplasty is a surgical option for an older patient with significant glenoid articular wear. Postoperatively the patient should be immobilized in neutral rotation for 6 weeks before initiation of therapy except in cases of simple arthroplasty, which can begin gentle passive motion immediately.

A final option is nonoperative treatment leaving the patient with a fixed dislocation. This is recommended in cases of prolonged dislocation, particularly in the elderly or low functional individuals or in cases of only minor disability.

In cases of traumatic posterior dislocation, poorer results are to be expected with increasing duration of dislocation, increasing size of a humeral head defect, increasing degree of deformity or arthritis, and the presence of concomitant injury. Complications include recurrence of dislocation, osteoarthritis secondary to trauma or abnormal joint forces from reconstruction, osteonecrosis, and loss of motion.

Recurrent Posterior Instability

Failure rates as high as 50% have been reported given the complex and multifactorial nature of recurrent posterior instability. In almost all cases, treatment of posterior instability begins with nonoperative measures unless symptoms of pain or dysfunction are present to a degree that warrants more immediate surgery. Surgery must be tailored to address each specific underlying component of instability. Physical therapy should include rotational and scapular strengthening with an emphasis on external rotation strengthening (particularly the infraspinatus) while avoiding impingement, voluntary episodes of instability, or positions that may result in subluxation while restoring normal shoulder motion and strength. Attention should also be given to muscular imbalances, weakness, or disturbances of normal coordinated motion. In general, nonoperative measures should be used for a minimum of 3 to 6 months before considering the patient a candidate for surgery, although in certain cases or causes of instability such as injury where nonoperative treatment has been shown to be less effective, the decision to proceed with surgery sooner is warranted.

Contraindications to surgery include voluntary instability owing to an underlying psychologic problem that is better addressed with psychotherapy, biofeedback, and muscle retraining. Patients with a poorly controlled seizure disorder require strict medical management. Patients with ligamentous hyperlaxity also represent a treatment challenge that is best addressed with extensive nonoperative management.

When operative management is chosen, it is essential to determine the degree and direction of instability and identify all bony and soft tissue abnormalities. Various procedures are available that address bony and soft tissue abnormalities and can be performed with either open or arthroscopic technique. Although more technically demanding, arthroscopic procedures have the advantage of reduced hospital stay, less postoperative pain, and improved cosmesis.

Open Procedures Addressing Bony Abnormalities

Posterior bone blocks are used in patients with congenital posterior dislocation, glenoid hypoplasia, and posterior bony defects. A posterior deltoid-splitting approach obviates the need for any tendon detachment and exposes the interval between the infraspinatus and teres minor, which is itself split, exposing the posterior capsule. A horizontal or T-shaped capsulotomy exposes the posterior glenohumeral

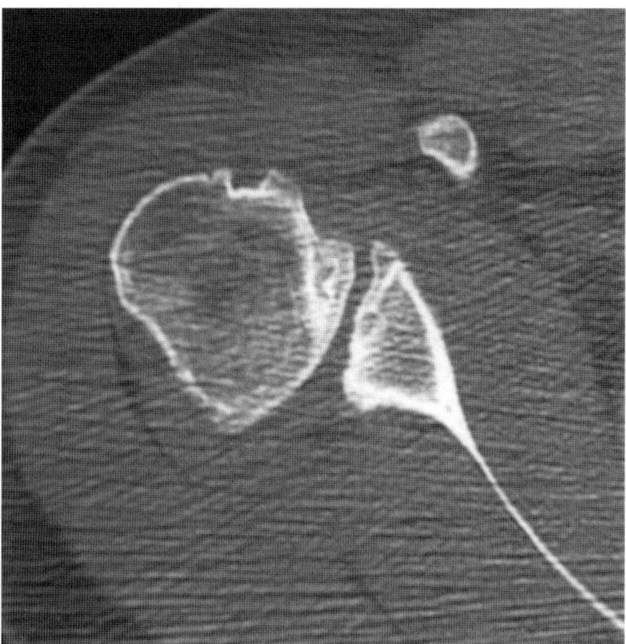

Figure 36-7 This is an axial CT scan demonstrating significant posterior glenoid bone deficiency, mild posterior subluxation, and early degenerative joint disease (DJD) in a 23-year-old RHD male who previously underwent an arthroscopic posterior labral repair, which has failed.

joint. An allograft bone block is secured with two screws to the posterior scapular neck at midlevel, projecting extracapsularly past the glenoid margin. Bone blocks are more often used in secondary procedures when primary soft tissue procedures have failed (Figs. 36-7 to 36-9).

In the case of excessive glenoid retroversion, an opening wedge osteotomy of the scapular neck or glenoid plasty can be used. This was originally performed using a posteroinferior acromion wedge of bone to fill the defect without the use of hardware for fixation. Results of this procedure have been mixed, partly because of the technically demanding nature and high complication rate, which includes glenoid articular fracture, nonunion, loss of graft position, osteonecrosis, degenerative arthritis, and resultant impingement.

Open Procedures Addressing Soft Tissue Abnormalities

A posterior-inferior capsular shift through a posterior approach has been used in patients with unidirectional, bidirectional (posterior and inferior), and multidirectional instability with a predominantly posterior component with good to excellent results regardless of direction or cause. Using a 60-degree oblique incision, the deltoid is split in a posterolateral raphe extending down no greater than 5 cm (to protect the axillary nerve) from the posterolateral corner of the acromion, and detached medially up to 4 cm for improved exposure. The infraspinatus is separated from the supraspinatus and teres minor and carefully elevated off the underlying capsule from medial to the glenoid

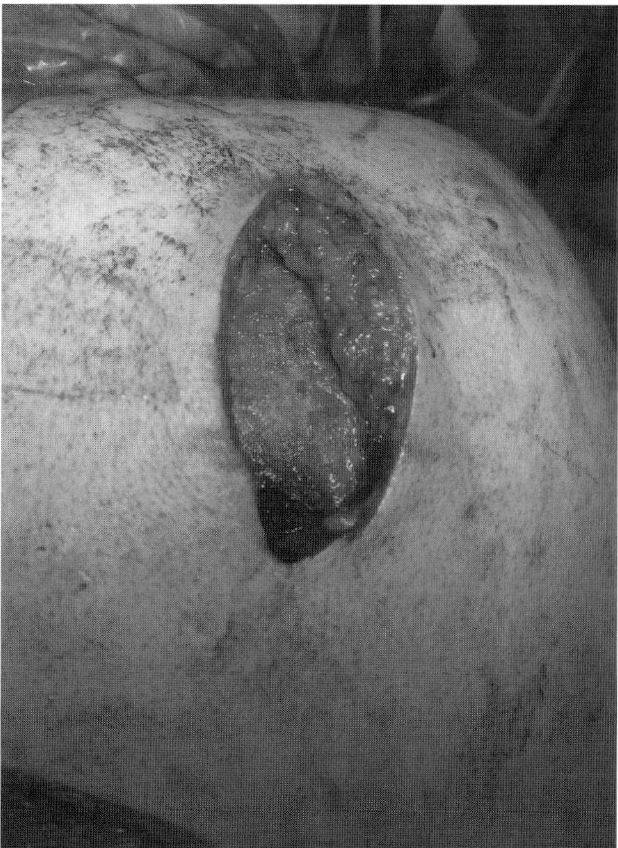

Figure 36-8 Intraoperative view of a posterior deltoid-splitting approach to the glenohumeral joint in the 23-year-old RHD male who previously underwent an arthroscopic posterior labral repair that had failed (same patient as in Fig. 36-7).

rim out laterally to its humeral insertion. The infraspinatus is then incised either obliquely creating two tendon flaps or vertically, if the tendon is attenuated, leaving a 1-cm stump on the greater tuberosity. The capsule is incised 1 cm medial to its humeral insertion, leaving a cuff parallel to the anatomic neck with nonabsorbable mobilizing sutures placed along the free medial edge. With increasing degrees of capsular laxity, a larger extent of inferior dissection, capsular incision, and shifting of inferior tissue superiorly should be performed. This is performed by making a horizontal capsular incision (T-fashion split), creating flaps inferiorly and superiorly. The superior flap is reattached to the cuff on the humerus shifting it inferiorly and then reinforced with attachment of the inferior flap shifting it superiorly and obliterating the inferior pouch. The infraspinatus is repaired placing the lateral portion deep to the medial portion, adding further reinforcement. Postoperatively the patient is immobilized for 4 to 6 weeks in neutral rotation with slight abduction prior to initiating therapy.

Repair of posterior labral injuries/reverse Bankart by open technique may be performed through a posterior deltoid-splitting approach with development of the interval between the infraspinatus and teres minor, and a vertical capsular incision to expose the joint. Suture anchor labral repair is then performed.

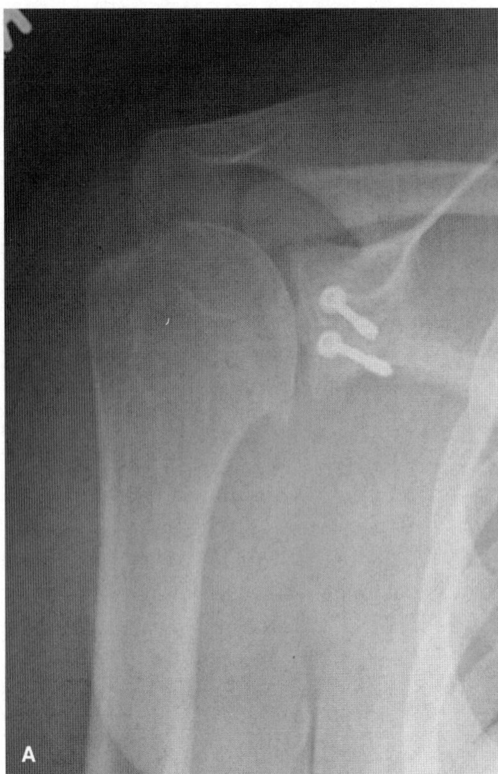

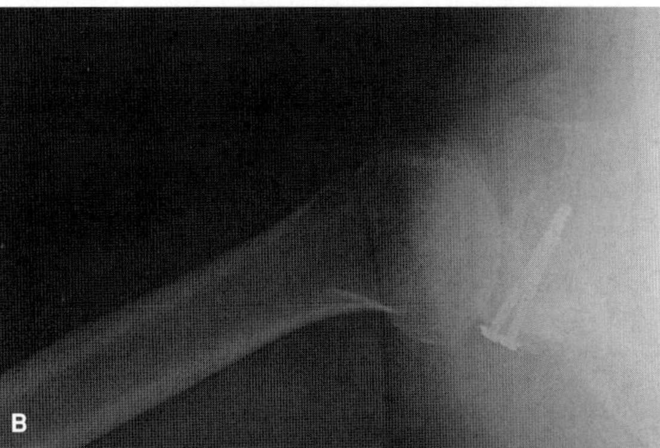

Figure 36-9 Postoperative true anteroposterior (AP) radiograph (**A**) and axillary (**B**) showing bone graft fixed with two screws and washers (same patient as in Figs. 36-7 and 36-8).

Arthroscopic Procedures

Arthroscopic approaches provide excellent visualization and are well suited for addressing the anatomy of the capsulolabral complex of the glenohumeral joint. Arthroscopic procedures are well developed for the repair of pathology specific to posterior instability and include reverse Bankart repair, capsular plication, and rotator interval closure, when indicated. Concurrent pathology such as rotator cuff tears, impingement, and SLAP lesions can be addressed at the same time. Regional or general anesthesia is used with patients in the lateral decubitus position and the arm in lateral traction.

The reverse Bankart lesion can be clearly visualized through a standard anterosuperior portal. Dual posterior portals provide access to the posterior inferior labrum, which can be repaired with suture anchors. The bone beneath the labrum should be decorticated to provide a bleeding bed, and anchors should be placed into the glenoid rim rather than the neck. The size of the lesion dictates the number of anchors necessary to provide secure fixation and restoration of the labral "bumper" (Figs. 36-10 and 36-11).

Posteroinferior capsular redundancy can be reduced with capsular plication using curved, corkscrew suture passers or crescent hooks after first abrading the capsule with a nonaggressive shaver. Nonabsorbable braided sutures are used, and capsular tissue is gathered toward the glenoid labrum (Figs. 36-12 and 36-13). Alternatively, if the posterior labrum is deficient or the capsular plication suture is felt to be pulling the labrum away from the glenoid, a suture anchor should be used for the plication.

Widened rotator interval closure begins with preparation of the capsule of that region with a rasp or shaver to elicit a bleeding response. Using a spinal needle, a braided suture is passed 1 cm medial to the humeral insertion of the supraspinatus, anterior to its anterior edge

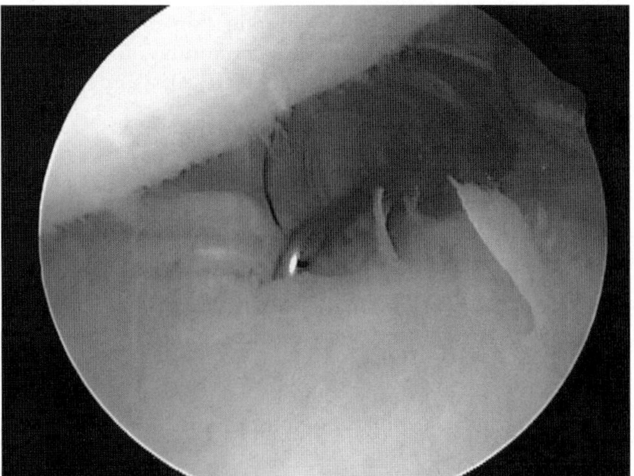

Figure 36-10 20 year-old RHD elite hockey player with right shoulder traumatic posterior labral tear. Anterosuperior viewing portal shows a posterior labral tear from 7 to 11 o'clock (probe is in tear at the 9 o'clock position).

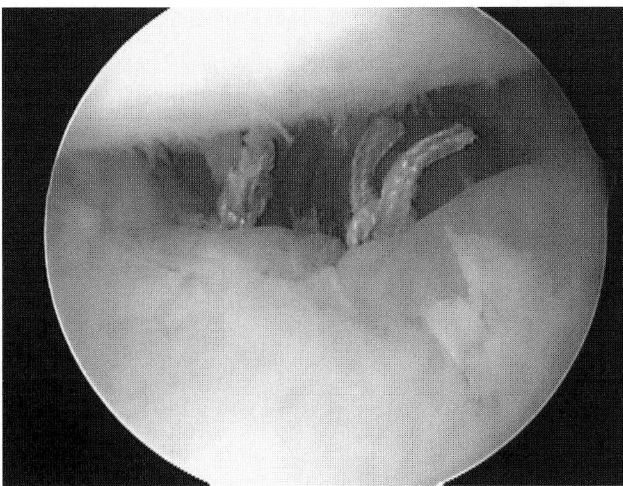

Figure 36-11 Anterosuperior viewing portal showing completed labral repair from 7 o'clock to 11 o'clock in same patient as in Figure 36-10.

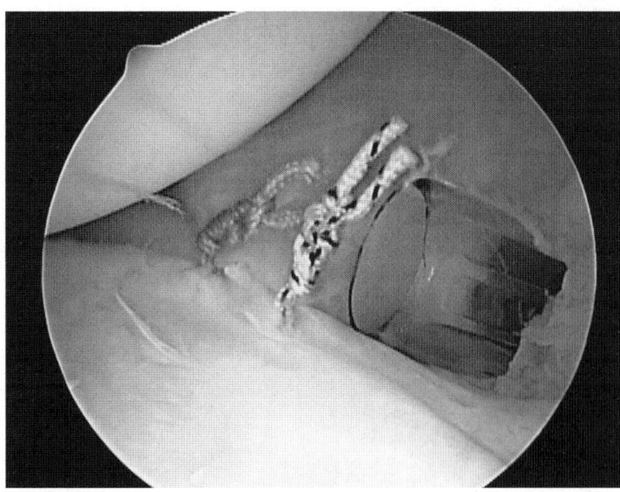

Figure 36-13 Anterosuperior viewing portal showing completed posterior capsular plication (same patient as in Fig. 36-12).

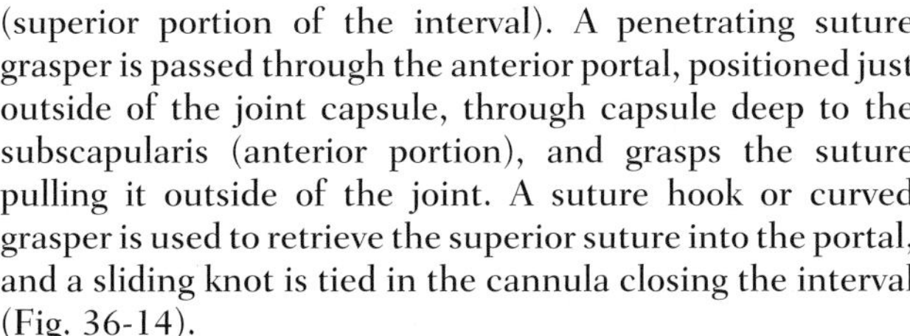

(superior portion of the interval). A penetrating suture grasper is passed through the anterior portal, positioned just outside of the joint capsule, through capsule deep to the subscapularis (anterior portion), and grasps the suture pulling it outside of the joint. A suture hook or curved grasper is used to retrieve the superior suture into the portal, and a sliding knot is tied in the cannula closing the interval (Fig. 36-14).

Postoperative care of patients following posterior arthroscopic repairs and stabilization procedures should begin with sling/brace immobilization with the arm in abduction and neutral to slight external rotation worn for 3 to 6 weeks full time depending on the type of repair and reliability of the patient. Gentle passive range of motion exercises can begin at 3 to 6 weeks followed by gradual strengthening with an emphasis on external rotation.

OUTCOMES AND CONCLUSION

Factors considered when evaluating outcomes include recurrence of instability, level of function and ability to perform activities of daily living (ADLs), return to previous activity, return to sport, pain, and general patient satisfaction. Scoring systems used to standardize and measure outcomes include the American Society of Shoulder and Elbow Surgeons (ASES) score, the simple shoulder test (SST), Rowe score, UCLA score, L'Insalata score, visual analog score, and SF-36 score.

With increased understanding of the anatomy and mechanics of shoulder instability, improved diagnostic imaging, and arthroscopic techniques tailored toward specific pathology, tremendous strides have been made in the management of posterior instability.

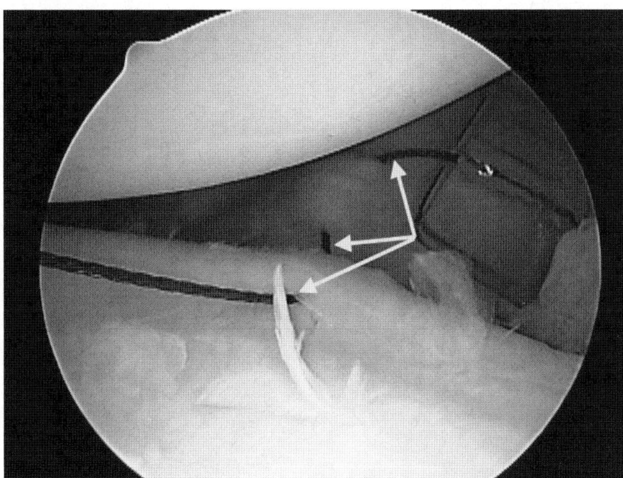

Figure 36-12 Anterosuperior viewing portal in a 15-year-old RHD female with multidirectional/posterior instability. The *arrows* point to a nitinol wire as it passes through the posteroinferior capsule into the intact labrum.

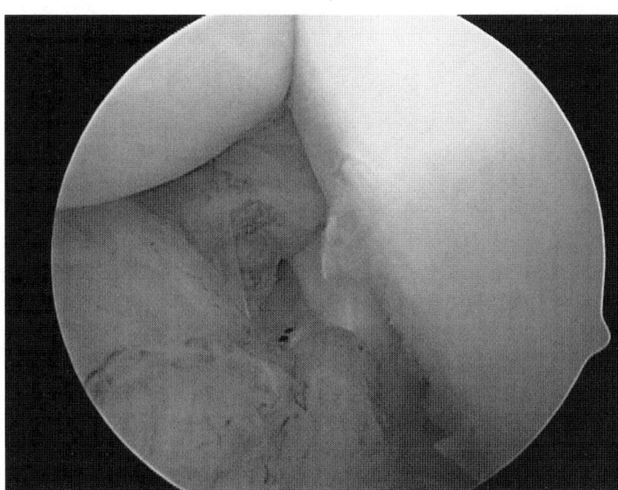

Figure 36-14 Rotator interval closure viewed from a posterior arthroscopic portal in a 17-year-old RHD female with multidirectional instability with posterior symptoms.

SUGGESTED READINGS

Heller KD, Forst J, Forst R, et al. Posterior dislocation of the shoulder: recommendation for a classification. *Arch Orthop Trauma Surg*. 1994;113:228–231.

Matsen FA 3rd, Titelman RM, Lippitt SB, et al. Glenohumeral instability. In: Rockwood CA Jr, Matsen FA 3rd, Wirth MA, et al., eds. *The Shoulder*. Vol 2. 3rd ed. Philadelphia: WB Saunders; 2004:655–794.

Robinson CM, Aderinto J. Posterior shoulder dislocations and fracture-dislocations. *J Bone Joint Surg Am*. 2005;87:639–650.

Robinson CM, Aderinto J. Recurrent posterior shoulder instability. *J Bone Joint Surg Am*. 2005;87:883–892.

ROTATOR CUFF IMPINGEMENT SYNDROME: DIAGNOSIS AND TREATMENT

CYRUS LASHGARI

Shoulder pain is the second most common musculoskeletal complaint after back pain encountered by the medical profession. Since Neer's description in 1972, subacromial impingement syndrome has become the most common shoulder diagnosis made by the orthopaedic surgeon. Despite its frequency, care must be taken to ensure the proper diagnosis is made and appropriate treatment instituted.

PATHOGENESIS

Etiology

The cause of rotator cuff pathology remains controversial. It is unclear if the spectrum of rotator cuff disease is a direct result of mechanical impingement or if intrinsic factors lead to cuff disease and secondarily cause changes within the coracoacromial arch. Neer believed that the rotator cuff impinges on the overlying CA arch, leading to repetitive microtrauma. Progressive extrinsic injury leads to eventual rotator cuff tears. Bigliani et al. showed that acromial morphology could worsen this extrinsic compression by narrowing the subacromial space. Acromions were divided into type I (flat), type II (curved), or type III (hooked). Hooked acromions were associated with 73% of the rotator cuff tears in their cadaver study. In a separate cadaver study, Flatow et al. showed that there was contact between the rotator cuff and acromion. This occurred over the supraspinatus and was more pronounced with type III acromions. Extrinsic compression worsens with a decrease in the subacromial space. This can occur from multiple additional causes such as acromioclavicular spurs, primary bursal swelling, or a laterally sloped acromion.

Abnormal motion of the humeral head with elevation, dynamic impingement, may worsen extrinsic compression. The rotator cuff functions to keep the humeral head centered on the glenoid as the arm is elevated. Several studies have shown that with an injured or weakened rotator cuff, the humeral head moves superiorly abutting the coracoacromial arch. Restoration of rotator cuff strength and function should decrease this dynamic compression.

Other investigators believe that intrinsic causes are more important in the development of rotator cuff pathology. Ogata and Uhthoff have described primary degenerative tendinopathy involving the rotator cuff and suggested that this may lead to tendon tears. Several studies have shown decreased vascularity in the area of the rotator cuff where tears are commonly seen. One study showed a differential pattern of vascularity between the bursal and articular side of the rotator cuff. The articular surface showed a decrease in blood supply relative to the bursal surface. This may help to explain why most partial rotator cuff tears occur on the articular side of the cuff. If extrinsic compression were the only or main cause of rotator cuff tears, it would stand to reason that the tears would be predominately bursal in origin. Although there is currently no consensus, it is probable that a combination of these factors leads to the development of rotator cuff disease.

Classification

Neer described three classes of impingement. These stages consisted of increasing damage to the rotator cuff and appeared age dependent. Further studies using MRI and ultrasound have confirmed an increasing rate of rotator cuff disease as patients age. Stage I consisted of edema and hemorrhage of the cuff and bursa. Stage II consisted of fibrosis and tendonitis of the rotator cuff, whereas stage III disease consisted of rotator cuff tearing. In practice, impingement can be classified according to the status of the rotator cuff. For those patients with intact rotator cuffs, nonoperative measures are exhausted before surgery is indicated. In patients with rotator cuff tears, surgical intervention should be discussed sooner, especially in patients younger than 65 years of age. In these patients, prolonged nonoperative therapy may lead to irreversible changes in the rotator cuff. These include muscle atrophy, fatty degeneration, changes in tendon morphology, and degenerative joint changes.

DIAGNOSIS

History

The diagnosis of subacromial impingement syndrome begins with a thorough history. Pain is the most common symptom. It is often described as a dull ache of the anterolateral shoulder radiating to the deltoid insertion. Pain is often worsened by overhead activities or extension of the arm behind the back. Activities with the arm at the side are usually pain free. Night pain often awakening the patient from sleep is a common complaint. Complaints such as stiffness, crepitus, or instability are less commonly associated with impingement syndrome and should alert the physician to the possibility of an alternate diagnosis. Older patients, in particular, should be evaluated for osteoarthritis. Patients younger than 40 years of age with shoulder pain often have instability leading to secondary impingement. Women between the ages of 40 and 60 years, diabetics, and those with thyroid disorders should be carefully evaluated for adhesive capsulitis.

Cervical spine disease commonly masquerades as shoulder pain. Pain radiating past the elbow, often associated with complaints of numbness and tingling, should raise concern about this diagnosis. A history of pain dependent more on neck than arm position also suggests a cervical cause. In contrast to patients with impingement syndrome, patients with cervical disc disease often state that their pain is better with their arm over their head. Pain into the upper trapezius is not necessarily related to the cervical spine. It is a common complaint in patients with shoulder disorders and is secondary to abnormal shoulder mechanics.

Most patients will describe a gradual onset of symptoms without a specific traumatic event. A recent onset of a new exercise routine or greater than normal physical activity such as heavy yard work often is described as the initiating event. Treatments initiated by the primary physician or patient should be documented. Activity modifications, medications, injections, and therapy are commonly tried before seeing the orthopaedic surgeon. The effect of these treatments is helpful in making the proper diagnosis. For example, a subacromial injection of cortisone or local anesthetic that relieves the pain is highly suggestive of impingement syndrome.

Physical Exam

The patient should be gowned so that both shoulders, including the scapulas, can be examined. The initial evaluation of the patient should include an examination of the cervical spine. Cervical spondylosis and radiculopathy often mimic intrinsic shoulder pathology. The physical exam includes motor and sensory testing of the entire upper extremity. Specific tests such as the Spurling (extension with rotation of the neck to the involved side) and Lhermitte (compression and flexion of the neck) maneuver are performed. Any reproduction of the patient's symptoms suggests that the cervical spine is at least partially involved. It must be remembered that both neck and shoulder pathology can coexist in the same patient.

The shoulder exam starts with inspection. Muscle wasting, suggestive of a chronic rotator cuff tear or peripheral nerve lesion, is documented. Range of motion is evaluated by standing behind the patient. This allows for evaluation of scapular rhythm and winging as active motion is evaluated. Forward elevation, external rotation in 90 degrees of abduction, external rotation at the side, and internal rotation are recorded both actively and passively. Although there often is a painful arc, the motion in patients with impingement syndrome is usually well preserved. Long-standing cases may show a mild decrease in motion, especially in internal rotation. A more profound loss of both active and passive motion in the shoulder suggests the diagnosis of adhesive capsulitis, assuming there is no significant glenohumeral arthritis.

Strength testing of the rotator cuff is performed next. Supraspinatus strength is examined using the Jobe test. The patient resists a downward force after the arm is placed in the plane of the scapula elevated to shoulder level with the thumb pointed toward the ground. The infraspinatus is tested with resisted external rotation with the arms at the side and elbows flexed to 90 degrees. The arms should be placed in internal rotation at the start of the test to isolate the infraspinatus. The teres minor is isolated with use of the horn blower's test. The arm is brought into 90 degrees of abduction and neutral rotation. The patient is then asked to rotate the shoulder externally to 90 degrees with the thumb pointed posteriorly. The subscapularis is tested either with the lift-off test or abdominal compression test. Patients with impingement syndrome generally have preserved strength although testing may elicit pain. This is especially true with the Jobe test. If there is significant pain, the patient may appear weak although the rotator cuff is intact.

Impingement signs are evaluated after strength testing. The Neer and Hawkins tests are most commonly performed. The Neer sign is performed by elevating the arm in the scapular plane while stabilizing the scapula. The patient complains of pain as the supraspinatus tendon impinges on the acromion usually above 70 degrees of elevation. The Hawkins sign is performed by internally rotating the arm with the arm in 90 degrees of forward flexion with the elbow flexed 90 degrees.

The exam is completed by testing for instability. In the young patient, instability can cause secondary impingement. The apprehension test is performed by bringing the arm into 90 degrees of abduction with the patient supine. Progressive external rotation is performed, trying to elicit apprehension as the patient feels the humeral head sliding anteriorly. The relocation test is then performed by applying a posteriorly directed force on the arm. The test is positive if there is relief of pain and/or apprehension. If instability is suspected as the cause of the impingement, the treatment will differ from that for primary subacromial impingement syndrome. Failure to appreciate mild instability is a leading cause of failed subacromial decompressions.

Differential injections help isolate the anatomic area responsible for the pain. The Neer impingement test consists of an injection of local anesthetic into the subacromial space. If the patient's pain is relieved or decreased, it is assumed that the subacromial space is a source of pain. If an injection of local anesthetic and/or cortisone into the subacromial space does not relieve a patient's symptoms, the diagnosis of impingement syndrome is questioned. In this setting, injections into the acromioclavicular joint or into the glenohumeral joint are helpful in evaluating other possible sources of pain.

Radiologic Testing

Standard radiographs of the shoulder should include an anteroposterior (AP) in internal rotation, scapular AP in external rotation, axillary, and supraspinatus outlet view. These films may reveal other causes of shoulder pain such as calcific tendonitis, osteoarthrosis of the glenohumeral or acromioclavicular joint, or an os acromiale. The supraspinatus outlet view is a lateral view with a 10-degree caudal tilt, affording a better view of acromial morphology. Typically there will be few abnormalities found in a patient with isolated subacromial impingement. Acromial spurring, sclerosis of the greater tuberosity, and subchondral cysts may be present.

Additional imaging includes plain film arthrogram, MRI, and ultrasound. These tests are often ordered to evaluate for tears of the rotator cuff. MRI gives the most additional information, allowing for evaluation of the labrum, AC joint, and biceps tendon. In well-trained hands, ultrasound is an inexpensive alternative for evaluation of the cuff. Although not

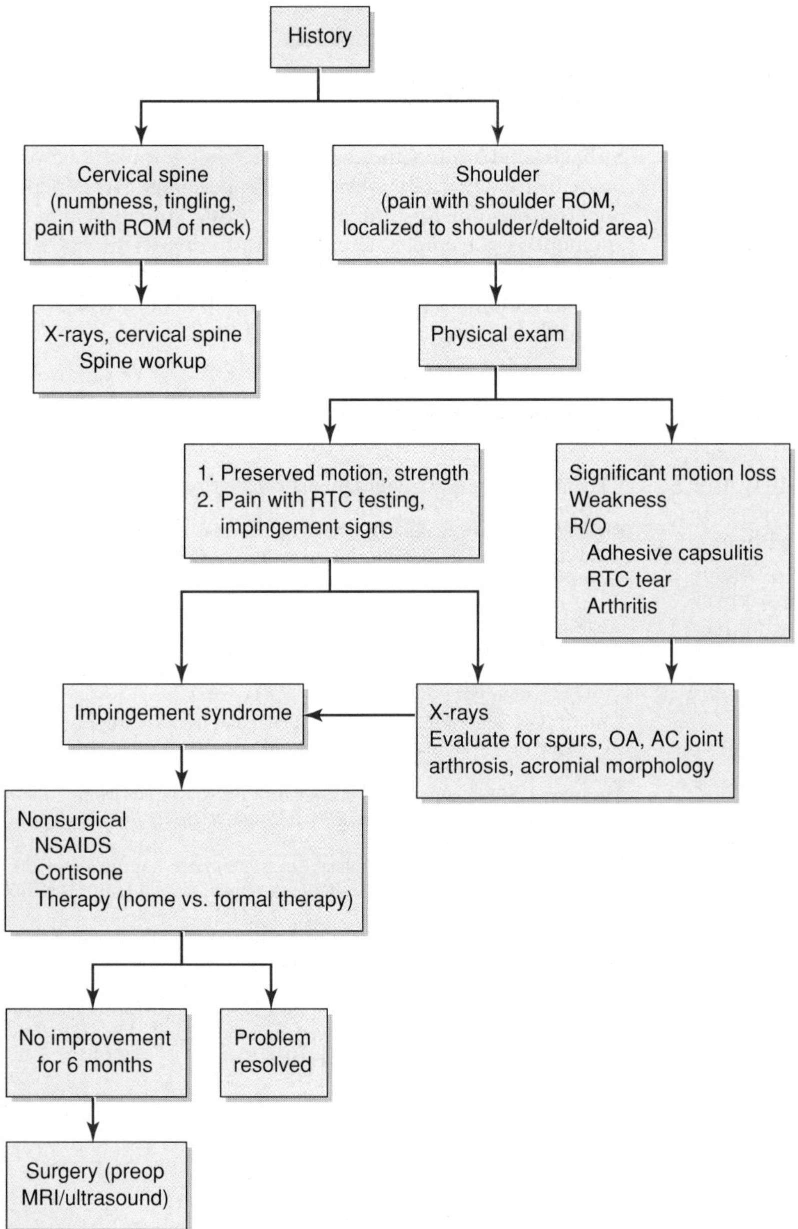

Figure 37-1 Diagnostic workup algorithm.

needed for the diagnosis and management of impingement syndrome, additional imaging is often obtained if nonoperative measures fail (Fig. 37-1).

TREATMENT

Nonsurgical Treatment

Historically, nonsurgical management has proved quite successful for subacromial impingement. Success rates of 70% to 80% have been seen across several studies. Options include activity modification, nonsteroidal anti-inflammatory drugs (NSAIDs), rehabilitation exercises, cortisone injections, and modalities such as ultrasound. Although these options are well established, few controlled trials have been done proving their efficacy.

NSAIDs, which have both anti-inflammatory and analgesic properties, are an integral part of most nonsurgical protocols. With the recent concern about cardiovascular side effects with these medications, it is advisable to try to limit their use to short periods (1 to 3 months) at the smallest effective dose. Acetaminophen can be tried as the first line of medication. If the pain is not well controlled with these medications, the use of cortisone injections into the subacromial space is indicated. Because of their deleterious effects on normal tissue, cortisone injections are used judiciously. In general, cortisone should be limited to three injections spaced at least 3 months apart. Steroid injections are particularly helpful in patients experiencing significant night pain.

Exercise is the most important aspect of nonsurgical therapy. After rest and medication have reduced the acute inflammation and pain, stretching and strengthening exercises can begin. The goal of stretching exercises is to restore a full range of motion through long, slow stretches with minimal pain. After range of motion is improved, strengthening of the rotator cuff and surrounding musculature can begin. Opinions differ as to the need for supervision by a physical therapist. Physical therapists may help those who need more encouragement and guidance. They also have the ability to use modalities such as ultrasound, phonophoresis, and iontophoresis to improve pain control. Despite these potential advantages, studies have shown no difference between supervised and unsupervised therapy.

Operative Treatment

If the patient's symptoms persist for 3 to 6 months despite appropriate nonsurgical treatment, operative intervention is indicated. Surgery consists of an anterior acromioplasty, bursectomy, and resection of the coracoacromial ligament. Routine resection of the distal clavicle is not recommended. Distal clavicle resection is indicated for patients with tenderness on exam or in those with inferior spurring of the AC joint that is thought to aggravate impingement. The goal of a subacromial decompression is to remove sufficient bone from the anterolateral acromion to create a type I, or flat, acromion. Similar results have been obtained using both open and arthroscopic techniques. Good to excellent results are seen in approximately 90% of patients with either method. The open acromioplasty remains an effective operation and is less likely to result in insufficient bone removal. An arthroscopic decompression allows inspection of the glenohumeral joint for additional pathology and decreases iatrogenic injury to the deltoid. The decision ultimately depends on surgeon experience. Postoperatively, NSAIDs and therapy are important to reduce residual inflammation and maximize return of function. The stretching and strengthening exercises used for nonoperative treatment are instituted in the early postoperative period. These should commence in the first few days after surgery.

CONCLUSIONS

Subacromial impingement syndrome is a common diagnosis made by the practicing physician. Proper diagnosis depends on a thorough history and physical exam. Nonsurgical management is extremely successful and consists of both relief of inflammation and rehabilitation. An arthroscopic or open acromioplasty is performed only after failure of a 3- to 6-month course of nonsurgical treatment.

SUGGESTED READINGS

Bigliani LU, Levine WN. Subacromial impingement syndrome. *J Bone Joint Surg Am*. 1997;79:1854–1868.

Bigliani LU, Morrison DS, April EW. The morphology of the acromion and its relationship to rotator cuff tears. *Orthop Trans*. 1986,10:228.

Ellma H. Arthroscopic subacromial decompression: analysis of one- to three-year results. *Arthroscopy*. 1987;3:173–181.

Flatow EL, Soslowsky LJ, Ticker JB, et al. Excursion of the rotator cuff under the acromion: patterns of subacromial contact. *Am J Sports Med*. 1994;22:779–788.

Liotard JP, Cochard P, Walch G. Critical analysis of the supraspinatus outlet view: rationale for a standard scapular Y-view. *J Shoulder Elbow Surg*. 1998;7:134–139.

Morrison DS, Frogameni AD, Woodworth P. Non-operative treatment of subacromial impingement syndrome. *J Bone Joint Surg Am*. 1997;79:732–737.

Neer CS II. Anterior acromioplasty for the chronic impingement syndrome in the shoulder: a preliminary report. *J Bone Joint Surg Am*. 1972;54:41–50.

Ogata S, Uhthoff HK. Acromial enthesopathy and rotator cuff tear: a radiologic and histologic postmortem investigation of the coracoacromial arch. *Clin Orthop*. 1990;254:39–48.

Spangehl MJ, Hawkins RH, McCormick RG, et al. Arthroscopic verus open acromioplasty: a prospective, randomized, blinded study. *J Shoulder Elbow Surg*. 2002;11:101–107.

PARTIAL THICKNESS ROTATOR CUFF TEARS: DIAGNOSIS AND TREATMENT

CARLOS A. GUANCHE

The natural history of partial-thickness rotator cuff tears is poorly understood. To begin with, two types of tears need to be considered. Specifically, there are bursal surface tears, whose history and treatment is relatively well-known and straightforward. The second type is an articular side tear, whose history, diagnosis, and treatment are not as clear-cut. It has only been since the advent of shoulder arthroscopy and increasing diagnostic abilities with MRI that we have been able to make the diagnosis. The few series available with respect to the treatment of this problem are sometimes contradictory. The largest issue is that the natural history of partial cuff tears is relatively unknown. Furthermore, as with many shoulder injuries, the patient becomes more symptomatic with increasing activity levels or demands placed on the injured shoulder. The treatment of this problem is certainly different in a professional baseball pitcher as compared with a middle-aged weekend athlete.

PATHOGENESIS

Pathophysiology

Human cadaveric studies have found that most partial-thickness tears are on the articular side. When partial-thickness tears are openly explored, significant delamination can be encountered, with the articular surface fibers demonstrating the greatest degree of damage. Most degenerative tears originate on the articular side of the supraspinatus tendon, near the insertion, and appear to be primarily from intrinsic tendinopathy and not secondary to anatomic variations or wear from contiguous structures. This finding may be owing to the poor blood supply of the articular side of the supraspinatus insertion. Codman first observed a hypovascular critical zone just proximal to the insertion of the supraspinatus tendon in 1934. It has subsequently been corroborated that the articular side of the supraspinatus insertion has only sparse vascularity, with almost no vessels; the bursal side, however, was well vascularized. This critical zone of ischemia on the articular side seems to correspond well with the common site of rupture of the tendon. The relative ischemia of this area may be one reason why the cuff is unable to repair itself.

The area of degenerative tendinosis occurs most often in this hypovascular zone. This area corresponds well with the crescent described by Burkhart. Immediately medial to this well-defined area of degeneration one can often see the rotator cable, a consistent thickening in the tendon. Typically, the tissue that makes up the cable and all tissue medial to that point is intrinsically healthy. The loss of this crescentic area is perhaps a normal part of aging, and its presence does not necessarily indicate a repairable lesion. Most patients can still elevate their arm with this defect since stress transmission occurs through the cable. This may explain why a significant percent of all tears of the rotator cuff are asymptomatic.

The supraspinatus, a small and relatively weak muscle, is in a key position and is therefore susceptible to overuse and injury. Given the hypovascularity of the tissues, it is not surprising that most tears originate in this tendon. When eccentric tensile overload occurs at a rate that is greater than the ability of the rotator cuff to repair itself, injury occurs. At some point weakness of the musculotendinous unit results in damage to the tendon and ultimately failure. Direct trauma to the shoulder may initiate the same process. A weak, fatigued, or injured rotator cuff is unable to oppose the superior pull of the deltoid effectively and keep the humeral head centered on the glenoid during elevation of the arm. This leads to inappropriate superior migration of the humeral head with active elevation of the arm, functionally narrowing the subacromial space. Continued dysfunction of the rotator cuff and further superior migration of the humeral head cause abutment against the undersurface of the acromion and the coracoacromial ligament, leading to signs of secondary impingement.

The secondary impingement may lead to reactive and degenerative osseous changes. This process of secondary impingement further damages the already injured and weakened cuff. Subacromial impingement does occur, but in most circumstances it is a secondary phenomenon.

Classification

Several classification schemes are available describing full-thickness rotator tears. Most focus on the size of the tear and offer some prognostic criteria following repair. The classification scheme used for partial-thickness tears is somewhat different in that it takes into account the status of both the articular and bursal sides of the tendon.

The scheme most commonly used is the Southern California Orthopedic Institute (SCOI) classification. The scheme separates tears into articular (A), bursal (B), and complete (C) types. The degree of tendon damage is further separated into degree of tearing on a numerical scale of 0 to 4. The grading begins with 0, which is a normal cuff, and culminates with grade 4 (Table 38-1). When recording a tear, all three areas are represented even if they are normal. For example, an A1/B2/C0 tear would be understood as a partial articular-sided tear with minimal fraying in a localized area with the bursal side having cuff fiber failure and bursal injury, extending <2 cm. Finally, despite the degree of injury on both sides, there is no complete tearing, hence the C0 designation.

In addition to the above classification, the more commonly seen entity has recently been termed a PASTA lesion, which is an acronym for a *p*artial *a*rticular *s*upraspinatus *t*endon *a*vulsion. These are the injuries that will be discussed more thoroughly in this chapter as they are typically more symptomatic than the bursal-side tears, which are more common in sedentary and typically older individuals.

TABLE 38-1 CLASSIFICATION OF PARTIAL ROTATOR CUFF TEARS

Tear Location	Grade	Description
A Articular	0	Normal cuff; no bursal changes
B Bursal	1	Minimal superficial bursal or synovial fraying (<1 cm)
C Complete	2	Fraying and failure of cuff fibers with synovial, bursal, or capsular injury (<2 cm)
	3	Fraying and fragmentation of tendon Entire tendon (<3 cm)
	4	Severe partial tear; includes flap tear Usually more than one tendon

DIAGNOSIS

History

The typical patient with a partial inner-surface tear is one who is relatively active in an overhead sport or a manual laborer. In most cases, the onset is insidious and does not present with much acute symptomatology. In many, the symptoms are initially vague and are more often stamina issues rather than inability to perform at a high level.

It is important to obtain an exhaustive history. Patients are often vague about the time of onset of symptoms and the inciting event. Pain needs to be evaluated for quality, location, and duration of symptoms. Actions that worsen symptoms and interventions that improve them are important variables. The timing of onset of pain (how many tosses and at what velocity before symptoms occur), the point in the throwing cycle at which symptoms are greatest, and past history of treatment and prior shoulder problems should be elicited.

The age of presentation in these patients is typically <45 years of age. In many overhead athletes, the history includes a lack of ability to participate at high levels for prolonged periods of time. A baseball pitcher, for example, would typically state that he is able to throw effectively for a few innings, but then his speed and control will start to decrease considerably more quickly than in the past.

Unlike many patients with classic rotator cuff pathology and subacromial impingement, these patients are unlikely to complain of significant night pain. They typically have no resting pain and are unlikely to need treatment if they do not participate in the offending activity.

Physical Examination

One of the most important aspects of the examination in any patient with shoulder pain is to evaluate both sides for symmetry (or lack thereof) and for scapulothoracic dyskinesia, which can be a subtle finding. Males should be examined with their entire upper body exposed, whereas women should be examined with either a tube top or a gown that allows visualization of both shoulders and scapulae. It is important to examine all of the anatomic areas of the shoulder when diagnosing a partial rotator cuff tear, especially as it relates to the possibility of subtle instability or labral tears. There is a high rate of concomitant labral injuries (especially Superior Labrum, Anterior to Posterior Tear [SLAP]) in patients with partial tears.

The physical examination of a patient with a partial cuff tear can be unimpressive, despite later finding a very significant tear on diagnostic imaging. Typically, the patient has a full passive and active range of motion with the exception perhaps of a limitation in internal rotation in high-level throwers. It is important to assess both shoulders for range of motion, especially at the extremes of internal and external rotation. Most patients do not have any significant scapulothoracic asymmetry.

Specific tests that may be positive in patients with significant partial tears are weakness with forward flexion, adduction, and internal rotation. This tends to put the leading edge of the supraspinatus on tension and is a sensitive indicator of continuity of this portion. Another test that may be positive is pain with 90 degrees of abduction with resistance. This test may actually reproduce the pain that many throwers experience in their motion. Since the typical complaints are of pain in the posterior aspect of the shoulder in the late cocking and early acceleration phases of throwing, placing the shoulder into 90 degrees of abduction, 15 to 20 degrees of forward flexion, and maximum external rotation will recreate the symptoms. A test is considered positive when it recreates complaints of pain that are well localized in the posterior aspect of the shoulder. This test has high sensitivity for diagnosis of partial-thickness undersurface tears of the rotator cuff or posterior labrum. The traditional supraspinatus examination with the arm forward flexed about 30 degrees and the hand in a neutral position is typically nondiagnostic in these patients.

With respect to areas of tenderness, the classic impingement signs are usually negative. There may be some focal tenderness over the greater tuberosity at the leading edge of the supraspinatus, but that is difficult to elicit in a well-muscled athlete.

Imaging

The standard radiographs that are obtained include a scapular anteroposterior (AP), an outlet view, and an axillary projection. Occasionally, a specific acromioclavicular joint view is also warranted. In most cases, the radiographs are normal. The most frequent positive findings are an area of greater tuberosity sclerosis or perhaps cysts over the area of the tear (Fig. 38-1). These areas usually correspond to the areas of tendon avulsion and indicate the chronicity and repetitive nature of the injury.

An arthrogram of the joint may be considered; however, it is typically not helpful in these partial tears. As with most arthrograms (and ultrasound), the technique is definitely operator dependent and the sensitivity varies depending on the experience of the technician.

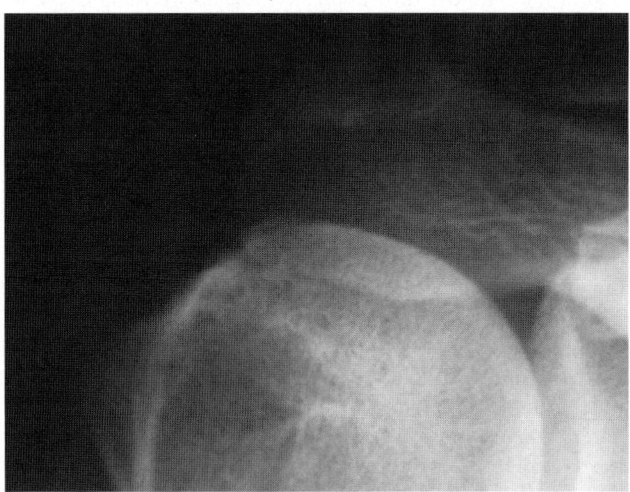

Figure 38-1 Radiograph depicting greater tuberosity sclerosis in a patient with a 75% full-thickness supraspinatus tear.

The most sensitive and specific examination is an MRI with a gadolinium arthrogram. These lesions are typically not seen on traditional MRI studies performed and as such should be highly suspected in a patient with the proper history and examination findings. Not only does the arthrogram portion improve the visualization of the rotator cuff pathology, but it also helps the evaluation of the labral structures that are frequently injured in these patients.

In addition to the standard MRI views, it is important to consider the inclusion of a series that positions the arm in an abducted and externally rotated position. It is not rare to see what appears to be a small and insignificant tear become a rather large tear with this maneuver (Fig. 38-2).

When a partial articular-sided tear is noted on an MRI, there is usually no significant retraction and, more important, no significant muscle atrophy or fatty infiltration. This is an important consideration, as either of these findings will significantly impact the patient's recovery following a surgical repair.

TREATMENT

Surgical Indications

Classically, the indications for repair of a partial-thickness tear have included one that is >50% of the full thickness of the involved tendon, with lesser tears requiring only debridement of the frayed tissue. Most studies have indicated that the supraspinatus footprint is between 12 and 16 mm long such that a tear >6 to 8 mm thick is an indication for surgery. The determination of the size of the tendon is difficult to make preoperatively based on MRI findings alone. It is therefore important to discuss this with each patient and make sure that the treatment alternatives are understood. Namely, that in tears that involve <25% of the footprint, a simple debridement and correction of any associated lesions may be all that is required. In addition, the determination of the degree of weakness preoperatively is important. In those patients in whom the clinical examination showed significant weakness and <25% of the tendon appears to be involved at the time of arthroscopy, the decision may be to repair the tear. The concept of individualizing the treatment based on the patient's age, activity level, and desire to return to the prior level is extremely important.

The most difficult part of the surgical decision in these patients is that the natural history of the problem is poorly understood. The typical young, active patient who is a repetitive thrower and is unable to participate at the desired activity level makes the problem easy to manage because any partial tear that makes throwing ineffective following a concerted conservative course of rotator cuff strengthening and pain control should undergo surgical repair. Patients who are more sedentary, or whose activity level is minimally affected, present a diagnostic dilemma, since the natural history of the progression of these partial tears into full-thickness tears is not completely known. However, cadaveric studies have shown that most partial-thickness tears

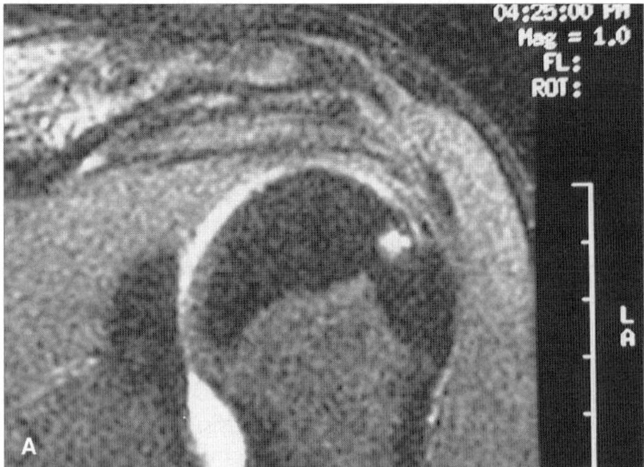

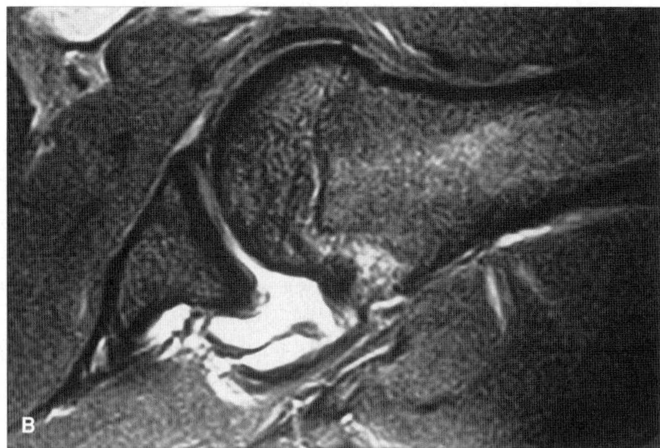

Figure 38-2 **A:** Coronal MRI (T2) view of a patient with clinical signs consistent with a partial rotator cuff tear. **B:** MRI (T2) view in abduction and external rotation depicting a near full-thickness tear of the supraspinatus.

are articular sided, and mechanical testing on these partial tears has led to complete disruption in a great percentage of samples. Although the correlation between cadaveric studies and in vivo pathophysiology is not always direct, it is important to consider this point in significant partial tears or in those unresponsive to conservative measures.

Surgical Contraindications

There are few true contraindications to surgical intervention in a patient who meets the criteria described above. One important consideration is that the patient must have full passive range of motion. There may be some minor limitations in active motion especially at the extremes of internal and external rotation. Any significant limitation, however, should be dealt with preoperatively with passive stretching. A significant limitation that is not resolved with aggressive conservative modalities preoperatively may require a capsular release. This is especially common in throwing athletes in whom the particular motion that is restricted is internal rotation.

Surgical Intervention

Options

The treatment of partial-thickness cuff tears has recently expanded as a result of the use of the arthroscope. With that in mind, most algorithms include the use of the arthroscope to make the diagnosis, especially those tears that are on the articular side. The treatment of outer surface tears can certainly be undertaken without the arthroscope with a traditional open technique, although as previously mentioned, there is a significant likelihood that a concomitant intra-articular surgical lesion exists, most commonly a labral tear. If the surgery is performed in an open fashion, the intra-articular visualization is at the very least compromised.

The recent literature supports the use of arthroscopic techniques that use suture anchors for solid cuff fixation. Two techniques are commonly used. One is the transtendon technique in which the remaining rotator cuff material is left intact and the tear is fixed with suture anchors placed through small incisions in the cuff. The other technique involves completion of the tear followed by arthroscopic repair (identical to what is performed in full thickness tears). The general guidelines for one technique over the other include the use of the transtendon technique in those tears where >75% of the tendon is intact. In tears where a larger portion of the tendon is involved, the tear is completed and a standard arthroscopic repair is performed. These are guidelines only, and the treatment should be based on the individual physician's experience with each technique.

Surgical Technique

The author's preferred technique involves the use of the lateral decubitus position for shoulder arthroscopy with hypotensive anesthesia. The transtendon repair technique is used in most cases, as this preserves a more significant portion of the normal rotator cuff and recreates the original footprint more effectively.

The procedure uses standard viewing portals, and the tear is delineated arthroscopically. The entire visualized cuff should be palpated and delineated for any significant intrasubstance delamination (Fig. 38-3). This includes debridement of the frayed edges and bony preparation of the footprint (Fig. 38-4). A spinal needle is now inserted from the lateral aspect of the joint into the area of the tear. The needle is then threaded with a large suture that can easily be found in the subacromial space. The subacromial space is then entered and the suture tag is found. A determination of the degree of bursal-sided tearing, if any, is made. If significant bursal tearing is noted, then a decision should be made to complete the tear and treat it in the standard fashion for a full-thickness tear.

If no significant bursal pathology is noted, a complete bursectomy is performed in anticipation of a transtendon repair and consequent suture tying in the subacromial space. If a complete bursectomy is not performed, significant difficulty will be encountered in the final stages of the repair as suture tying becomes very difficult without complete visualization. Once the subacromial space is cleared and any

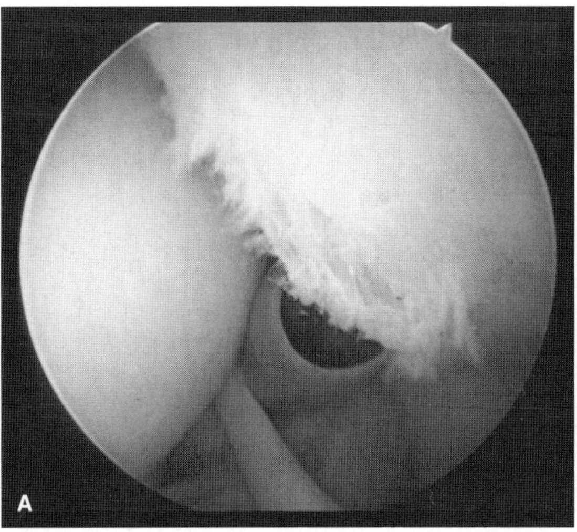

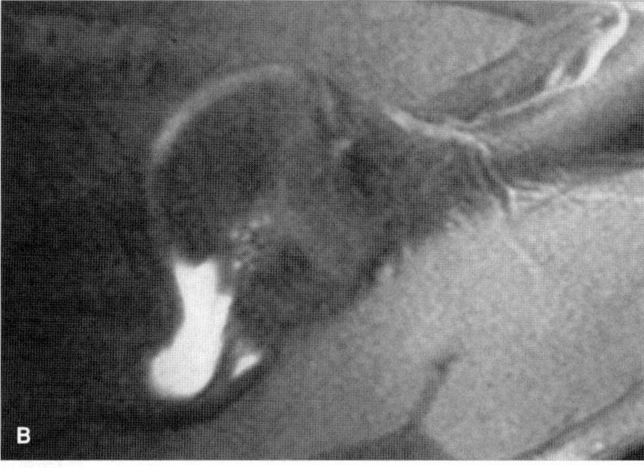

Figure 38-3 Intrasubstance delamination of a rotator cuff. **A:** MRI (T1) view of an inner surface delamination. **B:** Intra-articular visualization of this significant lesion.

osteophytes or coracoacromial pathology is addressed, the glenohumeral joint is then re-entered.

The joint is visualized from the posterior portal, and needle localization of the appropriate spot for suture anchor placement is now performed. In general, the traditional rule of thumb of one anchor per centimeter of tearing in the anterior to posterior dimension is followed. The appropriate number of anchors is then placed by making one longitudinal incision in the remaining cuff (parallel to the fibers of the tendon) just large enough to accommodate the suture anchor. In most cases, only one cuff incision is necessary, since the humerus can be rotated to position the anchors appropriately in the tuberosity. As the anchors are placed in the tuberosity, the sutures are pulled out of the anterior portal. All of the sutures are pulled out through this portal prior to beginning suture passing through the cuff.

Following completion of anchor insertion, the sutures are now passed through the tissue. Various suture-passing devices are available for this process, and they include needle-type devices with various curvatures and cannulated centers that allow suture shuttling through the appropriate point in the cuff. In addition, other penetrating devices allow for piercing the cuff tissue directly and grasping the suture (Fig. 38-5).

Anatomic cuff reattachment is the goal. The tendency with the technique is to advance a larger amount of cuff than is necessary, thus effectively overtensioning the cuff and leading to later excessive limitation of motion. It is important to gauge the amount of tissue that is taken with each suture and allow for a comfortable recreation of the footprint without undue tension following knot tying.

Once all of the sutures are passed, the subacromial space is again visualized from posterior and the knots are tied in a methodical fashion from anterior to posterior (Fig. 38-6). The basic principles of knot tying should be followed, namely a sliding locking knot that is backed up with reverse

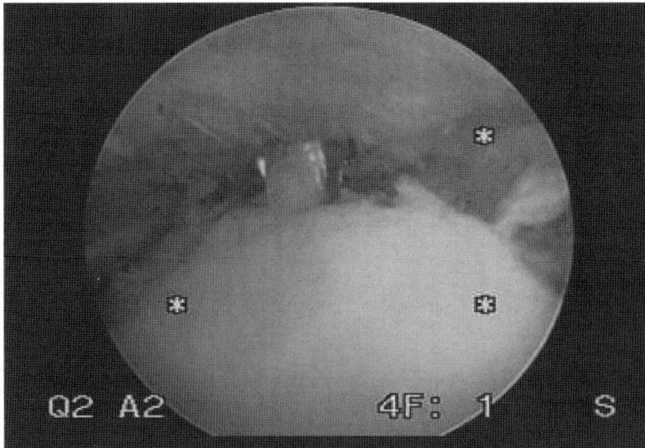

Figure 38-4 Preparation of the cuff tissue and the footprint of a partial-thickness tear. Right shoulder, posterior portal view. Note the anchor already in place at the anterior edge.

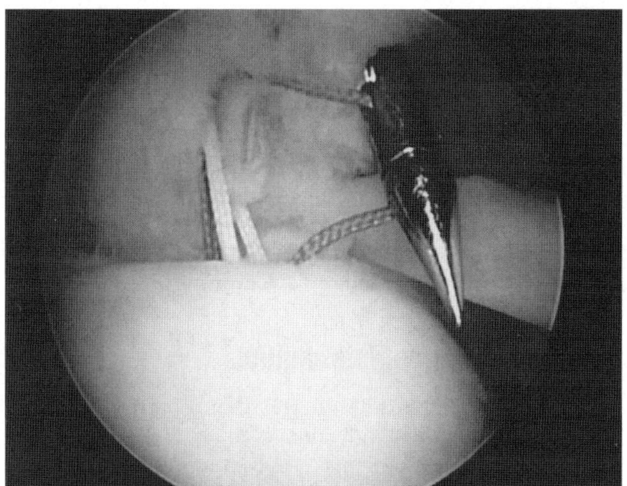

Figure 38-5 Suture penetrator being used for grasping a suture directly from the anchor after piercing the rotator cuff tissue.

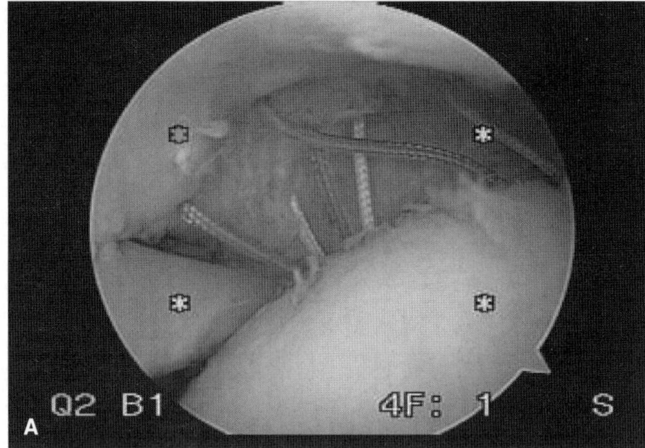

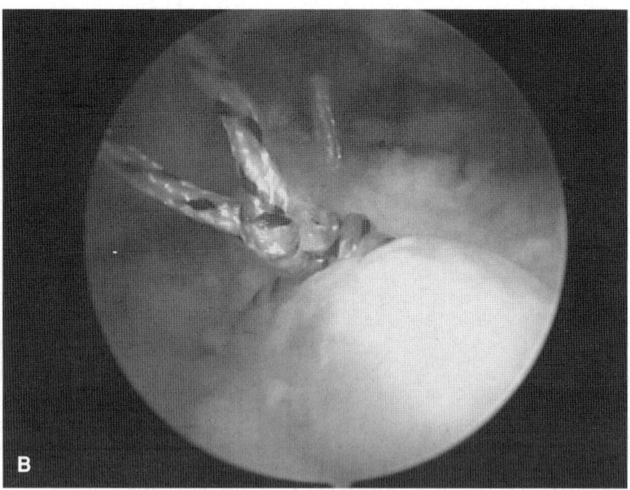

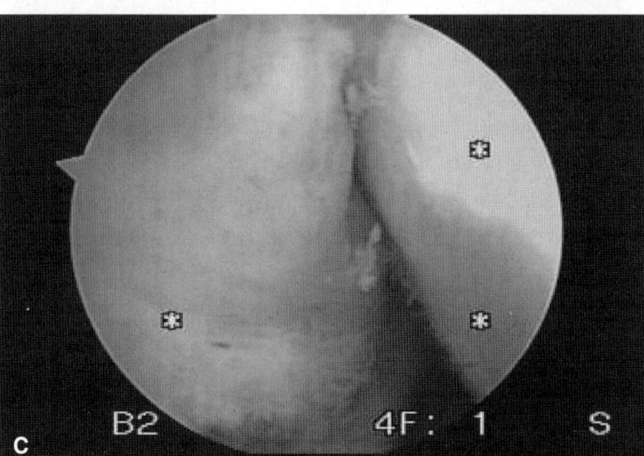

Figure 38-6 Sutures passed following anchor insertion (Right shoulder, posterior portal view). **A:** Intraarticular visualization of the final suture position. **B:** Subacromial visualization of the final sutures. **C:** Final intraarticular visualization of the cuff repair.

half hitches. In addition, only one pair of sutures should be in the portal while tying is taking place at any one time to avoid tangling of sutures.

Postoperative Rehabilitation

Following the surgical procedure, the patient is immobilized in a sling for 4 weeks with the institution of early elbow and hand range of motion exercises. During the second week, pendulum exercises are begun and gradually increased in range and frequency with a minimum of pain. The maximum forward flexion at this point (until 6 weeks postoperative) is kept to <90 degrees. At 6 weeks, the patient is allowed to begin active elevation and strengthening as tolerated. Typically a throwing program is instituted at 4 months. This is predicated on a complete range of motion and at near-complete (grade 4+/5) strength in all of the rotator cuff muscles and deltoid. Full, unrestricted activities including throwing are allowed at 6 months postoperatively.

Results of Surgical Intervention

In general, the literature indicates that a partial articular-sided tear in an active individual is likely to progress. Furthermore, simple acromioplasty does not predictably return the athlete to any semblance of his or her prior activity. The best results attained with partial-thickness tears have been in those cases where a repair has been performed. Several series delineate the arthroscopic evaluation and debridement of these tears with an acromioplasty. These have uniformly shown a lower rate of return to high-level activities as compared with series of repairs, regardless of the technique chosen. Up to 94% satisfactory results have been reported with arthroscopic decompression and mini-open rotator cuff repair.

In bursal-sided tears, however, the scenario is different in that many of these cases have a mechanical cause such as a prominent anterior acromion. In those cases, a debridement of the tear and subsequent acromioplasty may be of benefit in many patients. In general, the patients with this injury tend to be older and less active. Although degenerative labral tears are often encountered, these typically do not need any surgical fixation, unlike the patients with articular-side tears.

SUGGESTED READINGS

Burkhart SS. Arthroscopic debridement and decompression for selected rotator cuff tears. Clinical results, pathomechanics, and patient selection based on biomechanical parameters. *Orthop Clin North Am* 1993;24:111–123.

Fukuda H. The management of partial-thickness tears of the rotator cuff. *J Bone Joint Surg*. 2003;85B:3–11.

Lee SY, Lee JK. Horizontal component of partial-thickness tears of rotator cuff: imaging characteristics and comparison of ABER view with oblique coronal view at MR arthrography initial results. *Radiology*. 2002;224:470–476.

Lo IK, Burkhart SS. Transtendon arthroscopic repair of partial-thickness, articular surface tears of the rotator cuff. *Arthroscopy*. 2004;20:214–220.

Lohr JF, Uhthoff HK. The microvascular pattern of the supraspinatus tendon. *Clin Orthop*. 1990;254:35–38.

Lyons TR, Savoie FH, Field LD. Arthroscopic repair of partial-thickness tears of the rotator cuff. *Arthroscopy*. 2001;17:219–223.

Millstein ES, Snyder SJ. Arthroscopic management of partial, full thickness and complex rotator cuff tears: indications, techniques and complications. *Arthroscopy*. 2003;66:304–312.

Park JY, Chung KT, Yoo MJ. A serial comparison of arthroscopic repairs for partial- and full-thickness rotator cuff tears. *Arthroscopy*. 2004;20:705–711.

Park JY, Yoo MJ, Kim MH. Comparison of surgical outcome between bursal and articular partial thickness rotator cuff tears. *Orthopedics*. 2003;26:387–390.

Snyder SJ, Pachelli AF, Del Pizzo W, et al. Partial thickness rotator cuff tears: results of arthroscopic treatment. *Arthroscopy*. 1991;7:1–7.

ROTATOR CUFF TEARS: MINI-OPEN AND OPEN SURGICAL TREATMENT

ROGER G. POLLOCK

Pathology involving the subacromial soft tissues (the subacromial bursa and rotator cuff) constitutes the most common cause of shoulder pain. This pathology encompasses a spectrum of disease ranging from acute bursitis and tendinitis to chronic tendinitis and finally to tears of the rotator cuff, either partial thickness or full thickness. Considerable debate continues concerning the underlying cause of rotator cuff tears and also concerning their management. Treatment options for full-thickness rotator cuff tears include nonoperative treatment with exercises, subacromial decompression with debridement of the tear, and rotator cuff repair, either through arthroscopic, arthroscopically assisted (mini-open), or open surgical techniques. In addition, some massive rotator cuff tears are treated with tendon transfers, involving the use of latissimus dorsi, teres major, and/or pectoralis major tendons. This chapter will focus on mini-open and open repair of full-thickness rotator cuff tears.

PATHOGENESIS

The pathogenesis of rotator cuff tears likely involves both intrinsic tendon factors as well as the extratendinous anatomy of the subacromial space. Histologic studies of tendons have demonstrated degenerative changes in older specimens. Moreover, the tendon fibers undergo differential strains, with the articular-side fibers undergoing significantly greater tensile strain with the arm in abduction. This perhaps explains why tear initiation usually occurs on the undersurface or articular side of the tendon. Others have pointed to the relative avascularity of the "critical zone" of the supraspinatus as another intrinsic factor predisposing this region of the tendon to tear.

Others have emphasized the role of the extratendinous structures of the subacromial space, specifically, the coracoacromial arch in the pathogenesis of rotator cuff tears. Neer postulated that the overwhelming majority of rotator cuff tears were the result of attritional wear from excrescences on the undersurface of the anterior third of the acromion and to a lesser extent, the undersurface of the distal clavicle. Narrowing of the supraspinatus outlet by excrescences or spurs on the acromial undersurface resulted in frictional wear on the region of the supraspinatus, where most tears initiate. Several biomechanical studies have demonstrated that contact pressures between the acromial undersurface and the rotator cuff are maximal in this region of the supraspinatus with the shoulder abducted between 60 and 120 degrees. Moreover, cadaver studies have correlated acromial morphology with the incidence of rotator cuff tears and found that those with a type III or hooked morphology had the highest incidence of tears.

Trauma can play a role in the initiation or progression of rotator cuff tears. A hard fall can certainly result in tearing of the rotator cuff. An anterior dislocation in a patient older than 40 years of age can be associated with a rotator cuff tear. In younger patients, such dislocations result in stretching of the glenohumeral ligaments, avulsion of the anteroinferior labrum, or rarely, a fracture of the anteroinferior glenoid rim, but almost never in a full-thickness rotator cuff tear. A traumatic episode may also result in the progression of a previously existing rotator cuff tear, causing an acute onset of shoulder weakness. Such an acute extension of a chronic tear may turn an asymptomatic shoulder into one with acute pain and weakness. This is not infrequently seen in elderly patients.

Although trauma may be involved in the cause of rotator cuff tears, most tears probably are owing to attritional wear.

Full-thickness tears are rarely seen in those younger than 40 years of age and are likely caused by repetitive microtrauma involved with work and recreational sports activities. The incidence of full-thickness rotator cuff tears rises in those older than 40 years of age, and they occur more commonly in the dominant shoulder, supporting the notion that attrition is an important etiologic factor.

DIAGNOSIS

The diagnosis of subacromial pathology is made on the basis of a thorough history and physical examination of the shoulder. A subacromial injection of lidocaine can be used to confirm the diagnosis, and radiographs can provide supportive evidence and rule out other diagnoses. Staging of disease in the rotator cuff, ranging from tendinitis to partial tears to full-thickness tears can be precisely achieved through magnetic resonance imaging or ultrasonography.

Patients with rotator cuff pathology typically present with pain in the anterosuperior aspect of the shoulder. The pain usually radiates to the deltoid region, but not distally past the elbow. Pain, which is located predominantly in the posterior shoulder or trapezius region or which radiates into the forearm or hand or which is accompanied by paresthesias is more likely due to cervical radiculopathy than to subacromial pathology. In rotator cuff disease, the pain is usually increased with overhead use of the arm and with active abduction and reaching behind the body. Often the pain is increased at night with the supine position, perhaps because this increases compression of the inflamed tendon and bursa beneath the acromion. Patients may complain of a catching sensation and of shoulder weakness, particularly with activities performed above shoulder height. Frequently affected tasks include work activities that require lifting or repetitive overhead use and sports activities, such as tennis, golf, and swimming.

Several conditions involving the cervical spine and shoulder may present with symptoms similar to those of rotator cuff disease and should be considered in the differential diagnosis. Cervical radiculopathy, specifically a herniated cervical disc at the C5–C6 level, can present with pain in the deltoid and biceps regions. Acromioclavicular arthritis causes pain in the superior aspect of the shoulder and trapezial region and may coexist with rotator cuff disease. Adhesive capsulitis, particularly in its early prestiffness phase, may be mistaken for rotator cuff disease, as pain in the deltoid region is often the earliest symptom. Subtle glenohumeral instability may present as anterosuperior shoulder pain without frank episodes of subluxation or sensation of instability, particularly in young overhead athletes. These patients may have both an underlying instability problem and a secondary subacromial bursitis or tendinitis and may be difficult to diagnose precisely. Finally, calcific tendinitis can mimic a rotator cuff tear, as the anatomic distribution of pain is similar, and the intensity of pain may cause a pseudoparalysis, which can resemble the weakness seen with large rotator cuff tears. The history of an acute atraumatic onset and the presence of a calcific deposit on plain radiographs serve to differentiate these diagnoses.

Physical examination is usually quite helpful in the diagnosis of rotator cuff disease. In cases of chronic large or massive tears, simple inspection of the shoulder may suggest the diagnosis, as there is usually atrophy of the supraspinatus and infraspinatus muscles, and sometimes a visible rupture of the tendon of the long head of the biceps. There may be a diffuse swelling around the shoulder—a so-called fluid sign or a localized fluid collection at the acromioclavicular joint. Occasionally, with an acute traumatic tear, ecchymosis may be present. However, with smaller tears or more acute tears, the appearance of the shoulder is usually normal.

In rotator cuff disorders, there is frequently tenderness over the subacromial bursa and greater tuberosity. Approximately 10% to 15% of patients with a rotator cuff tear will also have symptomatic acromioclavicular arthritis, which is diagnosed clinically by tenderness directly over the acromioclavicular joint and by painful adduction of the shoulder. With full-thickness rotator cuff tears, subacromial crepitation can often be appreciated with passive range of motion of the shoulder. Usually, passive range of motion is preserved with rotator cuff tears, although a small percentage of shoulders with tears will develop stiffness. Active range of motion is often normal with smaller tears, but loss of active motion can occur with larger tears.

Shoulder strength, as measured with manual muscle testing, may be normal with partial-thickness tears and even with smaller full-thickness tears. However, larger tears usually produce shoulder weakness, which can be detected by resistance testing or in more severe cases, by lag signs or "drop-arm" signs. Thus, the patients may not be able to actively elevate or externally rotate the shoulder fully, producing a lag between their active and passive motion. In a similar manner, loss of infraspinatus function will cause a shoulder that is placed into an externally rotated position to fall into internal rotation, producing a drop-arm sign. Subscapularis deficiency results in an inability to lift the arm off the lumbar spine when it is placed into internal rotation, producing a positive "lift-off" sign, as described by Gerber.

Several other provocative tests are quite helpful in diagnosing rotator cuff problems. The Neer impingement sign, which is tested by stabilizing the patient's scapula while fully passively elevating the arm, is nearly always positive in patients with subacromial pathology. The Hawkins sign, tested by fully internally rotating the shoulder at 90 degrees of flexion, is also quite useful in detecting subacromial problems. Resisted testing of the supraspinatus, as popularized by Jobe, can further suggest rotator cuff pathology. Finally, the injection of 10 mL of 1% lidocaine into the subacromial space will reliably reduce or eliminate pain that is caused by subacromial pathology and can be helpful in confirming the diagnosis of a rotator cuff disorder.

Plain radiographs can provide anatomic data that support the diagnosis of a rotator cuff disorder. Excrescences on the acromion, greater tuberosity, and undersurface of the distal clavicle can be seen on an anteroposterior radiograph in a shoulder with rotator cuff pathology. Moreover, a diminished acromiohumeral interval is suggestive of a rotator cuff tear, and some would suggest that an acromiohumeral interval of <6 mm is indicative of an irreparable tear. In the supraspinatus outlet view, a lateral radiograph with a 10-degree caudal tilt, the morphology of the acromion, and any associated spurring can be clearly visualized. This information can be helpful in surgical planning, concerning the extent of the subacromial decompression that will be required in a particular shoulder. An axillary radiograph will reveal the presence of an unfused acromial epiphysis or os acromiale. Finally, plain radiographs are useful in ruling out other painful shoulder conditions, such as glenohumeral arthritis and calcific tendinitis.

Although a thorough history and physical examination supplemented by plain radiographs can allow the diagnosis of a rotator cuff or subacromial disorder, magnetic resonance imaging or ultrasonography can help to stage the problem accurately. These imaging techniques can differentiate between tendinitis, partial-thickness tears, and full-thickness tears of the rotator cuff. When a tear is present, these studies indicate which tendon or tendons are involved, the size of the tear, and the degree of tendon retraction. Magnetic resonance imaging is also quite useful in providing data about the rotator cuff muscles, such as information about the degree of muscle atrophy or fatty infiltration. Such structural information can help the surgeon choose an appropriate surgical technique for rotator cuff repair and provide insight about the reparability of a tear. In the United States, magnetic resonance imaging has replaced the arthrogram as the test of choice in most centers for staging rotator cuff disease. Ultrasonography, while relatively inexpensive and allowing bilateral examination in a cost-effective way, is less familiar to most North American surgeons and requires greater expertise to perform and interpret accurately.

TREATMENT

Treatment options for full-thickness rotator cuff tears include nonoperative treatment with exercises and various surgical techniques of repair. Nonoperative treatment has been shown to result in pain relief and functional improvement, but these results are less predictable than those of surgical repair and may deteriorate over time with tear extension. Older, more sedentary patients, who put less demand on the shoulder for overhead work or sports activities, appear to benefit more consistently from nonoperative treatment than younger, more active patients. Patients in their 70s and 80s are also more likely to present with chronic large or massive tears with a significant degree of muscle atrophy and fatty degeneration on magnetic resonance imaging. Such patients are less likely to achieve functional improvement after rotator cuff repair and are probably best managed with nonoperative treatment.

Younger, more active patients in their fifth, sixth, and seventh decades with a symptomatic full-thickness rotator cuff tear are best served by early rotator cuff repair. Numerous studies on the results of rotator cuff repair have reported a satisfactory outcome in 85% to 95% with predictable pain relief and functional improvement in most patients. Although complete healing of the tendons did not appear necessary to achieve satisfactory pain relief, the best functional results were seen in patients in whom the repair was intact at follow-up in studies by Harryman et al. and Gerber et al. Moreover, work by Yamaguchi et al. has suggested that the natural history of rotator cuff tears is extension of the tear in a considerable percentage of these tears. This information, combined with other recent data that demonstrate that muscle atrophy is only partially reversible and fatty infiltration of the muscles appears to be irreversible, would suggest that early repair of a symptomatic rotator cuff tear is the optimal treatment for an active, healthy patient.

The surgical techniques for rotator cuff repair continue to evolve. Since Neer's description of anterior acromioplasty in 1972, most of those techniques have combined subacromial decompression with tendon repair, although a few authors have recently questioned the use of acromioplasty. In addition to the traditional method of open rotator cuff repair, newer techniques combining arthroscopic acromioplasty with mini-open rotator cuff repair and completely arthroscopic repair have become more popular. For dealing with some of the massive irreparable tears, tendon transfer techniques and the use of synthetic grafts have been used. The remainder of this chapter will focus on the techniques of mini-open and open rotator cuff repair.

Arthroscopically Assisted or Mini-Open Repair

This technique combines arthroscopic subacromial decompression with open tendon repair through a small deltoid split. Since the anterior acromioplasty is performed arthroscopically, this technique allows preservation of the deltoid origin during the repair of the torn rotator cuff. Other advantages for this procedure compared with traditional open rotator cuff repair include lower perioperative morbidity and shorter hospital stays, superior cosmesis with smaller incisions, easier rehabilitation, and the ability to treat associated intra-articular pathology, such as labral tears or biceps lesions, during the arthroscopic portion of the procedure. In comparison with wholly arthroscopic repair, the mini-open procedure is technically easier to perform and has a lower learning curve.

Arthroscopically assisted or mini-open repair is most appropriate for small to medium-sized tears (i.e., <3 cm) without significant retraction. These tears usually involve the supraspinatus tendon alone or the supraspinatus and upper portion of the infraspinatus. Larger tears or those with extensive retraction can be treated with this technique, but are more easily treated with traditional open techniques, as these tears require more extensive tissue mobilization and transposition, which can be difficult to achieve through the limited exposure afforded by the small deltoid split. Subscapularis tears are also difficult to access through the mini-open approach and are usually treated using an open approach.

The procedure is performed with the patient in the beach-chair position under interscalene block regional anesthesia. Arthroscopic examination of the glenohumeral joint is carried out through a standard posterior portal. This allows for inspection of the intra-articular structures and treatment of associated pathology of the labrum or biceps tendon, as well as debridement of the undersurface of the rotator cuff, using arthroscopic instruments introduced

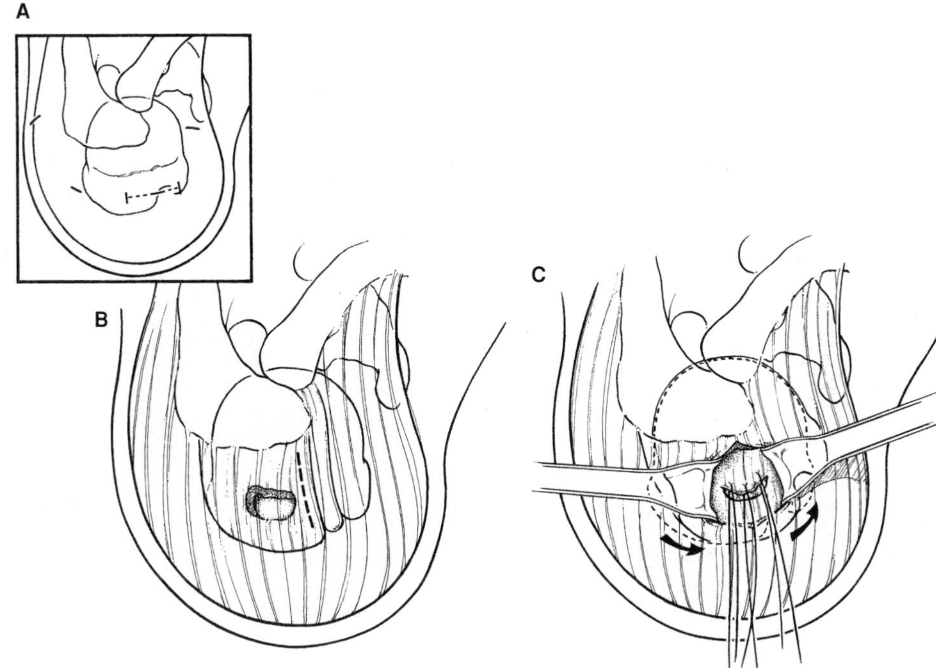

Figure 39-1 A: Limited 3- to 4-cm skin incision, which includes the anterolateral portal and is directed along the skin lines for cosmesis. B: Deltoid split (*dotted line*), starting from the anterolateral acromion and extending 4 cm distally. C: Arm rotation allows the tear to be positioned below the deltoid split. (From Post M, Bigliani LU, Flatow EL, et al. Rotator cuff repair. In: Post M, Bigliani LU, Flatow EL, et al., eds. *The Shoulder: Operative Technique*. Lippincott Williams & Wilkins; 1998, with permission.)

through a standard anterior portal. The arthroscope is then removed from the glenohumeral joint and is introduced into the subacromial space. An arthroscopic acromioplasty is performed to create a smooth undersurface of the anterior third of the acromion. As this technique has been extensively reviewed elsewhere in this text, we will focus on the details of the mini-open tendon repair.

After the arthroscopic acromioplasty has been completed, the arthroscope and burr are removed from the subacromial space. The anterolateral portal incision is extended to a total length of 3 to 4 cm and is directed horizontally along the skin lines (approximately parallel to the lateral border of the acromion) (Fig. 39-1A). This yields a more cosmetically pleasing scar than vertically oriented incisions. The subcutaneous tissue is incised and undermined to expose the deltoid fascia. The deltoid is then split from the anterolateral corner of the acromion to a point 4 to 5 cm distally, incorporating the previous puncture site through the deltoid in the split (Fig. 39-1B). Care is taken proximally not to release or avulse the deltoid from the anterior acromion and distally not to exceed 4 to 5 cm and thereby jeopardize the axillary nerve. Further bursectomy is then performed to allow better visualization of the torn rotator cuff. The torn portion of the rotator cuff can be delivered directly below the deltoid split by varying the rotation of the arm (Fig. 39-1C).

With the torn tendon now accessible for repair, sutures are placed into the tendon along the perimeter of the tear to assist with mobilization of the torn rotator cuff. A blunt periosteal elevator is used to release adhesions on both the articular and bursal surfaces of the cuff. The tendon is mobilized until it easily reaches its insertion on the greater tuberosity without significant tension. Occasionally, this may require a sharp release of the coracohumeral ligament at the base of the coracoid if this structure is tethering the retracted tendon. However, with most of the smaller tears selected for repair through this approach, mobilization is usually easily achieved without the need for sharp releases.

The region of the greater tuberosity that will receive the repaired rotator cuff is then prepared using a rongeur to remove any bony excrescences or fibrous tissue and to yield a bleeding bony base. Either suture anchor devices or sutures passed through bone tunnels in the greater tuberosity can be used to repair the cuff. It is this author's preference to use sutures passed through bone tunnels, as this technique allows more uniform compression of the tendon to the surface of the tuberosity than the suture anchor method, which provides more of a point contact type of fixation between the tendon and bone. One to three bone tunnels are then created, depending on the size of the tear to be repaired. The technique used by the author to create these tunnels in the greater tuberosity involves the use of a curved awl to start the tunnel proximally and then the use of a sharp trocar-tipped needle to pierce the lateral cortex of the tuberosity distally. Through each tunnel, two no. 1 or no. 2 braided nonabsorbable sutures are passed, thus doubling the number of sutures available for the repair. Each of the sutures is then passed through the torn tendon. The sutures are usually placed in simple fashion, although the modified Mason-Allen stitch is used for repairs of tissue of lesser quality. The sutures are tied with the arm at the side in neutral to slight internal rotation. After the tendon has been repaired, the deltoid split is repaired, and the skin is closed with a subcuticular repair.

Postoperatively, passive and assistive exercises are begun immediately to maintain the range of motion. Extension is deferred early on to avoid unduly stressing the tendon repair. A sling is used to prevent active use of the arm for approximately 6 weeks to protect the tendon repair. Active use for activities of daily living is allowed after 6 weeks, and resistive exercises are begun at 10 to 12 weeks postoperatively. Although the rehabilitation may proceed more easily and less painfully than after open repair (especially during the first few weeks), the rate of tendon healing to bone is not affected by the technique of repair. The biology of tendon healing still requires a period during which stresses across the repair must be minimized to avoid rerupture of the repaired tendon.

Open Rotator Cuff Repair

Since the first reported rotator cuff repair by Codman in 1911, open repair has been the standard method. During the first half of the twentieth century, the results of rotator cuff repair were unpredictable, probably largely owing to the acromionectomy procedures and transacromial approaches that were used. These procedures produced damage to the deltoid and alteration of its normal fulcrum, resulting in poor function and even inconsistent pain relief. Since the introduction of anterior acromioplasty by Neer and the abandonment of earlier acromionectomy techniques, the results of rotator cuff surgery have improved significantly, yielding satisfactory outcomes in 85% to 90% of patients.

A major advantage of open rotator cuff surgery is that it affords wide exposure for access to even massive tears of the rotator cuff. Such exposure is necessary when attempting to mobilize the chronically contracted tendons in a large or massive tear. The major disadvantage of this technique is that it involves incision of the anterior deltoid to gain exposure and to perform the anterior acromioplasty. This has the potential risk of deltoid dehiscence, though this complication is uncommon when the deltoid is repaired and protected properly in the early postoperative period. Greater perioperative morbidity, as measured by the need for narcotic analgesics and by longer hospital stays, is also cited as a relative disadvantage of open repair. There has been a shift to arthroscopically assisted rotator cuff repair for treating smaller tears and even more recently to arthroscopic repair of many tears. Although patient satisfaction and pain relief appear to be comparable for the results of open repair and those of arthroscopic repair, the structural results (i.e., anatomic healing of the repaired tendons to bone) of arthroscopic repair appear to be inferior to those of open repair for large and massive tears.

Open rotator cuff repair is performed with the patient in the semisitting or beach-chair position using regional interscalene block anesthesia. The patient is positioned so that the shoulder protrudes over the side of the operating table so that the arm can be extended and rotated during the procedure, particularly to gain access to retracted posterior cuff tendons. The shoulder is gently manipulated through a full passive range of motion to break up any capsular adhesions that occasionally may be present. An anterosuperior deltoid-splitting approach is used for the repair of most tears, although a deltopectoral approach is favored for isolated subscapularis tears. The preferred incision for most open repairs is a 6- to 7-cm incision, which starts over the lateral aspect of the acromion and proceeds to a point just lateral to the coracoid process. This yields a cosmetically acceptable scar, as the incision approximates the skin lines. A needle-tip electrocautery is used to incise the subcutaneous layer and to widely undermine this layer to expose the underlying deltoid fascia. The deltoid split starts anterior to the acromioclavicular joint and extends laterally 4 cm distal to the anterolateral corner of the acromion (Fig. 39-2A). A cuff of deltoid is left superiorly on the acromion to allow for a secure deltoid repair. This split in the deltoid is centered over the greater tuberosity to allow better exposure to the posterior cuff (Fig. 39-2B).

Subacromial decompression is next performed to remove any spurs or excrescences from the acromial undersurface. The coracoacromial ligament is released from the anterior aspect and undersurface of the acromion. This ligament is typically partially excised when there is a smaller tear but is preserved and later repaired back to the acromion in massive tears, where there is concern about the possibility of cuff failure and subsequent anterosuperior instability. After the anterior acromion has been exposed and adherent cuff and bursal tissue have been cleaned from its undersurface, a beveled osteotome (with the bevel facing upward) is used to perform an acromioplasty. The aim is to produce a smooth acromial undersurface, and the amount of bone removal varies according to the anatomy. By resecting only the downward projecting undersurface, effective decompression can be achieved with minimal shortening of the acromion. Osteophytes on the undersurface of the acromioclavicular joint are removed with a rongeur. Excision of the distal clavicle is performed only for preoperative acromioclavicular symptoms, and this is necessary in only 10% to 15% of cases. When this is necessary, the author prefers to resect the distal clavicle from below using a burr and rongeur so that the superior ligamentous envelope can be preserved to avoid microinstability of the acromioclavicular (AC) joint.

After the subacromial decompression, attention turns to mobilization and repair of the torn tendons. At this point, the characteristics of the tear are noted: size, shape, tendon involvement, degree of retraction, and quality of the tissue available for repair. The torn tendons are tagged with nonabsorbable sutures to assist with mobilization. A blunt periosteal elevator is used to release bursal adhesions, as well as to release adhesions between the tendons and capsule on the articular side. With acute tears, where there are no fixed contractures, mobilization proceeds quite easily. In large or massive chronic tears, these blunt releases may not be sufficient to restore mobile musculotendinous units to their insertion on the greater tuberosity. The torn tendon may be tethered by the adjacent intact tendon. Sharp release of the coracohumeral ligament at the base of the coracoid may assist with mobilization of the supraspinatus tendon. Additionally, as described by Bigliani, an "anterior interval slide" or sharp release of the interval between the supraspinatus and subscapularis tendons is performed when necessary (Fig. 39-2C). A similar release between the infraspinatus and supraspinatus is also occasionally needed.

The greater tuberosity is prepared by removing bony excrescences and residual fibrous tissue down to a bleeding bony base. The lesser tuberosity is similarly prepared if the subscapularis tendon is torn. Multiple bone tunnels are constructed, as previously described, using a sharp curved awl and a trocar-tipped needle. The location and number of tunnels varies according to the size of the tear. Through each

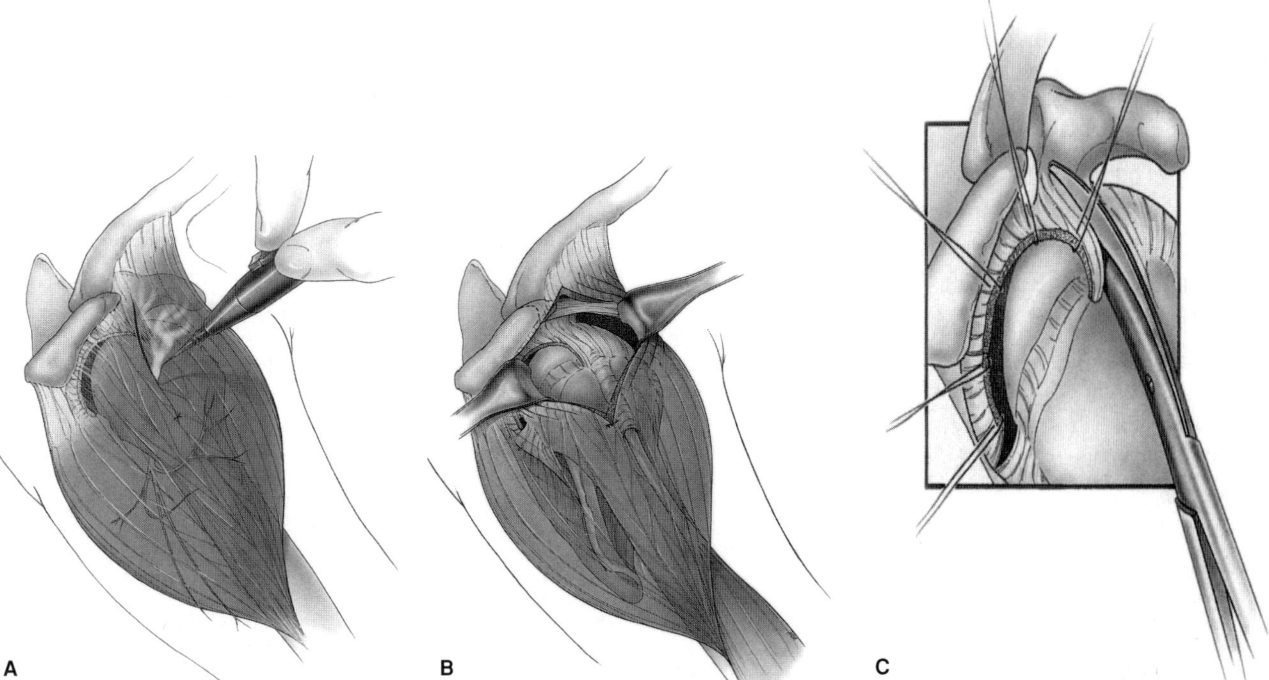

Figure 39-2 **A:** The deltoid split starts anterior to the acromioclavicular joint and extends in an anterolateral raphe for 4 cm distal to the anterolateral corner of the acromion. **B:** This deltoid split is centered over the greater tuberosity and affords good access to the torn tendons (especially posteriorly). **C:** A sharp release of the rotator interval and coracohumeral ligament to the base of the coracoid or "interval slide" assists with mobilization of a chronically retracted supraspinatus tendon. (From Post M, Bigliani LU, Flatow EL, et al. Rotator cuff repair. In: Post M, Bigliani LU, Flatow EL, et al., eds. *The Shoulder: Operative Technique*. Lippincott Williams & Wilkins; 1998, with permission.)

of the tunnels, two no. 1 or no. 2 braided nonabsorbable sutures are passed to maximize the number of sutures available for tendon-to-bone repair and to disperse the stresses in the repaired tendons. Simple sutures are preferred if the tendon is of stout quality, but modified Mason-Allen sutures may also be used if the tissue is of poorer quality. The sutures are tied with the arm at the side in slight flexion and neutral to slight internal rotation. Tendon-to-tendon sutures are passed to repair the intervals that have been released. If the biceps tendon is intact in its groove, it is left alone. If there is significant fraying of the tendon (>50% of the tendon thickness) or if it is subluxed, tenodesis is performed, and the intra-articular portion is excised. Using the techniques described, complete repair can usually be achieved. However, occasionally with three- and four-tendon tears, this is not possible, and partial repair is performed. In these rare cases, the emphasis is on restoring tissue both anteriorly and posteriorly, and there may be a residual defect superiorly. When the tendon repair has been completed, the split in the deltoid is repaired with no. 1 nonabsorbable braided sutures. A subcuticular skin closure is then performed.

Postoperatively, passive range of motion exercises are begun on the first postoperative day. These consist of pendulum exercises, as well as passive elevation in the scapular plane and passive external rotation (with the arm at the side). The degree of motion allowed depends on several factors, such as which tendons were involved, the tension on the repair, and the quality of the repaired tissue. With most tears, approximately 140 degrees of elevation and 40 degrees of external rotation are allowed in the early postoperative period. With subscapularis involvement, external rotation is usually limited to zero to 20 degrees. A sling is used for 6 weeks to prevent active use of the shoulder. More advanced stretching exercises, as well as light active use of the arm for activities of daily living, are added after 6 weeks. Resistive exercises are deferred for 3 months and are progressed gradually. Appropriate rehabilitation, which is supervised and directed by the surgeon, plays a crucial role in achieving a satisfactory outcome and avoiding complications, such as deltoid dehiscence and cuff tendon failure, after rotator cuff repair.

SUGGESTED READINGS

Adamson GJ, Tibone JE. Ten-year assessment of primary rotator cuff repairs. *J Shoulder Elbow Surg*. 1993;2:57–63.

Baker CL, Liu SH. Comparison of open and arthroscopically assisted rotator cuff repairs. *Am J Sports Med*. 1995;23:99–104.

Bassett RW, Cofield RH. Acute tears of the rotator cuff: the timing of surgical repair. *Clin Orthop*. 1983;175:18–24.

Bigliani LU. Rotator cuff repair. In: Post M, Bigliani LU, Flatow EL, et al., eds. *The Shoulder: Operative Technique*. Philadelphia: Williams and Wilkins; 1998:133–165.

Bigliani LU, Cordasco FA, McIlveen SJ, et al. Operative treatment of massive rotator cuff tears: long-term results. *J Shoulder Elbow Surg.* 1992;1:120–130.

Blevins FT, Warren RF, Cavo C, et al. Arthroscopic assisted rotator cuff repair: Results using a mini-open deltoid splitting approach. *Arthroscopy.* 1996;12:50–59.

Codman EA. *The Shoulder: Rupture of the Supraspinatus Tendon and Other Lesions in or about the Subacromial Bursa.* Boston: Thomas Todd; 1934.

Cofield RH, Parvizi J, Hoffmeyer PJ, et al. Surgical repair of chronic rotator cuff tears. A prospective long-term study. *J Bone Joint Surg.* 2001;83A:71–77.

Cofield RH. Rotator cuff disease of the shoulder. *J Bone Joint Surg.* 1985;67A:974–979.

Edwards TB, Walch G, Sirveaux F, et al. Repair of tears of the subscapularis. *J Bone Joint Surg.* 2005;87A:725–730.

Ellman H, Hanker G, Bayer M. Repair of the rotator cuff: End-result study of factors influencing reconstruction. *J Bone Joint Surg.* 1986;68A:1136–1144.

Galatz LM, Griggs S, Cameron BD, et al. Prospective longitudinal analysis of postoperative shoulder function: a ten-year follow-up study of full-thickness rotator cuff tears. *J Bone Joint Surg.* 2001;83A:1052–1056.

Gerber C, Fuchs B, Hodler J. The results of repair of massive tears of the rotator cuff. *J Bone Joint Surg.* 2000;82A:505–515.

Gerber C, Krushell RJ. Isolated rupture of the tendon of the subscapularis muscle. Clinical features in 16 cases. *J Bone Joint Surg.* 1991;73B:389–394.

Gerber C, Schneeberger AG, Beck M, et al. Mechanical strength of repairs of the rotator cuff. *J Bone Joint Surg.* 1994;76B: 371–380.

Harryman DT II, Mack LA, Wang KY, et al. Repairs of the rotator cuff. Correlation of functional results with integrity of the cuff. *J Bone Joint Surg.* 1991;73A:982–989.

Hawkins RJ, Misamore GW, Hobeika PE. Surgery for full-thickness rotator cuff tears. *J Bone Joint Surg.* 1985;67A:1349–1355.

Iannotti JP. Full-thickness rotator cuff tears: factors affecting surgical outcome. *J Am Acad Orthop Surg.* 1994;2:87–95.

Iannotti JP, Bernot MP, Kuhlman JR, et al. Postoperative assessment of shoulder function: a prospective study of full-thickness rotator cuff tears. *J Shoulder Elbow Surg.* 1996;5:449–457.

Levy HJ, Uribe JW, Delaney LG. Arthroscopic assisted rotator cuff repair: preliminary results. *Arthroscopy.* 1990;6:55–60.

Liu SH. Arthroscopically-assisted rotator-cuff repair. *J Bone Joint Surg.* 1994;76B:592–595.

McCallister WV, Parsons IM, Titelman RM, et al. Open rotator cuff repair without acromioplasty. *J Bone Joint Surg.* 2005;87A:1278–1283.

McLaughlin HL. Lesions of the musculotendinous cuff of the shoulder, I: the exposure and treatment of tears with retraction. *J Bone Joint Surg.* 1944;26:31–51.

Neer CS II. Anterior acromioplasty for the chronic impingement syndrome in the shoulder: a preliminary report. *J Bone Joint Surg.* 1972;54A:41–50.

Neer CS II. *Shoulder Reconstruction.* Philadelphia: WB Saunders; 1990:41–142.

Packer NP, Calvert PT, Bayley JI, et al. Operative treatment of chronic ruptures of the rotator cuff of the shoulder. *J Bone Joint Surg.* 1983;65B:171–175.

Paulos LE, Kody MH. Arthroscopically enhanced mini-approach to rotator cuff repair. *Am J Sports Medlite.* 1994;22:19–25.

Pollock RG, Flatow EL. Full-thickness tears: mini-open repair. *Orthop Clin North Am.* 1997;28:169–177.

Post M, Silver R, Singh M. Rotator cuff tear: diagnosis and treatment. *Clin Orthop.* 1983;173:78–92.

Sperling JW, Cofield RN, Schleck C. Rotator cuff repair in patients fifty years of age and younger. *J bone Joint Surg.* 2004;86A:2212–2215.

Weber SC, Schaefer R. "Mini-open" versus traditional open repair in the management of small and moderate size tears of the rotator cuff. *Arthroscopy.* 1993;9:365–366,.

Williams GR, Rockwood CA Jr, Bigliani LU, et al. Rotator cuff tears: why do we repair them? *J Bone Joint Surg.* 2004;86A:2764–2776.

Wolfgang GL. Surgical repair of tears of the rotator cuff of the shoulder: factors influencing the result. *J Bone Joint Surg.* 1974;56A:14–26.

Yamaguchi LE, Tetro AM, Blam O, et al. Natural history of asymptomatic rotator cuff tears: a longitudinal analysis of asymptomatic tears detected sonographically. *J Shoulder Elbow Surg.* 2001;10: 199–203.

ROTATOR CUFF TEAR: ARTHROSCOPIC TREATMENT

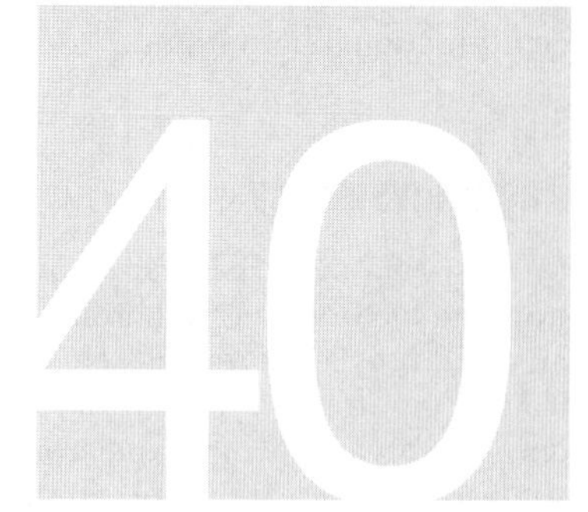

KYLE R. FLIK
ANDREAS H. GOMOLL
BRIAN J. COLE

Arthroscopic treatment of rotator cuff tears has become a routine procedure following a general trend toward using less invasive procedures. Proponents of this technique emphasize the decreased risk of complications such as infection, stiffness, and deltoid avulsions, whereas critics mention the lack of long-term studies, the controversy over the strength of fixation, and the technical challenge of all-arthroscopic repair of large tears for inexperienced practitioners. To help address the latter, this chapter will provide an overview of the indications, technique, and rehabilitation associated with arthroscopic rotator cuff repair.

PATHOGENESIS

Etiology

Although the exact pathogenesis is controversial, a combination of intrinsic and extrinsic factors is likely responsible for most rotator cuff tears. Intrinsic factors relate to the quality of the tendon substance itself, such as the chronic degeneration brought on by the relative hypoperfusion of a watershed area close to the insertion on the greater tuberosity, in conjunction with repetitive microtrauma.

Impingement ranks foremost among external factors implicated in rotator cuff tears. External or outlet impingement, the most common form, is caused by compression of the rotator cuff tendons as they pass underneath the coracoacromial arch. Narrowing of the subacromial space can be caused by the acromion itself as a result of arthritic changes of the acromioclavicular joint or by posttraumatic changes after proximal humerus fractures, especially with displacement of the greater tuberosity. In contrast, internal impingement is a controversial entity that has been described more recently and is thought to occur primarily in overhead and throwing athletes. Its anatomic correlate consists of undersurface fraying of the infraspinatus tendon where it contacts the posterior glenoid as the arm is placed in maximum abduction and external rotation, such as the late cocking phase of throwing. Although this contact may often be present physiologically, the repetitive injury and eccentric loading associated with throwing can lead to labral and rotator cuff tears. Last, and intrinsically related to internal impingement, is secondary or nonoutlet impingement. This is often described as a dynamic process in which subtle subluxation of the humeral head with activity can acutely narrow the subacromial space and thus lead to impingement symptoms. It is associated with mild glenohumeral instability but can also result from contracture of the posterior capsule, which causes obligate anterosuperior humeral head translation with forward flexion.

A thorough understanding of the etiology of rotator cuff tears enables the physician to formulate a treatment plan to address the specific pathology present in a particular patient.

Epidemiology

The point prevalence of shoulder pain has been estimated at 7% to 25% and the incidence at 10 per 1,000 per year, peaking at 25 per 1,000 per year among those 42 to 46 years of age. However, these are likely underestimates, as a large proportion of patients with rotator cuff tears remain asymptomatic. It is clear, nonetheless, that rotator cuff tears are strongly related to age; magnetic resonance imaging (MRI) scans of participants without shoulder pain reveal partial- and full-thickness rotator cuff tears in 4% of individuals younger than 40 years of age and in >50% older than 60 years. Furthermore, autopsy studies have demonstrated a prevalence of full-thickness rotator cuff tears of 6% in subjects younger than 60 years and 30% in those older than 60 years, although it was unknown how many of these had shoulder pain. Overall, the number of individuals with rotator cuff dysfunction is expected to grow with an aging population that is increasingly active and less willing to accept functional limitations.

Pathophysiology

In most rotator cuff tears, a combination of intrinsic and extrinsic factors leads to chronic tendon degeneration with eventual tensile failure. Rarely, acute tensile overload can lead to rupture of a healthy or minimally degenerated tendon. Most tears occur in and around the critical zone of the supraspinatus, an area between the bony insertion and musculotendinous junction, with relative hypoperfusion leading to increased susceptibility to damage. The natural history of rotator cuff dysfunction is not well understood. Prior investigations have demonstrated that 50% of individuals with asymptomatic tears developed pain within 5 years, although only 30% demonstrated increases in tear size. Studies investigating partial tears of the rotator cuff have demonstrated enlargement or progression to full-thickness tears in 80% of patients over a period of 2 years with nonoperative therapy. Once tears occur, there seems to be little to no evidence of spontaneous healing. A histopathologic study showed no signs of healing in pathologic specimens from partial-thickness tears. Furthermore, although shoulder complaints may be short lived, one study reported persistence or recurrence of symptoms in 40% to 50% of individuals 1 year after the initial presentation. It should also be understood that irreversible changes occur over time in the muscle tendon complex in the setting of rotator cuff detachment.

Classification

Partial tears generally involve <50% of the tendon thickness and do not lead to retraction of the muscle. Depending on the location within the rotator cuff tendon, partial-thickness tears can be classified as intrasubstance, bursal sided, or articular sided (undersurface), the latter constituting approximately 90% of partial tears. Weakness is uncommon in partial thickness tears but can arise from pain, which is often greater than in complete tears.

In contrast, full-thickness tears represent complete discontinuity of rotator cuff fibers resulting in communication between the articular and bursal spaces. The extent of the lesion on imaging studies is described in both anteroposterior and mediolateral directions. One centimeter is generally considered small, 1 to 3 cm medium, 3 to 5 cm large. and >5 cm massive. Tears that involve two or more tendons can also be classified as massive and require more complex reconstruction. In larger tears, chronically retracted muscles undergo fatty degeneration over time that may be irreversible and may make results of direct repair unsatisfactory.

Rotator cuff tears can be further classified based on tear configuration. Crescent-shaped, L-shaped, and U-shaped tears have been described, all of which require slight modifications in repair technique to achieve excellent fixation (see below).

DIAGNOSIS

Physical Examination and History

Clinical Features

Rotator cuff pain is frequently described as a dull ache of insidious onset extending over the lateral arm and shoulder. Overhead activities exacerbate the pain, and pain frequently increases at night and may awaken the individual from sleep. Weakness with the inability to abduct and elevate the arm is seen in more advanced cases; patients frequently describe difficulties combing hair, holding a hair dryer, and removing the wallet from their back pocket. Acute onset of weakness, especially in association with trauma, may indicate an acute tear.

The clinical examination of a candidate for arthroscopic rotator cuff repair follows the standard shoulder exam described in earlier chapters. As in any preoperative evaluation, assessment of associated pathology that could be encountered at the time of surgery is crucial. The biceps tendon, capsulolabral complex, acromioclavicular joint, acromion, and especially the subscapularis tendon are structures that may require additional interventions that could considerably prolong and complicate an all-arthroscopic procedure. Recognition of the size, shape, and tissue quality is crucial to a successful arthroscopic repair.

Radiologic Features

Radiography. In the anteroposterior (AP) view, joint space narrowing and osteophyte formation may indicate arthritis of the glenohumeral or acromioclavicular joints. Calcium deposits from calcifying tendonitis usually present just proximal to the rotator cuff insertion. Elevation of the humeral head on AP radiographs, especially when the subacromial space is decreased to less than <5 to 7 mm, has been associated with large rotator cuff tears. The axillary view is essential to exclude the possibility of a dislocation. This view also shows the joint space and helps identify the rare but occasionally symptomatic os acromiale, which is a persistent and ununited ossification center at the end of the acromion. The 30-degree caudal tilt view is useful to assess the condition of the acromioclavicular joint. Finally, the supraspinatus outlet view allows visualization of the bony structures of the scapulothoracic motion interface and shows acromial spurs or calcification of the coracoacromial ligament that might compress the underlying rotator cuff.

Ultrasound. Ultrasound is noninvasive, readily available, and inexpensive. Recent studies using arthroscopy or MRI for validation of ultrasound have demonstrated sensitivities of 58% to100% and specificities of 78% to 100% for full-thickness tears. It is less accurate in the detection of partial-thickness tears with sensitivities ranging from 25% to 94%.

MRI and MR Arthrography. Magnetic resonance imaging has sensitivities close to 100% for full-thickness tears and has all but replaced arthrography for the diagnosis for rotator cuff pathology. Moreover, the additional quantitative and qualitative information gleaned from this cross-sectional study aids in the surgical planning and prognosis. The combination of MRI and gadolinium arthrography further improves sensitivity, especially for the detection of partial tears, to >90%, and of labral pathology to >80%. Important concerns regarding MRI include the associated cost and high frequency of false-positives. Up to 30% of asymptomatic volunteers have findings of rotator cuff anomalies, and up to 50% show labral anomalies.

The surgeon should closely review all MRI series and images preoperatively to determine tear size and location, as well as tissue quality, since massive tears with retraction and fatty degeneration of the muscle might prove to be irreparable. Coronal images best show the supraspinatus and degree of tendon retraction, axial images best display subscapularis disruption, and sagittal images will give an estimate on the width of the cuff insertion that is disrupted.

TREATMENT

Nonoperative Treatment

A trial of nonoperative treatment is indicated in virtually all patients with rotator cuff pathology. One exception is the young patient presenting with acute weakness owing to a traumatic event. Conservative treatment includes subacromial steroid injections and anti-inflammatory medications to control pain in the acute period, followed by a physical therapy program designed to increase muscle strength and balance. This is best accomplished with attention to proper rehabilitation of the scapular stabilizers, the remaining intact rotator cuff, and the anterior deltoid.

Surgical Indications/Contraindications

The indications for arthroscopic rotator cuff repair follow those of open rotator cuff repair. The primary indication for surgical treatment is persistent pain unresponsive to nonoperative measures; poor function and diminished strength are secondary indications. The ideal surgical candidate is a compliant patient with adequate tendon quality who can follow a rigorous postoperative rehabilitation program. All patients should recognize that the results are dependent on many factors including tear size and retraction, tissue quality, muscle degeneration and atrophy, and overall health of the patient.

The few contraindications to arthroscopic rotator cuff repair include active or recent infection, medical comorbidities that make surgery or anesthesia unsafe, and advanced glenohumeral arthritis requiring arthroplasty. Relative contraindications may include significant fatty infiltration of the involved muscles and fixed superior migration of the humeral head with marked retraction of tendon edges on MRI.

Operative Treatment

Surgical Considerations

The goal of arthroscopic rotator cuff repair is to relieve pain and improve shoulder function while addressing all concomitant intra-articular pathology in a minimally invasive manner. Many technical aspects of arthroscopic rotator cuff surgery are evolving as our understanding of failure mechanisms and patient outcomes grows. Many issues remain controversial, such as the need for routine acromioplasty, the management of incomplete tears, optimal suture management, and anchor configuration—single row versus double row. Nonetheless, the successful arthroscopic treatment of rotator cuff tears depends on recognition of tear patterns, appropriate use of releases, secure fixation with restoration of the footprint under minimal tension, and proper rehabilitation.

Currently, most surgeons routinely perform an acromioplasty as part of the decompression prior to initiating repair. This may improve visualization in addition to reducing potential external compression of the cuff from the anterolateral acromion while affording space for the repaired tendon to clear the acromion during rotation. However, recent studies have suggested that routine performance of an acromioplasty may not be necessary. The primary technical concern while performing the acromioplasty relates to release of the coracoacromial (CA) ligament. A complete release of the ligament should be avoided, especially in large and massive rotator cuff tears, since it provides a restraint to superior escape of the humeral head in the rotator cuff deficient shoulder. An adequate acromioplasty, however, can easily be performed even without complete release of the CA ligament. Also, sparing the most anterior attachment of the CA ligament, as well as the deltoid fascia, helps to minimize fluid extravasation during subacromial arthroscopy.

Anesthetic Considerations

Arthroscopic rotator cuff repair is usually performed under general anesthesia with endotracheal intubation, laryngeal mask ventilation, regional anesthesia through an interscalene nerve block, or a combination thereof. The decision is made in collaboration with the patient and anesthesiologist. Regional anesthesia is beneficial especially for same-day surgical procedures since its analgesic effects commonly continue for several hours past discharge. Preemptive analgesia with nonsteroidal anti-inflammatories (NASAIDs) given the night before the operation is being used by an increasing number of surgeons and is usually continued for several days postoperatively. Concerns are emerging, however, regarding the potential inhibitory effects that NSAIDs might have on the early healing process.

Patient Positioning and Portal Placement

Based on the surgeon's preference, the patient is placed in either the beach-chair or lateral decubitus position. Although each position has unique advantages and limitations, both are acceptable choices for arthroscopic rotator cuff repair.

Portals useful in arthroscopic rotator cuff repair include standard posterior, anterior, anterolateral, and posterolateral portals (Fig. 40-1) as described in previous chapters. Anchor placement occasionally requires accessory portals that deviate from the standard portals described above. These portals should be kept as small as possible to minimize injury to the deltoid muscle and used only for percutaneous anchor placement without the use of a cannula. Another portal that we have recently described and find particularly

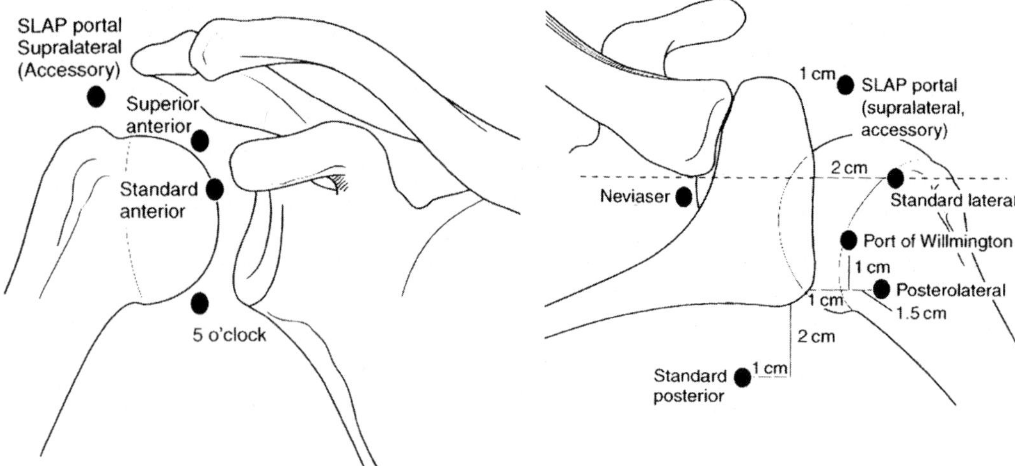

Figure 40-1 Standard portals in shoulder arthroscopy.

useful is the posteromedial portal, which is placed approximately 3 cm medial to the standard posterior portal and allows an in-line passage of a suture retrieving instrument (i.e., penetrating suture grasper).

Surgical Technique

Diagnostic Arthroscopy. A brief diagnostic arthroscopy is performed through standard anterior and posterior portals to evaluate potentially associated pathology. After the rotator cuff tear is visualized, it is often helpful to mark the exact location by passing a suture percutaneously through the tear into the subacromial space, especially in small tears, which can be difficult to visualize once the subacromial space is entered.

Subacromial Decompression. A bursectomy and limited acromioplasty is performed with an arthroscopic bur and radiofrequency ablation device to control bleeding. The rotator cuff tear is judiciously debrided simply to freshen the leading edge. The insertion site on the greater tuberosity (footprint) is cleaned of soft tissues and gently superficially debrided to create a bleeding subcortical surface.

Releases. Torn rotator cuff tendons often are contracted through their capsular attachments or are adherent to surrounding tissue. Releasing these attachments and adhesions with an electrothermal device or an arthroscopic elevator is crucial to obtaining full cuff mobilization. With a grasper or traction suture on the leading edge, the surgeon can evaluate the results of the performed release. If the tendon can be reduced to the footprint only by applying significant tension, further releases should be performed to allow for a tensionfree repair.

Releases should be performed between the cuff tendons and the undersurface of the acromion. Anterior releases in the rotator interval region can separate adhesions between the supraspinatus and the coracoid and subscapularis. Occasionally, posterior release between the supraspinatus and infraspinatus is required. In long-standing tears, the cuff may be adherent to the glenoid neck, and releasing the capsule adjacent to the superior and posterior labrum is particularly useful. However, the suprascapular nerve and vessels are at risk during this dissection, which should not extend further than 1 to 2 cm medial to the glenoid rim.

Tear Patterns. As mentioned earlier, several tear configurations have been described. Crescent-shaped tears are more commonly found acutely or subacutely and usually are easily mobilized and repaired directly to bone with suture anchors (Figure 40-2). U-shaped tears are usually larger and may require side-to-side repair (i.e., margin convergence) to reduce tear size and decrease tension on the leading edge, thus allowing for a more stable repair to the tuberosity (Figure 40-3). L-shaped tears are best addressed with a side-to-side repair of the longitudinal limb before securing the horizontal limb to bone with suture anchors (Figure 40-4). Side-to-side repairs are performed with free sutures that can be passed through the tendon substance with various instruments and techniques (Figure 40-5). Our preference is to use a straight penetrating suture grasper when working in the posterior two thirds of the cuff as well as during repair of the more medial extent of the side-to-side

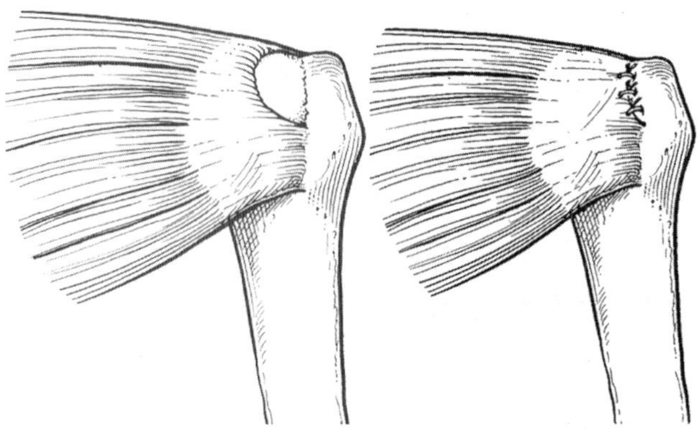

Figure 40-2 Crescent-shaped tear and repair.

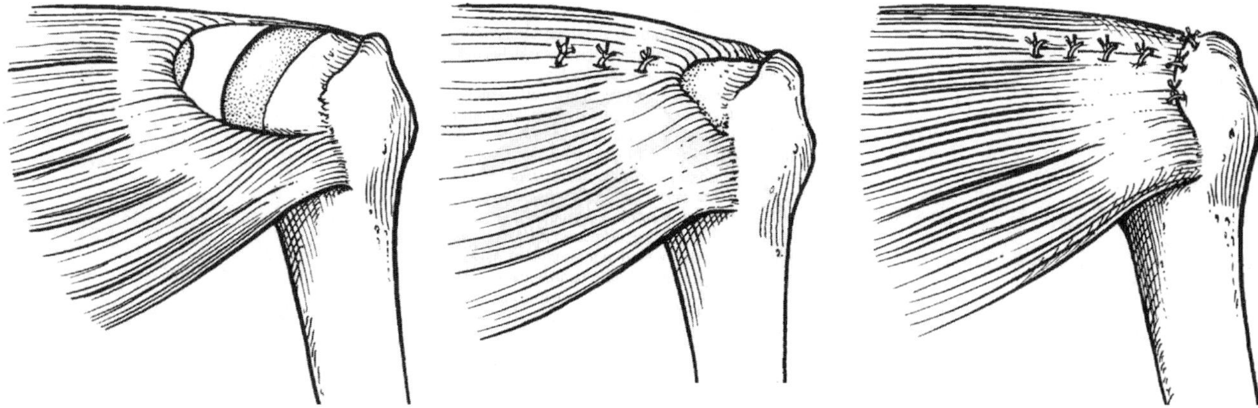

Figure 40-3 U-shaped tear and repair.

component of the tear. More laterally and anteriorly, a straight shuttle-type suture passing device is more effective.

Fixation. The actual repair of the tendon to the tuberosity can be performed with various techniques. The two most common portal configurations involve visualization through the lateral portal with instrumentation through the posterior or posteromedial portal (our preference), and vice versa. The first step is to prepare the footprint on the greater tuberosity to obtain an optimal environment for healing. Increasingly, surgeons refrain from extensive decortication during preparation of the footprint with an arthroscopic bur since it does not appear to improve healing and can compromise suture anchor fixation.

Arthroscopic repair of the rotator cuff tendon to the footprint uses suture anchors, which can be either bioabsorbable or metal, depending on surgeon preference. Advantages of bioabsorbable anchors include decreased artifacts on follow-up MRI and eventual resorption, potentially making revisions easier and reducing concerns over loose anchors that could damage the joint. Advantages of metal anchors include lower cost, decreased risk of anchor breakage during insertion, and lack of reactivity in the surrounding bone. Anchors are placed in the lateral aspect of the footprint for a single-row technique, or medially and laterally for a double-row technique in larger tears amenable to this anchor/suture configuration. The double-row technique reduces tension on the lateral anchors and secures the tendon to a larger bony surface.

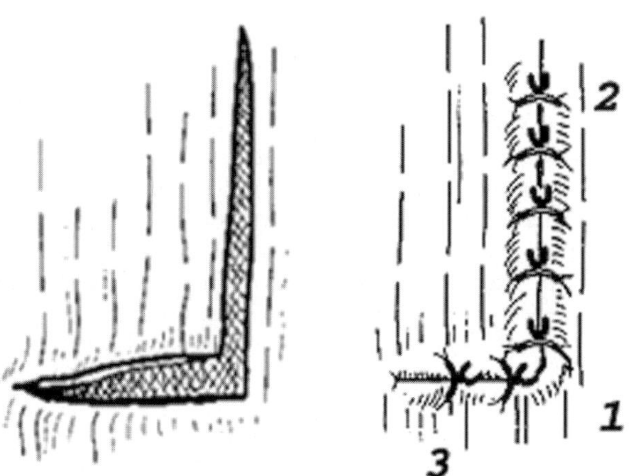

Figure 40-4 L-shaped tear and repair.

After anchors are placed, the suture on the anchor must be passed through the rotator cuff tendon. There are many devices on the market to facilitate this process; however, the senior author prefers working with low-profile penetrating suture graspers for the posterior cuff in combination with a 45-degree ipsilateral (i.e., right curve for right shoulder) curved suture shuttle device for the more anterior aspect of the tear. Alternatively, there are several excellent devices that can be passed with a loaded suture directly through the anterolateral or lateral portal (while viewing from posteriorly) and passed antegrade directly through the lateral tendon edge. Whenever shuttling or making use of the antegrade suture passing device, it is helpful to avoid having more than a single suture limb within the cannula at any given time to avoid entanglement.

It is important to consider the direction of tear retraction when placing sutures. Since most tears of the supraspinatus and infraspinatus tendons retract in a posteromedial fashion, sutures should be placed more posteriorly relative to the anchor to restore proper tendon orientation. Suture anchors should be placed in a methodical order to help with suture management, often from posterior to anterior. Sutures should be stored in unused cannulas to avoid entanglement, and only one suture should be kept in a working cannula during knot tying. We typically, whenever possible, place a central and medial anchor loaded with two sutures and retrieve all four limbs with a penetrating suture grasper placed through the posteromedial or posterior portal, creating two independent horizontal mattress sutures. Next, we place at least two additional anchors beginning more posterior and lateral to the first medial anchor already in position. The final anchor is placed typically just behind the bicipital groove in line with the second more laterally placed anchor.

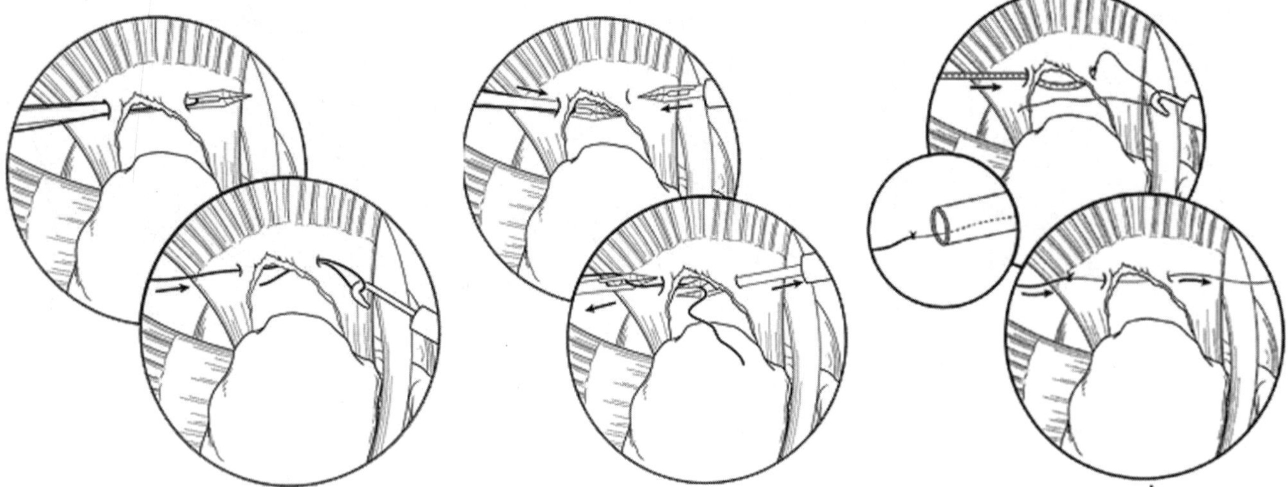

Figure 40-5 Side-to-side repair techniques for margin conversion sutures: antegrade (**left**), antegrade hand-off (**middle**), and antegrade shuttle (**right**) techniques.

Arthroscopic knot tying is a crucial technical aspect of a successful repair. Although many different sliding and nonsliding techniques have been described, the senior author prefers simple half hitches on alternating posts. This reliable and simple method does not require sliding of the suture through the tissue, which has been incriminated in suture cutout. Irrespective of the technique used, care must be taken to ensure that the knot tightly reduces the tendon to the anchor and bony bed of the footprint to allow healing.

Results and Outcome

Clinical outcomes after arthroscopic rotator cuff repair have been comparable to open reconstruction, despite the fact that radiologic investigations have demonstrated a comparatively higher rate of recurrent tears on MRI follow-up. Between 77% and 98% of patients are satisfied with their outcome after rotator cuff repair, with excellent pain relief and functional improvement in >80%. Benefits of arthroscopic repair versus open or mini-open techniques include smaller incisions with less soft tissue dissection, avoidance of deltoid detachment, improved visualization of the entire glenohumeral joint for evaluation and treatment of concomitant pathology, and decreased postoperative pain. However, arthroscopic repair has been associated with a significant rate of recurrent tears. Our own results have demonstrated a retear rate of ≤47% at 2 years on MRI examination. Nonetheless, clinical results do not seem to suffer in these patients. We have found significantly improved functional and pain scores, as well as improved strength, even in the setting of a recurrent tear, with patients rating their postsurgical shoulder at 85% of their normal contralateral side.

Complications are comparatively low, with infection reported in <1% of cases. Traction injuries of the brachial plexus occur as very rare complications when shoulder arthroscopy is performed in the lateral decubitus position, but are usually transient. The incidence of minor complications related to edema from fluid extravasation is unknown and is typically inconsequential; however, there have been reports of subcutaneous emphysema causing serious pulmonary complications during shoulder arthroscopy, which emphasizes the need for continued monitoring of the patient's shoulder and neck for excessive swelling or crepitus.

Postoperative Management

The postoperative rehabilitation program is one of the most important factors in achieving a good result. Postoperatively, patients are typically placed in a sling and a supportive abduction pillow, which is worn at all times, except for hygiene and therapeutic exercise. The rehabilitation program is divided into three phases, which are based on the progression of healing with increasing strength of the reconstruction:

In phase 1 (weeks 0 to 4), exercises are restricted to passive range of motion (ROM), with limits of motion based on intraoperative assessment of repair stability. Therapeutic exercises during this phase include pendulum exercises; elbow, wrist and hand ROM; grip strengthening; and isometric scapular stabilization.

During phase 2 (weeks 4 to 8), the sling is discontinued and ROM is progressed to 140 degrees of forward flexion, 40 degrees of external rotation, abduction to 60 to 80 degrees, and posterior capsular stretching to maintain or improve internal rotation. Therapeutic exercises are advanced to gentle active-assisted exercises in the supine position with progression to active exercises with resistance at 6 weeks. Deltoid and biceps strengthening is initiated, with the arm kept close to the side to minimize lever arm forces on the rotator cuff.

Phase 3 (approximately weeks 8 to 12) is characterized by progression to full motion as tolerated. Scapular strengthening is continued, and internal and external rotation isometric exercises are added to the program. During the final phase of rehabilitation, sport-specific activities are initiated, flexibility is maintained, and strengthening exercises are continued. Usually, formal physical therapy is discontinued after approximately 4 months, with return to unrestricted athletic activities at 6 months.

SUGGESTED READINGS

Berjano P, Gonzalez BG, Olmedo JF. et al. Complications in arthroscopic shoulder surgery. *Arthroscopy*. 1998;14:785–788.

Bigliani LU, Ticker JB, Flatow EL, et al. The relationship of acromial architecture to rotator cuff disease. *Clin Sports Med*. 1991;10:823–838.

Burkhart SS, Athanasiou KA, Wirth MA. Margin convergence: a method of reducing strain in massive rotator cuff tears. *Arthroscopy*. 1996;12:335–338.

Carpenter JE, Flanagan CL, Thomopoulos S, et al. The effects of overuse combined with intrinsic or extrinsic alterations in an animal model of rotator cuff tendinosis. *Am J Sports Med*. 1998;26:801–807.

Fuchs B, Weishaupt D, Zanetti M, et al. Fatty degeneration of the muscles of the rotator cuff: assessment by computed tomography versus magnetic resonance imaging. *J Shoulder Elbow Surg*. 1999;8:599–605.

Galatz LM, Ball CM, Teefey SA, et al. The outcome and repair integrity of completely arthroscopically repaired large and massive rotator cuff tears. *J Bone Joint Surg* Am. 2004;86A:219–224.

Gartsman GM, Khan M, Hammerman SM. Arthroscopic repair of full-thickness tears of the rotator cuff. *J Bone Joint Surg Am*. 1998;80:832–840.

Gartsman GM, O'Connor DP. Arthroscopic rotator cuff repair with and without arthroscopic subacromial decompression: a prospective, randomized study of one-year outcomes. *J Shoulder Elbow Surg*. 2004;13:424–426.

Goldberg BA, Lippitt SB, Matsen FA III. Improvement in comfort and function after cuff repair without acromioplasty. *Clin Orthop Relat Res*. 2001;390:142–150.

Kim SH, Ha KI, Park JH. et al. Arthroscopic versus mini-open salvage repair of the rotator cuff tear: outcome analysis at 2 to 6 years' follow-up. *Arthroscopy*. 2003;19:746–754.

Lau KY. Pneumomediastinum caused by subcutaneous emphysema in the shoulder. A rare complication of arthroscopy. *Chest*. 1993;103:1606–1607.

Lee HC, Dewan N, Crosby L. Subcutaneous emphysema, pneumomediastinum, and potentially life-threatening tension pneumothorax. Pulmonary complications from arthroscopic shoulder decompression. *Chest*. 1992;101:1265–1267.

Lehman C, Cuomo F, Kummer FJ, et al. The incidence of full thickness rotator cuff tears in a large cadaveric population. *Bull Hosp Jt Dis*. 1995;54(1):30–31.

Lo IK, Burkhart SS. Double-row arthroscopic rotator cuff repair: re-establishing the footprint of the rotator cuff. *Arthroscopy*. 2003;19:1035–1042.

Loutzenheiser TD, Harryman DT II, Yung SW, et al. Optimizing arthroscopic knots. *Arthroscopy*. 1995;11:199–206.

Potter HG, B. S. Magnetic imaging of the shoulder: a tailored approach. *Techniques Shoulder Elbow Surg*. 2005;6(1):43–56.

Schibany N, Zehetgruber H, Kainberger F, et al. Rotator cuff tears in asymptomatic individuals: a clinical and ultrasonographic screening study. *Eur J Radiol*. 2004;51(3):263–268.

Tempelhof S, Rupp S, Seil R. Age-related prevalence of rotator cuff tears in asymptomatic shoulders. *J Shoulder Elbow Surg*. 1999;8(4):296–299.

Wiener SN, Seitz WH Jr. Sonography of the shoulder in patients with tears of the rotator cuff: accuracy and value for selecting surgical options. *AJR Am J Roentgenol*. 1993;160:103–107; discussion 109–110.

Wilson F, Hinov V, Adams G. Arthroscopic repair of full-thickness tears of the rotator cuff: 2- to 14-year follow-up. *Arthroscopy*. 2002;18:136–144.

Yamaguchi K, Tetro AM, Blam O, et al. Natural history of asymptomatic rotator cuff tears: a longitudinal analysis of asymptomatic tears detected sonographically. *J Shoulder Elbow Surg*. 2001;10(3):199–203.

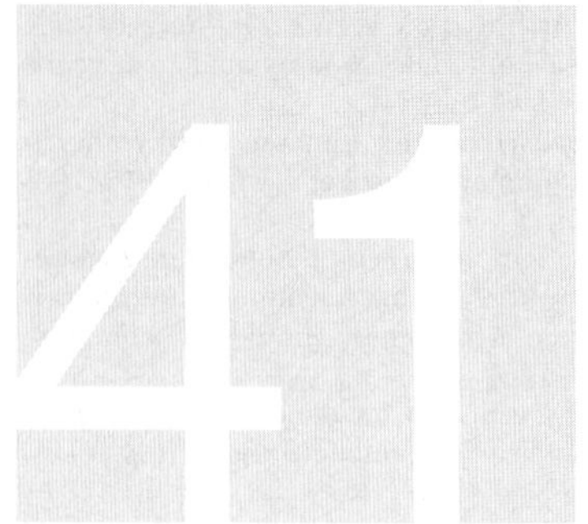

NERVE INJURIES ABOUT THE SHOULDER

SCOTT P. STEINMANN
GILBERT CSUJA

CLINICAL EVALUATION

History

Accurate recognition and diagnosis of potential neurologic injury about the shoulder is paramount for proper treatment of a patient's condition. In a patient presenting with complaints of shoulder pain or weakness, obtaining a thorough history should be the first step to establish an accurate diagnosis.

The patient should be questioned about pain, weakness, numbness, onset of symptoms, progression, timing of symptomatic episodes, and any improvement with time. The quality, level, and timing of pain are important factors to document. A visual scale to have the patient estimate his or her pain during the day and night, and compare this with the other noninvolved extremity may, be a useful adjunct.

In the emergency room setting, an accurate neurologic examination should be attempted. If all or part of the neurologic examination is unable to be completed, adequate documentation of this should be made. A cursory exam with documentation of "neurovascularly intact" may attract future litigation. Diagnosis of nerve injury may be delayed until the patient regains consciousness and becomes cooperative.

Physical Examination

The initial part of the neurologic exam of the shoulder and arm is examining the extremity for muscle atrophy. This can be done only with the shoulder completely exposed, to be able to view the shoulder and scapula.

An accurate neurologic examination should be able to be performed on any patient who is coherent, even in the setting of shoulder trauma. Starting the examination at the level of the fingers and hand is recommended, for most of this part of the exam should be able to be done with minimal discomfort to the patient. Assessing median, ulnar, and radial nerve motor and sensory functions should take little time and should include two-point discrimination measurements to both aspects of all fingers and thumb. Elbow flexion and extension can determine musculocutaneous nerve and high radial nerve function by testing for biceps, brachialis, brachioradialis, and triceps activity. Axillary nerve function is determined by testing shoulder abduction, specifically by looking at deltoid contraction with the arm at the patient's side. Loss of motor or sensory function in the distal extremity can also be helpful in locating the area of injury more proximally. If radial nerve dysfunction is seen distally in combination with axillary nerve injury (both nerves being branches of the posterior cord), this is an indication that the injury may have occurred at the level of the posterior cord of the brachial plexus.

More proximally, pectoralis major function tests lateral pectoral nerve (clavicular head) and medial pectoral nerve (sternal head) function. Latissimus dorsi is innervated by the thoracodorsal nerve and is tested by extending the arm, or contraction with coughing. Serratus anterior is supplied by the long thoracic nerve and is tested for by examining presence of winging while the patient forward flexes the arm such as in a wall push-up. The rhomboids are tested by scapular adduction and observing for muscle atrophy. The rhomboids, major and minor, are innervated by the dorsal scapular nerve.

Full arc abduction of the shoulder can be accomplished is some patients with both deltoid and supraspinatus separately. Supraspinatus and infraspinatus muscles are supplied by the suprascapular nerve and are tested by looking at external rotation strength and midrange abduction of the shoulder.

Examination of the neck should be considered an integral part of any shoulder and upper extremity examination. Just as brachial plexus injury can affect function of the muscles about the shoulder and arm, injury of the spinal cord and exiting nerve roots can do the same. Being able to illicit the patient's symptoms with flexion, extension of the neck, or with the Spurling maneuver indicates probable cervical radiculopathy. In upper motor neuron lesions, deep tendon reflexes may be hyperreflexic, there may be increased tone, and pathologic reflexes may be present.

Referred pain of cardiac or other intrathoracic origins such as gall bladder pain should be excluded as a cause of shoulder pain.

Much of the above shoulder examination is dependent on a healthy shoulder joint. It is often difficult to elicit whether the patient's pain (and weakness) on testing supraspinatus is caused by rotator cuff injury, internal joint pathology, or true neurologic injury. In these cases, lidocaine injection of the subacromial space may provide some benefit in decreasing pain to the area and obtaining a better examination.

Finally, patients with secondary gain issues commonly have nonphysiologic examination findings. However these patients cannot stop the latissimus from contracting while coughing when testing for latissimus function.

AXILLARY NERVE

The axillary nerve is a terminal branch of the posterior cord. It crosses over the anteroinferior aspect of the subscapularis muscle near its insertion, then turns posteriorly to cross the quadrilateral space, where it is in close contact with the inferior joint capsule. It has been reported to be as close as 10 mm inferior to the inferior glenoid labrum. When the nerve exits the quadrilateral space, it branches into two trunks. The posterior trunk branches to supply teres minor and posterior deltoid, then terminates as the superior lateral brachial cutaneous nerve. The anterior trunk travels subfascially, then enters the middle and anterior deltoid to innervate those muscles. The position of the anterior trunk is reported to be as close as 4 cm inferior to the anterolateral acromion. Internal topography studies of the axillary nerve show that on its exit from the posterior cord, the nerve is monofascicular, but by the time it exits the quadrangular space, the nerve has distinct fascicles. The deltoid motor fascicles run superolateral, and the teres minor and sensory fascicle run inferomedially.

Axillary nerve paralysis is the most common peripheral nerve injury to affect the shoulder. It is most commonly seen as a complication of shoulder dislocation, proximal humerus fracture, or blunt trauma to the shoulder. The literature reports 5% to 10% incidence of clear axillary nerve injury with glenohumeral dislocation. However, at least one study reports electromyography/nerve conduction study (EMG/NCS) findings in as many as 54% of dislocations, most patients being subclinical. Fortunately, most patients recover from their injury spontaneously. Patients who are at a higher risk of permanent injury are those older than 50 years of age and patients whose shoulder stays dislocated for >12 hours. The mechanism of injury is that of direct compression of the dislocated humeral head against the nerve. Because of the short length of the axillary nerve from its origin in the posterior cord of the brachial plexus and its attachment at the deltoid, traction injury may also result at the infraclavicular brachial plexus.

The axillary nerve may also be injured from blunt trauma to the shoulder without glenohumeral dislocation. Most reports of this kind of injury show a mechanism of posteriorly directed force from collisions in football and hockey with similar symptomatology; however, no isolated axillary nerve ruptures of this type were found reported (Fig. 41-1).

There is at least one report in the literature of rotator cuff tears associated with neuropathies. Of the 15 patients evaluated with this combination of injuries, 12 had EMG-demonstrable axillary nerve injury. Interestingly, only 2 of these 12 patients had decreased sensation over the lateral shoulder. This study reported that since the cause of nerve injury was thought to be a traction neurapraxia, treatment was recommended of rotator cuff repair followed by a monitored physical therapy protocol. Follow-up EMGs were reported to have shown significant nerve recovery in the study patients.

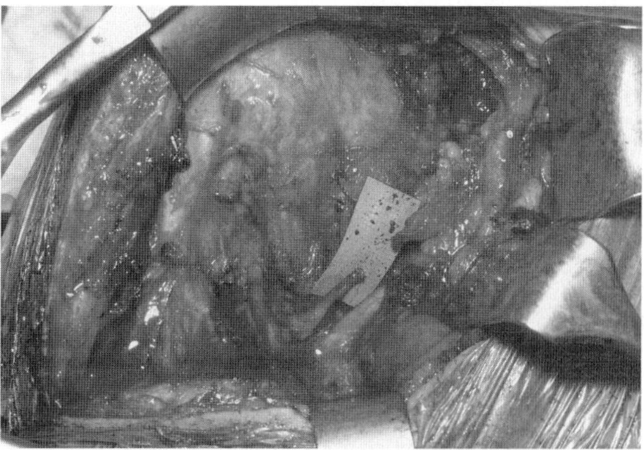

Figure 41-1 An 18-year-old male who dislocated his right shoulder 3 months prior, with no recovery of axillary nerve function. At surgery the axillary nerve was found to be torn. It was repaired with sural nerve grafts.

Quadrilateral nerve syndrome has been described as a compression of the axillary nerve (and posterior humeral circumflex artery) in the quadrilateral space. Symptoms may present as deltoid weakness, vague posterior shoulder pain, and tingling and numbness in lateral shoulder distribution. Compression of the nerve is presumed to be caused by anomalous fibrous bands, muscle hypertrophy, and mass effect. Treatment is mostly conservative, with most cases resolving spontaneously. Exploration and release of impinging structures are rarely needed.

Paralysis of the muscles innervated by the axillary nerve is also seen as one of many nerves injured in brachial plexus trauma. In these cases, avulsion or stretch injury of roots, trunks, or cords of the brachial plexus is the usual site of injury. Isolated axillary nerve injury in brachial plexus trauma has a reported incidence between 3% and 6% in the literature.

The axillary nerve is also at significant risk during some shoulder open and arthroscopic procedures (Fig. 41-2). These procedures include open rotator cuff repair, open and arthroscopic Bankart procedures, arthroscopic capsular release, arthroscopic thermal capsulodesis, open reduction internal fixation, and humeral nail placement for humeral head and neck fractures. The mechanism of injury varies to include traction injuries, incision or cautery of the nerve, screw placement through the nerve, and capturing the nerve with sutures intended to tighten the joint capsule. Incidence of iatrogenic nerve palsies after plate fixation is reported between 0% and 5%, whereas incidence of nerve injury after intramedullary nail placement is between 0% and 4%.

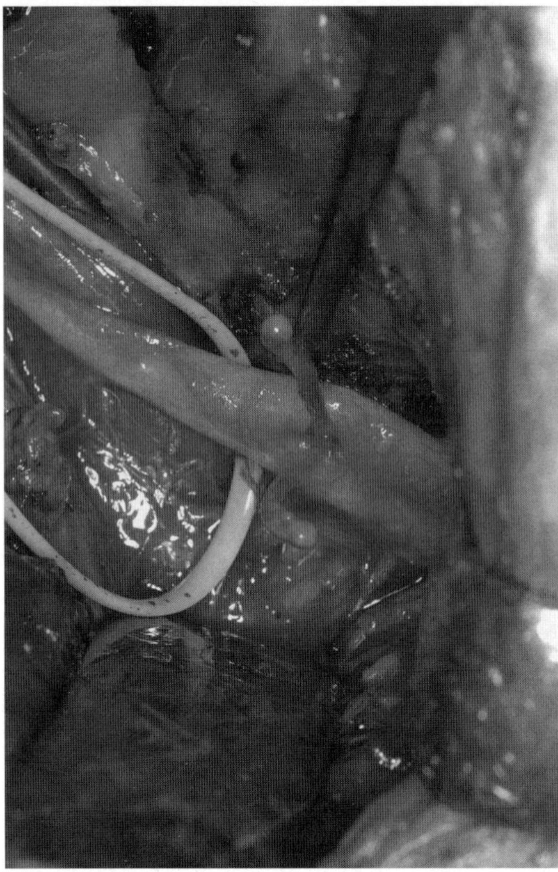

Figure 41-2 A 21-year-old man underwent prior arthroscopic instability repair. He awoke with severe axillary neuropathy. At surgical exploration, a suture was found compressing the axillary nerve. The suture can be seen dividing the axillary nerve. The suture was removed, and the patient achieved excellent recovery.

Although thermal capsular shrinkage procedures are on a sharp decline, the close proximity of the axillary nerve to the inferior glenohumeral joint capsule puts the nerve at a significant risk of injury owing to high temperatures. These injuries are thought to be caused by high temperatures in the shoulder joint with the nerve running as close as 1 cm to the inferior joint capsule. The reported incidence is 1% to 2% with spontaneous recovery in most cases.

As previously discussed, most axillary nerve injuries resulting from blunt trauma resolve spontaneously, so in these cases, it is recommended that nerve recovery should be observed for at least 3 months prior to considering surgical intervention. It is recommended that a baseline EMG/NCS be obtained at 3 to 4 weeks and repeated at 1 to 2 month intervals to assess nerve recovery. Physical therapy should be initiated to prevent loss of motion to the shoulder joint. There are no studies to show that electrical nerve or muscle stimulation speed recovery. If there are no signs of recovery by 6 months, surgical exploration with possible nerve grafting is indicated. Because of its short course through the axilla, cable grafting is the preferred choice of surgical repair. The axillary nerve is approached via a combined anterior/posterior incision. The nerve is identified anteriorly at its origin off the posterior cord and followed posteriorly through the quadrilateral space. It is then found posteriorly as it branches to innervate the deltoid and followed anteriorly. Neurolysis is done in cases where the nerve is shown to conduct with intraoperative direct electrical stimulation. Nerve grafting is done with preferred use of sural nerve graft if the nerve is ruptured, retracted, or if neuroma scarring is too great. Leechavengvongs reported nerve to long head triceps grafted to axillary nerve deltoid motor branches to reinnervate an otherwise nonrepairable axillary nerve with excellent results and rapid recovery.

Following surgical repair, the shoulder is immobilized in neutral abducted position for 2 to 3 weeks, followed by progressive active and active-assist therapy to regain shoulder range of motion. Maximal recovery of the nerve is expected at 12 to 18 months from surgery. One study with 25 patients with axillary nerve repair (most treated by sural nerve grafting) reported 23 patients obtaining M4 or M5 strength postoperatively. Neurotization of the nerve is usually done in massive brachial plexus trauma with thoracodorsal, spinal accessory, phrenic, and intercostal nerves. These patients have less optimal recovery.

SPINAL ACCESSORY NERVE

The spinal accessory nerve (cervical nerve [CN] XI) supplies motor function to the trapezius and sternocleidomastoid muscles, which is a major scapular stabilizer. It enters the neck through the jugular foramen and after passing through the sternocleidomastoid, it crosses the posterior cervical triangle obliquely to innervate the trapezius on its underside. The posterior cervical triangle is bordered anteriorly by the sternocleidomastoid, posteriorly by the trapezius and inferiorly by the clavicle. Although most motor function to the trapezius is derived from the spinal accessory nerve, at least some have dual innervation of the upper portion of the muscle from cervical roots 3 and 4.

The trapezius muscle takes its origins from the ligamentum nuchae superiorly and from the spinous processes of C7–T12. The muscle can be divided into three portions: upper, middle, and inferior. It is the upper portion of the muscle that originates from the ligamentum nuchae, rotating around to become the posterior border of the posterior cervical triangle, and finally attaching to the posterior aspect of the lateral third of the clavicle. This part of the muscle may have alternate innervation from cranial nerves 3 and 4 and may still remain functional after spinal accessory nerve injury. The upper portion elevates and upwardly rotates scapula. The middle portion of the muscle inserts on the medial acromion and the lateral aspect of the scapular spine and adducts and retracts the scapula. The most inferior portion of the muscle's origin is mostly thoracic spinous processes as far inferior as T12, and insertion is on the medial spine of the scapula. This portion mainly depresses and rotates the scapula downward. The spinal accessory nerve gives off branches to innervate these different parts sequentially, which is important in brachial plexus reconstruction for using the lower branches to neurotize injured nerves, without losing the elevating function of the upper trapezius and while preserving neck contour. In this situation, the rhomboids and serratus can partly compensate for the lost inferior sections with continued retraction of the scapula.

The trapezius muscle is the predominant stabilizer of the scapula, with its action of elevating, rotating, and retracting the shoulder blade. Loss of this function causes the shoulder to droop and allows the scapula to rotate downward, outward, and away from the midline. This causes winging of the scapula and decreases strength and range of motion in the planes of abduction and forward flexion. As the shoulder assumes this new position, subacromial impingement now becomes more likely, as does development of rotator cuff tendinopathy. Other shoulder stabilizers are overworked, which causes pain and spasm. The decreased range of motion can also result in a stiff shoulder and may advance to frank adhesive capsulitis. This, in turn, causes still active shoulder stabilizers and rotator cuff muscles to work even harder to compensate, worsening the patient's pain and spasm. In addition to the drooping shoulder, atrophy of upper trapezius fibers may cause a considerable change in the contours of the patient's neckline, which usually results in significant self-image problems.

Spinal accessory nerve injury, although initially seemingly benign, has significant morbidity, resulting in pain, disability, and a significantly altered physical appearance. Injury to the spinal accessory nerve can occur after penetrating trauma to the shoulder. Blunt trauma to the shoulder and neck region may also injure the nerve, causing trapezius palsy. However, the most common cause is iatrogenic laceration after cervical lymph node biopsy, which is reported to be as high as 3% to 8% in the literature.

The spinal accessory nerve is intimately involved with the cervical lymph nodes in the posterior triangle of the neck. During lymph node dissection, the nerve can easily be injured because of sharp laceration, clipping of nerve thought to be a vessel, or cautery of fibers.

The initial presentation of a patient with recent injury to the spinal accessory nerve is usually a painful shoulder with some decreased shoulder range of motion. Patients and treating physicians may attribute these complaints to postoperative pain. Initially the trapezius may show minimal wasting, and winging may not be appreciated. The levator scapulae muscle may be able to compensate and produce a normal-appearing shoulder shrug. Also, the possibility of a secondary innervation of the trapezius from upper cervical nerves may confuse the initial physical examination. As the trapezius becomes more atrophied, the appearance of the shoulder becomes more obvious, as discussed above.

The patient's history of recent surgical procedure and history of the above symptoms should make the astute physician think of the possibility of spinal accessory nerve injury. The condition is best diagnosed by EMG/NCS done, at the earliest, 3 to 4 weeks after injury. If the nerve injury is recognized within 6 months of the injury, the recommended plan is exploration with planned neurolysis versus repair of the nerve, either in primary fashion or with the use of (sural) nerve graft, depending on intraoperative findings. It is recommended to have intraoperative electrophysiologic testing available during the procedure. The preferred timing for surgery is as soon as possible after injury to the spinal accessory nerve for preservation of best nerve function; however, successful recovery of trapezius function has been reported as far out as 1 year.

In the more uncommon presentations of trapezius palsy resulting from blunt trauma, initial EMG/NCS should be done 3 to 4 weeks after injury as a baseline and the patient followed up every 2 to 3 months, looking for resolution of symptoms or improved EMG/NCS results. If no sign of recovery occurs by the 4- to 6-month time frame, surgical exploration is an option (Fig. 41-3).

Commonly, patients present late (>12 months from injury) with a history of multiple consultations without a clear diagnosis. After 12 months, primary repair of the nerve is generally not useful because of motor end plates degeneration. If the patient compensated well for his or

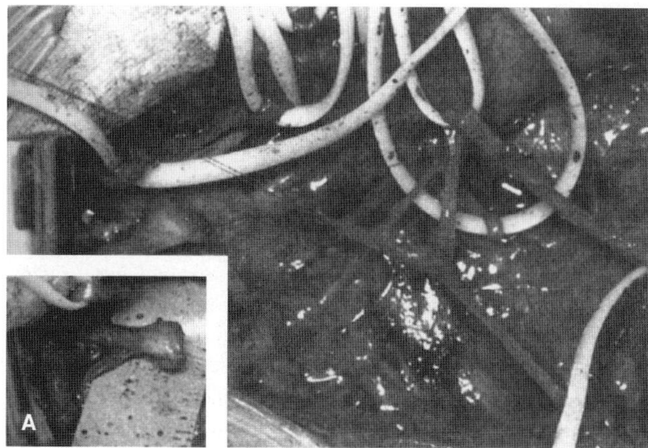

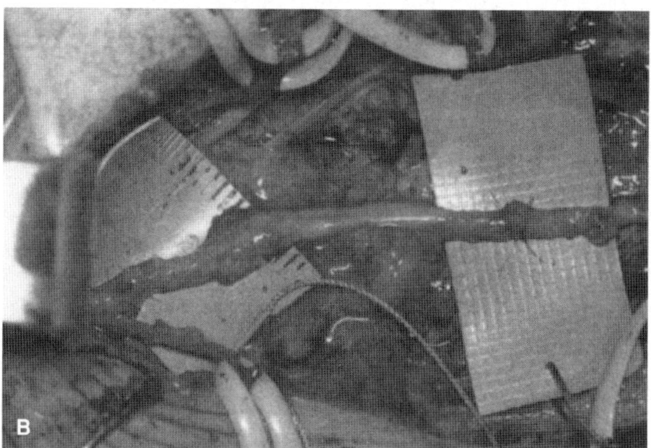

Figure 41-3 Spinal accessory nerve. (From Steinmann SP, Spinner RJ. Nerve problems about the shoulder. In: Rockwood CA Jr, ed. *The Shoulder*. Vol. 2. 3rd ed. Philadelphia: WB Saunders; 2004:1015, with permission.)

her condition, continued observation is a reasonable option. Some patients, however, have severe disability and are unable to function with their resultant level of function. Braces may be offered to these patients, but they tend to be cumbersome.

Many static stabilization procedures have been attempted in the past with modest results, for the large torsion forces on the scapula usually tend to stretch and tear such repairs. The current standard for trapezius reconstruction is the Eden-Lange procedure. This procedure involves dynamic transfer of the levator scapulae, rhomboid major, and rhomboid minor muscles. The levator is transferred to the lateral scapular spine, the rhomboid major as lateral as possible onto the infraspinatus fossa, and the rhomboid minor either to the scapular spine or the supraspinatus fossa. Multiple authors reported good results with this procedure. The salvage operations such as scapulothoracic fusion should be reserved for patients who either have failed all the above attempts at stabilization or have fascioscapulohumeral dystrophy with global loss of shoulder function. This is an operation with potentially very high complication rates.

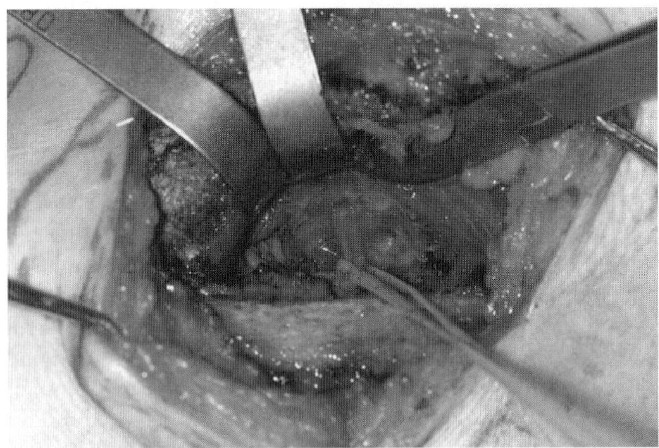

Figure 41-4 Suprascapular nerve compression. Nerve loop holds the suprascapular nerve being compressed by a large ganglion at the suprascapular notch in a 50-year-old man. The cyst was resected, and he achieved excellent recovery.

SUPRASCAPULAR NERVE

The suprascapular nerve is an important contributor to rotator cuff function. Its injury causes significant morbidity with loss of abduction and external rotation of the involved shoulder.

The suprascapular nerve takes its origin from the upper trunk of the brachial plexus; it courses through the posterior triangle of the neck following the omohyoid under the anterior border of the trapezius. The nerve enters the supraspinatus fossa through the suprascapular notch (under the superior transverse scapular ligament), where it gives off branches to innervate the supraspinatus muscle. Upon exiting the supraspinatus fossa through the spinoglenoid notch, the nerve splits off a sensory branch to innervate the posterior joint capsule and turns medial to innervate the infraspinatus muscle.

Major locations where the suprascapular nerve may be tethered are its origin off the upper trunk (the Erb point) and at the suprascapular notch, where it is noted to be relatively fixed. It may also be compressed at the level the spinoglenoid ligament as the nerve courses around the spine of the scapula. It is also here that the nerve may be as close as 20 mm to the superoposterior glenoid edge.

The suprascapular nerve can be injured as a result of blunt trauma sustained to the shoulder, often in occasional with a fracture of the scapula. A common cause of compression of the nerve is a ganglion cyst either at the suprascapular notch or at the spinoglenoid notch. The presumptive origin of these cysts is from degenerative glenoid labral tears (Fig. 41-4). The literature also cites many sports as potential predisposing factors for repetitive-type injury to the suprascapular nerve. The literature often cites volleyball players as the most commonly affected patients, but reports have also implicated baseball, tennis, and weight lifting as possible activities aggravating chronic injury. Parsonage-Turner syndrome is also a cause of idiopathic supraspinatus palsy. This condition has certain identifying characteristics and will be discussed later in the chapter.

Signs and symptoms of suprascapular nerve palsy are nearly identical to those of a rotator cuff tear initially. However, specific symptoms are dependent on the location of the injury or compression. When the injury level is at the suprascapular notch or proximally, patients complain of pain over the posterior and lateral aspects of the shoulder. They also note significant weakness of abduction and external rotation. When the site of injury is more distal, such as the spinoglenoid notch, there is usually less pain (owing to the fact that the sensory nerve may have split off the main nerve) and only loss of external rotation strength may be found. Later as significant muscle atrophy develops, the condition declares itself more clearly. Even then, supraspinatus atrophy is never observed owing to the bulk of the overlying trapezius.

MRI may rule out rotator cuff tear (RCT) as a cause and show fatty degeneration and atrophy of the involved muscles in the absence of massive RCT. Although acutely denervated muscles may not show any significant changes, MRI findings of subacute denervation are characterized by high signal intensity distributed homogeneously throughout the denervated muscle on T2-weighed images.

For cases of suprascapular neuropathy, where a compressive mass of the nerve is known, surgical exploration is recommended. Most ganglions at the spinoglenoid notch can be reached and debrided via shoulder arthroscopy, at which time the labral tear may also be debrided or repaired. A single ganglion noted on MRI with no neurologic involvement does not need operative resection. Repair of any associated symptomatic labral tear may be considered, but the ganglion itself does not need to be debrided. Repair of the labral tear will often cause the ganglion to resorb over time.

MUSCULOCUTANEOUS NERVE

The musculocutaneous nerve is a branch off the medial cord of the brachial plexus. It courses through the coracobrachialis in an oblique medial to lateral direction, entering the coracobrachialis approximately 5 cm below the coracoid. The nerve then travels in a lateral direction to send motor branches to first the biceps and then to the brachialis muscles. Distal to these branches, the nerve becomes the lateral antebrachial cutaneous nerve to supply the lateral forearm.

Musculocutaneous nerve injury is occasionally seen with glenohumeral dislocations and is occasionally seen as a result of penetrating trauma (such as knife wounds).

Most musculocutaneous nerve palsies present as a mixed motor and sensory situation with symptoms of weakness of elbow flexion and with pain and numbness along the radial forearm. However, a pure sensory syndrome of lateral antebrachial nerve compression may also be seen, with symptoms exacerbated by vigorous activity and elbow extension. The sensory nerve is thought to be compressed between the biceps and brachialis on its exit just lateral to the distal biceps tendon or by fascial bands in the antebrachial fossa. Treatment is usually conservative with rest, nonsteroidal anti-inflammatories, and posterior splint to limit hyperextension of the elbow.

If musculocutaneous nerve injury is suspected, either resulting from traumatic or from iatrogenic origin, and no recovery is seen by the 3 to 4-week mark postinjury, an EMG/NCS can be performed both for diagnostic purposes and to establish a baseline for following recovery of the nerve. Since most musculocutaneous nerve injuries are traction related versus sharp lacerations of the nerve, spontaneous recovery is expected within the first 3 to 6 months after initial injury. If no biceps recovery is seen by 6 months, or if initial injury is suspected to be a frank division of the nerve, surgical exploration should be performed. After exploration and neurolysis of the involved nerve segment where the nerve appears to be intact and intraoperative EMG shows conduction across the nerve segment involved, a further period of observation for recovery is recommended. If, however, neuroma scarring or complete laceration of the nerve is found, excision of scarred nerve segments with interpositional nerve grafting is the preferred treatment option.

In cases where the musculocutaneous nerve is injured as part of brachial plexus injury, or there may be no proximal segment to graft the nerve into, other reconstructive options for recovery of biceps function exist. The Oberlin transfer, which transfers one or two ulnar nerve (wrist flexion) fascicles to the motor branch to the biceps, is an excellent choice for rapid recovery of biceps function, owing to the short distance of reinnervation. Recovery of the biceps has been reported as soon as 3 months from the procedure, with ultimate biceps strength of M4 in >90% of patients. For patients who do not have the ulnar or median nerve available because of more extensive brachial plexus trauma, neurotization procedures from intercostals, spinal accessory, phrenic, and medial pectoral nerves may be an available option.

When patients are referred >1 year from their initial injury, the chance of successful muscle function recovery with nerve repairs and transfers is significantly decreased. For these patients, tendon transfer such as the Steindler flexorplasty is recommended. This procedure requires a functioning brachioradialis (radial nerve), which is transferred more proximally on the humerus with the plan of improving elbow flexion. Tendon transfers such as triceps, latissimus, and pectoralis major and minor are have also been described.

Another salvage technique of recovering elbow flexion is free muscle transfer. Many of these procedures have been performed with reasonable success, primarily using gracilis to supplement biceps function. This muscle has a proximal neurovascular pedicle and shape that is optimal for restoring biceps function. The proximal vessels are usually connected to the thoracoacromial trunk, with the obturator nerve branch connected to the spinal accessory nerve with sural graft extension. The proximal muscle is usually attached through bone sutures to the distal clavicle and acromion, while distally it is woven into biceps tendon.

LONG THORACIC NERVE

The long thoracic nerve is a pure motor nerve, formed from proximal contributions from cervical roots 5, 6, and 7. The nerve has a long course along the lateral thorax (26 cm) to its insertion on the serratus anterior. This muscle originates from the lateral aspect of the upper nine ribs and inserts along anteromedial scapula, with the inferior component of the muscle being the most important, inserting over the inferomedial corner of the scapula. This insertion is important in stabilizing the scapula on the chest wall and protracting the scapula in forward flexion and abduction. If this function is lost, scapular winging is seen with actions such as wall push-ups and overhead activities (Fig. 41-5). This winging is different than that caused by spinal accessory nerve injury in that, with the loss of serratus stabilization, the vertebral border and inferior pole of the scapula become more prominent This deformity becomes accentuated with forced forward flexion of the arm.

Patients affected by this injury complain of decreased forward flexion and abduction as well as pain and weakness about the shoulder. The pain is usually posterior and may result from spasm and overuse of other scapular stabilizers such as the rhomboids and levator scapulae. Complaints of initial severe pain followed by atrophy and winging is commonly seen in Parsonage-Turner syndrome.

Although plain radiographs should always be included in the diagnostic workup for any patient who presents with scapular winging, the best diagnostic test for long thoracic nerve injury is EMG/NCS. Radiographs, however, may detect the occasional osteochondroma that may cause compression of the nerve as well as other neoplasms inside and outside the thoracic cavity. CT scan and MRI are seldom useful except in cases of neoplasm or cervical disk herniation to make or refine the diagnosis.

Treatment of serratus anterior palsy is usually conservative, for most cases, idiopathic or resulting from closed

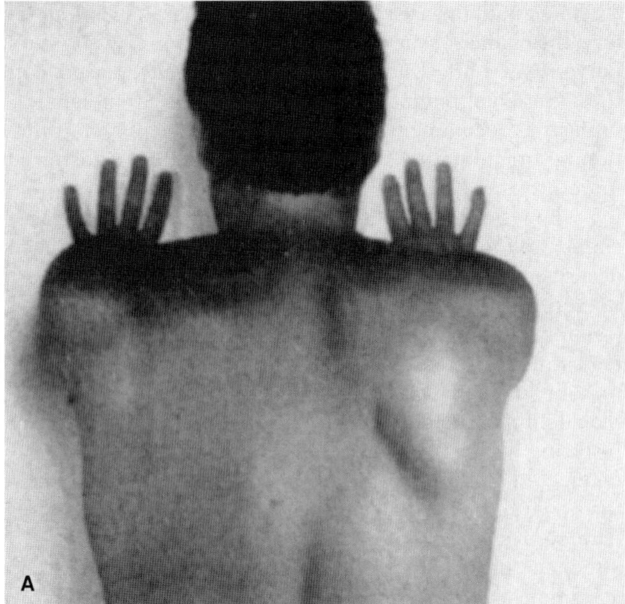

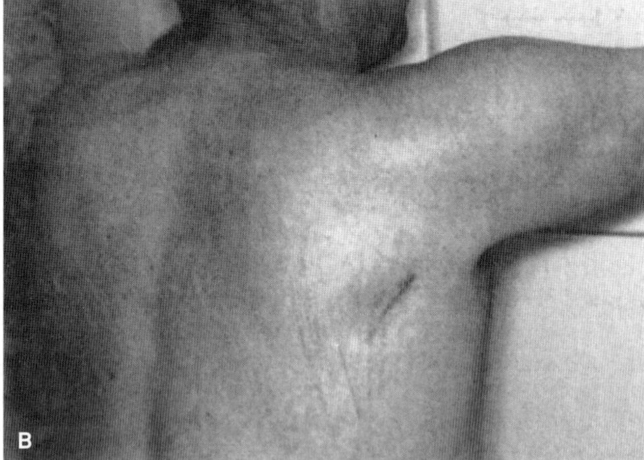

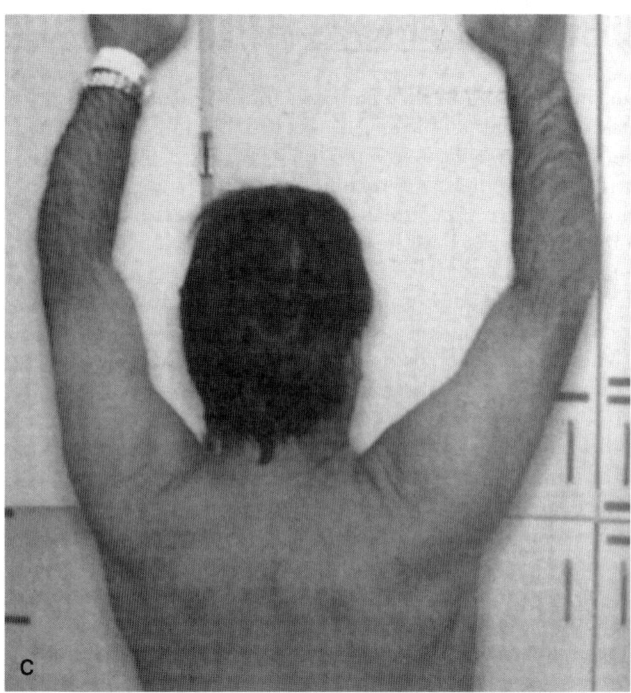

Figure 41-5 Long thoracic nerve palsy. A complete long thoracic nerve paralysis from Parsonage-Turner syndrome developed in this 36-year-old man. His winged scapula did not improve after 3 years. He had persistent pain in his shoulder and disability when performing overhead maneuvers. **A:** Prominent right scapula winging is noted preoperatively. **B:** Postoperatively, the winging has disappeared after pectoralis major transfer. The posterior incision has healed well. **C:** Postoperatively, his shoulder arc of motion has improved as well. (From Steinmann SP, Spinner RJ. Nerve problems about the shoulder. In: Rockwood CA Jr, ed. *The Shoulder*. Vol. 2. 3rd ed. Philadelphia: WB Saunders; 2004:1016, with permission.)

injury, resolve spontaneously. Physical therapy is initiated to preserve motion and for shoulder-strengthening exercises. Braces are not considered effective. If there is no improvement seen clinically or with EMG/NCS after 9 months, and the patient is severely affected by his or her loss of scapular protraction or by pain, operative intervention in the form of muscle transfers is a potential option.

The preferred procedure is pectoralis major sternal head muscle transfer via tendon interposition graft to the scapula. Graft choices are autograft or allograft and include fascia lata or hamstring tendons. Allograft Achilles tendon is a great option, as its proximal portion drapes over the pectoralis muscle and tendon and its distal tendon portion provides strong attachment to the scapula.

Scapulothoracic fusion is usually reserved for patients who failed tendon transfer procedures and continue to be severely disabled by their condition and for patients with multimuscle atrophy and weakness such as patients with fascioscapulohumeral dystrophy. This procedure has a high reported complication rate and may be disabling in itself owing to severely decreased shoulder motion and variable pain relief.

PARSONAGE-TURNER SYNDROME

Parsonage-Turner syndrome, also known as brachial neuritis, is thought to be an uncommon condition. Men are more likely to be affected, with a reported male-to-female ratio ranging between 2:1 and 11:1. Age of presentation is variable, but most patients present in the third to seventh decades of life.

The cause of this condition remains unclear but is thought to be inflammatory or immune mediated. Brachial neuritis is described following a viral illness, immunization, surgery, extreme exercise, and pregnancy. There is also thought to be an inherited form of the syndrome known as hereditary neuralgic amyotrophy. Patients affected with this disorder usually present at an earlier age and may have recurrent episodes of what typically appears to be Parsonage-Turner syndrome.

Onset of the syndrome is somewhat typical in that patients describe an initial onset of severe shoulder pain with no apparent cause. The pain is commonly described as intense and burning in quality and may last from days to weeks. This painful episode is followed by progressive muscle atrophy with accompanying weakness and sensory loss. Fewer patients with atypical presentation complain of motor and sensory loss but are fortunate enough not to have the initial painful onset. Muscles innervated by C5 and C6 are most commonly involved, and the most typically affected nerves include the suprascapular, axillary, long thoracic, anterior interosseous, and radial nerves. Brachial neuritis can affect individual nerves or involve many nerves of the brachial plexus and the cervical region (such as the spinal accessory nerve) at the same time. Approximately 10% of the cases have bilateral presentation.

The diagnosis of Parsonage-Turner syndrome is primarily made on history, a thorough physical examination, and ruling out other conditions that may be responsible for the patient's symptoms. Some orthopaedic conditions that may have similar presentations and symptoms include herniated cervical disk, perilabral ganglia, rotator cuff tear, impingement syndrome, shoulder bursitis, calcific tendonitis, and adhesive capsulitis. Neurologic conditions that may mimic this condition include entrapment syndromes also known as inflammatory demyelinating polyneuropathy, transverse myelitis, and mononeuritis multiplex. EMG/NCS will identify nerves and muscles involved and will initially show acute denervation, with fibrillation and positive waves seen at the 3- to 4-week mark. MRI is useful more to exclude other diagnoses and will typically show a picture of selective involved muscle atrophy with increased signal on T2-weighed scans.

As in the case of other idiopathic nerve syndromes such as Bell palsy, most patients show spontaneous improvement with time. However, recovery can be variable, with most patients having residual effects such as winging. Most patients recover within 3 to 6 months, but complete recovery may take >12 months. Treatment is supportive, with nonsteroidal anti-inflammatory medications and other analgesics. The use of steroids and immunoglobulin therapy has not been shown to be effective. Physical therapy is recommended to regain range of motion and to strengthen shoulder girdle muscles. As in all other cases of permanent deficits described earlier in this chapter, tendon transfers may be of use to treat long-term disability.

SUGGESTED READINGS

Adams JE, Steinmann SP. Nerve injuries about the elbow. *J Hand Surg*. 2006;31A:303–313.

Antoniou J, Tae SK, Williams GR, et al. Suprascapular neuropathy. Variability in the diagnosis, treatment and outcome. *Clin Orthop*. 2001;386:131–138.

Bigliani LU, Compito CA, Duralde XA, et al. Transfer of the levator scapulae, rhomboid major, and rhomboid minor for paralysis of the trapezius. *J Bone Joint Surg*. 1996;78A:1534–1540.

Bigliani LU, Perez-Sanz JR, Wolfe IN. Treatment of trapezius paralysis. *J Bone Joint Surg*. 1985;67A:871–877.

Burkhead WZ, Scheinberg RR, Box G. Surgical anatomy of the axillary nerve. *J Shoulder Elbow Surg*. 1992;1:31–36.

Chuang DC, Yeh MC, Wei PC. Intercostal nerve transfer of the musculocutaneous nerve in avulsed brachial plexus injuries: Evaluation of 66 patients. *J Hand Surg*. 1992;17A:822–828.

Connor PM, Yamaguchi K, Manifold SG, et al. Split pectoralis major transfer for serratus anterior palsy. *Clin Orthop*. 1997;341:134–142.

Flatow EL, Bigliani LU. Tips of the trade. Locating and protecting the axillary nerve in shoulder surgery. The tug test. *Orthop Rev*. 1992;21:503–505.

Jobe C, Kropp WE, Wood VE. The spinal accessory nerve in a trapezius splitting approach. *J Shoulder Elbow Surg*. 1996;5:206–208.

Leechavengvongs S, Witoonchart K, Uerpairojkit C, et al. Nerve transfer to biceps muscle using a part of the ulnar nerve in brachial plexus injury (upper arm type): a report of 32 cases. *J Hand Surg*. 1998;23A:711–716.

Marmor L. Paralysis of the serratus anterior due to electric shock relieved by transplantation of the pectoralis major muscle. A case report. *J Bone Joint Surg*. 1983;45A:156–160.

Misamore GW, Lehman DE. Parsonage-Turner syndrome (acute brachial neuritis). *J Bone Joint Surg*. 1996;78A:1405–1408.

Oberlin C, Beal D, Leerhavengvongs S, et al. Nerve transfer to bicepsmuscle using part of ulnar nerve for C5-C6 avulsion of the brachial plexus: anatomical study and report of four cases. *J Hand Surg*. 1994;19A:232–237.

Parsonage MJ, Turner JW. Neuralgic amyotrophy. *Lancet*. 1943;1: 532–535.

Steinmann SP, Moran EA. Axillary nerve injury. Diagnosis and treatment. *J Am Acad Orthop Surg*. 2001;9(5):328–335.

Steinmann SP, Spinner RJ. Nerve problems about the shoulder. In: Rockwood CA Jr, ed. *The Shoulder*. Vol. 2. 3rd ed. Philadelphia: WB Saunders; 2004:1009–1031.

Steinmann SP, Wood MB. Pectoralis major transfer for serratus anterior paralysis. *J Shoulder Elbow Surg*. 2003;12:555–560.

Wong KL, Williams GR. Complications of thermal capsulorrhaphy of the shoulder. *J Bone Joint Surg*. 2001;83A(suppl 2):151–155.

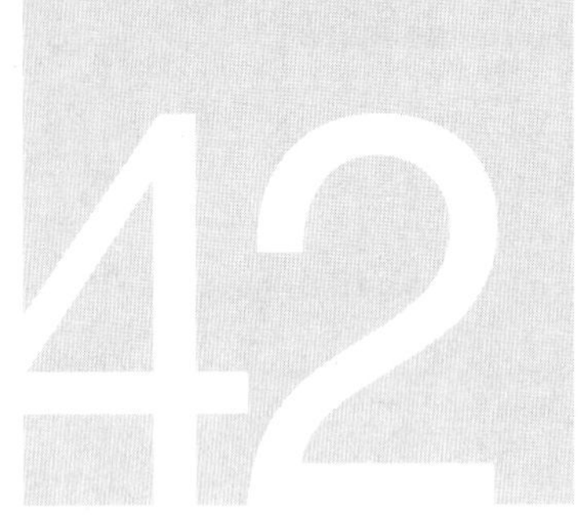

CHRONIC MASSIVE ROTATOR CUFF TEARS: EVALUATION AND MANAGEMENT

ANDREW GREEN

Chronic massive rotator cuff tears present a great treatment challenge. Because of unique pathologic anatomic features, they must be considered distinct from both smaller chronic tears and acute traumatic massive rotator cuff tears. For the purposes of this review, chronic massive rotator cuff tearing implies that there has been long-standing pathology, not necessarily with concurrent symptoms, leading to the presentation of a patient with a massive rotator cuff tear and substantial rotator cuff muscle atrophy. This implies that the tear is difficult to repair primarily, if not sometimes irreparable. With an aging population and increasing functional expectations, it is likely that we will encounter this difficult problem with increasing frequency.

Various treatment options are available including pain management, nonoperative rehabilitation, subacromial debridement, biceps tenodesis or tenotomy, rotator cuff repair, and rotator cuff reconstruction, all of which have some demonstrated efficacy. The goals and expectations of the treatment of this difficult problem must be clearly understood and defined to maximize the outcome. Determining the best treatment for an individual patient with a chronic massive rotator cuff tear can be difficult. There are no randomized prospective studies that compare nonoperative and operative treatment, nor are there any studies that compare the various surgical options. The purpose of this review is to present a current understanding of chronic massive rotator cuff tears and discuss the evaluation and management of patients with chronic massive rotator cuff tears.

PATHOGENESIS

Etiology and Pathophysiology

The cause of rotator cuff tears has been the subject of extensive debate, and there are several factors that are implicated in the development of rotator cuff tears. Interestingly, the presence of a tear does not a priori render a shoulder symptomatic. Studies of large numbers of patients with symptomatic rotator cuff tears note that the size of a tear does not directly correlate with self-reported symptoms.

The cause of rotator cuff tears is usually categorized as either intrinsic or extrinsic. Intrinsic factors relate to pathology of the rotator cuff muscles and tendons. This includes degenerative changes that occur with aging, tendon overload, and relative hypovascularity of the anterior aspect of the supraspinatus tendon. Extrinsic factors include subacromial impingement, glenohumeral instability, and unstable os acromiale. Patients with chronic massive rotator cuff tears usually do not have a history of significant shoulder trauma. In occasional cases there is a remote history of trauma that may have caused the tearing. The context of the onset of symptoms is an important consideration. Although many patients with chronic massive rotator cuff tears have an insidious onset of symptoms with gradual worsening, some report a more acute onset of symptoms sometimes related to a traumatic event.

TABLE 42-1 ROTATOR CUFF TEAR SIZE CLASSIFICATION

Small tear	<1 cm
Medium tear	1–3 cm
Large tear	3–5 cm
Massive tear	>5 cm

Epidemiology

Patients with chronic massive rotator cuff tears are usually older. This is consistent with the results of studies that demonstrate that there is an increasing prevalence of rotator cuff tears even in asymptomatic individuals with advancing age. Less frequently, younger patients, often males with a history of substantial labor or physical activity involving the upper extremities, present with chronic massive rotator cuff tears.

Classification

Rotator cuff tears are usually classified according to the chronicity and size of the tear. The chronicity of a rotator cuff tear can refer to either the duration of symptoms or the duration of pathology. There are several approaches to classifying the size of rotator cuff tears. The most commonly used approach is based on the dimensions of the tear (Table 42-1). Rotator cuff tears can also be classified according to the number of tendons that are involved, with massive tears involving at least two complete tendons.Additionally, the extent of tendon retraction and the tissue quality are important factors that are not generally accounted for by the various size-based classification systems. Nevertheless, muscle quality is especially important in the context of larger rotator cuff tears. Muscle quality can be appreciated on physical examination as atrophy of the spinati muscles, as well as on CT and MR imaging. Based on CT and MR imaging, the rotator cuff muscles are graded as stage 0 (completely normal), stage 1 (some fatty streaks), stage 2 (marked fatty infiltration but more muscle than fat), stage 3 (as much fat as muscle), or stage 4 (more fat than muscle).

Important Points

- Tear size
- Number of tendons involved
- Tendon retraction
- Rotator cuff muscle status

DIAGNOSIS

Physical Examination and History

Clinical Features

Patients with chronic massive rotator cuff tears typically present with pain and shoulder dysfunction and tend to be older than the average patient with a rotator cuff tear. Less commonly, younger patients present with chronic massive rotator cuff tears. Chronic massive rotator cuff tears can present in three different clinical settings. Although most patients present with an insidious onset of shoulder pain and dysfunction, some present with a history of a previous significant traumatic injury that caused the tear or a recent traumatic event that aggravated an underlying pre-existing rotator cuff tear. Patients with the latter presentation, acute-on-chronic tears, present in two clinical scenarios. The first includes patients with pre-existing chronic symptomatic rotator cuff tearing who sustain an injury that causes an acute extension of the tear. The second group has pre-existing asymptomatic rotator cuff tears and an acute injury that results in the onset of shoulder pain. In either case, there was pre-existing rotator cuff tearing. After an acute traumatic injury, patients may be unable to actively elevate their arm. In some cases there is extensive anterior arm ecchymosis. The important point is that patients who deny pre-existing symptoms but have the typical clinical features of chronic rotator cuff tearing; spinatus atrophy, external rotation weakness, and characteristic plain radiographic findings are likely to have had pre-existing rotator cuff tearing.

The status of the rotator cuff can usually be accurately determined with a detailed physical examination. Any evaluation for shoulder pathology should also include examination of the cervical spine and a focused neurologic evaluation. Cervical spondylosis, stenosis, and radiculopathy can cause shoulder pain that mimics the pain of rotator cuff pathology. Shoulder girdle weakness can also be the result of brachial plexus disorders (Parsonage-Turner syndrome and brachial neuritis, or tumor) or suprascapular neuropathy. Last, the presentation of chronic septic arthritis can mimic a chronic massive rotator cuff tear and should not be forgotten when evaluating patients. Table 42-2 lists differential diagnosis disorders.

Visual inspection of the patient provides important anatomic information. Several findings are consistent with chronic massive rotator cuff tearing. These include anterior superior subluxation and prominence of the humeral head, infraspinatus and supraspinatus atrophy, and chronic rupture of the proximal tendon of the long head of the biceps. Supraspinatus atrophy is more difficult to detect beneath the trapezius muscle. In many cases massive rotator cuff tears can be detected as a palpable defect at the supraspinatus insertion at the anterior lateral aspect of the shoulder. Swelling owing to subdeltoid synovial fluid can also be present. Deltoid detachment is rare but is usually visible as a defect at the anterior aspect of the origin of the middle deltoid.

TABLE 42-2 DIFFERENTIAL DIAGNOSIS FOR CHRONIC MASSIVE ROTATOR CUFF TEAR

Cervical spondylosis
Brachial plexus injury
Parsonage-Turner syndrome/brachial plexitis
Pancoast tumor
Suprascapular neuropathy
Rotator cuff tear arthropathy
Septic arthritis

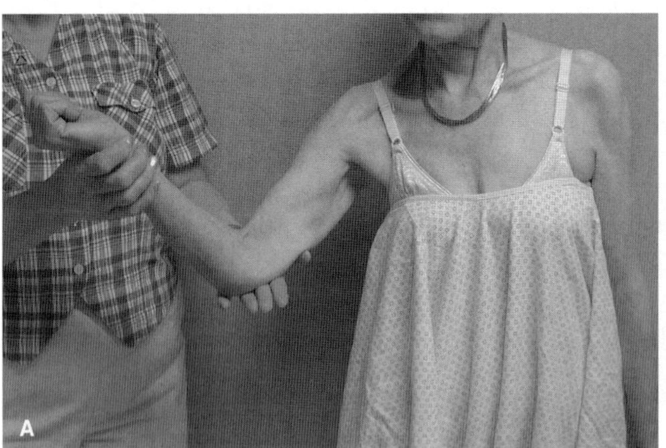

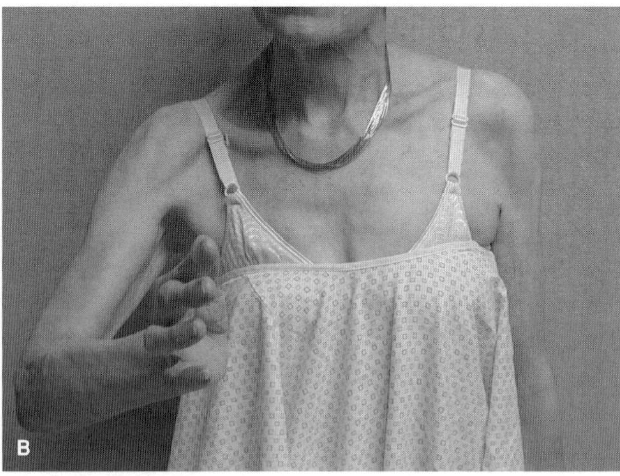

Figure 42-1 The right shoulder has an external rotation lag sign in this patient with a massive rotator cuff tear. **A:** The arm can be passively externally rotated. **B:** The patient cannot actively externally rotate the arm. (From Green A. Chronic massive rotator cuff tears: evaluation and management. *J Am Acad Orthop Surg*. 2003;11:321–331, with permission.)

Active and passive shoulder motion is assessed in scapular plane elevation, external rotation with the arm at the side and in 90 degrees abduction, internal rotation behind the back and at 90 degrees abduction, and across-chest adduction. When motion is assessed, the scapulohumeral rhythm is also assessed. Several studies have noted alterations in scapulohumeral rhythm in the presence of shoulder pathology. Significant loss of passive shoulder motion is uncommon in the presence of a massive rotator cuff tear. Nevertheless, patients can have subtle loss of motion in specific directions that can contribute to symptoms. It is important to recognize shoulder stiffness in the presence of rotator cuff tear for two reasons. First, strength is more difficult to evaluate when there is substantial stiffness. Second, the cause of the stiffness (adhesive capsulitis, capsular contracture, or glenohumeral arthritis) may be the cause of the patient's symptoms. Despite severe rotator cuff deficiency, some of these patients have good elevation strength owing to compensatory deltoid strength. Consequently, many patients with chronic massive rotator cuff tears have full active shoulder elevation. Patients with significant deltoid weakness may be unable to actively elevate their arm.

External rotation weakness is characteristic of chronic massive rotator cuff tears. Elevation weakness is a less consistent finding. Some patients have sufficient deltoid strength to mask the absence of supraspinatus strength. The Jobe empty can test, which assesses strength with the shoulder elevated about 90 degrees and internally rotated with the thumb pointing downward, will usually cause pain and elicit weakness. Pain can also be the cause of inability to elevate the arm. A subacromial injection with 10 centiliters (100 mL) of 1% lidocaine can eliminate the pain and allow a better assessment of rotator cuff strength.

Rotational weakness is often easiest to elicit. External rotation weakness and external rotation lag are signs of massive rotator cuff tearing that involves the infraspinatus tendon (Fig. 42-1). An external rotation lag sign is elicited by passively positioning the arm in maximal external rotation. When there is marked weakness, the patient is unable to hold the arm in this position and the hand falls toward the abdomen. The horn blower's sign, inability to externally rotate the elevated arm, also demonstrates severe infraspinatus weakness. Associated subscapularis tearing is less common but may also be present. Patients with chronic atraumatic subscapularis tearing have internal rotation weakness, variable excessive passive external rotation, and a positive lift-off test or belly-press maneuver[6] (Fig. 42-2).

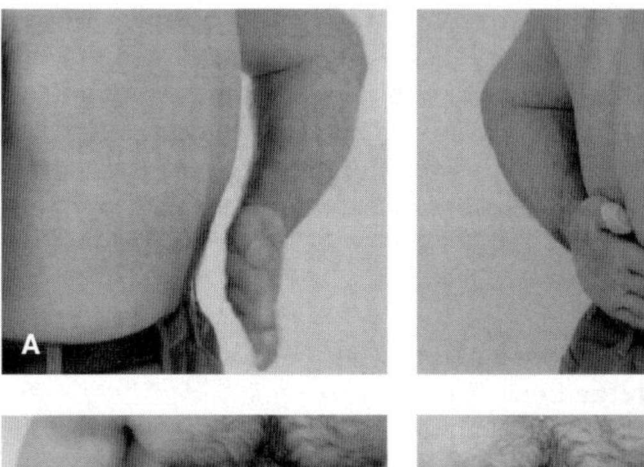

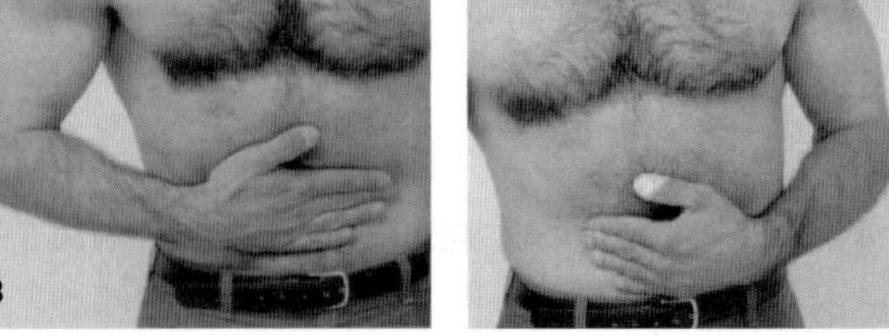

Figure 42-2 **A:** A positive lift-off maneuver in a patient with a subscapularis tendon tear of the left shoulder. **B:** A positive belly-press test of the left shoulder in the same patient. Note the posterior position of the left elbow. (From Lyons RP, Green A. Subscapularis tendon tears. *J Am Acad Orthop Surg*. 2005;13:353–363, with permission.)

The lift-off test is difficult to perform when there is pain or limited shoulder motion that prevents positioning of the arm and hand behind the back. Unfortunately, subscapularis tears are often overlooked or ignored by inexperienced examiners, both surgeons and radiologists.

Various physical examination maneuvers and signs are performed and assessed to evaluate patients with rotator cuff disorders. Park et al. evaluated eight physical examination tests. The combination of the painful arc sign, drop-arm sign, and infraspinatus muscle test produced the best posttest probability (91%) for full-thickness rotator cuff tears, especially in patients older than 60 years of age.

The combination of a detailed history and thorough physical examination often provides sufficient information to establish a diagnosis of massive rotator cuff tearing. Imaging studies provide information to confirm the diagnosis and assist in treatment selection.

Important Points—Physical Examination

- Spinati atrophy
- Anterior superior humeral head position
- Rupture of the proximal tendon of the long head of biceps
- Weak external rotation

Radiologic Features

Plain Radiographic Evaluation. A complete evaluation of the shoulder includes a series of five plain radiographs. These views include a true anteroposterior, anteroposterior in internal and external rotation, axillary lateral, and outlet. Although plain radiographs do not visualize soft tissues, they demonstrate skeletal and osseous changes that suggest the presence of rotator cuff pathology and are particularly helpful in assessing patients with chronic massive rotator cuff tears (Fig. 42-3).

Elevation of the humeral head relative to the glenoid and narrowing of the acromiohumeral space are findings that are consistent with long-standing rotator cuff pathology (Fig. 42-4). It has been suggested that an acromiohumeral space <7 mm is consistent with a rotator cuff tear and that when the space is <5 mm, there is a massive tear. Erosion or rounding off of the greater tuberosity (femoralization) is typical of long-standing massive rotator cuff tearing. Similarly, long-standing contact of the greater tuberosity with the acromion can lead to the formation of a facet on the underside of the lateral acromion as well as spurring and excrescences on the greater tuberosity that can be visualized on anterior posterior radiographs. The true anteroposterior and axillary lateral radiographs can also demonstrate glenohumeral arthritis. The axillary lateral view also demonstrates the relative anteroposterior position of the humeral

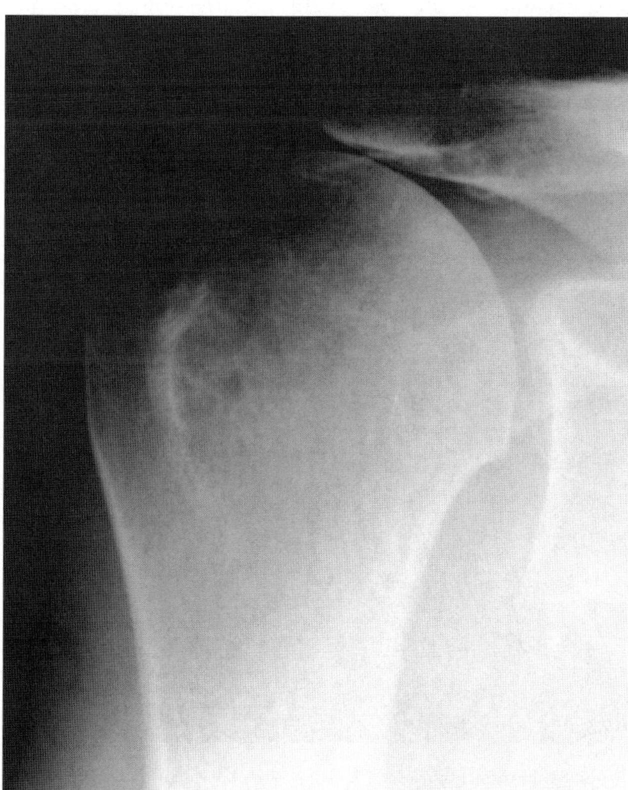

Figure 42-3 True anterior posterior radiograph of a shoulder with a chronic massive rotator cuff tear. Although, there is reduction of the acromial humeral space and the humeral head is elevated relative to the glenoid, there is no glenohumeral arthritis.

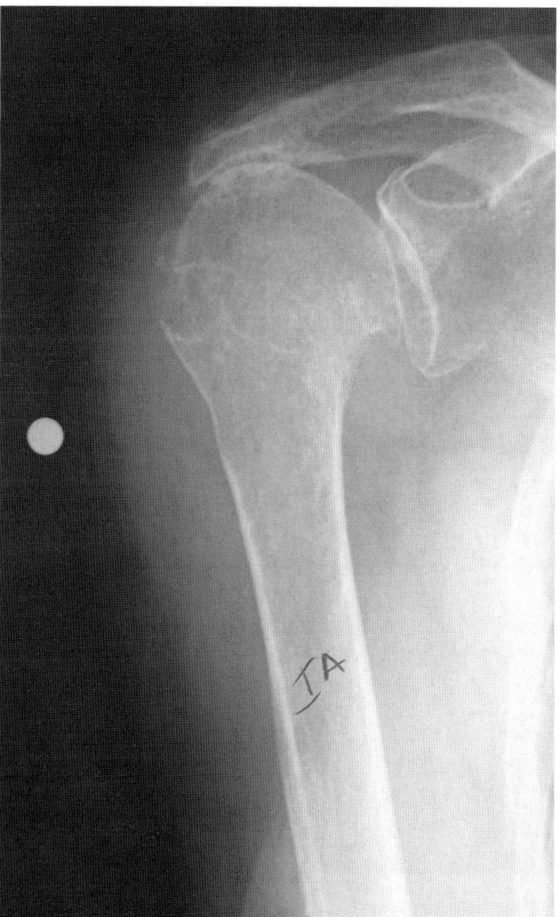

Figure 42-4 True anterior posterior radiograph of a shoulder with rotator cuff tear arthropathy. There is no acromiohumeral space, there are degenerative changes of the glenohumeral joint, and the greater tuberosity is rounded off.

head. Anterior subluxation on an axillary lateral radiograph is consistent with anterior superior instability or subscapularis tendon tear. The outlet view is used to demonstrate the acromial morphology.

The typical radiographic findings of rotator cuff tear arthropathy include loss of the glenohumeral joint space, elevation of the humeral head, erosion and rounding off of the greater tuberosity, and articulation of the humeral head with the acromion (Fig. 42-4). It is important to recognize the presence of significant glenohumeral arthritis as it is a relative contraindication to rotator cuff repair and reconstruction.

Important Points—Plain Radiographs

- Superior humeral head subluxation
- Acromial humeral space narrowing
- Femoralization of the humeral head

Advanced Imaging of the Rotator Cuff. Historically, arthrography is cited as the gold standard for the diagnosis of rotator cuff tearing. However, newer imaging modalities such as ultrasonography and MRI provide better information and have replaced arthrography as the imaging tests of choice for rotator cuff pathology.

Acceptance of ultrasonography for imaging the rotator cuff has been variable. Centers with extensive experience report high rates of sensitivity and specificity. Other centers are not able to confirm these findings. Although some of the variability is related to inexperience, some is also related to differing diagnostic criteria. More recent technologic advances are encouraging a re-evaluation of the value of ultrasonography for imaging the rotator cuff. This includes use of ultrasound by the examining physician.

Magnetic resonance imaging is the current state of the art for imaging the rotator cuff. It can be highly accurate and demonstrates detailed anatomic information, including tear size and muscle quality. The latter information can help establish the chronicity of the rotator cuff tearing and the potential functional status of the cuff. Goutallier et al, reported that higher grades of presurgical fatty degeneration of the rotator cuff muscles are associated with inferior outcomes.

The coronal oblique magnetic resonance images are primarily used to evaluate the supraspinatus tendon and muscle. The extent of retraction and the size and quality of the supraspinatus muscle can be determined (Fig. 42-5A). Fatty replacement of the supraspinatus muscle in the supraspinatus fossa indicates chronic pathology. The size of the supraspinatus tear in the anterior-to-posterior direction can be assessed by noting the tear on sequential images. The sagittal oblique images demonstrate the anterior-to-posterior extent of tearing as well as the quality of all of the rotator cuff muscles (Fig. 42-5B). The axial images can demonstrate the biceps tendon, as well as subscapularis, infraspinatus and teres minor tearing and muscle quality. Axial T2 images are essential for a complete magnetic resonance imaging (MRI) evaluation of the shoulder.

MRI is also helpful in cases of other less-common disorders that can mimic massive rotator cuff tearing. Specifically, patients with external rotation weakness should be evaluated with MRI. Suprascapular nerve palsy, spinoglenoid notch cysts with compression of the infraspinatus branch of the suprascapular nerve, and cervical spine disorders are examples of such disorders. Myopathic changes on MRI are more consistent with neurologic abnormality.

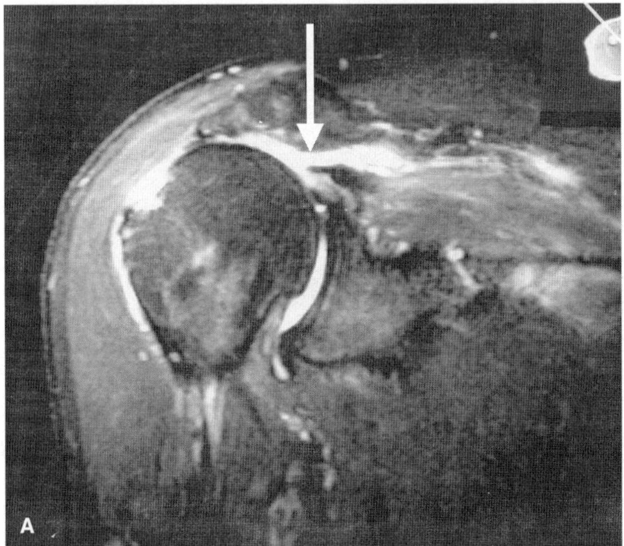

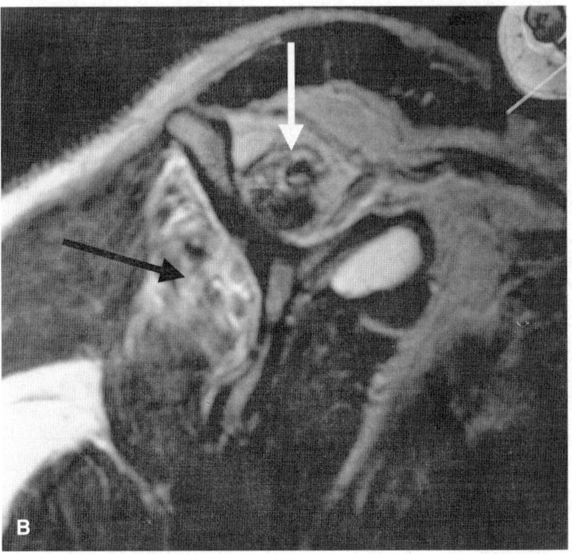

Figure 42-5 MRI scans of the right shoulder of a 64-year-old male with a chronic rotator cuff tear. **A:** T2 coronal oblique image demonstrates the supraspinatus tendon tear, atrophy of the muscle, and fatty replacement in the supraspinatus fossa. The supraspinatus tendon (*arrows*) is at the glenoid. **B:** T1 sagittal oblique image demonstrates fatty replacement in the supraspinatus fossa and lipoatrophy of the infraspinatus muscle. (From Green A. Chronic massive rotator cuff tears: evaluation and management. *J Am Acad Orthop Surg*. 2003;11:321–331, with permission.)

MR arthrography is not usually required for routine evaluation of the rotator cuff. However, it can be helpful in imaging the rotator cuff after surgery when it is difficult to differentiate scar tissue from tendon.

Although many studies have confirmed the accuracy of magnetic resonance imaging of the rotator cuff, the specific indications for MRI are rarely addressed. Overuse of MRI is a pervasive problem, and careful clinical evaluation can help to define the appropriate usage of this excellent imaging technique. In most cases the diagnosis of a chronic massive rotator cuff tear can be made with a careful history and physical examination alone. MRI is clearly indicated early in the evaluation of shoulder pain and dysfunction after an acute traumatic injury.

TREATMENT

The successful outcome of treatment of chronic massive rotator cuff tearing depends on selecting the best treatment option for the specific case at hand. Chronic massive rotator cuff tears present in various patients, and treatment options include nonoperative methods, surgical debridement, repair, and reconstruction. Studies have reported high success rates with each of these approaches. In some cases, more than one of the options may be appropriate. Thus, careful consideration of many factors is important, and treatment should be individualized to the case at hand.

Nonoperative Treatment

Many patients with chronic massive rotator cuff tears can be successfully treated without surgery. The rationale behind nonoperative treatment is that some individuals have asymptomatic rotator cuff tears and never present for evaluation and treatment. Activity modification, oral nonsteroidal anti-inflammatory medications, and corticosteroid injections can help some individuals manage their symptoms. Studies of nonoperative treatment of full-thickness rotator cuff tear note improvement in about 50% to 85% of patients.The duration of symptoms seems to correlate with the long-term success of nonoperative treatment.

Some authors have noted that repeated corticosteroid injections have a detrimental effect on the rotator cuff and articular surfaces. In addition, some studies note a negative correlation between the results of rotator cuff repair and the number of preoperative corticosteroid injections. Other studies suggest that the association is less clear-cut. Injections can be very helpful in the initial phases of physical therapy and rehabilitation. With less pain, patients are better able to participate in a rehabilitation program. Nevertheless, repeated corticosteroid injections should be avoided.

The focus of physical therapy is the restoration of shoulder motion and strengthening of the intact portions of the rotator cuff and the periscapular and deltoid muscles. Passive motion is improved with stretching exercises. Strengthening of the internal and external rotators is best achieved with resisted exercises performed with the arms below chest level. Deltoid strengthening should be initiated in the supine position with the effects of gravity minimized and then progressed to an upright seated or standing position. In addition, scapular muscle strengthening can enhance the function of a weak rotator cuff. There are various techniques for strengthening, including isometric, isotonic, and isokinetic exercises. Strengthening should be progressed gradually and within the patient's comfort level.

Patients with atraumatic onset of pain and with marked spinati atrophy, evidence of chronic rotator cuff tearing, are ideal candidates for nonoperative treatment. In many such cases it is unlikely that the massive rotator cuff tear will be repairable. Thus, nonoperative management should be the first line of treatment.

Operative Treatment

Operative treatment of chronic massive rotator cuff tears encompasses a spectrum of complexity ranging from minimally invasive arthroscopic approaches to major reconstructive surgery. There are advocates for all options but few objective data to guide selection.

Open and Arthroscopic Treatment Without Rotator Cuff Repair

Some authors advocate subacromial decompression and rotator cuff debridement as treatment for massive irreparable rotator cuff tears.The rationale behind subacromial smoothing and rotator cuff debridement includes our knowledge that there are asymptomatic individuals with rotator cuff tears, and the fact that a substantial proportion of patients who have a satisfactory result from a repair of a massive rotator cuff tear have persistent rotator cuff defects after the repair.

Debridement and acromioplasty is best suited for lower-demand individuals. More active individuals who fail nonoperative treatment are probably better served with attempted rotator cuff repair. Some authors report that the results of debridement of full-thickness rotator cuff tears deteriorate with time.

Although most rotator cuff tears are at least partially repairable, in some cases the tear is either not repairable or repair would be unlikely to substantially alter shoulder function. The ideal candidate for debridement is an individual with shoulder pain who has good elevation strength, can actively elevate the arm overhead, and can externally rotate the arm with gravity eliminated. This suggests that there is good shoulder kinematics and that the internal and external rotators are balanced.

Either an open or arthroscopic approach can be used for subacromial debridement. The arthroscopic approach has the advantage of an easier and more rapid rehabilitation because the deltoid origin is preserved. Acromial smoothing as opposed to formal acromioplasty is performed to remove undersurface spurring and rough excrescences. Similarly, the greater tuberosity is smoothed; a so-called reverse acromioplasty arthroscopic subacromial decompression. Thus, the coracoacromial arch is maintained by avoiding an excessive acromioplasty and by preserving the coracoacromial ligament. This helps to prevent loss of the restraint to superior humeral head subluxation that the intact coracoacromial arch provides.

Biceps tenotomy or tenodesis is recommended as an adjunct to arthroscopic debridement of chronic massive rotator cuff tears. If there is subluxation or dislocation of the tendon of the long head of the biceps or partial tearing, this can be an effective procedure to alleviate shoulder pain associated with chronic massive rotator cuff tears. In the older patient, arthroscopic tenotomy is a minimally invasive procedure that does not require the postoperative immobilization or protection that a tenodesis requires.

Factors associated with a poor prognosis with arthroscopic treatment of chronic massive rotator cuff tears include preoperative superior migration of the humeral head, the presence of subscapularis tearing or weakness, the presence of glenohumeral arthritis, and decreased range of motion. Most authors point out that although the short-term results of arthroscopic treatment are encouraging, the long-term results often deteriorate.

Rotator Cuff Repair

Many studies and reviews have presented the techniques and the results of rotator cuff repair. Most recent studies of rotator cuff repair have reported successful outcome in 80% to 90% of cases.The traditional goal of rotator cuff repair is to repair the rotator cuff tendons to the proximal humerus and to decompress the subacromial space without disrupting the coracoacromial arch. The role of acromioplasty has been recently questioned, and some authors do not routinely perform it as part of a rotator cuff repair. Repair of chronic massive rotator cuff tears is particularly difficult because of tendon substance loss, retraction, scarring, and poor mechanical properties. Several techniques and maneuvers are used to mobilize the rotator cuff tendons and facilitate the repair. Traditional open techniques, mini-open, and all arthroscopic repairs have been advocated. Determining the feasibility of a repair is of primary importance as not all chronic massive rotator cuff tears are repairable.

Open Rotator Cuff Repair. A skin incision is made over the top of the lateral third of the acromion in the Langer lines. This is a very cosmetic incision and can be extended anteriorly to permit a deltopectoral approach if required to repair a concomitant subscapularis tear. The skin and subcutaneous tissue are elevated as full-thickness flaps to expose the acromion and the origins of the anterior and middle heads of the deltoid muscle. The anterior deltoid is elevated off the anterior acromion, and the deltoid fibers are split laterally just posterior to the deltoid raphe for about 3 to 4 cm. In doing this, the coracoacromial ligament is released from the acromion but not resected. This approach allows ample access to the subacromial and subdeltoid spaces, as well as the supraspinatus, infraspinatus, and teres minor tendons.

The goal of anterior acromioplasty is to flatten the undersurface of the anterior acromion, decompress the subacromial space, and create a smooth acromial surface, without disrupting the coracoacromial arch. Spurring on the undersurface of the distal clavicle is also removed. Care is taken to avoid excessive resection, especially shortening of the acromion to prevent anterior superior instability.

Subacromial and subdeltoid adhesions are released, and excess bursal tissue can be excised to allow visualization of the rotator cuff tear. Adhesions under the anterior deltoid are often more tenacious and require more formal dissection to clearly visualize the rotator cuff interval and subscapularis tendon.

The subscapularis tendon is inspected for tearing. Tears of the upper third of the subscapularis tendon can often be repaired through this exposure. More extensive tears may require a separate deltopectoral approach. Similarly, the biceps tendon is visualized both within the glenohumeral joint and by pulling the more distal aspect up from the biceps groove.

Next the supraspinatus and infraspinatus tendon edges are identified and traction sutures are placed. In contrast to cases of acute massive tears that can usually be easily mobilized to the tuberosity, additional steps are required to mobilize chronic massive tears. Fascial adhesions superficial to the supraspinatus and infraspinatus muscles are bluntly released. Releasing the rotator cuff interval and the coracohumeral ligament at the base of the coracoid helps to mobilize the supraspinatus tendon. Capsular releases superiorly and posteriorly will also improve mobility (Fig. 42-6). Occasionally, the interval between the supraspinatus and infraspinatus tendons, the so-called posterior interval, is released to allow differential mobilization of the supraspinatus and infraspinatus tendons (Fig. 42-7). The limit of mobilization of the supraspinatus and infraspinatus muscles is determined by the extent to which the suprascapular nerve can be mobilized. The standard anterosuperior approach allows only 1 cm of lateral advancement of the tendons whereas the mobilization of the supraspinatus muscle from the supraspinatus fossa of the scapula permits $\leq$3 cm of lateral advancement.

Once the rotator cuff is fully mobilized, the insertion site on the proximal humerus is prepared by decorticating the bone just lateral to the articular surface. Tendon reattachment can be accomplished by passing no. 2 braided nonabsorbable sutures through transosseous tunnels or by using suture anchors. Many suture techniques are available. The Mason-Allen suture technique is usually recommended. Augmentation of the bone of the greater tuberosity with small plates or washer-type devices is advocated when there is substantial osteopenia to improve the strength of the suture bone interface

After the rotator cuff repair is completed, the anterior deltoid origin is reattached to the anterior acromion with nonabsorbable sutures passed through drill holes in the acromion. This repair is reinforced with additional nonabsorbable sutures. A secure repair of the deltoid is critical to avoid postoperative deltoid avulsion. Again, the coracoacromial ligament is preserved and essentially reattached to the acromion as part of the deltoid repair.

The rotator cuff should be repairable with the arm at the side. A repair with excessive tension is likely to fail.If this is not possible, a partial repair is performed or rotator cuff reconstruction is considered. Burkhart has espoused the concept of partial repair that re-establishes the cable construct of the rotator cuff.This is in part achieved by repairing the cuff defect side to side. In many cases the infraspinatus can be mobilized laterally and superiorly to be

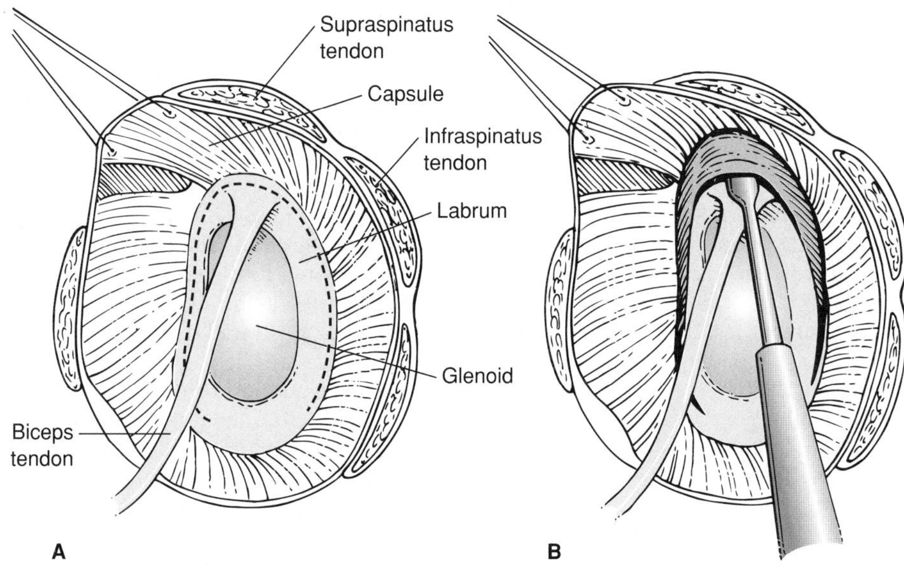

Figure 42-6 A, B: Glenohumeral capsular releases to mobilize the rotator cuff. (From Green A. Chronic massive rotator cuff tears: evaluation and management. *J Am Acad Orthop Surg.* 2003;11:321–331, with permission.)

repaired to the greater tuberosity. Although some authors have advocated reattachment of the rotator cuff more medially into the articular surface, this is not a widely accepted technique.

Mini-Open Rotator Cuff Repair. Mini-open rotator cuff repair combines some of the advantages of arthroscopic and open surgery. Advocates of mini-open rotator cuff repair stress that there is less deltoid morbidity than with an open repair. This claim is controversial. The access through the deltoid split is more limited than with an open repair and may lead to more aggressive deltoid retraction. Consequently, the mini-open technique should be applied carefully when repairing massive tears. Additionally, the rate of postoperative infection appears to be higher after mini-open rotator cuff repair.

Arthroscopic Rotator Cuff Repair. All-arthroscopic rotator cuff repairs are quickly becoming the preferred technique for rotator cuff repair. As the technique has evolved, it has been applied to larger rotator cuff tears. Although the early functional outcomes appear similar to the outcomes of open repairs, the incidence of persistent or recurrent tear is higher for all-arthroscopic repairs. All-arthroscopic techniques attempt to perform all of the essential steps of an open repair to mobilize and repair the rotator cuff. New techniques are being developed to improve the fixation and tendon apposition.

Partial Rotator Cuff Repair. Partial rotator cuff repair is an alternative that lies between debridement and complete rotator cuff repair. This generally refers to repair of the infraspinatus. Margin convergence without tendon-to-bone repair is also advocated. It is thought that this restores the anterior-to-posterior stabilizing characteristics of the rotator cuff. Partial rotator cuff repair can be performed with open or arthroscopic techniques.

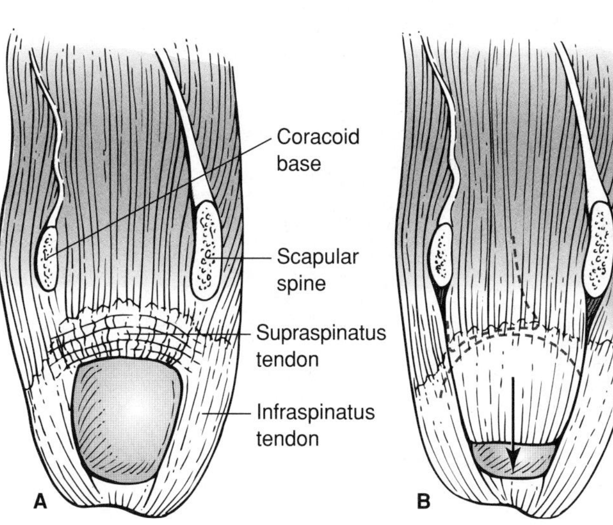

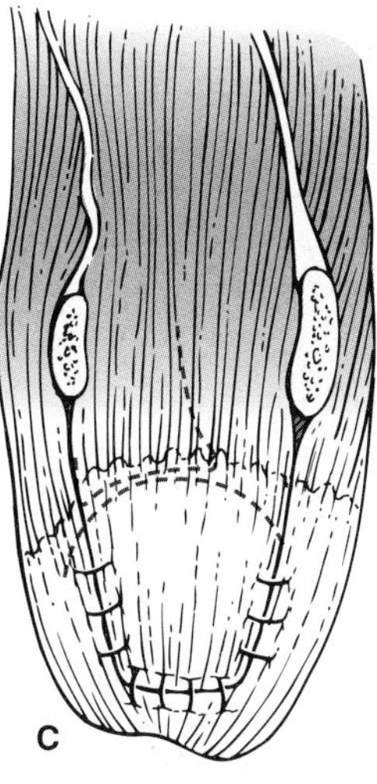

C

Figure 42-7 Anterior and posterior rotator cuff interval releases to mobilize a large tear of supraspinatus and infraspinatus tendons. A: *Dotted lines* indicate the releases. B: Supraspinatus tendon mobilized separate from infraspinatus. C: Tendon sutured into place for the repair. (From Green A. Chronic massive rotator cuff tears: evaluation and management. *J Am Acad Orthop Surg.* 2003;11:321–331, with permission.)

Postoperative Rehabilitation After Rotator Cuff Repair

The postoperative recovery and rehabilitation is lengthy. The repair is protected with an arm sling or abduction immobilizer for 6 to 8 weeks. Abduction positioning is used to relieve tension on a repair that can be accomplished with the arm at the side, but not to allow repair of an irreparable tear. Passive stretching exercises to regain shoulder motion are begun the day after surgery. After repair of chronic massive tears, passive internal rotation and horizontal adduction are avoided for the first 6 weeks to protect the infraspinatus repair. Light active use and active assisted range of motion is initiated after 6 weeks. Formal strengthening is delayed until 12 weeks after surgery. The overall recovery can take >12 months. Overly aggressive early rehabilitation, especially strengthening, has been implicated as a cause of failure.

Results of Repair of Chronic Massive Rotator Cuff Tear

There are few studies that specifically analyze the results of repair of massive rotator cuff tears. Most studies combine the repairs of a spectrum of tear sizes and find that the results of repair of larger tears are inferior to the results of repair of smaller tears. The results of the repair of chronic massive rotator cuff tears vary. Most patients have significant reduction in pain and some functional improvement. Harryman et al. and Gerber found that repair integrity rather than the original tear size best correlated with the functional outcome of rotator cuff repair. Bigliani et al. evaluated the long-term results of repair of chronic massive rotator cuff tears and reported 85% good and excellent results. Bjorkenheim et al. found that the results of repair of large and massive rotator cuff tears were markedly inferior to the results of repair of smaller tears. Most recently, Jost et al. studied the clinical outcome after failed healing of rotator cuff repairs. They found that the outcome was significantly correlated with the size of the postoperative tear and the extent of fatty degeneration of the infraspinatus and subscapularis muscles. They also found that the size of the tear at follow-up was related to the size of the original tear; larger persistent tears were associated with larger initial tears. Goutallier et al. demonstrated that recurrent tear was greater for tendons whose muscle showed fatty degeneration >grade 1. Fatty degeneration of the infraspinatus or subscapularis muscles had an influence on supraspinatus tendon outcome. Rokito et al. found that all of their patients were satisfied after repair of a chronic large or massive rotator cuff tear, that >1 year was required for restoration of strength, and that the final strength was less than in the contralateral shoulder. Duralde and Bair reported good and excellent results in 67% of patients who had partial rotator cuff repair.

Rotator Cuff Reconstruction

Various approaches have been described to reconstruct irreparable massive rotator cuff tears. These include transfers of the rotator cuff tendons, other muscle and tendon transfers, and tissue and synthetic substitution and augmentation. These procedures attempt to restore the function of the rotator cuff muscles and tendons.

Subscapularis transfer is used to achieve complete rotator cuff repair when repair of the supraspinatus and

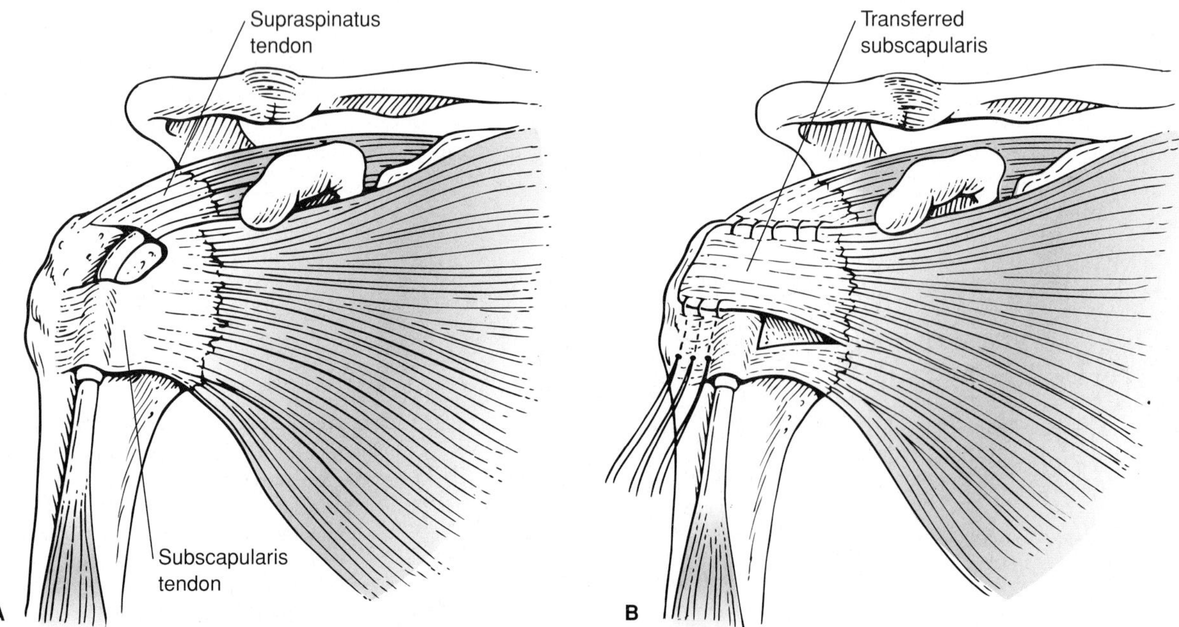

Figure 42-8 Subscapularis transfer. **A:** The upper portion is elevated off of the anterior capsule and transferred superiorly. **B:** Note that the inferior muscular insertion is left intact. (From Green A. Chronic massive rotator cuff tears: evaluation and management. *J Am Acad Orthop Surg*. 2003;11:321–331, with permission.)

infraspinatus leaves a residual superior defect. The upper third of the subscapularis tendon is separated from the anterior capsule and is then transferred superiorly (Fig. 42-8). Most series do not commonly report using subscapularis transfer. Subscapularis transfer does have the risk of causing internal rotation weakness or internal rotation contracture.

Debeyre et al. first described lateral advancement of the supraspinatus muscle and found that the results of repair of larger rotator cuff tears were improved by this procedure. Ha'eri and Wiley also reported good results with lateral advancement of the supraspinatus muscle. In addition, they found that the muscle was not denervated by the procedure. Although Warner et al. demonstrated that the supraspinatus could be safely mobilized up to 3 cm laterally, formal lateral advancement of the supraspinatus muscle is not widely performed.

Latissimus dorsi transfer is used to substitute for loss of the infraspinatus and supraspinatus tendons (Fig. 42-9). The transfer uses a healthy and strong muscle to restore external rotation and head depression forces that are lost in chronic massive rotator cuff tears. Gerber found that the

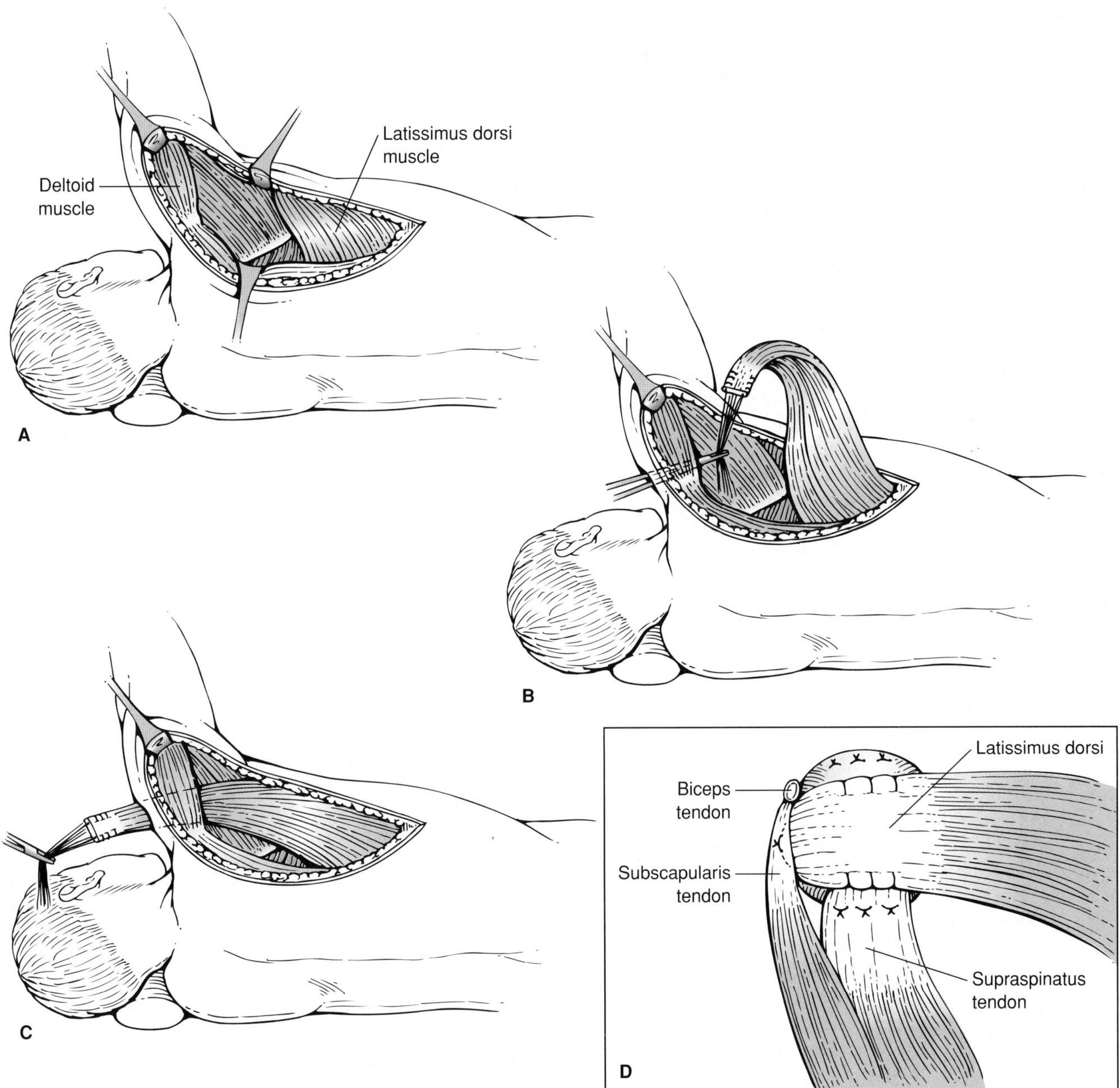

Figure 42-9 Latissimus dorsi transfer for massive irreparable rotator cuff tear. **A:** The latissimus dorsi muscle and tendon are dissected. **B:** The latissimus dorsi tendon is released from the humerus, and sutures are placed into the tendon. **C:** The tendon is passed inferior to the posterior deltoid and the acromion to the superior wound. **D:** The transferred tendon is sutured to the edge of the mobilized but deficient cuff edge and the greater tuberosity. (Modified from Green A. Chronic massive rotator cuff tears: evaluation and management. *J Am Acad Orthop Surg*. 2003;11:321–331, with permission.)

results of latissimus dorsi transfer for massive rotator cuff tear were better if the subscapularis tendon was intact. Iannotti et al. report that patients with better preoperative elevation and external rotator function have better results. Miniaci and MacLeod reported 82% satisfactory results after latissimus dorsi transfer in patients with previously failed operative treatment of massive rotator cuff repair. Other reports have not been as favorable. The results of primary latissimus dorsi transfer appear to be superior to the results of salvage for failed rotator cuff repair.

Other reconstructive procedures have been described but are infrequently reported. These include teres minor transfer, deltoid muscular flap transfer, and trapezius transfer. Although all of these procedures attempt to substitute for the absence of supraspinatus function, they do not address or restore the balance between the anterior and posterior force couples of the rotator cuff.

Tissue substitution or augmentation with material synthetics, autologous and autogenous tissue grafts, and xenograft material has been attempted. The results have been limited, and these techniques are not broadly used. Neviaser et al. reported >80% good and excellent results when they used freeze-dried rotator cuff to repair chronic massive rotator cuff tears. Aside from the potential for foreign body reaction to synthetics or tissue rejection, these techniques do not replace the atrophic and weakened rotator cuff muscles that are typically present with chronic massive rotator cuff tears. Recently, several biologic tissue implants, including xenograft tissue, have been developed to augment rotator cuff repairs. The effect of these implants on outcome is unclear. Despite promising findings in animal rotator cuff repair models, concerns remain about tissue compatibility. Early human clinical studies have not reproduced the same successful findings. Inflammatory reactions after small intestinal submucosal tissue augmentation were recently reported and may be owing to retained cells and DNA.

Glenohumeral Arthrodesis

Glenohumeral arthrodesis is not a commonly performed procedure. Arthrodesis can be performed for painful chronic massive irreparable rotator cuff tears if the goal is a strong, stable shoulder girdle. This may be appropriate for the painful shoulder with anterior superior dislocation because of loss of the coracoacromial arch. However, rotator cuff reconstruction is preferred if the articular surfaces are intact. Otherwise, shoulder arthrodesis may actually result in undesirable loss of upper extremity function below the chest level. Arthrodesis is also difficult to achieve in the typical osteopenic elderly patient who presents with chronic massive rotator cuff tearing. Arntz et al. reported that the results of humeral head replacement for rotator cuff tear arthropathy were better than arthrodesis.

SUMMARY

Chronic massive rotator cuff tears can cause substantial shoulder pain and dysfunction. Several treatment options are appropriate in different clinical settings. Consequently, careful patient evaluation and treatment selection are critically important. Many patients with chronic massive rotator cuff tears can be treated nonoperatively. The goals of surgical treatment must be considered in the context of the individual patient and the complexity of the procedure itself as well as the postoperative recovery and rehabilitation. In some cases, a complete primary repair is possible whereas in others only a partial repair can be achieved. Reconstruction of the rotator cuff is most appropriate for younger, more active patients for whom functional restoration is important. Latissimus dorsi transfer is the preferred reconstructive option for active individuals who are disabled by shoulder pain and weakness of elevation and external rotation and have good deltoid strength. Most of the other reconstructive options have more limited indications and have not been conclusively shown to be superior to debridement procedures. Older, inactive patients, especially those with significant medical comorbidities, are better served by less complicated management approaches that provide pain relief.

SUGGESTED READINGS

Aldridge JM III, Atkinson TS, Mallon WJ. Combined pectoralis major and latissimus dorsi tendon transfer for massive rotator cuff deficiency. *J Shoulder Elbow Surg*. 2004;13:621–629.

Arntz CT, Jackins S, Matsen III FA. Surgical management of complex irreparable cuff deficiency. *J Arthroplasty*. 1991;6:363–370.

Bassett RW, Cofield RH. Acute tears of the rotator cuff: the timing of surgical repair. *Clin Orthop*. 1983;175:18–24.

Bigliani LU, Cordasco FA, McIlveen SJ, et al. Operative repair of massive rotator cuff tears: long-term results. *J Shoulder Elbow Surg*. 1992;1:120–130.

Bjorkenheim J, Paavolainen P, Ahovuo J, et al. Surgical repair of the rotator cuff and surrounding tissues: factors influencing the results. *Clin Orthop*. 1988;236:148–153.

Bokor DJ, Hawkins RH, Huckell GH, et al. Results of nonoperative management of full thickness tears of the rotator cuff. *Clin Orthop*. 1993;294:103–110.

Bradley MP, Tung G, Green A. Overutilization of shoulder magnetic resonance imaging as a diagnostic screening tool in patients with chronic shoulder pain. *J Shoulder Elbow Surg*. 2005;14:233–237.

Burkhart SS, Nottage WM, Ogilvie-Harris DJ, et al. Partial repair of irreparable rotator cuff tears. *Arthroscopy*. 1994:363–370.

Burkhart SS. Arthroscopic treatment of massive rotator cuff tears. Clinical results and biomechanical rationale. *Clin Orthop*. 1991;267:45–56.

Clare DJ, Wirth MA, Groh GI, et al. Shoulder arthrodesis. *J Bone Joint Surg Am*. 2001;83A:593–600.

Codman EA. *The Shoulder: Rupture of the Supraspinatus Tendon and Other Lesions in or about the Subacromial Bursa*. Boston: Thomas Todd; 1934.

Cofield RH, Briggs BT. Glenohumeral arthrodesis. *J Bone Joint Surg*. 1979;61:668–677.

Cofield RH. Rotator cuff disease of the shoulder. *J Bone Joint Surg*. 1985; 67-A:974–979.

Cofield RH. Subscapular muscle transposition for repair of chronic rotator cuff tears. *Surg Gynecol Obstet*. 1982;154:667–672.

Debeyre J, Patte D, Elmelik E. Repair of ruptures of the rotator cuff of the shoulder with a note on advancement of the supraspinatus muscle. *J Bone Joint Surg*. 1965;47-B:36–42.

Dierickx C, Vanhoof H. Massive rotator cuff tears treated by a deltoid muscular inlay flap. *Acta Orthop Belgica*. 1994;60:94–100.

Duralde XA, Bair B. Massive rotator cuff tears: the result of partial rotator cuff repair. *J Shoulder Elbow Surg*. 2005;14:121–127.

Fenlin JM Jr, Chase JM, Rushton SA, et al. Tuberoplasty: creation of an acromiohumeral articulation—a treatment option for massive,

irreparable rotator cuff tears. *J Shoulder Elbow Surg*. 2002;11:136–142.
Galatz LM, Ball CM, Teefey SA, et al. The outcome and repair integrity of completely arthroscopically repaired large and massive rotator cuff tears. *J Bone Joint Surg*. 2004;86A:219–224.
Gartsman GM. Massive, irreparable tears of the rotator cuff. Results of operative debridement and subacromial decompression. *J Bone Joint Surg*. 1997;79-A:715–721.
Gazielly DF. Deltoid muscular flap transfer for massive defects of the rotator cuff. In: Burkhead WZ Jr, ed. *Rotator Cuff Disorders*. Baltimore: Williams & Wilkins; 1996:356–367.
Gerber C, Fuchs B, Hodler J. The results of repair of massive tears of the rotator cuff. *J Bone Joint Surg*. 2000;82-A:505–515.
Gerber C, Krushell RJ. Isolated rupture of the tendon of the subscapularis muscle. Clinical features in 16 cases. *J Bone Joint Surg*. 1991;73-B:389–394.
Gerber C, Maquieira G, Espinosa N. Latissimus dorsi transfer for the treatment of irreparable rotator cuff tears. *J Bone Joint Surg Am*. 2006;88:113–120.
Gerber C, Schneeberger AG, Beck M, et al. Mechanical strength of repairs of the rotator cuff. *J Bone Joint Su*. 1994;76-B:371–380.
Gerber C. Massive rotator cuff tears. In: Iannotti JP, Williams GR, eds. *Disorders of the Shoulder*. Philadelphia: Lippincott, Williams & Wilkins; 1999:57–93.
Goutallier D, Postel JM, Bernageau J, et al. Fatty muscle degeneration in cuff ruptures. Pre- and postoperative evaluation by CT scan. *Clin Orthop Relat Res*. 1994;304:78–83.
Goutallier D, Postel JM, Gleyze P, et al. Influence of cuff muscle fatty degeneration on anatomic and functional outcomes after simple suture of full-thickness tears. *J Shoulder Elbow Surg*. 2003;12:550–554.
Ha'eri GB, Wiley AM. Advancement of the supraspinatus in the repair of ruptures of the rotator cuff. *J Bone Joint Surg*. 1981; 63-A:232–238.
Harryman DT, Mack LA, Wang KY, et al. Repairs of the rotator cuff: correlation of functional results with integrity of the cuff. *J Bone Joint Surg*. 1991;73-A:982–989.
Herrera MF, Bauer G, Reynolds F, et al. Infection after mini-open rotator cuff repair. *J Shoulder Elbow Surg*. 2002;11:605–608.
Iannnotti JP, Ciccone J, Buss DD, et al. Accuracy of office-based ultrasonography of the shoulder for the diagnosis of rotator cuff tears. *J Bone Joint Surg*. 2005;87-A:1305–1311.
Iannotti JP, Hennigan S, Herzog R, et al. Latissimus dorsi tendon transfer for irreparable posterosuperior rotator cuff tears. Factors affecting outcome. *J Bone Joint Surg Am*. 2006;88:342–348.
Iannotti JP, Zlatkin MD, Esterhai JL, et al. Magnetic resonance imaging of the shoulder: sensitivity, specificity, and predictive value. *J Bone Joint Surg*. 1991;73-A:17–29.
Jost B, Pfirrmann CWA, Gerber C. Clinical outcome and structural failure of rotator cuff repairs. *J Bone Joint Surg*. 2000;82-A:304–313.
Klepps S, Bishop J, Lin J, et al. Prospective evaluation of the effect of rotator cuff integrity on the outcome of open rotator cuff repairs. *Am J Sports Med*. 2004;32:1716–1722.
Klinger HM, Steckel H, Ernstberger T, et al. Arthroscopic debridement of massive rotator cuff tears: negative prognostic factors. *Arch Orthop Trauma Surg*. 2005;125(4):261–266.
Levy O, Pritsch M, Oran A, et al. A wide and versatile combined surgical approach to the shoulder. *J Shoulder Elbow Surg*. 1999;8:658–659.
Malcarney HL, Bonar F, Murrell GA. Early inflammatory reaction after rotator cuff repair with a porcine small intestine submucosal implant: a report of 4 cases. *Am J Sports Med*. 2005;33:907–911.
McCallister WV, Parsons IM, Titelman RM, et al. Open rotator cuff repair without acromioplasty. *J Bone Joint Surg Am*. 2005;87:1278–1283.
Miniaci A, MacLeod M. Transfer of the latissimus dorsi muscle after failed repair of a massive tear of the rotator cuff: a two to five-year review. *J Bone Joint Surg*. 1999;81-A:1120–1127.
Nagy L, Koch PP, Gerber C. Functional analysis of shoulder arthrodesis. *J Shoulder Elbow Surg*. 2004;13:386–395.
Neviaser JS, Neviaser RJ, Neviaser TJ. The repair of chronic massive ruptures of the rotator cuff of the shoulder by use of a freeze dried rotator cuff. *J Bone Joint Surg*. 1978;60-A:681–684.
Ozaki J, Fujimoto S, Masuhara K, et al. Reconstruction of chronic massive rotator cuff tears with synthetic materials. *Clin Orthop*. 1986;202:173–183.
Paavolainen P. Teres minor transfer. In: Burkhead WZ Jr, ed. *Rotator Cuff Disorders*. Baltimore: Williams & Wilkins; 1996:342–348.
Park HB, Yokota A, Gill HS, et al. Diagnostic accuracy of clinical tests for the different degrees of subacromial impingement syndrome. *J Bone Joint Surg Am*. 2005;87:1446–1455.
Reilly P, Bull AM, Amis AA, et al. Passive tension and gap formation of rotator cuff repairs. *J Shoulder Elbow Surg*. 2004;13:664–667.
Rockwood CA Jr, Williams GR Jr, Burkhead WZ Jr. Debridement of degenerative, irreparable lesions of the rotator cuff. *J Bone Joint Sur*. 1995;77-A:857–866.
Rokito AS, Cuomo F, Gallagher MA, et al. Long-term functional outcome of repair of large and massive chronic tears of the rotator cuff. *J Bone Joint Surg*. 1999;81-A:991–997.
Scheibel M, Lichtenberg S, Habermeyer P. Reversed arthroscopic subacromial decompression for massive rotator cuff tears. *J Shoulder Elbow Surg*. 2004;13:272–278.
Sclamberg SG, Tibone JE, Itamura JM, et al. Six-month magnetic resonance imaging follow-up of large and massive rotator cuff repairs reinforced with porcine small intestinal submucosa. *J Shoulder Elbow Surg*. 2004;13:538–541.
Teefey SA, Hasan SA, Middleton WD, et al. Ultrasonography of the rotator cuff. A comparison of ultrasonographic and arthroscopic findings in one hundred consecutive cases. *J Bone Joint Surg*. 2000;82-A:498–504.
Tung GA, Yoo DC, Levine SM, et al. Subscapularis tendon tear: primary and associated signs on MRI. *J Comput Assist Tomogr*. 2001;25:417–424.
Walch G, Boulahia A, Calderone S, et al. The "dropping" and "hornblower's" signs in evaluation of rotator-cuff tears. *J Bone Joint Surg Br*. 1998;80:624–628.
Walch G, Edwards TB, Boulahia A, et al. Arthroscopic tenotomy of the long head of the biceps in the treatment of rotator cuff tears: clinical and radiographic results of 307 cases. *J Shoulder Elbow Surg*. 2005;14(3):238–246.
Warner JJ, Parsons IM IV. Latissimus dorsi tendon transfer: a comparative analysis of primary and salvage reconstruction of massive, irreparable rotator cuff tears. *J Shoulder Elbow Surg*. 2001;10:514–521.
Warner JJP, Krushell RJ, Masquelet A, et al. Anatomy and relationships of the suprascapular nerve: anatomical constraints to mobilization of the supraspinatus and infraspinatus muscles in the management of massive rotator cuff tears. *J Bone Joint Surg*. 1992;74-A: 36–45.
Weiner DS, Macnab I. Superior migration of the humeral head. A radiological aid in the diagnosis of tears of the rotator cuff. *J Bone Joint Surg Br*. 1970;52:524–527.
Zheng MH, Chen J, Kirilak Y, et al. Porcine small intestine submucosa (SIS) is not an acellular collagenous matrix and contains porcine DNA: possible implications in human implantation. *J Biomed Mater Res B Appl Biomater*. 2005;73(1):61–67.
Zvijac JE, Levy HJ, Lemak LJ. Arthroscopic subacromial decompression in the treatment of full thickness rotator cuff tears: a 3 to 6 year follow-up. *Arthroscopy*. 1994;10:518–523.

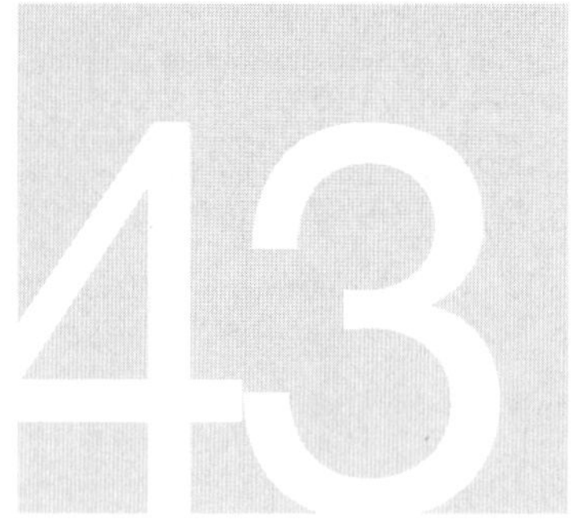

GLENOHUMERAL ARTHRITIS: RHEUMATOID

JOAQUIN SANCHEZ-SOTELO

Rheumatoid arthritis (RA) is a chronic, systemic inflammatory disorder with an estimated worldwide prevalence of about 1%. Its prevalence increases starting in the third decade of life; 5% of the population older than 70 years develops RA. Musculoskeletal involvement in RA is characterized by the formation of an erosive synovitis that results in continued bone, cartilage, and soft tissue degradation.

The shoulder is involved in many patients with longstanding RA (Fig. 43-1); some authors have estimated shoulder involvement in about 60% of rheumatoid patients. The condition may affect all the synovial joints of the shoulder region—glenohumeral, acromioclavicular, and sternoclavicular—and the scapulothoracic articulation may become secondarily affected by periscapular fibrosis (Table 43-1). Associated soft tissue involvement is common, and many patients (between 25% and 50% depending on the series) with rheumatoid involvement of the shoulder eventually develop rotator cuff compromise. When the cervical spine is affected, patients may complain of referred pain to the shoulder region.

It is important to remember that pharmacologic treatment of rheumatoid arthritis has continued to improve, and the presentation of patients with RA has changed somewhat owing to the effect of these medications. Some of them are powerful modulators of the immune system that may substantially increase the risk of infection if they are not discontinued prior to surgery. The possibility of rheumatoid involvement and infection coexistence should be taken into consideration. Some patients may also develop shoulder symptoms related to steroid-induced humeral head osteonecrosis.

The purpose of this chapter is to review the evaluation and surgical treatment of glenohumeral rheumatoid arthritis. Physical therapy and steroid injections also play a role in the treatment of shoulder RA. However, multiple steroid injections should be avoided, as they may have a deleterious effect on connective tissue structures. Most physicians suggest limiting injections to three and repeating injections only when significant improvement resulted from the previous injection.

ORTHOPEDIC EVALUATION OF THE RHEUMATOID SHOULDER

Rheumatoid involvement of the shoulder is characterized by pain associated with various degrees of stiffness, weakness, and deformity. Most patients are referred to the orthopedic surgeon for evaluation and treatment of glenohumeral joint involvement. However, the acromioclavicular, sternoclavicular, and scapulothoracic articulations should be evaluated systematically, as failure to address them may lead to incomplete improvement. It is important to assess active and passive range of motion as well as rotator cuff atrophy and strength.

In addition, the shoulder region should be viewed in the context of other joints involved in the upper and lower extremity. Hip, knee, foot, or ankle problems may need to be addressed first if they are symptomatic enough, as well as to decrease the load of crutches or a walker on the upper extremity, especially if rotator cuff repair will be required. Hand and elbow involvement should also be taken into consideration not only to address the most symptomatic joint first and delineate an overall surgical plan for the upper extremity but also to leave room for shoulder and elbow stems should shoulder and elbow arthroplasty both be needed. Finally, all patients undergoing surgical intervention should be evaluated for atlantoaxial instability and temporomandibular involvement (Fig. 43-2).

Radiographic features at presentation will change depending on the stage and severity of rheumatoid involvement. Patients with early synovitis may have minimal radiographic changes, but most patients do present joint line narrowing, osteopenia, and various amounts of erosion and bone loss at the humeral head, glenoid, and coracoacromial arch (Fig. 43-1). Proximal humeral migration may indicate cuff attenuation or tearing.

Glenoid bone stock should be carefully evaluated in every patient with glenohumeral rheumatoid arthritis (Fig. 43-3). Some times plain radiographs clearly show preserved bone stock, but in cases with advanced medial glenoid erosion, a

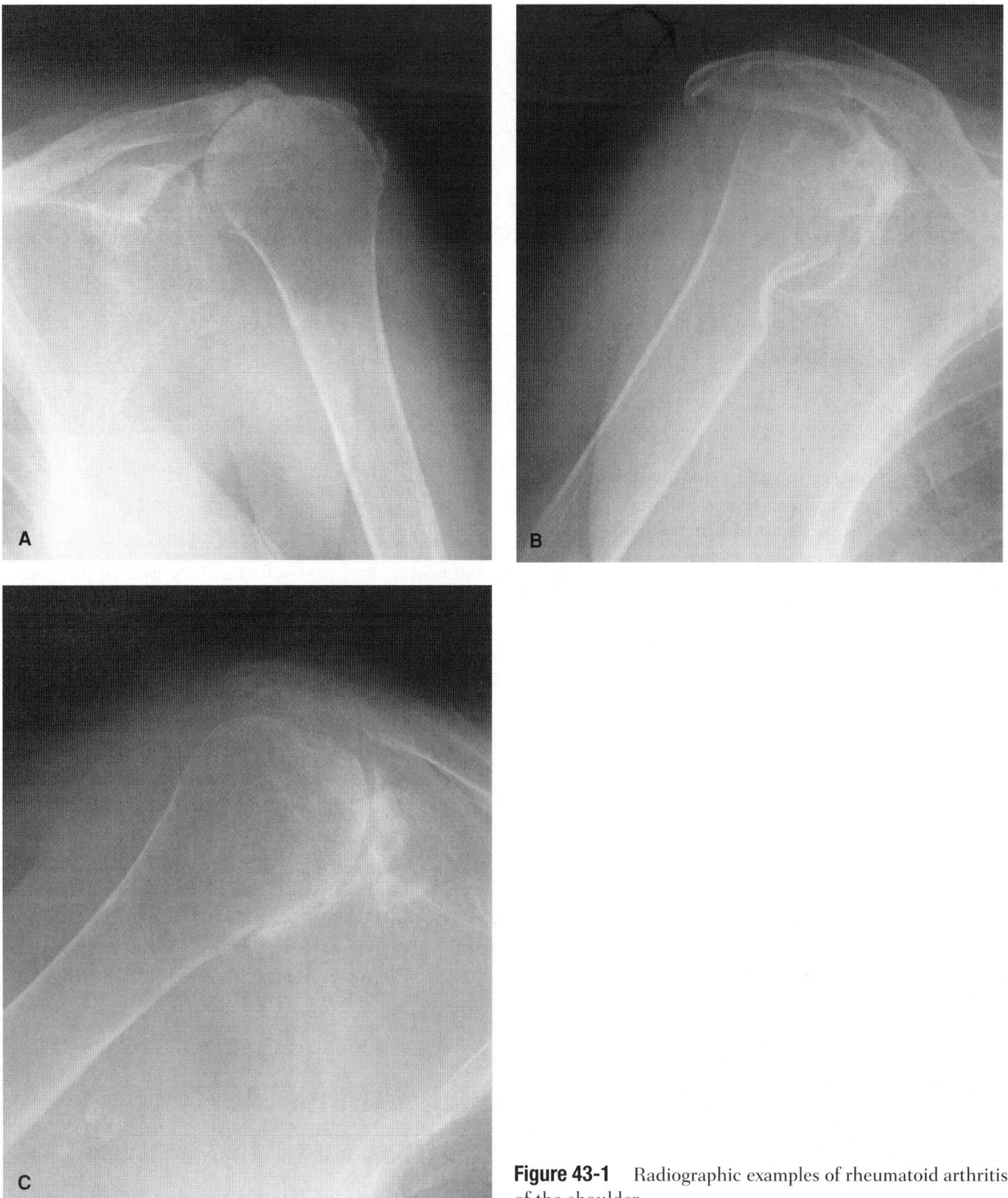

Figure 43-1 Radiographic examples of rheumatoid arthritis of the shoulder.

CT scan may be helpful for preoperative planning. Shoulder MR should be considered in patients with clinical evidence of rotator cuff involvement but is not needed in every case.

SHOULDER SYNOVECTOMY

Arthroscopic synovectomy may be indicated in patients with synovitis when the glenohumeral arthritis is not severe enough to warrant shoulder arthroplasty. The indications for synovectomy have decreased as the effectiveness of medical treatment has increased. The severity of synovitis may be evaluated with either MR or arthrography.

This procedure is attractive for several reasons. Arthroscopic surgery provides global access to the entire joint with minimal morbidity, allows a relatively quick recovery, and is associated with a low complication rate. In addition, it provides access not only to the glenohumeral joint but also to the subacromial space and acromioclavicular joint if needed. Associated rotator pathology may be addressed at the time of arthroscopy. Finally, it does not burn any bridges for a later arthroplasty unless it is complicated by a permanent nerve injury or deep infection.

TABLE 43-1 SPECTRUM OF SHOULDER PATHOLOGY IN RHEUMATOID ARTHRITIS

- Glenohumeral joint
  - Synovitis
  - Arthritis
  - Sepsis
  - Steroid-induced osteonecrosis
- Subacromial bursitis
- Rotator cuff tears
- Acromioclavicular joint synovitis and arthritis
- Sternoclavicular joint synovitis and arthritis
- Scapulothoracic fibrosis
- Referred pain (cervical spine affected)

A complete glenohumeral synovectomy often requires use of at least three portals, as the axillary recess is difficult to reach from the standard posterior and anterosuperior portals. Patients with associated capsule contracture and floating cartilage flaps may benefit from contracture release and cartilage debridement, respectively. Subacromial bursectomy may be required as an isolated or associated procedure; acromioplasty and resection of the coracoacromial ligament are not recommended to avoid weakening of the coracoacromial arch, which may become problematic should cuff attenuation or tearing occur.

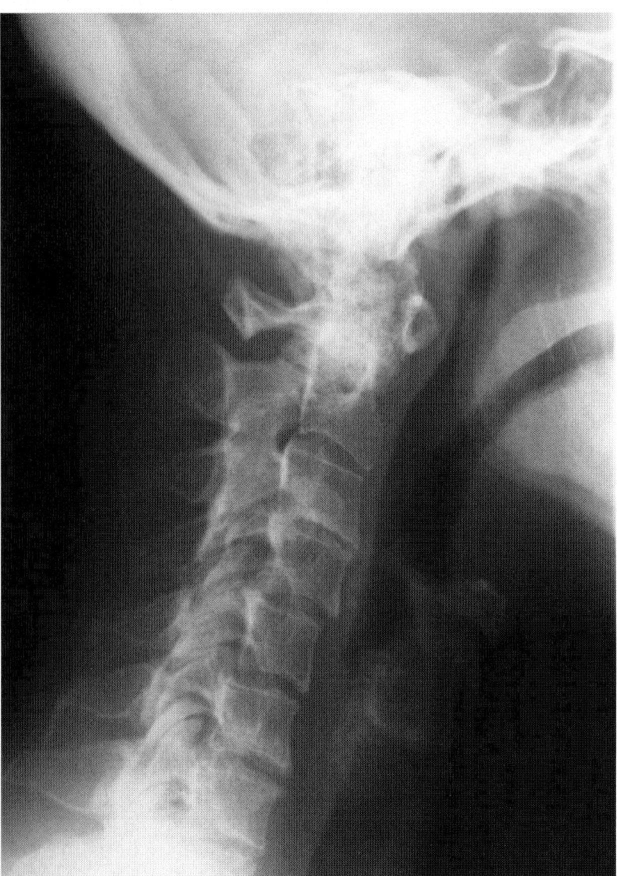

Figure 43-2 Atlantoaxial instability is present commonly in patients with RA and may complicate anesthesia.

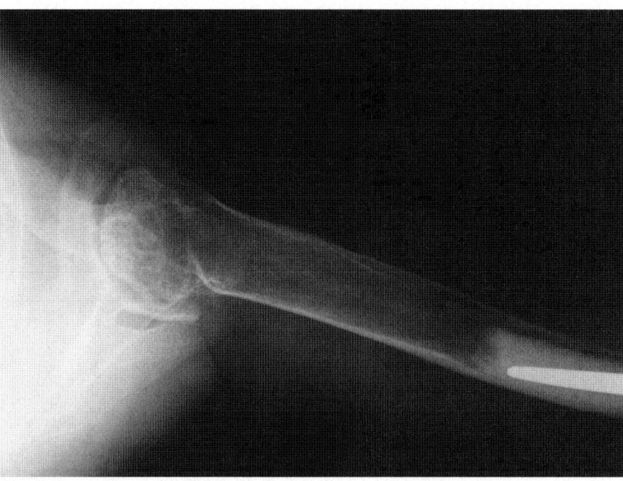

Figure 43-3 Progressive glenoid bone loss may compromise the ability to implant a glenoid component.

Shoulder synovectomy and subacromial bursectomy are more reliable in terms of pain relief than restoration of motion. Interestingly, published reports on the effectiveness of arthroscopic shoulder synovectomy for RA are sparse. Although synovectomy has been proposed to delay progressive joint deterioration, this prophylactic effect has been difficult to prove in clinical practice. The Mayo Clinic experience on arthroscopic shoulder synovectomy was recently reviewed. Sixteen shoulders were followed for a mean of 5.5 years after synovectomy; improvement in pain was noted in 13 patients, with less predictable improvement in motion. Most patients with radiographic follow-up showed disease progression, and worse results were obtained in those patients with more severe radiographic changes at presentation.

SHOULDER ARTHROPLASTY

Implant Selection and Surgical Technique

Shoulder arthroplasty is indicated to relieve pain and improve function in patients with symptomatic glenohumeral arthritis that will not respond to other treatment options. Although orthopedic surgeons generally advise delaying joint arthroplasty in other locations or conditions as much as possible, it may be advisable to recommend shoulder arthroplasty sooner rather than later in rheumatoid patients before glenoid bone loss, contractures, and rotator cuff tearing compromise the ability to use a glenoid component or to improve motion and strength.

Nonconstrained total shoulder arthroplasty seems to provide the best results in terms of pain relief and functional restoration. However, glenoid component implantation is contraindicated if glenoid bone stock is insufficient or there is an associated large and irreparable rotator cuff tear. Good results have been reported with both resurfacing and standard humeral components. Uncemented tissue-ingrowth humeral components can be used if the metaphyseal bone is intact and if it is possible to achieve adequate diaphyseal contact and fit. However, cemented fixation is advisable in many instances, realizing the potential complications of cement removal from the humeral shaft in rheumatoid patients should revision surgery be needed. When cement is used, it is wise to use antibiotic-loaded polymethylmethacrylate. The use of a reverse shoulder arthroplasty in rheumatoid patients with extensive cuff tearing is controversial; it may provide surprisingly good functional results initially, but the glenoid is oftentimes too osteopenic to allow secure and long-lasting fixation of the glenoid implant.

Several technical aspects should be contemplated at the time of shoulder arthroplasty (Table 43-2). The skin is usually extremely fragile. Local osteopenia may facilitate the occurrence of intraoperative fractures; humeral rotation for exposure should be done carefully, and extension of the deltopectoral approach by deltoid detachment from the acromion and spine of the scapula (the so-called anteromedial approach) is recommended to reduce the risk of fracture in the presence of severe osteopenia and contractures. The rotator cuff should be systematically evaluated and prepared for repair when tears are found. The coracoacromial arch should be preserved intact as a stabilizing mechanism against anterosuperior subluxation in the event of rotator cuff failure.

Although preoperative radiographs and CT scan provide useful information to determine the feasibility of glenoid implantation, the final decision is made at the time of surgery. A hole may be drilled at the glenoid center to estimate the thickness of remaining bone stock; usually, a component can be safely placed if there is at least 2 cm of depth. Central bone loss is more common than peripheral bone loss; however, when segmental bone loss is present, consideration may be given to structural bone graft. A pegged glenoid component is used if possible, as it seems to allow better implant/cement/bone interface (Fig. 43-4); however, keeled glenoid components may allow implantation in situations where loss of bone stock will not allow secure placement of a pegged glenoid component. When glenoid bone stock is insufficient, shoulder hemiarthroplasty is the preferred option.

Humeral head size is selected based on the patient's humeral size as well as stability and motion. When the joint is contracted, it may be necessary to select a smaller humeral head to maintain functional motion. On the other hand, patients with attenuated soft tissues may require a larger humeral head to fill the joint space in the presence of a stretched capsule and rotator cuff tendons.

The rare patient with rheumatoid arthritis whose severe cuff involvement is not associated with severe glenoid bone loss may benefit from a reverse shoulder arthroplasty. The same precautions in terms of exposure and avoidance of undue stresses to decrease the risk of fracture should be taken into consideration. Glenoid reaming should be done carefully, because the glenoid can be easily fractured by a sudden torque if the reamer is trapped against irregular bone.

Postoperative physical therapy follows the general guidelines of shoulder arthroplasty, with sequential passive, active-assisted, and strengthening exercises. Patients who require an associated rotator cuff repair should not start active use of the shoulder for at least 6 weeks. Patients with severely compromised soft tissues and cuff benefit from a limited-goals type of program., Some authors recommend letting the patient immediately return to activities of daily living after a reverse arthroplasty; in patients with rheumatoid arthritis, it is probably best to delay immediate activity for the first 4 weeks with the use of a sling.

TABLE 43-2 SHOULDER ARTHROPLASTY IN RA: TECHNICAL CONSIDERATIONS

- Early rather than late surgery may improve outcome
- High-risk intraoperative fractures
  - Consider anteromedial approach
- High incidence of rotator cuff attenuation and tears
  - Preserve coracoacromial arch
  - Repair associated rotator cuff tears if possible
- Glenoid bone loss
  - Preoperative CT scan
  - Intraoperative assessment
  - Better outcome when glenoid component implanted
    - Insufficient glenoid bone stock
    - Irreparable cuff tear
  - Humeral stem
  - Selective uncemented fixation
  - Beware if current or future elbow replacement
    - Cement restrictor
    - Shorter stems
    - Consider resurfacing (bone stock permitting)
- Humeral head size based more on soft tissue tension than humerus size
- Address associated acromioclavicular/sternoclavicular pathology
- Postoperative rehabilitation
  - Standard vs. limited-goals program
  - Scapulothoracic fibrosis may limit range of motion

Results

Shoulder arthroplasty is associated with pain relief in most rheumatoid patients; functional improvements have not been consistently reported in the literature. When a glenoid component can be safely implanted, total shoulder arthroplasty is associated with a better outcome than with humeral head replacement. Likewise, when an associated cuff tear is found, concomitant cuff repair significantly improves postoperative clinical shoulder scores compared with those of patients in whom tears are not repaired.

The results of a multicenter prospective study were recently published. Thirty-six hemiarthroplasties and 25 total shoulder arthroplasties were followed for a mean of 3 years. The underlying diagnosis was rheumatoid arthritis in 53 shoulders and other inflammatory conditions in the remaining shoulders. Shoulder arthroplasty was associated with a significant improvement in pain and quality

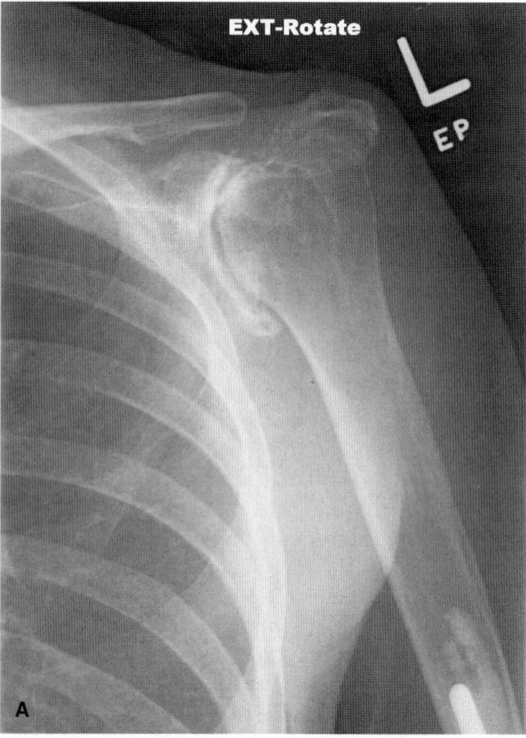

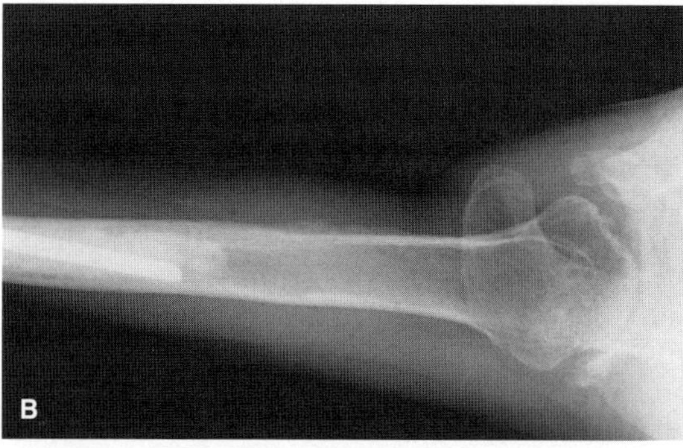

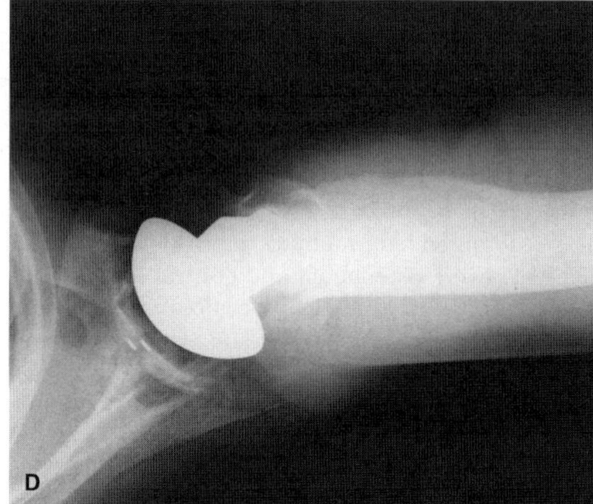

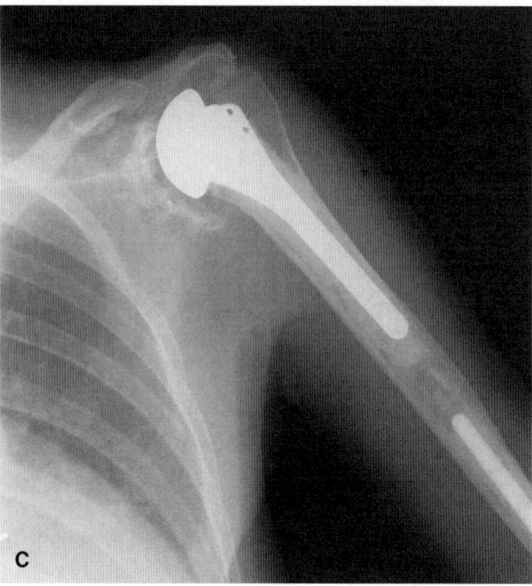

Figure 43-4 Preoperative (**A**, **B**) and postoperative (**C**, **D**) radiographs of a patient with severe rheumatoid involvement that required total shoulder arthroplasty. Glenoid bone loss was not severe enough to prevent implantation of a glenoid component. The tip of an elbow humeral component can be appreciated below the cemented shoulder humeral stem.

of life. Motion was also improved, to a mean of 90 degrees with hemiarthroplasty and 115 degrees with total shoulder arthroplasty. Complications included four periprosthetic fractures (two intraoperative), glenoid loosening in two shoulders, and progressive glenoid erosion in four hemiarthroplasties. Other authors have reported a high incidence of rotator cuff tears occurring after shoulder arthroplasty in RA, as well as higher rates of glenoid loosening with longer follow-up.

Resurfacing humeral components avoid the use of a stem, which facilitates the use of stemmed elbow replacement as well as shoulder revision surgery should this become needed. However, humeral head erosion commonly seen in rheumatoid arthritis may compromise fixation of resurfacing components. In addition, glenoid exposure is compromised by the retained humeral head. The published experience of a single institution with this type of component has been satisfactory. These authors studied 33 hemiarthroplasties and 42 total shoulder arthroplasties and reported significant improvements in pain relief, an average flexion gain of about 50 degrees, a high rate of satisfactory results, and only three reoperations for component loosening or progressive glenoid erosion after hemiarthroplasty.

Reverse shoulder arthroplasty may be considered for patients with glenohumeral arthritis, an associated irreparable cuff tear, and pseudoparalysis. General concerns about glenoid component failure are especially concerning in RA owing to glenoid erosion and osteopenia. Many authors consider RA a relative contraindication for reverse arthroplasty. In a small series of eight rheumatoid shoulders treated with a reverse arthroplasty, the average Constant score improved from 17 to 63 points; there were two cases of glenoid loosening, and three failed acromion osteosynthesis. These findings emphasize the functional improvement that can be expected after reverse arthroplasty as well as the high rate of mechanical failure and other complications.

ROTATOR CUFF REPAIR

Isolated cuff repair in patients with rheumatoid arthritis is not very commonly required. Most patients with a cuff tear have associated glenohumeral arthritis and undergo shoulder arthroplasty and cuff repair in the same surgical intervention. However, rheumatoid patients will occasionally present with symptomatic rotator cuff tear and minimal articular changes, and when nonoperative treatment fails, they may be candidates for rotator cuff repair.

The repair of the rotator cuff in rheumatoid patients may be challenging. Some patients have associated stiffness. In addition, the friable nature of the cuff and humeral head osteopenia may compromise the security of open and arthroscopic techniques. Acromioclavicular erosion may debilitate the coracoacromial arch; if acromioplasty is needed, it should be performed carefully, and every effort should be made to preserve the coracoacromial arch.

There is limited published information about the outcome of cuff repair in RA. The Mayo Clinic experience was recently reviewed. Twenty-three repairs were followed for a mean of 10 years or until revision. Tears were partial thickness in nine cases; full-thickness tears were categorized as medium in nine cases, large in four, and massive in one. Surgery provided significant improvements in pain, but motion and strength remained mostly unchanged. No improvement was reported in five cases, three of which underwent reoperation. Full-thickness tears tended to be associated with worse function after surgery. Although pain relief and patient satisfaction may be achieved after surgical repair of rotator cuff tears, functional gains should not be expected when the tear is full thickness.

THE ACROMIOCLAVICULAR AND STERNOCLAVICULAR JOINTS

When acromioclavicular joint (ACJ) arthritis does not respond to nonoperative treatment, consideration should be given to ACJ synovectomy and resection of the distal end of the clavicle, which may be performed open or arthroscopically. Involvement of the sternoclavicular joint may require synovectomy and rarely resection of the medial end of the clavicle.

SUGGESTED READINGS

Barrett WP, Thornhill TS, Thomas WH, et al. Nonconstrained total shoulder arthroplasty in patients with polyarticular rheumatoid arthritis. *J Arthroplasty*. 1989;4:91–96.

Collins DN, Harryman DT II, Wirth MA. Shoulder arthroplasty for the treatment of inflammatory arthritis. *J Bone Joint Surg* 2004;86A:2489–2496.

Figgie HE III, Inglis AE, Goldberg VM, et al. An analysis of factors affecting the long-term results of total shoulder arthroplasty in inflammatory arthritis. *J Arthroplasty*. 1988;3(2):123–130.

Friedman RJ, Thornhill TS, Thomas WH, et al. Non-constrained total shoulder replacement in patients who have rheumatoid arthritis and class-IV function. *J Bone Joint Surg*. 1989;71A:494–498.

Kelly IG. Unconstrained shoulder arthroplasty in rheumatoid arthritis. *Clin Orthop*. 1994;307:94–102.

Koorevaar RC, Merkies ND, de Waal Malefijt MC, et al. Shoulder hemiarthroplasty in rheumatoid arthritis. 19 cases reexamined after 1-17 years. *Acta Orthop Scand*. 1997;68(3):243–245.

Lehtinen JT, Kaarela K, Belt EA, et al. Incidence of glenohumeral joint involvement in seropositive rheumatoid arthritis. A 15 year endpoint study. *J Rheumatol*. 2000;27(2):347–350.

McCoy SR, Warren RF, Bade HA III, et al. Total shoulder arthroplasty in rheumatoid arthritis. *J Arthroplasty*. 1989;4(2):105–113.

Rittmeister M, Kerschbaumer F. Grammont reverse total shoulder arthroplasty in patients with rheumatoid arthritis and nonreconstructable rotator cuff lesions. *J Shoulder Elbow Surg*. 2001;10:17–22.

Rozing PM, Brand R. Rotator cuff repair during shoulder arthroplasty in rheumatoid arthritis. *J Arthroplasty*. 1998;13(3):311–319.

Smith AM, Sperling JW, Cofield RH. Rotator cuff repair in patients with rheumatoid arthritis. *J Bone Joint Surg*. 2005;87A:1782–1787.

Sneppen O, Fruensgaard S, Johannsen HV, et al. Total shoulder replacement in rheumatoid arthritis: proximal migration and loosening. *J Shoulder Elbow Surg*. 1996;5(1):47–52.

Sojbjerg JO, Frich LH, Johannsen HV, et al. Late results of total shoulder replacement in patients with rheumatoid arthritis. *Clin Orthop*. 1999;366:39–45.

Stewart MP, Kelly IG. Total shoulder replacement in rheumatoid disease: 7- to 13-year follow-up of 37 joints. *J Bone Joint Surg*. 1997;79B:68–72.

Thomas BJ, Amstutz HC, Cracchiolo A. Shoulder arthroplasty for rheumatoid arthritis. *Clin Orthop*. 1991;265:125–128.

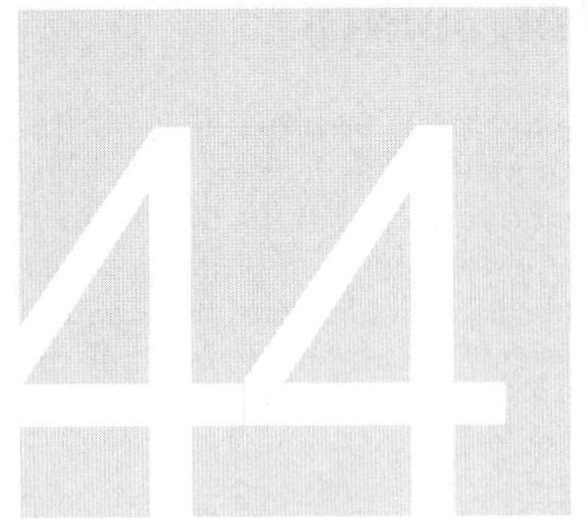

GLENOHUMERAL ARTHRITIS: OSTEOARTHRITIS

JOHN W. SPERLING

Osteoarthritis is recognized as the most common type of glenohumeral arthritis. It is characterized by a progressive arthropathy with loss of articular cartilage and hypertrophic changes in the subchondral bone. In treating the patient with glenohumeral osteoarthritis, multiple facets need to be incorporated to formulate a successful treatment plan. The process begins with a thorough understanding of the severity of the patient's symptoms, functional demands, and ability to comply with postoperative restrictions. Appropriate imaging studies, in conjunction with a careful examination, allow the physician to outline a proper treatment plan for the patient.

PATHOGENESIS

Osteoarthritis of the shoulder is significantly less common than that of the hip or knee. There is a progressive increase in the incidence with increasing age. Subclinical stages of osteoarthritis may exist for decades. Subchondral cysts may be present in both the humeral head as well as the glenoid. The typical pathologic findings of osteoarthritis include thinning or complete loss of cartilage on the humeral head. In addition, the humeral head may flatten with progressive sclerotic changes. Osteophytes frequently develop at the margin of the articular surface in a circumferential pattern. These osteophytes may increase tension on the capsule with resultant loss of shoulder motion.

One of the characteristics that differentiates osteoarthritis from rheumatoid arthritis and other inflammatory types of glenohumeral arthritis is the typical preservation of the rotator cuff. Multiple studies have demonstrated that the rotator cuff is intact in 90% to 95% of patients with osteoarthritis.

Also typical of osteoarthritis is the posterior glenoid wear pattern frequently present. This disease pattern results in posterior glenoid wear with associated posterior humeral subluxation. There is progressive stretching of the posterior capsule with thickening and contracture of the anterior capsule.

PATIENT EVALUATION

History

Evaluation of the patient with glenohumeral arthritis begins with taking a thorough history. It is critically important to understand the severity of the patient's symptoms and functional demands. It is essential to understand the primary complaint of the patient—is it weakness, pain, or loss of motion?

One should determine how long the shoulder pain has been present as well as whether there was a specific traumatic event. Patients are asked to rate their pain on a 1 to 10 scale at rest, with activities, and at night. Alleviating and aggravating factors are determined. Patients are asked to specifically localize the pain. Does the pain occur in the superior-lateral aspect of the shoulder? Does the pain occur in a radicular pattern down the arm, possibly consistent with a neurologic cause?

One should ask about prior evaluations and treatment. What studies have been performed in the past and what were the results? Has the patient had a trial of physical therapy? Has the patient had prior injections? If so, what was the location and response? Has there been prior shoulder surgery? If so, what was the indication, postoperative therapy, and outcome? Were there any problems with wound healing?

REVIEW OF SYSTEMS

A focused review of systems should be documented. Is there a history of metabolic or rheumatologic disease? Does the patient have a history of other joint involvement, and in what order should they be addressed? Is there a history of neurologic symptoms or neck pain?

One needs to determine whether there is a history of cough, shortness of breath, or weight loss. Although uncommon, patients may present with shoulder pain as a symptom of lung cancer. A list of medications and associated medical problems should also be compiled to assist with planning of medical clearance prior to surgery.

Physical Examination

The first step in the physical examination is inspection with evaluation for atrophy and appearance of prior incisions. One examines for atrophy associated with long-standing rotator cuff disease as well as evidence of deltoid deficiency. Palpation begins at the cervical spine. Cervical motion is evaluated, and testing for potential cervical radiculopathy is performed with a Spurling test. Examination is bilateral and should include the wrist, elbow, and shoulder. Examination of the upper extremities includes assessment of reflexes, strength, and sensation.

Shoulder range of motion and strength is carefully assessed. Active and passive shoulder abduction is recorded. One needs to determine whether there is a component of anterior-superior humeral head escape or altered scapular motion with shoulder elevation. External rotation and internal rotation are recorded. Typically, shoulder strength is graded on a 1 to 5 scale for internal rotation, external rotation, flexion, extension, and abduction. Deltoid and periscapular muscles are also tested.

Radiographic Studies

Three shoulder views are routinely obtained: an axillary view and 40- degree posterior oblique views with internal and external rotation. On the anteroposterior (AP) view, one evaluates both the medial-lateral and superior-inferior acromiohumeral distance. Among patients with glenoid erosion, there is a decrease in the amount of humeral head offset from the lateral border of the acromion. Specifically, among patients with significant glenoid erosion, the lateral border of the humeral head is medial to the lateral edge of the acromion. In patients with rotator cuff deficiency, which is less common in osteoarthritis, there may be superior subluxation of the humeral head with a decrease in the acromial-humeral distance. One caveat is that with posterior subluxation that is frequently present in osteoarthritis, there can be the false appearance of superior humeral head subluxation.

The AP radiographs are also helpful in determining the overall degree of osteopenia, thickness of the cortices, and size of the humeral canal. Serial radiographs taken over time will allow one to confirm the diagnosis of osteoarthritis compared with other diagnoses that may include rheumatoid arthritis, osteonecrosis, cuff tear arthropathy, and traumatic arthritis. The axillary view allows assessment of glenoid erosion and glenohumeral subluxation. CT scans have become an extremely valuable tool in evaluating the patient prior to consideration of operative intervention, especially total shoulder arthroplasty. In the setting of glenoid erosion, CT scans provide important information concerning glenoid version and quantifying the amount of bone loss (Fig. 44-1). Three-dimensional CT is a new development that can further assist in evaluating the humerus and glenoid.

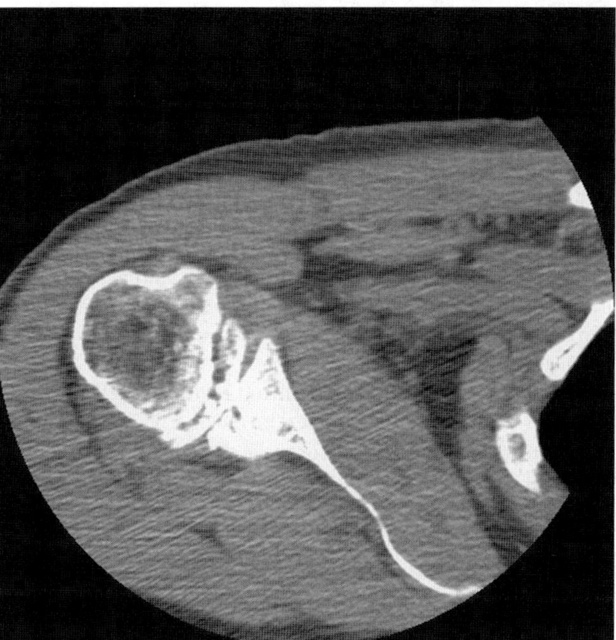

Figure 44-1 Preoperative CT scan used to evaluate degree of glenoid erosion.

TREATMENT

After integrating the information obtained from the history, physical exam, and imaging studies, one determines the specific diagnosis and can present treatment options to the patient. In the setting of glenohumeral arthritis, conservative therapy plays an important role in the early stages of disease. Nonsteroidal anti-inflammatories and intra-articular steroid and/or hyaluronic acid injections may provide temporary pain relief. A physical therapy program that focuses on restoring and maintaining range of motion and strength may be tried. Heat and cold therapy as well as ultrasound may reduce the inflammatory response and provide pain relief.

Although many patients with early shoulder osteoarthritis can be successfully treated with nonoperative modalities, patients with more advanced disease may require surgical intervention. In determining the most appropriate treatment, it is critical to clearly understand the patient's goals. Patients must be accepting of the postoperative restrictions and comply with the rehabilitation. The gold standard for severe osteoarthritis is total shoulder arthroplasty; however, in the young active patient or those patients who are unable to accept the restrictions associated with a prosthesis, this option may not be suitable. In these select cases, arthroscopic treatment or interposition arthroplasty may provide symptomatic relief.

Arthroscopic Treatment

The ideal candidate for arthroscopic debridement is a young, active, high-demand patient with isolated Outerbridge grade I to III chondral lesions. In addition, ideal candidates have congruent joint surfaces and minimal osteophyte formation. A thorough arthroscopic lavage may help remove inflammatory enzymes and proteins from the joint fluid. In addition, debridement of surface irregularities, displaced chondral flaps, and labral tears with removal of loose bodies may alleviate mechanical symptoms. Capsular contractures can also be released to help restore motion.

There have been limited reported results of arthroscopic treatment of arthritis. Ogilvie-Harris and Wiley were the first to report results of arthroscopic debridement for glenohumeral arthritis. The authors reported that 60% of patients with mild disease had improvement; however only 30% of patients with moderate to severe disease had relief. Weinstein et al. evaluated the extent and duration of pain relief after arthroscopic debridement for stages I to III glenohumeral arthritis. Among the 25 patients with a mean follow-up of 34 months, there were 2 excellent, 18 good, and 5 unsatisfactory results. A trend was noted toward worse results with increasing severity of cartilage changes. The authors also reported that 10 of 12 patients with marked preoperative stiffness had significant improvement of motion. Patients with large osteophytes and/or nonconcentric joints had worse results.

Cameron et al. reported on arthroscopic debridement and capsular release among patients with Outerbridge grade IV lesions. There were 45 patients with a minimum 2-year follow-up. Patient satisfaction scores improved significantly with 87% of patients indicating they would have the surgery again. Osteochondral lesions >2 cm^2 were associated with earlier return of pain and failure of the procedure.

Biologic Resurfacing

In the setting of osteoarthritis, biologic resurfacing of the glenoid alone or in combination with hemiarthroplasty has been reported to provide good pain relief. Traditionally these patients, especially heavy laborers, have been considered candidates for glenohumeral fusion. Although fusion results are satisfactory in 80% of cases, persistent scapulothoracic muscle pain and significant loss of motion make this an unattractive option for many active patients.

Techniques described usually involve an open approach; however, an all-arthroscopic resurfacing technique has recently been published. The goals of interposition arthroplasty and hybrid interposition arthroplasty are pain relief and restoration of function while preserving bone stock for future procedures. Several different materials have been described for use as an interposition material including anterior capsule, fascia lata autograft, and allografts of Achilles tendon, lateral meniscus, dura mater, and purified porcine submucosa.

Hybrid arthroplasty combining biologic resurfacing of the glenoid and hemiarthroplasty was first described by Burkhead and Hutton in 1995. A recent review of Burkhead's long-term results (5 to 13 years) of 26 shoulders that underwent interposition arthroplasty demonstrated excellent results in 12 of 26 (46%), 9 of 26 a satisfactory result (35%), and 5 of 26 an unsatisfactory result (19%) using Neer's criteria.

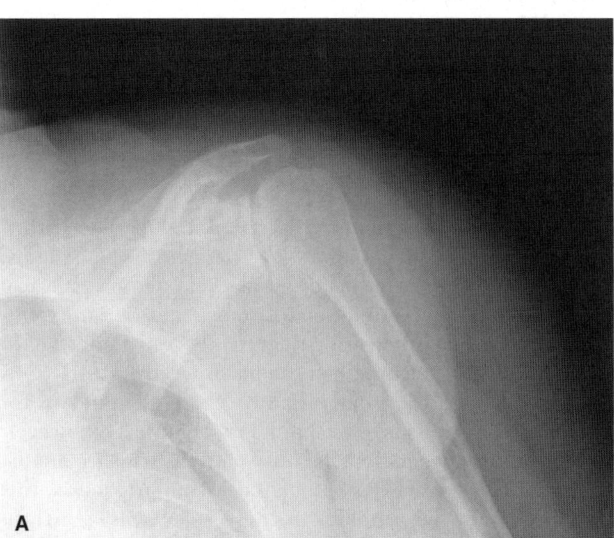

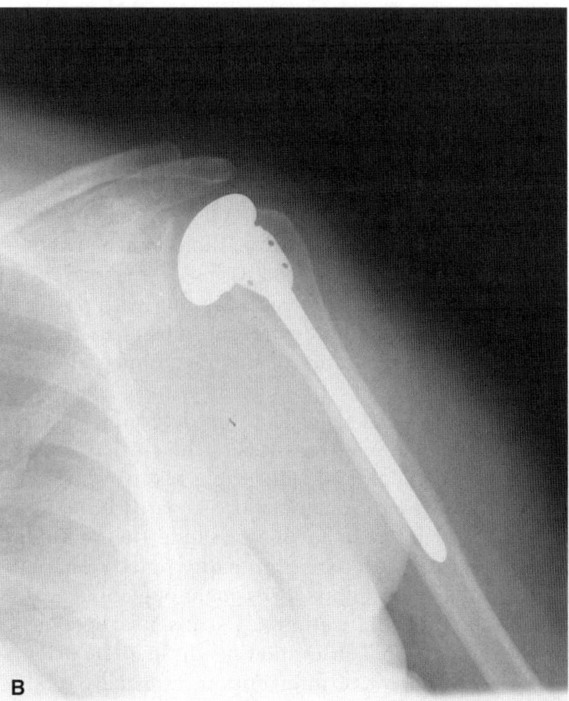

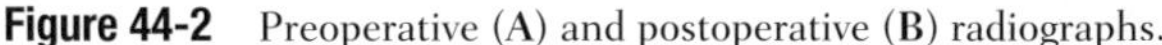

Figure 44-2 Preoperative (A) and postoperative (B) radiographs.

Shoulder Arthroplasty

Total shoulder arthroplasty is the gold standard treatment for osteoarthritis of the shoulder (Fig. 44-2). Several studies have been published that demonstrate the superiority of total shoulder arthroplasty compared with hemiarthroplasty for osteoarthritis of the shoulder. The chance of good to excellent pain relief with total shoulder arthroplasty is >90% whereas it is 80% to 85% with hemiarthroplasty.

In addition to retrospective reviews, prospective studies have been performed demonstrating superior pain relief with total shoulder arthroplasty. Gartsman et al. performed a prospective study of 51 shoulders with osteoarthritis, a concentric glenoid, and an intact rotator cuff. The shoulders were randomly assigned to hemiarthroplasty or total shoulder arthroplasty (TSA). Total shoulder arthroplasty had significantly better pain relief. In addition, there were no revisions in the TSA group and three revisions in the hemiarthroplasty group for painful glenoid arthritis.

Conclusion

Arthroscopic debridement for glenohumeral arthritis may be indicated in young active patients with mild to moderate disease or in carefully selected patients with advanced disease who do not want prosthetic replacement. Debridement of chondral and labral lesions, loose body removal, and capsular releases are the goals of arthroscopic treatment. Long-term results of arthroscopic debridement are unknown, but in patients with mild disease, short-term results are encouraging. Biologic resurfacing of the glenoid alone, or in combination with hemiarthroplasty, may provide a reasonable option in the young patient with glenohumeral arthritis. Total shoulder arthroplasty, however, remains the gold standard for treatment of end-stage glenohumeral osteoarthritis.

SUGGESTED READINGS

Brislin KJ, Savoie FH III, Field LD, et al. Surgical treatment for glenohumeral arthritis in the young patient. *Tech Shoulder Elbow Surg.* 2004;5:165–169.

Burkhead WZ, Hutton KS. Biologic resurfacing of the glenoid with hemiarthroplasty of the shoulder. *J Shoulder Elbow Surg.* 1995;4:263–270.

Cameron BD, Galatz LM, Ramsey ML, et al. Non-prosthetic management of grade IV osteochondral lesions of the glenohumeral joint. *J Shoulder Elbow Surg.* 2002;11:25–32.

Cofield RH. Shoulder arthrodesis and resection arthroplasty of the shoulder. *Instr Course Lect.* 1985;34:268–277.

Gartsman GM, Roddey TS, Hammerman SM. Shoulder arthroplasty with or without resurfacing of the glenoid in patients who have osteoarthritis. *J Bone Joint Surg.* 2000;82:26–34.

Nowinski RJ, Burkhead WZ Jr. Hemiarthroplasty with biologic glenoid resurfacing: 5–13 year outcomes. 70th Annual Meeting, New Orleans, LA, February 5–9, 2003.

Ogilvie-Harris DJ, Wiley AM. Arthroscopic surgery of the shoulder: a general appraisal. *J Bone Joint Surg.* 1986;68B:201–207.

Weinstein DM, Bucchieri JS, Pollock RG, et al. Arthroscopic debridement of the shoulder for osteoarthritis. *Arthroscopy.* 2000;16:471–476.

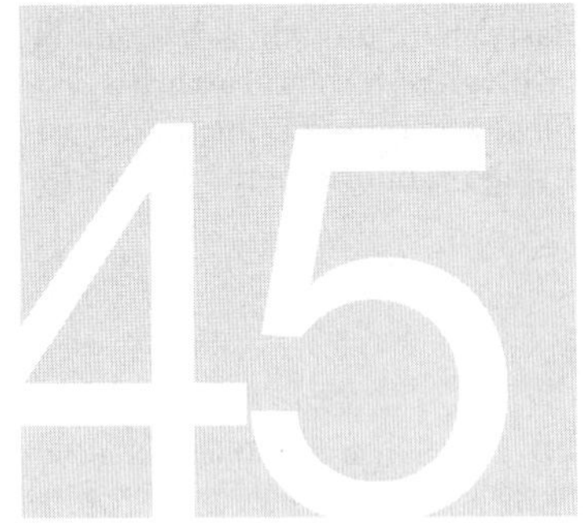

ROTATOR CUFF TEAR ARTHROPATHY

GREGORY P. NICHOLSON

Rotator cuff–deficient shoulders with degenerative joint disease are a treatment challenge. Most patients will present primarily because of shoulder pain. Shoulder function can be variable even with significant chronic rotator cuff deficiency. The arthritic condition of the shoulder owing to a chronic rotator cuff tear has been termed "cuff tear arthropathy." This is characterized clinically by pain and poor active motion but with near-normal passive motion. It is most common in women older than the age of 62 years. Many patients are unaware of the condition until the onset of pain. Operative intervention presents a challenge because of the lack of rotator cuff and the degenerative changes present.

PATHOGENESIS

Etiology

Cuff tear arthropathy (CTA) is an age-related disease. Rotator cuff fiber failure occurs as a result of degenerative processes. This occurs over a period of time. The body adapts as the humeral head elevates through the defect in the rotator cuff and contacts the acromion. The coracoacromial (CA) arch becomes the new fulcrum for the humeral head. Osseous adaptive changes on the humeral head occur with rounding off of the greater tuberosity. The acromion becomes concave, and a new acromiohumeral articulation forms. The patient may have surprisingly little pain, good function, and not know of the condition. The nonphysiologic contact of the humeral head on the acromion and superior glenoid can lead to repeated cartilage and osseous wear with fluid production. Pain and crepitus and loss of function can occur. With further bony erosion and progressive cuff damage, shoulder function may deteriorate.

A seemingly minor trauma can precipitate symptoms in the shoulder. Extension of the pre-existing rotator cuff tear can disrupt the balance of the shoulder that has developed. This can lead to significant pain and loss of function. The degenerative condition was present, but the trauma exposed the vulnerability of the shoulder.

Epidemiology

It is unknown how many patients with rotator cuff tears progress into cuff deficiency and arthropathy. MRI, ultrasound, and cadaver studies have reported rotator cuff tears in the elderly population to be more prevalent with each decade. Some report the presence of rotator cuff tears in 50% of the population older than 70 years of age. Most of these are asymptomatic. There are some estimates that 4% to 5% of patients with rotator cuff tears may progress to a symptomatic CTA from a degenerative cuff tear that is irreparable. Certainly most rotator cuff tears will not progress to a CTA clinical picture. In most series most patients with CTA are women older than 62 years of age. Thus it is a disease that is most prevalent in the seventh and eighth decade of life.

Pathophysiology

Because of the muscle imbalance and superior elevation of the humeral head, and loss of cuff function, there is a progressive degeneration of both rotator cuff substance and bone structure from the humeral head and acromion. The acromion becomes sclerotic and concave. The greater tuberosity becomes rounded off. There is an "acetabularization" of the acromion and a "femoralization" of the humeral head. The superior glenoid also is subjected to increased force from the elevated humeral head. The subacromial bursa becomes thickened and fibrotic. The arthropathic process creates an environment of fluid production, enzyme production, and further degenerative changes.

There are no classification schemes with which to grade the severity of the functional loss, pain, or radiographic changes. There are no studies to correlate the severity of radiographic changes with shoulder function or pain. This makes it difficult to communicate about disease severity, treatment options, and success or failure.

DIAGNOSIS

Physical Examination and History

Clinical Features

The patient history is important. History of previous surgery around the shoulder, especially earlier attempts at rotator cuff repair with coracoacromial arch violation, is important to know. A history of trauma such as previous falls, dislocations, or fractures needs to be known. History of inflammatory arthritis, previous infections, gout, and the number of previous steroid injections is important to document. Also the type of medication the patient is on, especially antimetabolites or corticosteroids, is extremely important to document.

Patients will typically present with a progressive loss of motion and strength, with increasing pain. Night pain is common. The ability to use the hand away from the body can be compromised. The patient will have an internal rotation drop sign as the forearm falls into internal rotation when trying to reach or hold out in a handshake-type position. The other presentation will be a minor trauma that results in a significant amount of pain and shoulder dysfunction. The relatively small insult exposes the vulnerability of the affected shoulder.

Physical examination will typically reveal poor active motion and near-normal passive motion (Table 45-1). Visual inspection from behind the patient will reveal degrees of atrophy of the supraspinatus and infraspinatus. There may be a fluid-filled appearance under the deltoid owing to excessive fluid production. Strength testing will elicit weakness in external rotation. Crepitus with both active and passive motion may be noted. All of these findings may be seen with surprisingly little pain. The patients who have very poor active elevation ability (<45 degrees), using mostly a shoulder shrug, and very little if any pain, are termed "pseudoparalytic." This is a functionally disabling condition. Anterior superior instability with the humeral head riding out from underneath the coracoacromial arch with attempted elevation is important to note.

Radiologic Features

Imaging studies with plain x-ray views are essential (Fig. 45-1). The views obtained should be a true anteroposterior (AP) of the glenohumeral joint, an axillary view, and a scapular Y view (Table 45-2). In patients without advanced osseous changes, a CT scan or MRI scan can be considered. This will give a quantitative and qualitative impression of the size and location of the rotator cuff tear and, more important, the status of the rotator cuff muscle bellies. These studies can provide the surgeon with an assessment for the reparability of a rotator cuff tear. They can also provide qualitative information about the status of the muscle bellies of the cuff muscles. Most patients with advanced rotator cuff tear arthropathy with adaptive and degenerative changes seen on plain films will not require advanced imaging studies such as CT scan or MRI, however.

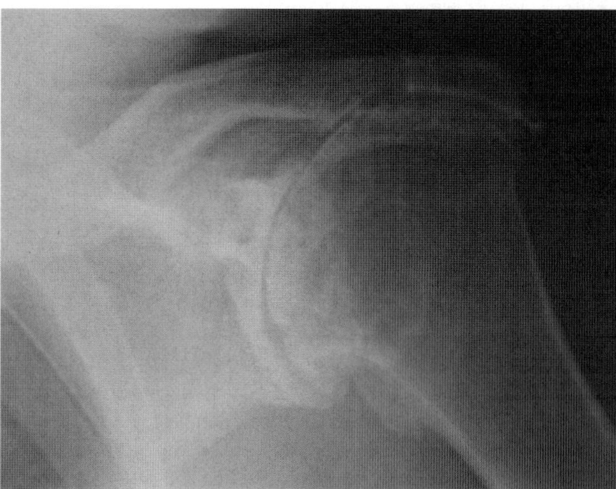

Figure 45-1 Anteroposterior radiograph of a left shoulder with characteristic cuff tear arthropathy changes: humeral head elevation, adaptive changes on the acromion, and greater tuberosity. There are degenerative joint changes in the glenohumeral joint.

Radiographically there can be seen a pattern of more superior wear with significant adaptive changes and concavity of the acromion. There can be more of a centralized wear pattern between the humeral head and significant loss of glenoid bone stock. There can also be seen a more massive destructive arthropathy between the humeral head, glenoid, and acromion. It is unclear if these are three different points on the time line of degeneration, or if the shoulder responds differently with differing degenerative patterns to the chronic cuff deficiency. There has been no validated staging or classification of these radiographic changes or of clinical function. To make matters more confusing, not every shoulder with an irreparable rotator cuff tear goes on to painful, symptomatic cuff tear arthropathy.

TABLE 45-1 CLINICAL FEATURES OF CUFF TEAR ARTHROPATHY
Poor active elevation
Near-normal passive elevation
Pain
Crepitus from coracoacromial arch
Fluid under deltoid

TABLE 45-2 RADIOGRAPHIC FEATURES OF CUFF TEAR ARTHROPATHY
Humeral head elevation (acromiohumeral narrowing)
Concavity of acromion ("acetabulization")
Rounding off of greater tuberosity ("femoralization")
Glenohumeral wear (usually superior glenoid wear)
Later stages: collapse of humeral head congruity

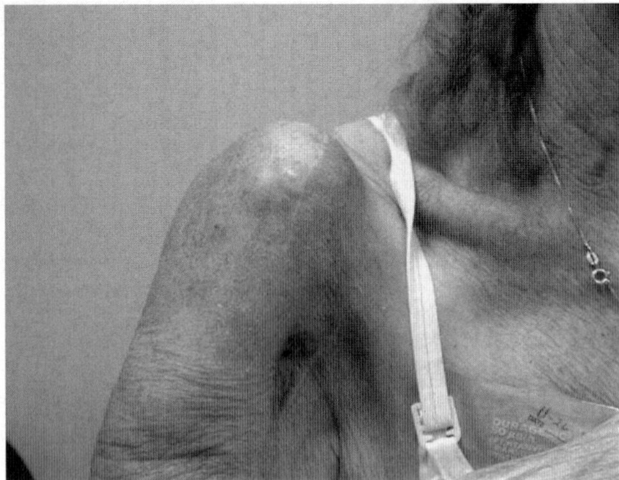

Figure 45-2 This patient exhibits anterosuperior instability with attempted active elevation. There was previous rotator cuff repair failure with coracoacromial arch violation. Hemiarthroplasty will not correct the anterosuperior instability. A reverse shoulder replacement is a better option.

Differential Diagnosis

With the characteristic features of end-stage CTA, it is not hard to make the diagnosis based on history, physical exam, and radiologic findings. Other conditions also need to be considered. The cause of the rotator cuff deficiency leading to the arthritis and shoulder dysfunction is important to know. Other diagnostic possibilities include rheumatoid arthritis, neuropathic arthropathy, septic arthritis, and failed rotator cuff repair with loss of coracoacromial arch containment. Rheumatoid arthritis will usually have multiple joint involvement. Neuropathic arthropathy is most commonly caused by syringomyelia. An MRI of the cervical spine will aid in the diagnosis. Rotator cuff repair failure with anterosuperior instability will be apparent by history of previous surgery, physical exam, and MRI. The patients with multiple failed rotator cuff repair will manifest anterosuperior instability with attempted elevation (Fig. 45-2). The degenerative changes on the humerus, acromion, and glenoid will not be as advanced as those seen with CTA. Function is poor and pain is significant in this population with cuff deficiency and joint injury.

Thus the workup for cuff deficiency with arthritis involves history, physical examination, standard radiographs, blood work to rule out infection or rheumatoid arthritis, and routine blood work. Joint aspiration is rarely indicated unless septic arthritis is suspected.

TREATMENT

Nonoperative

Conservative management would include a corticosteroid injection to decrease the inflammation and fluid production and to control the pain and allow the patient to rehabilitate. Physical therapy should focus on the structures that are left, which are typically some of the external rotators, some of the internal rotators, and the anterior deltoid. These exercises can be done at home. They should be done without pain, and isometrics and closed chain technique is easiest in the elderly population. This can help patients gain another 5, 10, or 15 degrees of motion and stability. This can be a significant gain for these patients with regard to using the hand away from the body. If pain relief can be maintained, patients can be quite satisfied with these gains. Realistic expectations for active motion, strength, and function should be emphasized to the patient.

Operative Treatment

The primary indication for surgical intervention is pain relief. As stated earlier, the active forward elevation and shoulder function ability of patients in this disease process can be somewhat variable. Some patients have almost no pain but extremely poor function with the inability to actively elevate above the horizontal or even use the hand away from the body at waist height. This patient is much more of a challenge because they have a painless pseudoparalysis of the shoulder. Hemiarthroplasty will not restore active elevation ability in a patient who has pseudoparalysis. Any surgery on cuff tear arthropathy is a limited-goals procedure for pain relief and improved function of the shoulder for activities of daily living. The ability to actively elevate above the horizontal will be unpredictable.

For the patient who has pain that is unresponsive to conservative management and has had no previous coracoacromial arch surgery, and who has active elevation ability of 60 degrees or better, the best treatment option for rotator cuff tear arthropathy seems to be hemiarthroplasty. There is no advantage to total shoulder arthroplasty with resurfacing of the glenoid in an unconstrained shoulder design. Bipolar shoulder hemiarthroplasty has poorer active elevation ability than hemiarthroplasty. Arthrodesis is poorly tolerated in the elderly population and is not recommended.

Hemiarthroplasty has shown the ability to predictably relieve pain in cuff tear arthropathy. Functional ability, specifically active elevation, has been less predictable, however. At best, patients and surgeons should expect active elevation on the average to be approximately 90 degrees. With longer follow-up, hemiarthroplasty has shown progressive bone changes in the acromion and glenoid. These changes have correlated with increasing pain and decreasing function. It is unclear why some patients do better than others with regard to active elevation and shoulder function. No prognostic factor has been identified to correlate with a better functional result. However, it is quite clear that poorer results are associated with those patients who had prior rotator cuff surgery and coracoacromial arch violation. If there has been coracoacromial arch violation, hemiarthroplasty is not indicated, as anterosuperior instability will result.

Reverse shoulder arthroplasty was approved for use in the United States in 2004. It had been used in Europe for >8 years. The reverse shoulder arthroplasty is indicated for cuff deficiency and joint injury when no other satisfactory option is available (Table 45-3). Specific indications

TABLE 45-3 INDICATION FOR REVERSE SHOULDER ARTHROPLASTY

Irreparable cuff deficiency
Pain
Poor active elevation (<60 degrees)
Anterosuperior instability or coracoacromial arch violation
Preferably age >65
Adequate glenoid bone stock
Functioning deltoid
No other satisfactory option exists

include CTA with a pseudoparalysis clinical picture. If there is extremely poor active elevation, hemiarthroplasty will not predictably restore elevation ability. If there has been previous coracoacromial arch violation or there is anterosuperior instability of the humeral head, then reverse is a better option. If there is a failed hemiarthroplasty for CTA or fracture, then reverse is a better option. In age-matched populations with CTA and no previous surgery, the reverse arthroplasty achieved an average of 40 degrees greater active forward elevation compared with hemiarthroplasty. The reverse provides for the potential for better active elevation ability. However, both internal and external rotation can be limited owing to the constraint of the reverse design.

Reverse shoulder arthroplasty is indicated for those patients who have had multiple failed rotator cuff repair attempts with violation of the coracoacromial arch and present with pain, poor function, and anterior superior instability. It should also be considered in those patients with pseudoparalysis and extremely poor active motion. Those patients with an extremely thin acromion or an acromial insufficiency fracture should also be considered candidates for reverse shoulder arthroplasty.

Operative Technique

The operative technique for arthroplasty in cuff tear arthropathy begins with a thorough preoperative evaluation. The vast majorities of these patients are elderly, older than 62 years of age, and have comorbidities. Positioning is important. The patient should be moved to the lateral edge of the operating room table. The operative arm should be able to be brought off the side of the table for gentle extension, external rotation, and adduction to dislocate the humeral head forward. The head and neck need to be supported. The shoulder and arm are draped free for maximum flexibility and position.

A deltopectoral approach is used so as not to violate the anterior deltoid. The cephalic vein can be taken laterally with the deltoid or medially with the pectoralis major according to the surgeon's preference. Extensive bursal material will be encountered under the deltoid and under the clavipectoral fascia lateral to the strap muscles off the coracoid. This material should be debrided. The subscapularis should be incised off the lesser tuberosity. The subscapularis should be tagged with sutures and reflected medially.

At this point, the humeral head is very gently dislocated. These patients are typically females older than 65 years of age with osteopenic bone. Great care should be taken to gently distract the arm and put a flat retractor behind the humeral head; with extension, adduction, and external rotation the humeral head is brought forward. The humeral head should be osteotomized with an oscillating saw. Careful reaming of the humeral canal should be performed owing to osteopenic bone. In the vast majority of these cases, the humeral stem is cemented into place. Also, cement will stabilize the proximal aspect of the humerus and support sutures that are placed through the anterior anatomic neck for subscapularis reattachment.

Humeral prosthetic head size and position are chosen. General guidelines can be thought of as choosing a humeral head size that will fill the existing coracoacromial arch (Fig. 45-3). It is helpful to have a prosthetic head that allows approximately 50% of posterior translation on the glenoid. With the arm in approximately 70 degrees of abduction, at least 40 degrees of internal rotation of the arm should occur.

The subscapularis is repaired to the lesser tuberosity after relocation of the new prosthesis in the joint. A drain may or may not be used underneath the deltoid. In many patients, because of the amount of bursal material and fluid production that needed to be debrided, there can be significant dead space. A drain for 24 hours may prevent a collection of a hematoma. The deltopectoral interval is then

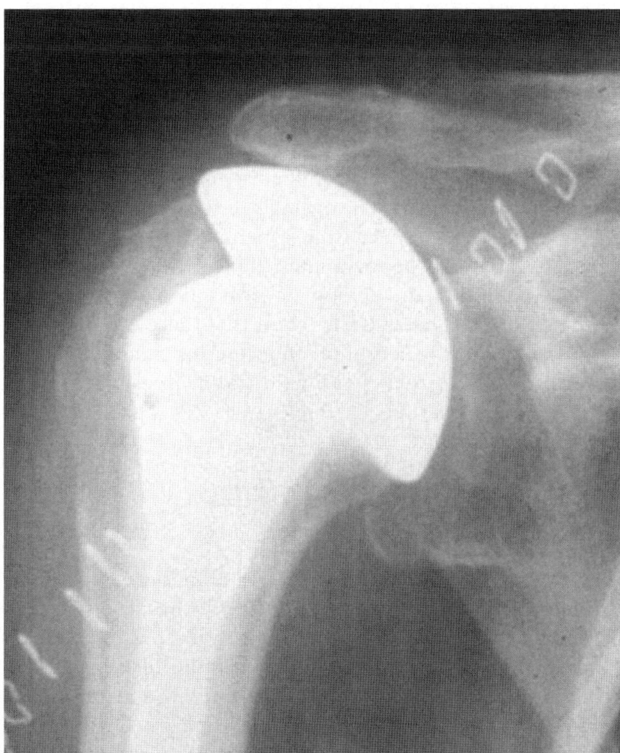

Figure 45-3 Hemiarthroplasty for cuff tear arthropathy. Note that the prosthetic head size fills the arch of the upper glenoid and coracoacromial arch without overstuffing the joint.

tacked closed with absorbable sutures. The subcutaneous tissue is closed with absorbable sutures and then the skin closed by surgeon preference. A supportive sling and swathe device can be applied.

Aftercare

Patients after hemiarthroplasty for cuff tear arthropathy should be supported in a sling. Passive range of motion should begin on the first postoperative day with pendulum exercises. Passive external rotation with a limit of 30 degrees, passive forward elevation with a limit of approximately 90 degrees, and pulley exercises should be instituted. The patient is encouraged to use the hand, wrist, and elbow for activities of daily living within the sling. After 1 month, the sling can be discontinued and active assisted range of motion can begin. Isometric strengthening for the muscle groups that are still workable are instituted. These include the external rotators, all three heads of the deltoid, and the scapular rotators. At the end of 2 months, light resistive exercises with resistive exercise bands should be instituted for the external rotators, the internal rotators, and all three heads of the deltoid. Patients should be informed both preoperatively and postoperatively that this will be a prolonged and slow rehabilitation. They will not reach their best or maximum potential for approximately 6 months after the operation.

Results to be Expected from Hemiarthroplasty for Cuff Tear Arthropathy

Multiple studies have documented the predictable pain relief that hemiarthroplasty can provide to patients who have unremitting pain from the degenerative changes of arthritis with cuff deficiency. This has also been shown to be the most consistent when there have not been previous attempts at rotator cuff repair or acromioplasty/coracoacromial arch violation type surgery. The average active forward elevation that patients can expect from a hemiarthroplasty for cuff tear arthropathy is approximately 90 degrees. Most studies have 2-year follow-up, but longer-term follow-up studies are being reported. These studies show that there is progressive bony erosion of the acromion and superior glenoid and that these erosions correlate with pain and decreasing function over the longer periods of time.

Operative Technique for Reverse Shoulder Arthroplasty

The operative technique for reverse shoulder arthroplasty is through the deltopectoral approach. It has also been described through the superior approach by incising the deltoid off the anterior acromion and repairing the deltoid. The technical considerations are to obtain exposure to the glenoid that is not needed in hemiarthroplasty. The humeral head is resected, and the glenoid component is placed in the inferior aspect of the glenoid. The inferior capsule needs to be elevated off the glenoid rim and the glenoid component placed inferiorly. The component should be placed at neutral or at best a slight inferior tilt. These technical tips can avoid scapular notching inferiorly. The humeral component is placed in approximately 10 degrees of retroversion. The myofascial sleeve tension should allow the humeral component to reduce under the glenoid with a 1- to 2-mm push-pull action. The strap muscles will be under tension. The humerus should be cemented.

Aftercare for the reverse is similar to the hemiarthroplasty; however, the author rarely has patients do formal therapy after a reverse shoulder arthroplasty. A sling is used for 3 to 4 weeks. Patients are allowed to do activities of daily living in the sling immediately. Closed chain exercises for the anterior deltoid and isometrics for external and internal rotation are begun. The reverse will allow the scapula to function more efficiently, and patients progress very well on their own with surgeon direction.

In a comparison study with follow-up >3 years follow-up, patients with no prior shoulder surgery and CTA were treated either with hemiarthroplasty or reverse shoulder arthroplasty. The patients with reverse shoulder arthroplasty had 40 degrees greater active forward elevation for an average of 138 degrees, and the Constant score was 20 points higher than for those patients with hemiarthroplasty. There were no cases of glenoid loosening requiring revision. The hemiarthroplasties had more than one third of the cases with progressive bone erosion in the superior glenoid and acromion with increasing pain.

Complications

Complications of hemiarthroplasty for cuff deficiency begin with the fact that these are elderly patients and have

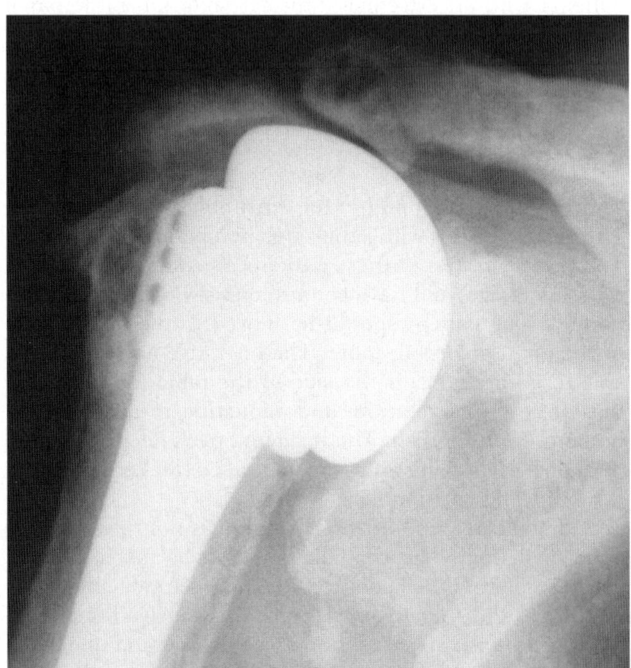

Figure 45-4 Hemiarthroplasty with progressive superior glenoid erosion. Increasing pain and decreasing function were noted by the patient.

comorbidities. Medical problems can be exacerbated by surgery in the elderly. The unpredictable function results, especially with regard to strength and active forward elevation, make it imperative that a discussion occurs with the patient to avoid unrealistic expectations. One of the complications that has recently been seen after 4- to 5-year follow-up is the bone erosion that is progressive at the superior glenoid and the undersurface of the acromion that correlates with increasing pain and decreasing function (Fig.45- 4).

Complications of the reverse arthroplasty include dislocation, hematoma formation, infection, implant failure, and scapular notching inferior to the glenoid component. The complication rate is higher than with hemiarthroplasty, but these complications do not seem to affect the results of the operation. Glenoid loosening has been rare, but is a concern with longer-term follow-up.

SUMMARY

Cuff tear arthroplasty is a disabling condition of the shoulder found in elderly patients. It is variable in its presentation with regard to the extent of degenerative osseous change in the glenoid, humeral head, and acromion. It is variable in its presentation with regard to preoperative active elevation ability and pain level. The overriding indication for operative intervention in cuff tear arthropathy is pain relief.

SUGGESTED READINGS

Boulahia A, Edwards TB, Walch G, et al. Early results of a reverse design prosthesis in the treatment of arthritis of the shoulder in elderly patients with a large rotator cuff tear. *Orthopedics*. 2002;25:129–133.

Favard L, Lautmann S, Sirveaux F, et al. Hemiarthroplasty versus reverse arthroplasty in the treatment of osteoarthritis with massive rotator cuff tear. In: Walch G, Boileau P, Mole D, eds. *2000 Shoulder Prostheses . . . Two to Ten Year Follow-up*. Montpelier, France: Sauramps Medical; 2001:261–268.

Neer CS II, Craig EV, Fukuda H. Cuff-tear arthropathy. *J Bone Joint Surg*. 1983;65A:1232–1244.

Pollock RG, Deliz ED, McIlveen SJ, et al. Prosthetic replacement in rotator cuff-deficient shoulders. *J Shoulder Elbow Surg*. 1992;1:173–186.

Sanchez-Sotelo J, Cofield RH, Rowland CM. Shoulder hemiarthroplasty for glenohumeral arthritis associated with severe rotator cuff deficiency. *J Bone Joint Surg*. 2001;83A:1814–1822.

Werner CML, Steinmann PA, Gilbart M, et al. Treatment of painful pseudoparesis due to irreparable rotator cuff dysfunction with the Delta III reverse-ball-and-socket total shoulder prosthesis. *J Bone Joint Surg*. 2005;87A:1776–1786.

Zuckerman JD, Scott AJ, Gallagher MA. Hemiarthroplasty for cuff tear arthropathy. *J Shoulder Elbow Surg*. 2000;9:169–172.

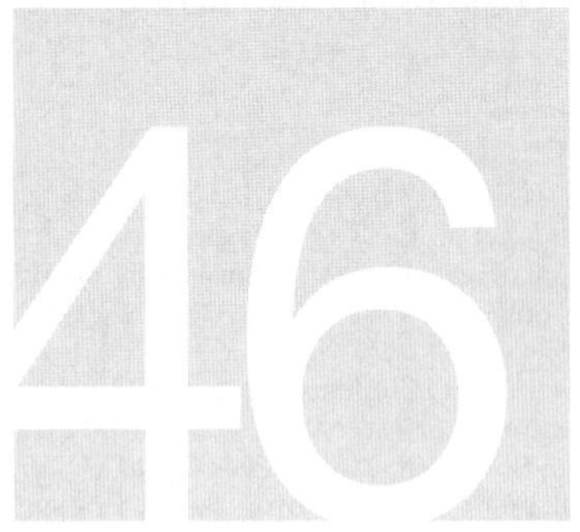

FROZEN SHOULDER

MICHELE T. GLASGOW

Frozen shoulder is defined as "a condition characterized by functional restriction of both active and passive motion." Zuckerman et al. further classified frozen shoulder into primary and secondary groups. Primary frozen shoulder was considered idiopathic. Secondary frozen shoulder was divided into intrinsic, extrinsic, and systemic subtypes (Table 46-1). More specific, quantitative definitions have been sought. Diagnostic criteria have included duration of symptoms, loss of motion, and radiographic evaluation. Significant variability in the diagnostic criteria has made treatment and outcome studies difficult to compare (Table 46-2).

PATHOGENESIS

Etiology

Primary, or idiopathic, frozen shoulder has by definition no clear cause. There are, at best, associations that link underlying disease processes to loss of soft tissue compliance. A cellular basis for disease has been speculated. Deficiencies in cellular immunity, identified in some studies, have been thought to result in an autoimmune disease resulting in capsular contracture. However, reports have not been consistent among investigators, and this proposed cause remains controversial.

Chromosomal abnormalities have been suggested, and shoulder capsule tissue culture analysis has demonstrated trisomy seven and eight in seven patients with frozen shoulder. Trisomy seven has been identified in the tissue of the Dupuytren contracture suggesting a similar common pathway. In addition, cellular mechanisms related to metalloproteinases, enzymes that control collagen remodeling, and cytokines have been implicated.

Secondary frozen shoulder may be caused by surgery, fracture, nonsurgical soft tissue trauma such as rotator cuff tear or contusion, tendonitis, and arthritis. These are considered causes of secondary frozen shoulder that are intrinsic to the shoulder joint itself. Extrinsic conditions may occur with secondary frozen shoulder. These include neurologic injuries from head trauma, brain surgery or cerebrovascular accident, cervical radiculitis, brachial plexopathy, thoracic outlet syndrome, and peripheral nerve palsy. Antiepileptic treatment with phenobarbitone has been associated with frozen shoulder. Other associated conditions include cardiac disease and cardiac surgery, thoracic tumors such as bronchogenic carcinoma and Pancoast tumor. Desmoid tumors of the shoulder girdle presenting as frozen shoulder have been recently reported. Systemic disease may also be associated with secondary frozen shoulder. These diseases include diabetes, hypothyroidism, hyperthyroidism, polymyalgia rheumatica, myositis, and many other systemic illnesses.

Systemic diseases may stimulate cellular changes within the shoulder joint capsule. Advanced glycosylation end products (AGEs) accumulate in the basement membranes of diabetics. The accumulation of AGEs results in irreversible cross-links between adjacent protein molecules. This appears related to acquired defects in vascular compliance in diabetics and may reflect a common pathway that leads to arthrofibrosis in the diabetic population. Association of frozen shoulder with diabetes, thyroid disease (both hypothyroidism and hyperthyroidism), hyperlipidemia, and other systemic illnesses is clearly seen. The exact mechanism(s) that lead to capsular restriction have yet to be delineated definitively.

Epidemiology

Frozen shoulder is noted to have a prevalence of 2% to 5% in the general population. It is generally considered more common in women than men, but this is not consistent across all studies. The age presentation is most commonly 40 to 60 years. However, it may occur earlier in long-standing insulin-dependent diabetics. Incidence of frozen shoulder in diabetics has been reported from 10% to as high as 35%. Diabetics with frozen shoulder are more likely to have additional organ involvement.

Recurrence in the same shoulder and concurrent bilateral disease are unusual in the general population, but may occur in diabetics. Both shoulders may be affected in 6% to 34% of patients across multiple studies. Diabetics appear to be more likely to develop bilateral stiffness ($\leq$40%).

TABLE 46-1 PRIMARY AND SECONDARY FROZEN SHOULDER

Primary frozen shoulder
 Idiopathic

Secondary frozen shoulder
 Intrinsic: Shoulder fracture, tendonitis, rotator cuff tear, degenerative joint disease
 Extrinsic: Neurologic—radiculopathy, head trauma, complex regional pain syndrome, Parkinson, cardiovascular accident, humeral fractures
 Systemic: Diabetes, thyroid disease, myositis/polymyalgia rheumatica

Pathophysiology

Pathophysiology is a final end pathway of fibrosis and decreased capsular compliance. Loss of external rotation with associated scarring and contracture of the rotator interval capsule, coracohumeral, and superior glenohumeral ligaments is pathognomic of frozen shoulder.

Idiopathic frozen shoulder is defined in three phases. These phases are the following:

- The initial phase ("freezing phase") is marked by insidious onset of pain of increasing severity. This lasts from a few weeks up to 9 months. It is associated with the loss of active and passive motion. Arthroscopy and histology studies demonstrate acute synovitis (Fig. 46-1).
- The second phase ("frozen phase") is associated with less pain. The hallmark of this phase is global shoulder stiffness. Comfort for activities of daily living is achieved within the patient's limited range. The duration of this phase may be 3 to ≥12 months. Pathologic specimens demonstrate extensive fibrosis with high cellular populations of fibroblasts and myofibroblasts.
- The *final phase* ("thawing phase") is characterized by return of motion toward normal over a period of 5 to 26 months on average. This phase, however, has been cited in the literature to extend as far as 8 to 10 years following the onset of symptoms. Outcome studies regarding the natural history of the thawing phase are clouded by lack of consistent study inclusion criteria. Methodology frequently has been retrospective and without control groups. Patient numbers have generally been small, and frequently studies have included mixed treatments and causes. Despite this, reports suggest persistent mild pain and/or stiffness in ≤50% of patients. At mean follow-up, Binder, Bulgen and colleagues reported little functional impairment in 40 out of an initial study group of 42 patients. However, 45% of patients continued to have pain and/or restricted range of motion.

TABLE 46-2 CLINICAL DIAGNOSIS OF FROZEN SHOULDER

1. **Duration of symptoms:** 3 weeks to >3 months
2. **Range of motion** (as percentage of normal side): >50% loss of passive external rotation or abduction
3. **Range of motion** (absolute restriction): limitation of 30 degrees or more in two or more planes
4. **Normal radiographs** (idiopathic frozen shoulder)

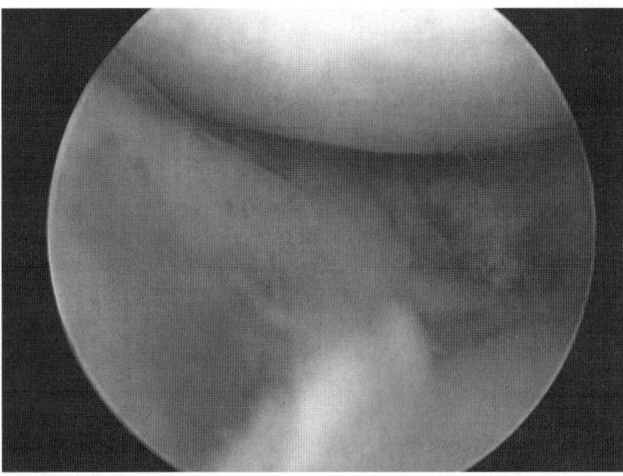

Figure 46-1 Joint synovitis encountered at arthroscopy.

DIAGNOSIS

History

Idiopathic frozen shoulder is characterized by three phases of clinical presentation. The physician is challenged to identify the stage and evaluate the patient for other causes or associated disease processes. Concurrent bilateral involvement is relatively uncommon. Initial presentation of concurrent bilateral frozen shoulder may suggest systemic disease. It is incumbent on the clinician at all stages to evaluate for possible associated conditions. This necessitates a careful and thorough general medical history.

Idiopathic frozen shoulder in the initial phase is characterized by pain without history of significant trauma. Aching unrelieved by rest and worsening at night is frequent. Loss of range of motion is pathognomic. The patient may present with protective posturing of the arm in an adducted internally rotated position against the body. The physical examination is generally notable for severe pain with range of motion. X-ray films taken at this time are generally negative, though there may be slight osteopenia.

In phase II (frozen phase) the patient reports less pain. Significant motion restriction is noted with pain generally at the extremes of available motion. There is functional restriction of activities of daily living. Night pain remains common.

Phase III (thawing phase) is characterized by variable activity limitations associated with loss of range of motion. Generally over the course of observation, both range of motion and night pain demonstrate gradual improvement. Despite improvement, studies suggest that motion remains limited relative to the contralateral normal extremity in ≥50% of patients.

Physical Examination

Global assessment of the neck and bilateral shoulder complexes as well as the upper extremity is essential. Exam of the shoulder should include the following:

- Inspection and palpation of the neck and shoulder to include both the glenohumeral and scapulothoracic articulations
- Cervical spine range of motion with the Spurling test
- Assessment of range of motion according to the American Shoulder and Elbow Surgeons (ASES) standard format. Motion arcs of the affected and unaffected shoulder are recorded for the following:
  - Forward elevation in the sagittal plane
  - External rotation at the side (ERS)
  - External rotation at 90 degrees of coronal abduction if possible (ERA)
  - Internal rotation at 90 degrees of coronal abduction if possible (IRA)
  - Cross-body adduction measuring the difference from the antecubital fossa to the opposite shoulder (XBA)
  - Internal rotation/extension up the back (IRB)
- Strength is recorded for forward elevation, abduction, and external and internal rotation. Ancillary strength testing may include belly press. The lift-off test may be difficult to assess if significant posterior capsular contracture and/or pain does not allow adequate glenohumeral internal rotation. Additional active tests may include the supraspinatus stress test and the Whipple test.

  A distal upper extremity exam should be performed to assess range of motion and strength. This will assist in evaluating for secondary neurologic conditions (i.e., cervical radiculopathy, complex regional pain syndrome, brachial plexopathy, and others).

Radiography

Plain Radiography

Anterior-posterior views are suggested in internal and external rotation. Outlet and true axillary views complete the shoulder series. Radiographs are inspected for fracture, tumor, calcific tendonitis, arthritis, and subacromial spurring.

Arthrography

Presently this is not commonly used. Arthrographic findings have failed to show correlations with clinical outcome.

MRI With or Without Intra-Articular Contrast

MRI imaging may be useful in the evaluation of the rotator cuff and bony anatomy in a patient with weakness or unusual presentation. Common findings in frozen shoulder are thickening of the coracohumeral ligament and rotator interval capsule. Synovitic abnormalities at the top of the subscapularis tendon and volume loss at the axillary recess are noted.

Ancillary Diagnostic Testing

Blood Studies

Generally, blood work is not needed for the evaluation and treatment of frozen shoulder. The clinician may elect to order selective tests if an underlying systemic disease or infection is suspected.

Electromyography

Testing is indicated in selected cases where neurogenic causes of shoulder motion loss are suspected.

TREATMENT

Conservative, Nonsurgical Measures

Conservative, nonsurgical measures have been demonstrated to be successful.

Physical Therapy

Gentle, firm stretching has been reportedly effective in the relief of pain and restoration of motion in 90% of patients. Physical therapy may be done at home with monthly visits to the therapist and surgeon, or more extensive formal evaluation and treatment may be performed as indicated. Basic exercises include supine active assisted forward elevation, supine external rotation with a stick, cross-body adduction, and standing towel exercises for internal rotation up the back. Multiple repetitions are performed and held for firm end field stretch without pain. The hallmark of stretching in frozen shoulder is repetition of exercises multiple times throughout the day. Prospective studies suggest "supervised neglect," described as supportive therapy and exercises within the pain limit, produced superior 24-month outcome compared with vigorous stretching. Techniques of translational manipulations or glides may also be used by the therapist. Range of motion and visual analog pain scores have been noted to improve with this technique using regional anesthesia.

Anti-Inflammatories and Analgesics

Anti-inflammatories and analgesics have been demonstrated to assist with pain relief. Patients who used analgesics and exercise were shown to have greater improvement than with exercise alone. Short-course oral prednisolone was shown to have short-term benefit over placebo with regard to pain and motion at 3-week follow-up. Benefits compared with placebo were not maintained beyond 6 weeks.

Injections

Literature with regard to the use of injection is controversial. Results of intra-articular injections are difficult to interpret because they are frequently associated with other treatment modalities. In patients with painful stiffness, a 50% improvement in pain scores associated with injection has been reported. Bulgen et al. reported early improvement in pain and range of motion with no long-term advantage in comparing patients receiving intra-articular injection with an untreated control group. Intra-articular glucocorticoid injection with and without joint distension was compared prospectively. Intra-articular lidocaine (19 mL volume) and 20 mg of triamcinolone hexacetonide was compared with triamcinolone hexacetonide alone. Injection was confirmed by ultrasound and repeated with an end point of a maximum of six weekly injections or no symptoms. Pain measured by visual analog scale was no different between groups, but the distension group showed improvement in range of motion. Comparison with normal controls or opposite shoulder evaluation was not provided.

Despite controversy, data suggest that intraarticular glucocorticoid injection may assist in pain relief in frozen shoulder. Thus, injection may facilitate early rehabilitation.

Operative Treatment

Manipulation Under Anesthesia

Indications for manipulations under anesthesia include 3 months of worsening symptoms despite compliance with home exercise or failure to improve motion over 6 months of treatment. Loew et al. have reported on 30 consecutive patients with primary frozen shoulder resistant to analgesics and therapy for 6 months. They noted excellent restoration of range of motion with manipulation. Manipulation was performed gently following their standard protocol. This included the following:

- General anesthesia in a supine position
- Measurement of premanipulation range of motion
- Manipulation with the humerus held close to the axilla to diminish lever arm effect
- Forward elevation and internal rotation with light traction
- Cross-body adduction to stress and release the posterior capsular contracture
- External rotation stretch from neutral (ERS)
- External rotation at 90 degrees of scapular abduction

Postmanipulation arthroscopy performed by Loew et al. demonstrated capsular ruptures anteriorly (24 of 30), posteriorly (16 of 30), and superiorly (11 of 30). Four patients had acute superior labral anterior posterior (SLAP) tears. Four patients had anterior labral detachments; one of which was osteochondral. Three patients had partial tears of the subscapularis tendon, and two had middle glenohumeral ligament tears.

Manipulation may also be done under regional anesthesia or after local anesthetic intra-articular distension. Harryman and Lazarus describe a protocol for manipulation under anesthesia. Their protocol is as follows:

- Sagittal plane elevation with observation for crepitant lysis of scar
- Cross-body adduction
- Abducted internal rotation followed by internal rotation with the arm adducted
- Internal rotation up the back if the patient is awake and cooperative
- External rotation in 90 degrees of coronal abduction followed by external rotation after carefully lowering the arm to an adducted position

Postsurgically, the use of regional anesthesia has benefit in that it allows for painless patient cooperation in the instruction and reinforcement of the postsurgical stretching program. Stretches are repeated multiple times daily following hospital discharge with emphasis on achieving forward elevation, rotation, and posterior capsular stretching. Postmanipulation intra-articular injections with steroids may be used to diminish postsurgical inflammation and pain. Injection, however, has not been shown to enhance outcome.

Disadvantages of manipulation under anesthesia include the obvious inability to visualize intra-articular pathology available with arthroscopy. A cumulative 1% complication rate has been reported. Complications include rotator cuff tear, fracture, nerve palsy, and dislocation. Insulin-dependent diabetics have poor outcomes with regard to maintenance of range of motion following manipulation. The overall recurrent stiffness rate is between 5% and 20% including diabetic and nondiabetic patients.

Open Release

Indications for open release include postsurgical stiffness with glenohumeral scarring, muscle contracture, and excessive extra-articular scarring. An open approach is indicated when lengthening of the subscapularis is required following an anterior instability procedure. Resection of spurs and heterotopic bone may also be performed efficiently via an open approach.

A limited deltopectoral exposure or deltoid-splitting incision may be used for release of the rotator interval capsule and coracohumeral ligament. This may be combined with gentle manipulation to restore motion.

Drawbacks of open release include poor accessibility to the posterior capsule from this anterior approach. If it is necessary to release the middle and inferior glenohumeral ligaments, a subscapularis take-down may be necessary. This necessitates restriction of rehabilitation postsurgically to protect the subscapularis repair. Open release followed by manipulation under anesthesia has been shown to improve range of motion and pain relief with mean follow-up approaching 7 years in some studies.

Arthroscopic Release

Arthroscopy allows visualization of the glenohumeral joint. Inflamed synovium may be resected with a shaver and capsular release performed with arthroscopic basket or cautery.

Indications for arthroscopic capsular release include the following:

- Inability to achieve full range of motion with gentle manipulation under anesthesia
- Consideration in insulin-dependent diabetics with resistant contractures
- Patients with significant osteopenia in whom there is a concern of fracture with manipulation
- Postsurgical and posttraumatic stiff shoulder where recurrent fracture or soft tissue injury may occur with manipulation

The technique for arthroscopic release may involve multiple glenohumeral portals. A high posterior portal may be positioned just cephalad to the standard posterior portal. Entry into the joint may be difficult secondary to scarring and contracture. The blunt trocar is advanced into the joint carefully to avoid iatrogenic articular injury. A secondary anterior portal is selected just superior to the rolled board of the subscapularis. This may be localized using a spinal needle from an outside-in technique. The cannula enters the joint slightly laterally along the upper border of the subscapularis.

Diagnostic arthroscopy is performed to record any associated pathology. If the biceps is scarred and immobile, it is tenotomized at the glenoid rim.

Harryman and Lazarus recommend synovectomy followed by posterior capsular resection first. They note that fluid extravasation posteriorly is limited by the infraspinatus muscle. They recommend using arthroscopic basket forceps to spread the muscle off the capsule. A posterior superior followed by direct posterior and posterior inferior release are performed. A rotary shaver is used to resect the edges of the capsular release.

In progressing to the inferior capsule, a 70-degree arthroscope may be used from the front or the arthroscope alternatively may be positioned in the posterior superior portal. An additional posterior portal is positioned approximately 2 cm caudal and 1 cm lateral to the high posterior portal. A spinal needle can be used to localize the best position such that the approach is parallel to the floor of the axillary pouch. The capsule is incised outside the labrum and close to the glenoid. The axillary nerve passes obliquely anteromedial to posterolateral along the inferior margin of the capsule. Authors suggest that an arthroscopic basket forceps be used to spread the extracapsular tissue off the inferior capsule prior to incising the capsule. This is preferred to avoid axillary nerve injury.

Working from the anterior portal, a rotator interval release with attention to the coracohumeral and superior glenohumeral ligament is performed. The anterior superior release is performed above the biceps and labrum. The coracoacromial ligament and conjoined tendon are visualized from the posterior intra-articular arthroscopy portal. Attention is turned to release of the middle glenohumeral ligament (Fig. 46-2) and anterior aspect of the inferior glenohumeral ligament connecting the release inferiorly. Debris may be resected with a motorized shaver. The blades of the shaver are positioned away from the axillary nerve and rotator cuff with judicious use of suction.

Other authors have used bipolar cautery to perform releases. At the inferior pouch, maintaining close apposition

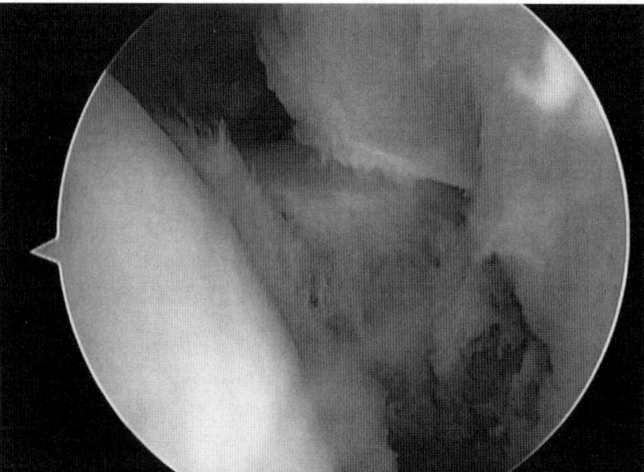

Figure 46-2 Anterior capsular release. Middle glenohumeral ligament has been incised revealing subscapularis tendon.

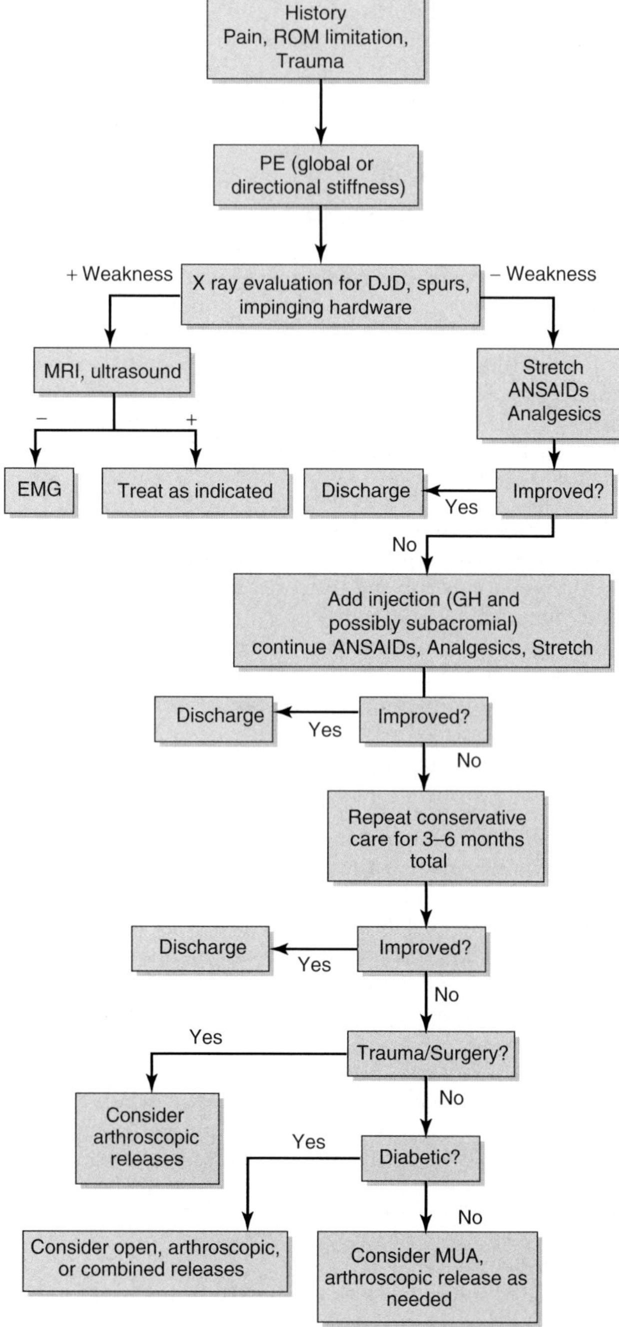

Figure 46-3 Algorithm for treatment of frozen shoulder. ROM, range of motion; PE, physical examination; DJD, degenerative joint disease; MRI, magnetic resonance imaging; NSAIDs, nonsteroidal anti-inflammatory drugs; EMG, electromyogram; GH, glenohumeral; MUA, manipulation under anesthesia.

to the inferior glenoid neck protects the axillary nerve. General anesthesia is preferred. If the deltoid is stimulated, the bipolar direction is changed. Maintaining the cautery along the glenoid rim and using accessory portals for improved access in the axillary pouch is helpful.

Subacromial arthroscopy for release of scar may be performed. Idiopathic frozen shoulder pathology is classically a primary intra-articular capsular fibrotic process, and subacromial findings may be limited. However, in the posttraumatic stiff shoulder, significant subacromial adhesions may be present, necessitating extensive debridement. Acromioplasty is performed if there is abrasion of the undersurface of the coracoacromial ligament or significant spurring.

The arthroscopic equipment is then withdrawn. Gentle manipulation to assess range of motion is performed. An intra-articular steroid may be used.

Postsurgical management includes physical therapy immediately. Interscalene anesthesia can be helpful, and the patient may be discharged with a home exercise program. Postsurgical admission may be beneficial if pain control or medical factors are of concern. Continuous interscalene anesthesia may also be used to facilitate early and frequent range of motion.

Results of arthroscopic release for frozen shoulder have been reported extensively throughout the literature. Studies have generally found significant increase in both Constant scores and ASES scores. Ogilvie-Harris et al. noted in a comparative series of 20 patients undergoing manipulation under anesthesia and 20 patients undergoing arthroscopic release that range of motion was similar but surgical arthroscopic release provided better function and pain relief overall at a mean follow-up of 2 to 5 years.

Potential complications of arthroscopic capsular release include risks and complications inherent to surgical procedures including infection, bleeding, and nerve injury. One report of transient axillary neurapraxia was found. Postoperative instability has not been noted. Persistent stiffness has been reported. Despite 50% of their patients demonstrating persistent stiffness in internal rotation, Segmuller et al. demonstrated 88% satisfactory outcome. Two of three patients dissatisfied with their final outcome were diabetic. In stratifying groups based on causes, patients with idiopathic frozen shoulder appear to do better than those with secondary posttraumatic or postsurgical stiffness. Diabetics have been demonstrated to do initially worse in terms of motion and pain relief with comparable final outcomes to those of patients without diabetes.

Overall, arthroscopic capsular release is a technically demanding procedure, but is generally a safe procedure with few complications noted in the literature (Fig. 46-3).

SUGGESTED READINGS

Buchbinder R, Hoving JL, Green S, et al. Short course prednisolone for adhesive capsulitis (frozen shoulder or painful stiff shoulder): a randomized, double blind, placebo controlled trial. *Ann Rheum Dis*. 2004;63:1460–1469.

Binder AL, Bulgen DY, Hazelman BL, et al. Frozen shoulder: a long-term prospective study. *Ann Rheum Dis* 1984;43:361–364.

Bulgen DY, Binder AI, Hazelman BL. Frozen shoulder: prospective clinical study with an evaluation of three treatment regimens. *Ann Rheum Dis*. 1984;43:353–360.

Chambler AFW, Carr AJ. Aspects of current management. The role of surgery in frozen shoulder. *J Bone Joint Surg Br*. 2003;85-B:789–795.

Gam AN, Schydlowsky P, Rossel I. Treatment of "frozen shoulder" with distention and glucocorticoid compared with glucocorticoid alone: a randomized controlled trial. *Scand J Rheumatol*. 1998;6:425–430.

Griggs SM, Ahn A, Green A. Idiopathic adhesive capsulitis. a prospective functional outcome study of non-operative treatments. *J Bone Joint Surg Am*. 2000;82:1398–1407.

Harryman DT, Lazarus MD. The stiff shoulder. In: Rockwood CA, Matsen FA, Wirth MA, et al., eds. *The Shoulder*. 3rd ed. Philadelphia: WB Saunders; 2004:1121–1172.

Loew M, Heichel TO, Lehner B. Intraarticular lesions in primary frozen shoulder after manipulation under general anesthesia. *J Shoulder Elbow Surg*. 2005;14:16–21.

Ogilvie-Harris DJ, Biggs DJ, Fitsialos DP, et al. The resistant frozen shoulder. Manipulation versus arthroscopic release. *Clin Orthop Relat Res* 1995;319:238–248.

Placzek JD, Roubal PJ, Freeman DC, et al. Long term effectiveness of translational manipulation for adhesive capsulitis. *Clin Orthop*. 1998;356:181–191.

Segmuller HE, Taylor DE, Hogan CS, et al. Arthroscopic treatment of adhesive capsulitis. *J Shoulder Elbow Surg*. 1995;4:403–408.

Shaffer B, Tibone JE, Kerlan RK. Frozen shoulder: a long-term follow-up. *J Bone Joint Surg Am*. 1992;74:738–846.

Zuckerman JD, Cuomo F, Rokito F. Definition and classification of frozen shoulder: a consensus approach. *J Shoulder Elbow Surg*. 1994;4:572.

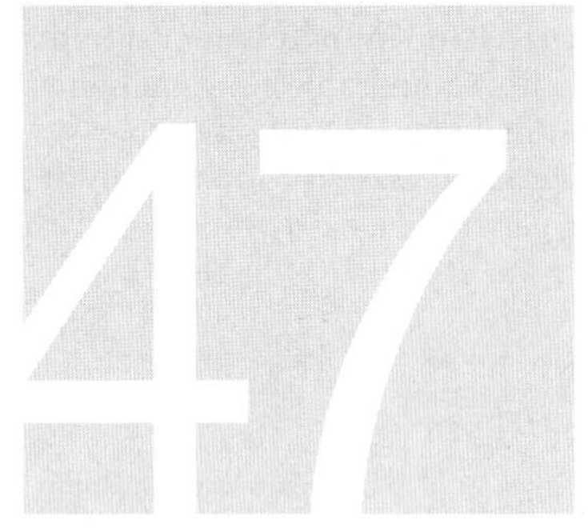

PHYSICAL EVALUATION OF THE ELBOW

SRINATH KAMINENI

CLINICAL HISTORY

A careful history is of the utmost importance since it can lead to the diagnosis in most cases. Before focusing on the main complaint, it is important to determine some basic information about your patient. With each piece of information obtained, the investigator should always continually be triaging some differential diagnoses. The patient's *age* allows an early distinction between possible congenital or developmental conditions when young, e.g., congenitally dislocated radial head presenting in a child unable to fully supinate the forearm in extension as compared with a greater tendency for degenerative pathologies in the elderly. Some pathologies (e.g., lateral epicondylitis) occur in the middle of an average life span, between 20 and 60 years, but not at the extremes beyond this range. The *occupation* may point toward some obvious diagnoses—e.g., the baseball pitcher is more prone to medial collateral ligament injury and valgus extension overload syndrome, whereas a manual laborer may present with primary degenerative arthrosis. Those in occupations involving a lot of weight bearing on the elbows—e.g., plumbers, carpenters, and gardeners—may show a tendency for olecranon bursitis. Which is the *dominant arm* (right, left, or ambidextrous), and is it the arm presenting with the current problem?

Primary Presenting Complaint

The most common primary symptom, the presenting complaint, is pain. Also note any secondary complaints, which may or may not be directly linked with the primary complaint; elbow pain with numbness of the hand as occurs in median nerve entrapment at the elbow is an example of linked symptoms. Which of the symptoms is most troublesome to the patient, with respect to being most disabling to his or her function? Ask for a subjective prioritization.

The following characteristics of pain are important to investigate:

1. *Location*—Ask the patient to be precise and delineate the painful area with a single finger to map its extent where possible. Sometimes the pain is vague and poorly defined, as in a rheumatoid elbow with articular and periarticular pain (Table 47-1).
2. *Periodicity*—Is the pain constant or intermittent, spontaneous or associated with specific activities?
3. *Severity*—Sometimes sequential visual analogue scores are useful for tracking the progression of pain on different office visits and after any intervention.
4. *Quality*—Pain can be described in many ways, notably as sharp, dull, deep-seated, aching, stabbing, locking with loose bodies, grating with a degenerative joint, apprehension of an unstable joint, and so on.
5. *Timing*—Is the pain worse in the morning, suggestive of rheumatoid disease; in the evening, suggestive of degenerative disease; or at night, which may suggest chronic granulomatous or neoplastic pathologies.
6. *Radiation*—Does the pain radiate proximally or distally into the anatomically relevant muscle groups (e.g., tennis elbow of ECRB degenerative cause can radiate distally into the forearm to the distribution of the extensor mass musculature), or does the pain radiate into a dermatomal distribution? For example, ulnar nerve entrapment between the two heads of flexor carpi ulnaris can cause radiating pain along the medial forearm to the ring and little fingers, median nerve entrapment between the two heads of pronator teres causes radiating pain into the radial 3.5 digits of the hand, and cervical osteoarthritis can cause radiating pain or numbness into the whole hand. Also bear in mind that pain at the elbow can originate from the neck, necessitating a cervical spine examination.
7. *Duration*—How long has the pain been present and troubling the patient?
8. *Relieving factors*—Osteoarthritis pain improves with rest, rheumatoid arthritis is not particularly relieved by rest

TABLE 47-1 LOCATION OF PAIN IN RELATION TO COMMON DIFFERENTIAL DIAGNOSES

Location of Pain	Differential Diagnoses
Medial elbow	Medial epicondylitis (golfer's elbow), flexor-pronator sprain, Little Leaguer's elbow, ulna collateral ligament sprain, cubital tunnel syndrome (posteromedial)
Anterior elbow	Biceps rupture, bicipital tendonitis, median nerve compression/ pronator syndrome
Lateral elbow	Lateral epicondylitis/tennis elbow, radial head fracture, osteochondral fracture, radiocapitellar chondromalacia/osteochondritis desiccans, posterior interosseous nerve (PIN) compression syndrome, radial plica syndrome
Posterior elbow	Olecranon osteophytosis (throwing athletes), triceps tendinitis/rupture, olecranon bursitis, ulna neuritis (posteromedial)
Poorly localized	Periarticular pain/circumferential pain–rheumatoid arthritis; lateral—PIN entrapment

but with analgesics and anti-inflammatory medications, and an acute traumatic soft tissue injury (ligament sprain) is helped by cooling with an ice bag.

9. *Aggravating factors*—Using an osteoarthritic joint worsens the pain, wrist extension against resistance aggravates tennis elbow, and wrist flexion against resistance aggravates golfer's elbow.

Mechanism of Injury/Pathology

The mechanism of injury/pathology should also be sought from the patient. This is often the most fruitful part of the history taking. If there was a specific injury to account for the current complaint, the direction, magnitude, and timing of the forces involved should be examined. Distinguish between a single event (e.g., an eccentric single contraction of the biceps during a football tackle leading to an acute distal biceps rupture) or multiple events (e.g., multiple painful episodes during biceps curls while weight lifting, leading to a partial biceps rupture). Some pathologies arise as a result of overuse, which may seem unimportant to the patient—e.g., a prolonged period of gardening or sports followed by tennis elbow after 2 days. During the time of injury or unusual event(s), did the patient observe any noises or other symptoms—a pop suggestive of a ligament sprain or rupture, a click as in an elbow instability, locking of the joint owing to a trapped loose body or instability, immediate swelling of a hematoma, or a delayed swelling of a traumatic or inflammatory effusion?

Litigation

Is there any intention of or pending legal action concerning the complaint being presented? Although not all-inclusive, pending litigation may adversely affect the patient's perception of the problem with an alteration of the portrayal of the clinical symptoms and signs.

Patient's Perception

What does the patient understand of the presenting problem, what advice has been given previously, and what is the patient's perception of the final outcome? Understanding the patient's perception at the time of presentation gives valuable insight into the potential for a good outcome.

PHYSICAL EXAMINATION

A standard method of examination proceeds along a standard algorithm: inspection, active motion, passive motion, and relevant imaging. During the physical examination, the affected side should be compared with the contralateral (normal) side.

Inspection

The *carrying angle* is the angle of the forearm relative to the arm when the upper limb is in a neutral position next to the body (fully extended and supinated). Age, sex, and racial variations should be considered; normal is 5 to 10 degrees in males; 10 to 15 degrees in females.[1] If the carrying angle is outside the normal range, the observable deformity (posttraumatic or growth disturbance—cubitus varus or gun stock deformity of <5 to 10 degrees [Fig. 47-1] or cubitus valgus >15 degrees), bearing in mind that all "deformity"

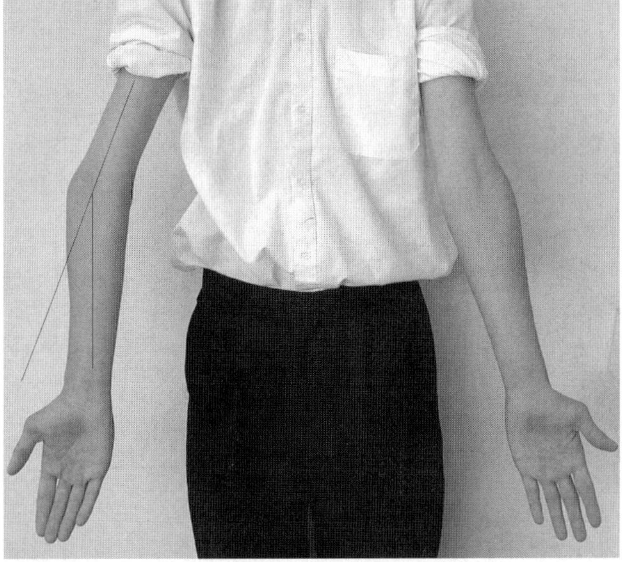

Figure 47-1 An 18-year-old man with a 20-degree cubitus varus deformity following a childhood malunited supracondylar distal humeral fracture.

TABLE 47-2 LOCATION OF SWELLING IN RELATION TO COMMON DIFFERENTIAL DIAGNOSES

Location of Swelling	Differential Diagnoses
Medial elbow	Subluxing ulnar nerve with elbow flexion, prominent medial epicondyle from childhood avulsion malunion, ganglion in the cubital tunnel
Anterior elbow	Retracted muscle belly of distal biceps tendon ruptures (Figs. 47-2, 47-3), antecubital ganglion, anteriorly dislocated radial head
Lateral elbow	Joint effusion, dislocated/fracture radial head (RH) (developmental/traumatic) (Fig. 47-4), caput magna of RH osteoarthritis
Posterior elbow	Olecranon bursitis (student's elbow)—septic bursitis is more painful than nonseptic/chronic bursitis, rheumatoid arthritis nodules (Fig. 47-5), retracted triceps rupture

may not be pathologic (normal racial or sexual variation). The skin color can be instructive in some conditions and should be compared with the contralateral nonpathologic limb; for example, an anterior ecchymosis as a result of a biceps rupture will be unilateral, and skin changes as a result of chronic psoriasis can be bilateral. Some skin changes can be nonpathologic but should be noted, e.g., port-wine stains, strawberry nevi, grey slate marks, and so on. Following trauma or some surgeries reflex sympathetic dystrophy can often lead to reddened skin that is shiny and painful.

Swellings can occur in any part of the elbow, and their fundamental characteristics help to diagnose the underlying pathology. Basic characteristics to define are the exact location and size. Other characteristics require palpation and are outlined below. *Scars* can be either traumatic or iatrogenic/surgical. The size and shape of the scar is noteworthy and can be helpful for planning future surgeries. Also note the quality of the scar, which can indicate the patient's healing response; for example, a keloid scar may

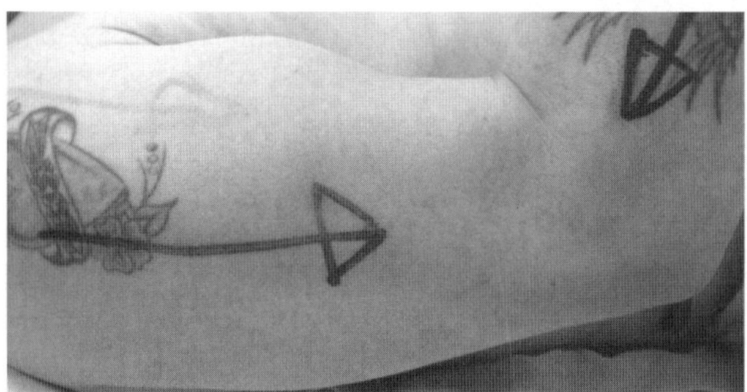

Figure 47-2 Distal biceps tendon rupture with proximal migration of the muscle belly (Popeye sign).

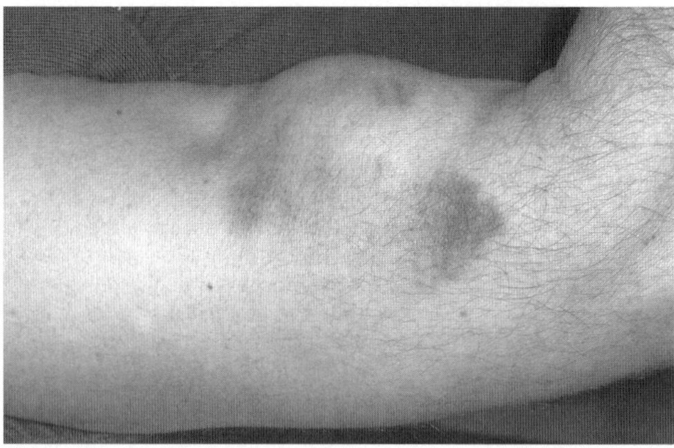

Figure 47-3 Proximal biceps tendon rupture with distal migration of the muscle belly with associated bruising (Popeye sign).

indicate a vigorous scar response and the potential for elbow capsular contracture, whereas a paper-thin scar may indicate a poor healing response, of relevance to ligamentous ruptures requiring repair. Finally note any *muscle wasting*. In the forearm that has undergone a Volkman ischemic contracture, owing to compartment syndrome, the forearm musculature can be markedly wasted (Fig. 47-6). In the hand, the wasting of interosseous muscles/hypothenar eminence may be indicative of ulnar nerve compression in the cubital or Guyon tunnel; and wasting of the thenar eminence may indicate median nerve entrapment between the two heads of pronator teres (pronator syndrome) or may indicate nerve compression in the carpal tunnel (carpal tunnel syndrome) (Table 47-2).

Motion

Active Range of Motion

Normal elbow motion is an arc of motion from 0 degrees (full extension) to 145 degrees (full flexion). Loss of extension can be a sensitive indicator of intra-articular pathology and can signal an acute event (e.g., intra-articular effusion [synovial or hematoma] or a chronic event (e.g., degenerative arthrosis with anterior capsular contracture). Loss of flexion can be a consequence of posterior capsular contracture.

The normal forearm axial rotational arc of motion is 70 to 90 degrees (pronation, palm down), 80 to 90 degrees (supination, palm up). When assessing forearm rotation, the examiner should ensure that the patient's elbow is flexed to 90 degrees and positioned next to the trunk, thereby avoiding shoulder abduction or adduction. These latter motions can falsely alter forearm motion, with shoulder abduction compensating for a restriction in pronation and shoulder abduction compensating for supination restriction. Thumb and hand motion relative to the distal radioulnar joint can also lead to a false sense of motion of the forearm axis.

Passive Range of Motion

If the active range of motion is incomplete, passive range of motion testing will highlight a difference since pain often inhibits the active range. If active and passive ranges are

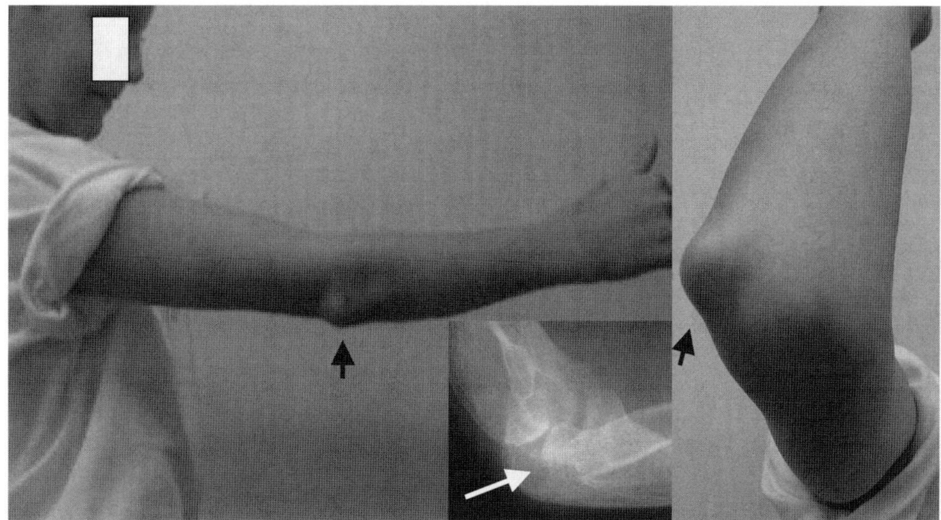

Figure 47-4 Developmental dislocation of the radial head, producing a lateral swelling and restriction of prosupination.

complete, the latter can be used to gain information about both the midarc and end-arc of the motion. The primary information that is sought regarding the mid-arc of motion is whether or not there is crepitus, which is suggestive of chondral degenerative pathology. This assessment can be enhanced by asking the patient to actively resist the passive motion, thereby increasing the joint reactive forces and accentuating signs originating from the bearing surfaces.

Gently pressuring the joint beyond the normal arc will provide information about the restraint to greater motion, but this test can be painful if done with excess zeal. During this assessment, one should continually consider whether the end point to the passive motion is rigid as in bony contact, or less rigid or soft implying a soft tissue cause of the end point (Table 47-3). With forced end-arc flexion, approximation of the forearm to arm musculature prevents greater flexion, whereas in thin patients the coronoid process may abut the coronoid fossa. In end-arc extension, there is the bony abutment between the olecranon process and its reciprocal fossa. In a normal joint such forced end-arc testing

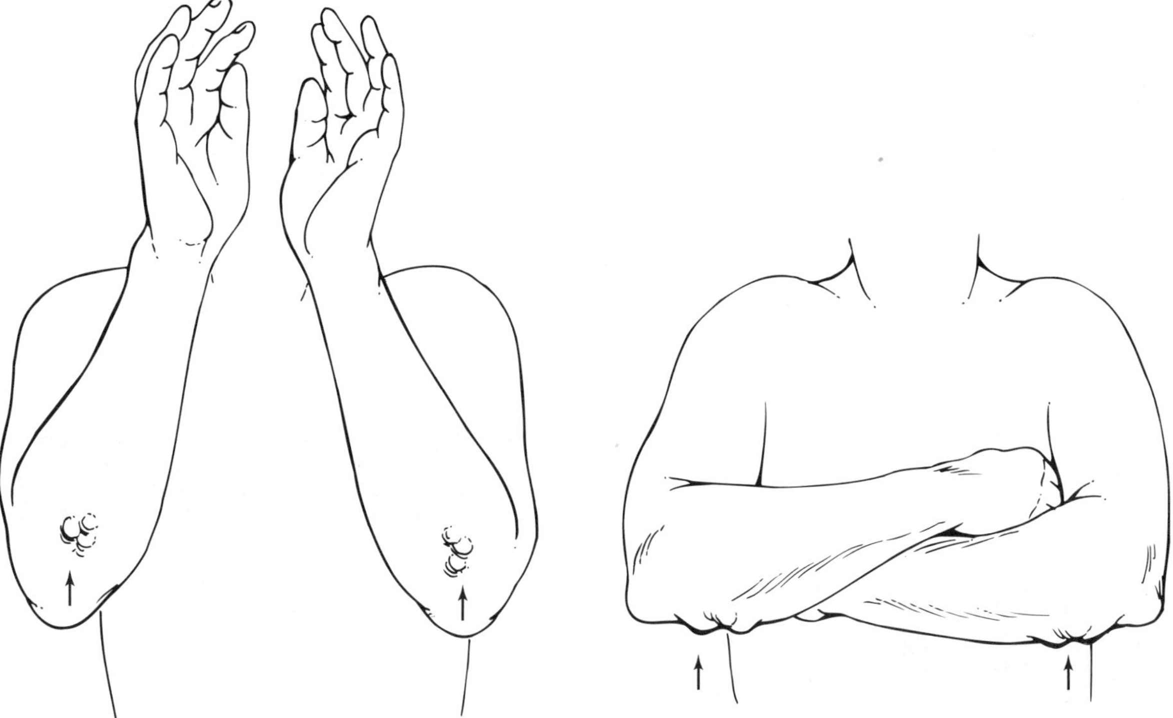

Figure 47-5 Typical position for rheumatoid nodules on the subcutaneous borders of the forearms (**illustration**), with a background **photograph** of severe rheumatoid swellings.

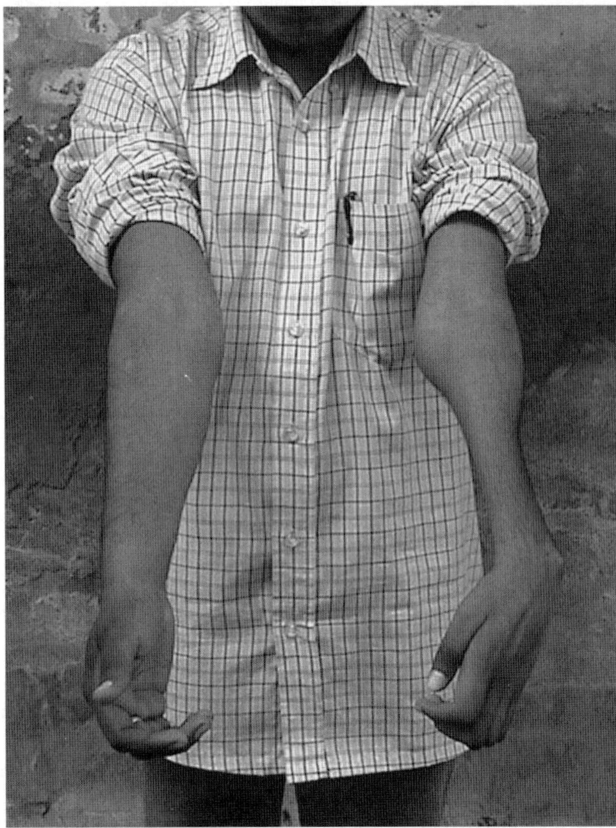

Figure 47-6 Volkman ischemic contracture of left forearm after an elbow fracture dislocation, treated in plaster cast. Forearm muscles have necrosed, and fibrotic scar tissue remains.

is not painful, but pain may be encountered with pathologic changes in osteophytosis and loose bodies.

For forearm rotation testing, the distal humerus should be immobilized and motion should be achieved by rotation of the forearm at the distal radioulnar joint. A common mistake is to hold the patient's hand to test for forearm rotation, which serves to build in an error to the rotation values so gained, since wrist joint laxity can be $\leq$15 degrees and more in patients with rheumatoid arthritis. Forced end-arc pronation and supination are normally resisted by forearm muscular stretching, although in thin subjects bony abutment can occur between the radius and ulna.

Isometric Strength Testing

For muscle strength testing, the elbow should be supported in 80 to 110 degrees of flexion with the forearm in neutral rotation. If tested either in greater extension or greater flexion, the maximum strength decreases to 75%.[3] The examiner should support the flexed elbow in the cupped palm of one hand with the other hand holding the distal forearm to produce resistance to motion. When attempting to grade the power of muscles or to longitudinally track changes in their strength, a grading system is useful, notably the MRC muscle strength grading system (Table 47-4). This method of testing is for isometric strength, but the clinical history should guide the examiner to also test for eccentric and concentric contractions where appropriate, first without resistance then with resistance. The specific movements to be tested are elbow flexion and extension, forearm pronation and supination, and wrist flexion and extension. The latter two movements are relevant to the examination of the elbow since most of the muscles driving these actions cross the elbow joint and can be symptomatic at the elbow.

TABLE 47-3 DIFFERENTIAL DIAGNOSES ASSOCIATED WITH PASSIVE MOTION

Motion Tenderness	Differential Diagnoses
Extension/ hyperextension	**Anterior pain with full extension**—anterior capsular strain/tear, brachialis/biceps partial rupture **Anterior pain with loss of extension**—anterior capsular contracture, biceps/brachialis contracture **Posterior pain with full extension**—olecranon osteophyte impingement (valgus extension overload syndrome)[2]
Flexion/ hyperflexion	**Anterior pain**—coronoid with or without osteophyte impingement in coronoid fossa, caput magna of radial head impingement in radial fossa **Anterior pain with numbness at 120–135 degrees flexion**—supracondylar process compression of MN **Posterior pain**—triceps tendonitis **Posterior pain with loss of full flexion**—posterior/posteromedial capsular contracture, large effusion/hemarthrosis, ulna neuritis or ulnar nerve impingement on osteophytes or ganglion
Pronation	Developmental/traumatic dislocation of radial head, interosseous membrane contracture, forearm bone(s) malunion, golfer's elbow, pronator syndrome
Supination	Developmental/traumatic dislocation of radial head, interosseous membrane contracture, forearm bone(s) malunion, tennis elbow, supinator syndrome

TABLE 47-4 MRC GRADING OF MUSCLE STRENGTH

Grade	Motion
5	Normal motion against maximal resistance
4	Normal motion against moderate resistance
3	Normal motion against gravity and minimal resistance
2	Normal motion with gravity eliminated
1	Flicker of motion only
0	No palpable muscle contraction

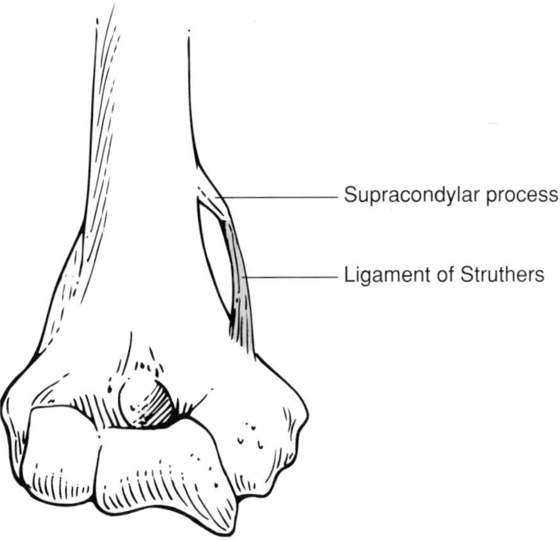

Figure 47-7 Medial supracondylar process and ligament of Struthers, sources of median nerve compression.

Functional Evaluation

The elbow, in combination with the shoulder, functions to place the hand where needed to manipulate the environment. Whereas the shoulder motion defines a sphere centered on the glenohumeral joint, the elbow allows the hand to move in and out to the extremity of the sphere, along the radii of the sphere.[4] To perform most activities of daily living, a full range of elbow motion is *not* necessary, and this is possible with a sagittal flexion arc from 30 to 130 degrees and forearm rotational arc of 50 degrees pronation and 50 degrees supination. A comprehensive assessment should include 15 activities of daily living that primarily test the flexion arc and 15 activities that test the forearm rotational arc of motion (Fig. 47-11). However, assessing the elbow function can be adequately and consistently performed using an overall evaluation scoring system, the Mayo Elbow Performance Score,[4] in which five activities of daily living are addressed (Table 47-5).

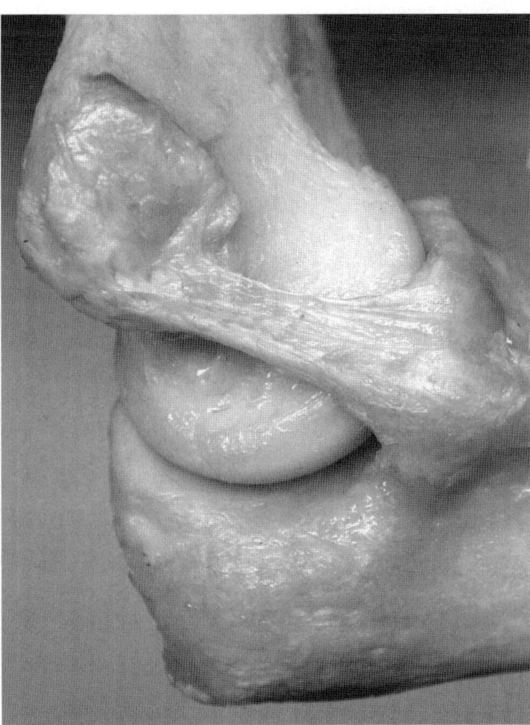

Figure 47-8 Cadaveric dissection demonstrating the origin of the anterior medial collateral ligament (AMCL) at the anteroinferior aspect of medial epicondyle and the insertion at the sublime tubercle of the proximal ulna.

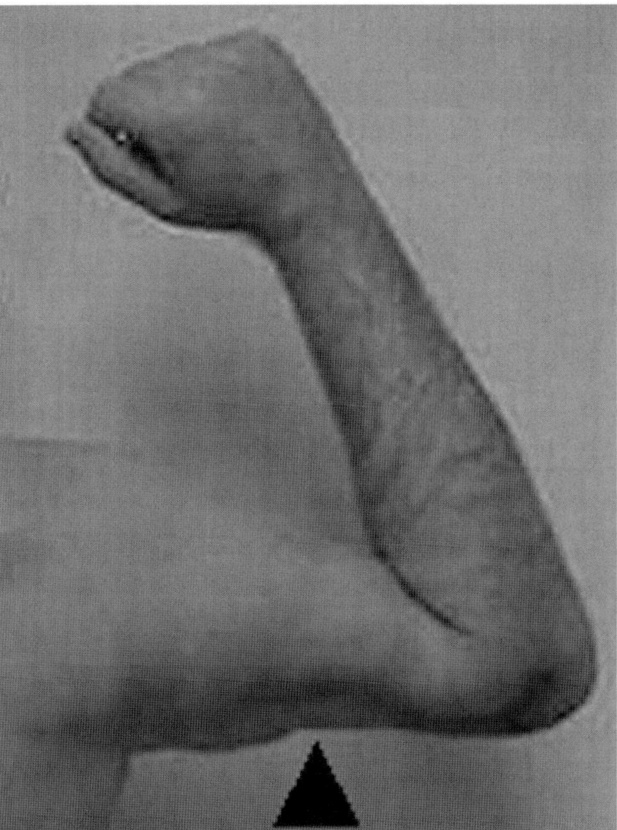

Figure 47-9 Triceps rupture with a consequent inability to extend the elbow against gravity.

Special Elbow Tests

The clinical history and the generic tests detailed above will enable the examiner to decide whether specific pathology related tests are required for further clarity of the presenting complaint. The tests outlined below in this section are not mandatory for all patients, but only for those about whom the examiner has a level of suspicion regarding the diagnosis. These special and specific tests fall broadly into three categories: (i) ligamentous instability tests, (ii) inflammation tests, and (iii) neurology-based tests.

Ligamentous Instability Tests

The arm is maintained in full extension with one hand supporting the elbow and the other producing a valgus or varus

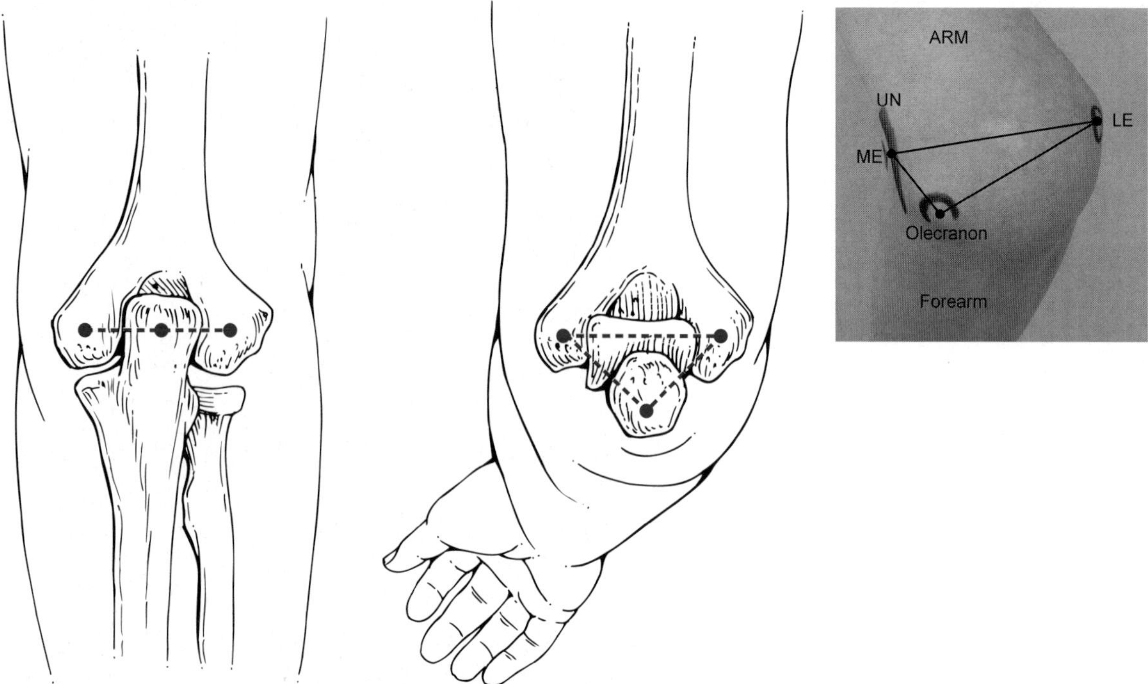

Figure 47-10 Normal posterior alignment is present when the olecranon forms a straight line with the two epicondyles with the elbow extended. An equilateral triangle is formed when the elbow is flexed to 90 degrees. **Inset photograph** demonstrates malalignment of these bony points owing to a malunited supracondylar humeral fracture. ARM, ;LE, lateral epicondyle; ME, medial epicondyle; UN, ulnar nerve.

torque on the distal radioulnar joint. In this position the olecranon process is closed packed in the reciprocal fossa and may conceal less severe ligamentous injuries.

To reduce the effect of bony restraint to valgus or varus deformation, the elbow is flexed to 20 to 30 degrees, which allows less severe ligamentous injuries to be uncovered. The difficulty with testing valgus/varus stability in this position is that the humerus rotates outside the examiner's control, thereby introducing an error to the extent of any instability detected. Hence when testing in slight elbow flexion, the

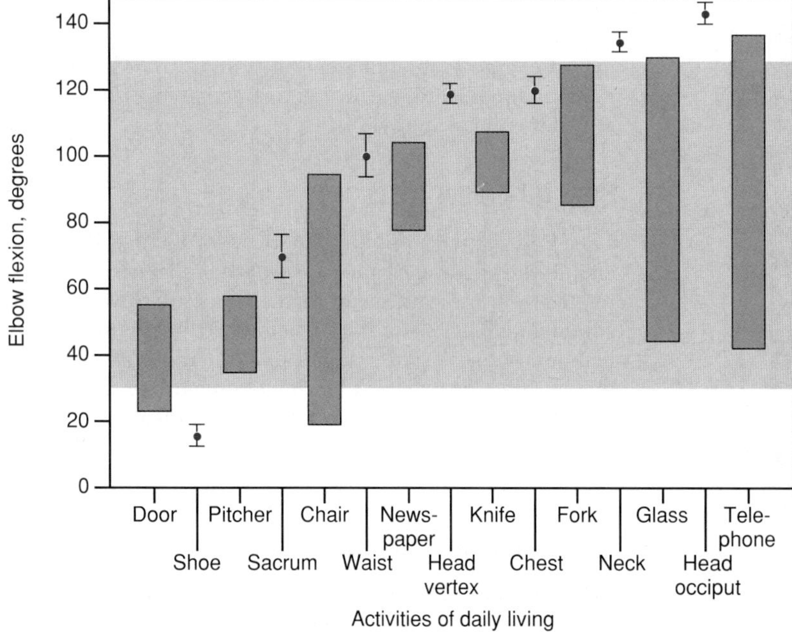

Figure 47-11 Fifteen activities of daily living. Those that can be achieved within a 100-degree arc of flexion (30 degrees–130 degrees) are in the central grey area.

TABLE 47-5 THE MAYO ELBOW PERFORMANCE SCORE

Function	Points	Definition (Points)
Pain	45	None (45) Mild (30) Moderate (15) Severe (0)
Motion	20	Arc >100 degrees (20) Arc 50–100 degrees (15) Arc <50 degrees (5)
Stability	10	Stable (10) Moderate instability (5) Gross instability (0)
Function	25	Comb hair (5) Feed (5) Perform hygiene (5) Don shirt (5) Don shoes (5)
Total	100	

From Morrey BF, An KN, Chao EY. Functional evaluation of the elbow. In: Morrey BF, ed.. *The Elbow and Its Disorders*. 2nd ed. Philadelphia: WB Saunders; 1993.

effect of the shoulder is minimized by placing it in either full external rotation for valgus stress testing or full internal rotation for varus stress testing[5] (Fig. 47-12). When considering what constitutes a positive test result, either increasesin laxity compared with the normal contralateral limb or an increase in pain is a relevant finding. However, be wary of the contralaterally lax "normal" elbow when comparing with the known pathologic side.

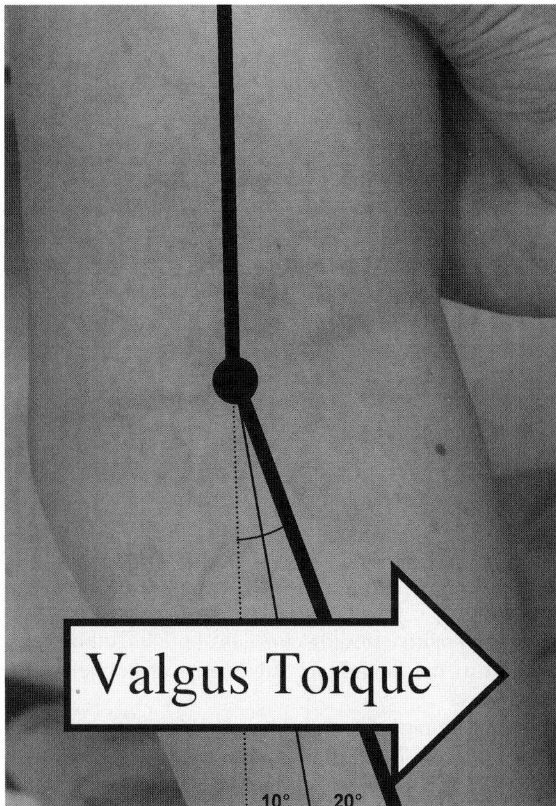

Figure 47-12 Valgus stability testing in a fully extended elbow. The arm is stabilized, and the forearm is moved in the plane of testing.

TABLE 47-6 DIFFERENTIAL DIAGNOSES FOR NERVE DYSFUNCTION ABOUT THE ELBOW

Nerve	Pathologic Cause for Dysfunction
Ulna	Medial olecranon/trochlea osteophyte/ganglion impingement, subluxing nerve, or long-standing cubitus valgus causing tardy palsy, flexor carpi ulnaris (FCU) hypertrophy in athletes, scarred nerve following elbow trauma, nerve swelling owing to trauma/pregnancy
Radial	Entrapment in callus of healing humeral fracture; posterior interosseous nerve (PIN) entrapment owing to fibrous bands, recurrent vessels leash of Henry, extensor carpi radialis brevis (ECRB), arcade of Frohse, supinator distal border
Median	Compression by the ligament of Struthers[a] proximal to the elbow; compression between the two heads of the pronator teres (pronator syndrome)
Lateral antebrachial cutaneous nerve (LACN)	Compressive neuropathy in athletes with forced repetitive pronation

Biceps reflex, innervation C5>C6; brachioradialis reflex, innervation C6>C5; triceps reflex, innervation C7–C8.
[a]von Schroeder HP, Scheker LR. Redefining the "Arcade of Struthers." *J Hand Surg [Am]*. 2003;28:1018–1021.

In the *moving valgus stress test*, the examiner places, and maintains thoughout the test, a constant valgus torque on a fully flexed elbow, which is then rapidly fully extended (Fig. 47-13). This is essentially a motion version of the common

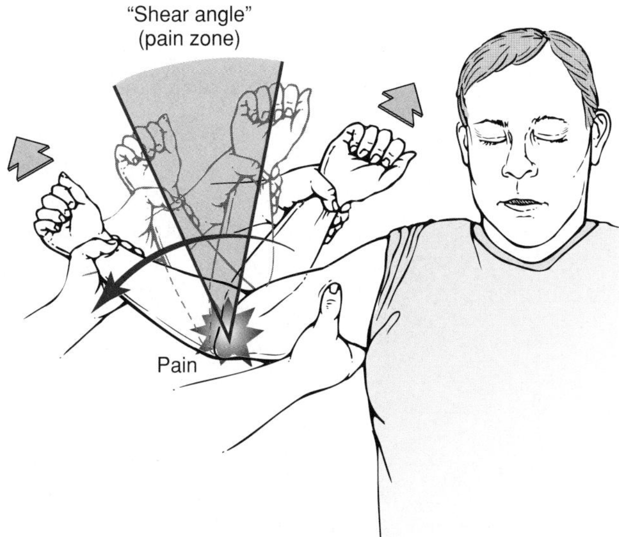

Figure 47-13 The moving valgus stress test for identifying medial collateral ligament (MCL) injuries.

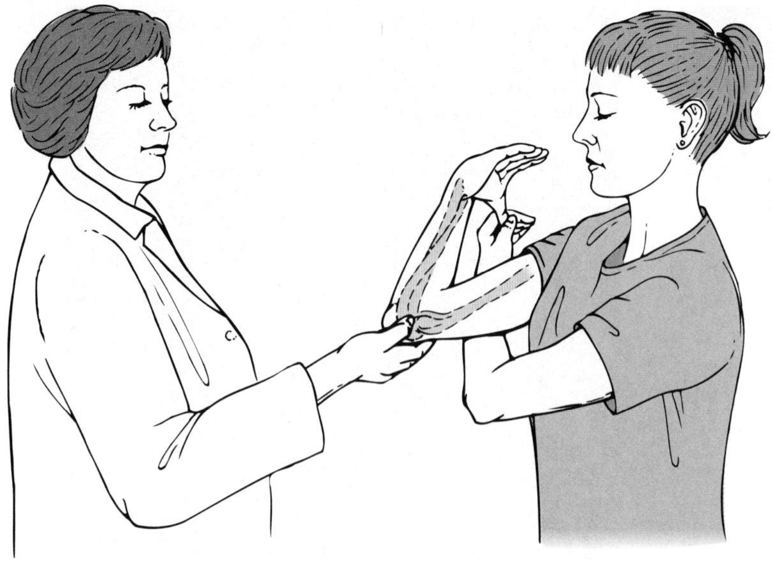

Figure 47-14 The milking test for identifying anterior medial collateral ligament (AMCL) injuries in continuity.

milking test. A positive finding consists of medial elbow pain predominant in the flexion arc shear zone of between 120 and 70 degrees.[6]

In the *milking test*, the examiner or the patient pulls the thumb of the pathologic limb with a valgus torque, with the elbow flexed between full 130 and 70 degrees[7,8] (Fig. 47-14). Pain is produced at the site of the medial collateral ligament, anterior band. This test is especially sensitive when there is a medial collateral ligament injury.

The *posterolateral rotatory instability test*, also referred to as the *pivot shift maneuver*, tests for insufficiency of the lateral collateral ligament complex.[9] The patient is positioned supine on a couch (Fig. 47-15). The radial head is seen to sublux/dislocate when the supinated forearm is axially compressed and stressed with a valgus torque and passively fully extended from 30-degree flexion. The radial head relocates with a clunk with flexion from full extension to 30-degree flexion (Fig. 47-15). This test is rarely positive in the awake patient but is quite helpful to perform while the patient is under anesthesia. In the awake patient, the push-up test may prove more patient friendly, with the patient requested to push up from a seated position, with the hands firmly pushing on the chair arms. The patient's hands should be in full supination. The patient will report pain or will not use the affected side to push up from the chair.

Inflammatory Tests

In *resisted wrist extension* (lateral epicondylitis), the examiner resists the patient's effort to extend a flexed wrist while maintaining an extended elbow, pronated forearm, and radially deviated wrist. Pain originating from the lateral epicondyle constitutes a positive test.

In *passive wrist flexion* (lateral epicondylitis), the examiner fully flexes the patient's wrist, with a pronated forearm, and extends the elbow from a flexed starting position.

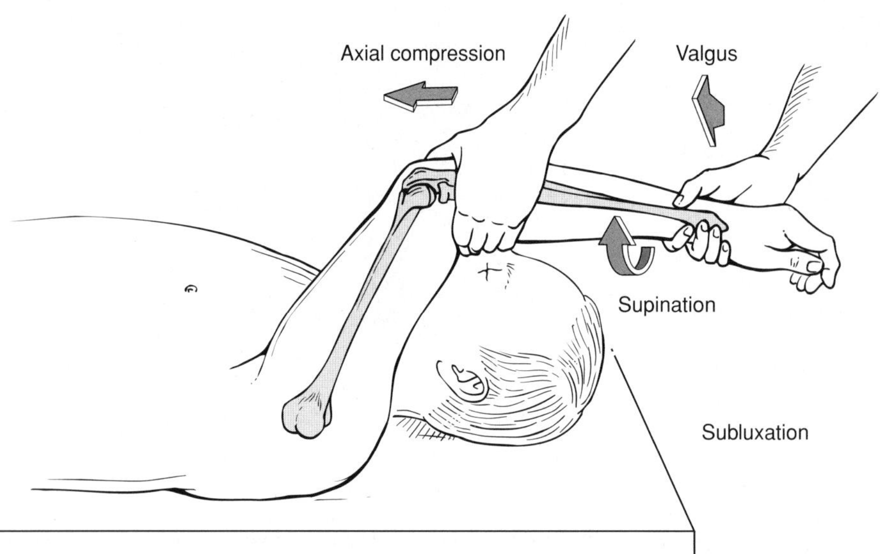

Figure 47-15 Posterolateral instability test-degree starting flexed position. The posterior subluxed radial head will reduce with a clunk.

A painful response can also emanate from radial nerve compression, requiring electrodiagnosis.

In *resisted middle finger extension* (lateral epicondylitis), resistance to the patient's attempt to maintain extension of the middle finger proximal interphalangeal joint causes pain at the lateral epicondyle. This tests the involvement of the extensor digitorum communis in the lateral epicondylar symptoms.

In *resisted wrist flexion* (medial epicondylitis), the examiner resists the patient's attempt to flex a fully extended wrist, with a supinated forearm and extended elbow. A positive result constitutes pain at the medial epicondyle.

In *passive wrist extension* (medial epicondylitis), with the patient's wrist flexed, the forearm fully pronated, and the elbow flexed to 15 degrees, the examiner performs wrist extension, forearm supination, and elbow extension simultaneously. Pain emanating from the medial epicondyle constitutes a positive result.

Neurology-Based Tests

Three major mixed nerves and cutaneous nerves need formal assessment, along with the dermatomal sensory distributions and motor end organs. The sensation of these dermatomes and cutaneous nerves should be performed as a matter of routine. The major mixed nerves acting on the elbow are the ulnar, radial, and median nerves.

The *ulnar nerve* can be palpated behind the medial epicondyle, and any irritability should be noted. A small percentage of normal subjects demonstrate subluxing ulnar nerves, which can be felt to sublux over the medial epicondyle during flexion and relocate during extension. In some, this finding is associated with irritability and some degree of ulnar nerve dysfunction. Sensation is tested with light touch and pin-prick testing of the little finger and ulnar half of the ring finger. Motor function is tested by the examiner, resisting the patient's attempt to spread apart the patient's fully extended fingers, a function of the ulnar nerve innervated interosseous muscles of the hand. However, *Martin-Gruber anastomosis* may produce normal interosseous muscle function in the presence of an ulnar nerve lesion at the elbow and should be borne in mind. This anatomic anomaly provides motor fibers for interosseous muscle innervation from the median nerve; these fibers enter the ulnar nerve in the forearm, distal to the cubital tunnel. Normally the innervation is entirely from the ulnar nerve, without interruption from the C8 and T1 spinal origin.

In the *Tinel test* (cubital tunnel syndrome), gentle tapping of the ulnar nerve, as it lies on the posterior aspect of the medial epicondyle, should not cause a tingling sensation in the forearm's ulnar nerve innervated territory and the little finger and ulnar half of the ring finger in the normal subject. When this test is positive, the indication is that there is nerve regenerative activity occurring at the test site, and hence, this is a useful test for tracking the progress of a recovering nerve. Care should be taken not to percuss the nerve too vigorously, since the Tinel sign will be positive even in normal subjects, leading to misdiagnosis. Another source of testing error can be a Guyon tunnel compression of the ulnar nerve at the wrist, which should be sought separately.

The *elbow hyperflexion test* (cubital tunnel syndrome) consists of maintaining full elbow flexion with wrist extension for 3 minutes.[10] A positive finding constitutes pain, numbness, and ulnar nerve distribution tingling owing to this positionally induced nerve ischemia in the cubital tunnel.

The *Froment test* is a test of ulnar nerve motor dysfunction. The examiner pulls strongly on a sheet of paper that the patient is asked to hold firmly between the thumb and index finger. A positive test consists of the paper being withdrawn by the examiner, since the ulnar nerve innervated adductor pollicis and flexor pollicis brevis deep head are unable to maintain good pinch strength with thumb metacarpophalangeal joint (MCPJ) flexion and interphalangeal joint (IPJ) extension. With ulnar nerve (UN) dysfunction, the thumb MCPJ becomes hyperextended and the IPJ flexes in an attempt to maintain the pinch grip.

The *radial nerve* is not an easily palpable nerve, but can be palpated 1 to 2 cm distal to the anterior radiocapitellar joint while pronating and supinating the forearm. This motion allows the nerve to pass under the examiner's digit and causes symptoms of pain when the nerve is pathologically compressed. Sensory dysfunction of the main radial nerve trunk (proximal to the elbow) or the superficial radial nerve (distal to the elbow after bifurcation of the main nerve) leads to tingling or paresthesia of the first dorsal web space. Motor dysfunction at the elbow leads to a wrist drop owing to loss of innervation of the wrist extensors in the forearm.

In the *resisted forearm supination test* (radial tunnel syndrome), pain is reproduced when the examiner resists the patient's attempt at supinating the forearm. This is an important test to carry out when one of the differential diagnoses is tennis elbow because of the infrequent but recognized possibility that the two pathologies coexist.

The *median nerve* supplies the cutaneous innervation to the radial three and a half digits, along with the ulnar half of the volar forearm. It can be compressed by anomalous anatomy, notably the ligament of Struthers, a ligament that passes from the humeral shaft to the medial epicondyle in 1% of the population.[11] Since the brachial artery accompanies the nerve on occasion, there may be concurrent symptoms of vascular compromise. The lacertus fibrosus can also be a source for median nerve compression, and resisted supination from a starting position of supination can cause pain in the median nerve distribution. The other common site for median nerve compression is the carpal tunnel of the wrist, but this latter does not cause any paresthesia of the forearm, as is the case with more proximal compressions. Motor signs of median nerve compression include weakness of forearm pronation (pronator teres), wrist flexion and abduction (flexor carpi radialis), and flexion of the thumb IPJ (flexor pollicis longus). Thenar eminence wasting may also be observed in long-standing cases.

For the *resisted forearm pronation test* (pronator teres syndrome), the examiner resists the patient's attempt to pronate the forearm with a flexed and extended elbow. The reproduction of tingling and paresthesia in the median nerve distribution in the forearm and hand constitutes a positive result.

In the *resisted middle finger flexion test* (FDS compression of Median nerve), when the examiner resists the patient's attempt to flex the middle finger from a starting position of extension, a pathologic flexor digitorum superficialis fibrous arc can cause compression and distal signs as above.

With the *Kiloh-Nevin sign* (anterior interosseous nerve syndrome), when the patient is asked to form a tip-to-tip pinch with the thumb and index finger, making an *O* sign, the patient can form only a pulp-to-pulp pinch, reminiscent of a raindrop. The median nerve/anterior interosseous nerve, when compressed between the two heads of pronator teres, interrupts the motor innervation to the flexor pollicis longus and the radial half of the flexor digitorum profundus, with the subsequent inability to flex the terminal joints of the thumb and index finger.[12]

The *lateral antebrachial cutaneous nerve* (LACN) is the sensory terminus of the musculocutaneous nerve. Its sensory distribution is the radial half of the forearm between the elbow and wrist. When pathologic, a Tinel sign can be elicited with percussion of the nerve immediately lateral to the biceps tendon in the elbow flexion crease.

Abbreviations

AMCL–Anterior medial collateral ligament
DDRH–Developmental dislocation of radial head
DIY–Do it yourself
ECRB–Extensor carpi radialis brevis
EDC–Extensor digitorum communis
EMG–Electromyogram
GE–Golfer's elbow
IA–Intra-articular
IPJ–Interphalangeal joint
LB–Loose body
LCL–Lateral collateral ligament
MCPJ–Metacarpophalangeal joint
MN–Median nerve
NCV–Nerve conduction study
OA–Osteoarthritis
PIN–Posterior interosseous nerve
RA–Rheumatoid arthritis
RCJ–Radiocapitellar joint
RSD–Reflex sympathetic dystrophy
TE–Tennis elbow
UN–Ulnar nerve
ΔΔ–Differential diagnosis

REFERENCES

1. An KN, Morrey BF, Chao EY. Carrying angle of the human elbow joint. *J Orthop Res*. 1984;1:369–378.
2. Andrews JR, Wilk RE, Satter White YE, et al. Physical examination of the thrower's elbow. *J Orthop Sports Phys Ther*. 1993;17(6):296–304.
3. Kapandji AI. *The Physiology of Joints*. New York: Churchill Livingstone; 1970. *Upper Limb*; vol 1.
4. Morrey BF, An KN, Chao EY. Functional evaluation of the elbow. In: Morrey BF, ed.. *The Elbow and Its Disorders*. 2nd ed. Philadelphia: WB Saunders; 1993.
5. Regan WD, Morrey BF. The physical evaluation of the elbow. In: Morrey BF, ed. *The elbow and Its Disorders*. 2nd ed. Philadelphia: WB Saunders; 1993.
6. O'Driscoll SW, Lawton RL, Smith AM. The "moving valgus stress test" for medial collateral ligament tears of the elbow. *Am J Sports Med*. 2005;33:231–239.
7. Elattrache NS, Jobe FW. Treatment of ulnar collateral ligament injuries in athletes. In: Morrey BF, ed. *Master Techniques in Orthopaedic Surgery—The Elbow*. Vol. 1. 2nd ed. Philadelphia: Lippincott, Williams & Wilkins; 2002:229–247.
8. Jobe FW, Elattrache NS. Diagnosis and treatment of ulnar collateral ligament injuries in athletes. In: Morrey BF, ed. *The Elbow and Its Disorders*. 3rd ed. Philadelphia: WB Saunders; 2000:549–555.
9. O'Driscoll SW, Bell DF, Morrey BF. Posterolateral rotatory instability of the elbow. *J Bone Joint Surg Am*. 1991;73:440–446.
10. Buehler MJ, Thayer DT. The elbow flexion test. A clinical test for the cubital tunnel syndrome. *Clin Orthop Relat Res*. 1988;233:213–216.
11. von Schroeder HP, Scheker LR. Redefining the "Arcade of Struthers". *J Hand Surg [Am]*. 2003;28:1018–1021.
12. Rask MR. Anterior interosseous nerve entrapment: (Kiloh-Nevin syndrome) report of seven cases. *Clin Orthop Relat Res*. 1979;142:176–181.

IMAGING OF THE ELBOW

JEFFREY C. KING

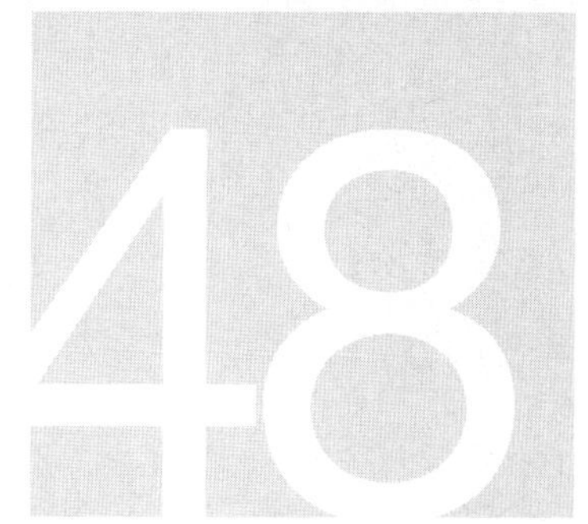

The elbow joint is a complex structure with three separate intracapsular articulations. These are highly congruent joints with multiplanar, noncollinear surfaces that make imaging difficult. The relatively small amount of overlying soft tissue and the ease of positioning, however, aid in imaging efforts. As with other joints, multiple imaging tools are available. The most commonly used include plain radiographs, computed tomography, and magnetic resonance imaging. Arthrography is often a useful adjunct to these studies, but is less commonly used alone. Ultrasound may be helpful in some situations where dynamic images are required. Plain tomography and xeroradiography have largely been replaced by newer, better studies and are mentioned here for the sake of completeness.

This chapter will review current imaging modalities for the elbow, including appropriate techniques and parameters. Guidelines to assist in choosing the appropriate test for specific clinical situations will be discussed.

PLAIN RADIOGRAPHS

Anteroposterior (AP) and lateral radiographs remain the workhorses of elbow imaging. The AP view (Fig. 48-1A) demonstrates the distal humeral articular surface, medial and lateral epicondyles, radial head and neck, and most of the proximal ulna, excluding clear views of the coronoid and olecranon processes. The ulnohumeral and radiocapitellar joint spaces are well seen and can demonstrate widening or narrowing depending on the clinical condition. The lateral radiograph (Fig. 48-1B) clearly shows the coronoid and olecranon processes, as well as the associated fossa. The radial head overlies the coronoid, but should still allow adequate visualization of both structures. Adequacy of the lateral view can be determined by the target sign of three concentrically larger circles seen in the distal end of the humerus. These rings represent, from inside out, the minimum dimension of the trochlea, the capitellum, and the medial rim of the trochlea. Malrotation by as little as 5 degrees will disrupt this appearance. Anterior and posterior fat pads can be seen in situations of intra-articular distension (Fig. 48-2). The supinator fat stripe can be displaced by swelling associated with radial head fractures.

The AP view is obtained with the elbow fully extended on an appropriately sized image receptor. The arm is parallel with the plate, and the forearm is in supination. The beam is directed perpendicular to the midpoint of the elbow joint, and the joint is centered on the film. The lateral view is obtained with the shoulder abducted to 90 degrees, the arm parallel to the plate, and the forearm in full supination. The beam is directed perpendicular to the elbow joint, or ideally at a 7-degree caudal angle to replicate the carrying angle.

In situations where full extension of the elbow is not possible, the AP view can be compromised (Fig. 48-3). A single AP view obtained through a flexed elbow is of little value. In this situation, two views—an AP view of the proximal forearm and an AP view of the distal humerus—should be obtained.

The forearm view is obtained with the forearm placed flat and the elbow joint centered on the plate. A greater degree of flexion deformity will require increased kilovoltage (Kvp) to allow adequate penetration to demonstrate bony detail. The humerus view is obtained with the distal humerus flat on the plate with the elbow centered. The forearm should be supported for comfort. The beam is directed perpendicular to the elbow joint.

Additional views are obtained to visualize specific features of the elbow anatomy. The internal (medial) oblique view improves visualization of the trochlea, olecranon, and coronoid. The external (lateral) oblique view improves visualization of the radiocapitellar joint, radioulnar joint, medial epicondyle, and coronoid tubercle.

The internal oblique view is obtained with the arm positioned initially as for an AP view. The arm is then rotated internally 45 degrees. The beam is directed perpendicular to the plate and elbow joint. The external oblique view is obtained by rotating the arm externally 45 degrees.

The radial head is better visualized with the radial head view and lateral radial head rotation positions. The radial head view (Fig. 48-4) minimizes the overlap of the radial head and coronoid, improving visualization of radial head and capitellar pathology. Visualization of the fat pads is enhanced as well. The lateral rotation positions demonstrate

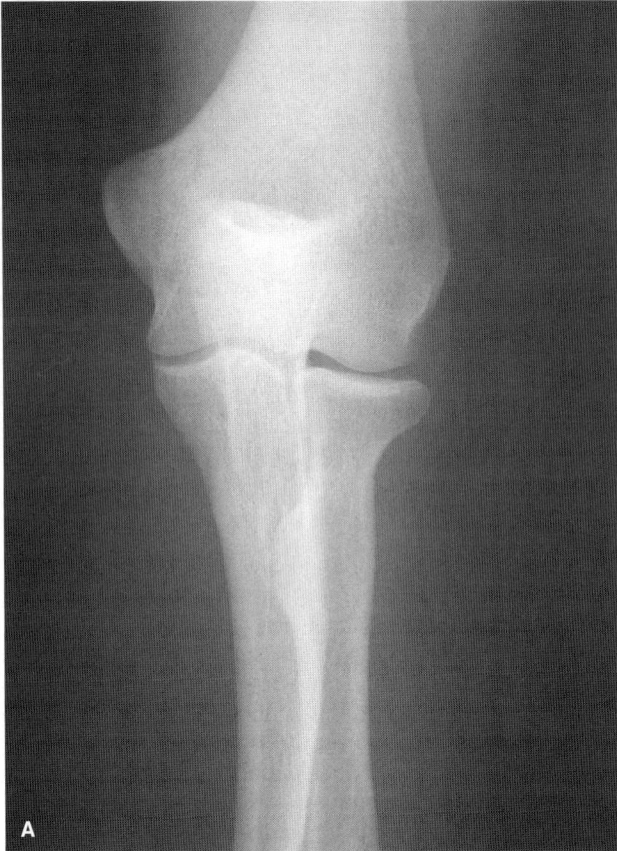

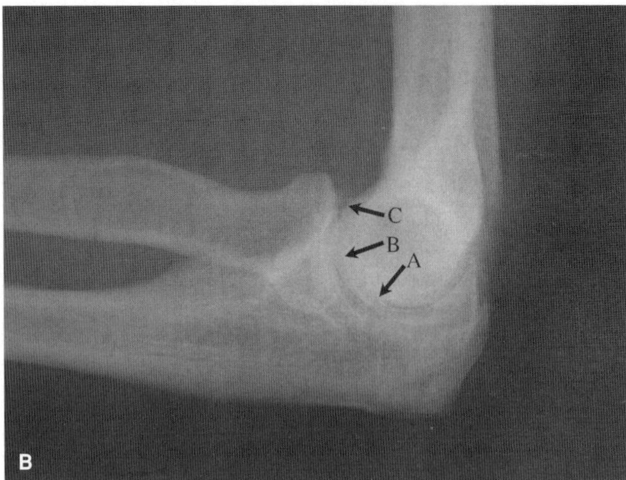

Figure 48-1 A: Anterior-posterior (AP) view of the elbow in full extension. B: Lateral view of the elbow. Note concentric circles representing, from the center out, (*A*) trochlear sulcus, (*B*) capitellum, and (*C*) medial wall of the trochlea.

the radial head in profile throughout its full available arc of motion. The radial tuberosity is the most obvious indicator of the position of forearm rotation. The coronoid is viewed without superimposition with the coronoid-trochlea position.

The radial head view is obtained by positioning the elbow in the standard lateral position and angling the beam 45 degrees cephalad, parallel to the long axis of the humerus. The lateral rotation positions require standard lateral position of the elbow and perpendicular beam position. The forearm is then positioned in hypersupination, midsupination, midpronation, and hyperpronation. The coronoid-trochlea image is obtained by positioning similar to the radial head view, but angling the beam 45 degrees caudal.

There are several special axial views of the elbow. These include the axial olecranon projection view, which enhances the visualization of the olecranon margins and associated spurs; also, the cubital tunnel view demonstrates any bony abnormalities or encroachment on the ulnar nerve in the cubital tunnel.

The axial olecranon projection view is obtained with the proximal dorsal forearm flat against the plate, full supination, and maximal elbow flexion with the humerus overlying the forearm. The beam is angled 20 degrees toward the hand along the long axis of the forearm. The cubital tunnel view is obtained by placing the humerus flat on the plate, maximal flexion of the elbow, and 15 degrees of external rotation of the arm. The beam is directed perpendicular to the plate and elbow joint.

Finally, a gravity stress view may be used for evaluation of valgus instability. This technique can minimize apprehension but requires patient relaxation and cooperation to avoid a false-negative result. Gravity-induced valgus instability is demonstrated by widening of the joint space of the medial side of the joint.

This is a cross-table view, with the patient supine and the arm abducted 90 degrees away from the side. The arm is externally rotated, the thumb pointing to the floor. The

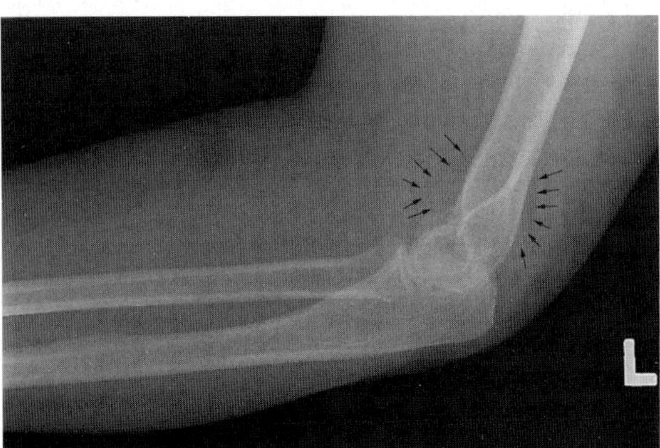

Figure 48-2 Lateral view of the elbow with occult radial head fracture. Note the elevated anterior and visible posterior fat pads (*black arrows*).

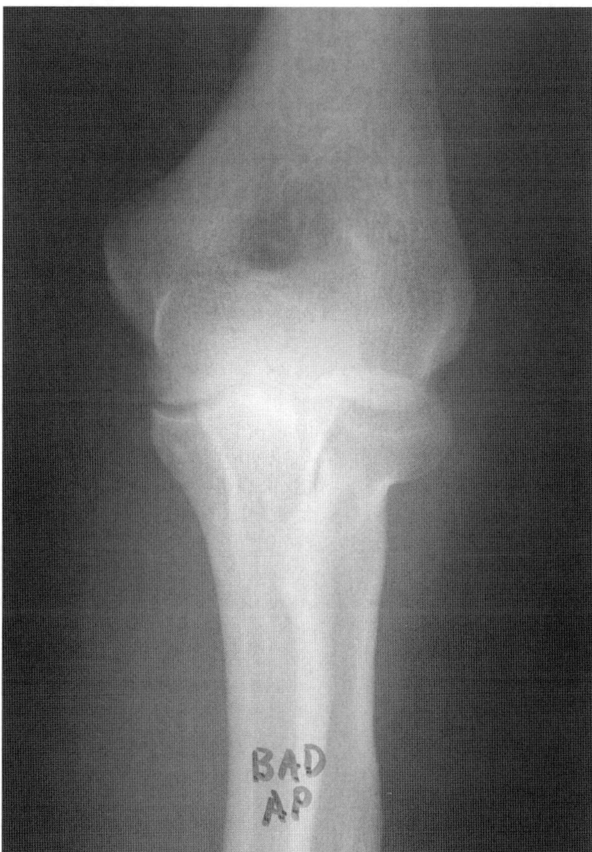

Figure 48-3 Poor-quality anterior-posterior view of the elbow. Flexed position creates overlap of structures and inadequate visualization of bony detail.

elbow is flexed 15 degrees. The plate is oriented vertically and placed dorsal to the elbow. The beam is directed horizontally, perpendicular to the elbow joint.

Plain Radiograph Interpretation

Specific osseous structures and relationships should be systematically reviewed and irregularities noted, and when indicated, additional views or studies obtained. On all views the radial head should line up with the capitellum. The radiocapitellar and ulnohumeral joint space should be symmetric on the AP view; the coronoid-trochlear and the olecranon-trochlear joint spaces should be symmetric on the lateral view. Visualization of the anterior and posterior fat pads on the lateral radiograph (Fig. 48-2) is a reliable sign of intra-articular fluid collection, most common with trauma or inflammation. Occult fracture should be sought when accompanied by a history of trauma. Finally, for all of the utility of plain radiographs, they still present a two-dimensional representation of a three-dimensional structure. The ability of computed tomography and magnetic resonance imaging to present the elbow anatomy in three dimensions underscores their importance as an adjunct to the diligent history taking and careful physical examination in the diagnosis of elbow pathology.

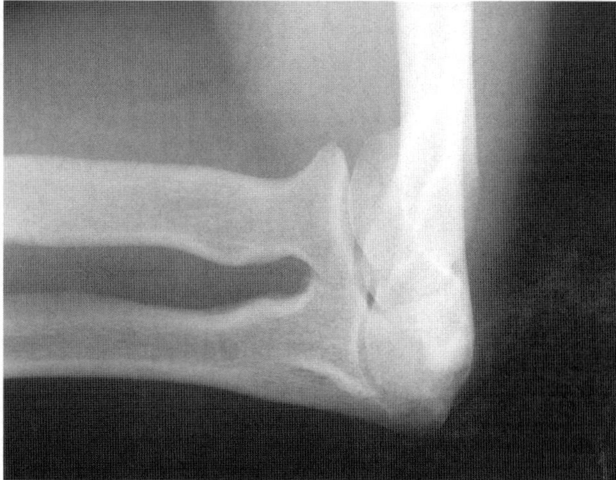

Figure 48-4 Radial head view. Overlap of the coronoid is minimized, improving visualization of the radial head and capitellum.

COMPUTED TOMOGRAPHY

Computed tomography (CT) has largely supplanted the use of plain tomography in this country. CT has the advantage of clearer images and multiplanar views over plain tomography, although metal artifact remains a limitation. Three-dimensional rendering of the elbow joint is possible as well (Fig. 48-5). The decreased slice thickness and helical image acquisition of the newest scanners provide for improved clarity of reconstructed images. Nonaffected bones can be digitally subtracted to allow improved visualization of the involved area (Fig. 48-6). This is especially helpful in complex coronoid fractures as well as for preop planning for elbow malunion surgery. The injection of radio-opaque dye with or without air (single- or double-contrast arthrogram) provides more sensitive evaluation of cartilaginous loose bodies and the status of the articular cartilage. The author believes that

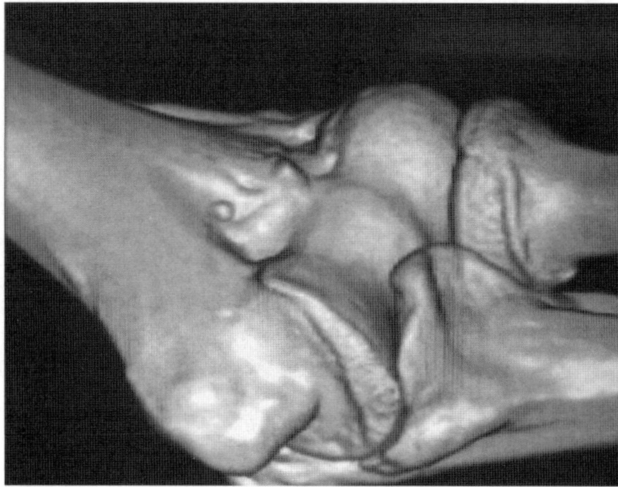

Figure 48-5 Three-dimensional reconstruction of the elbow joint. Coronoid spur and anterior loose body are well seen.

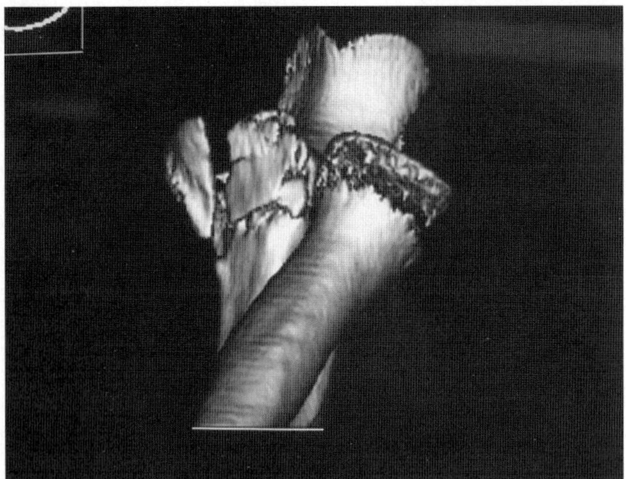

Figure 48-6 Three-dimensional reconstruction of the elbow joint with digital removal of the humerus. The comminuted coronoid fracture is clearly seen. The abnormality of the radial head represents artifact rather than radial head/neck fracture.

CT arthrogram provides the best evaluation for loose bodies in the elbow with catching and/or locking, although other literature demonstrates no advantage of CT arthrogram over MRI evaluation.

MAGNETIC RESONANCE IMAGING

Magnetic resonance imaging (MRI) provides the highest-quality images of the soft tissues about the elbow. As more imaging protocols emerge, the utility of this technology broadens. MRI should be used, however, to test a specific hypothesis, developed by the history and clinical examination, rather than as a "fishing expedition" on any and all painful elbows. The nature of the suspected problem determines the positioning and imaging protocols used to evaluate the elbow. Common indications include collateral ligament injuries (Fig. 48-7A, B), osteochondritis desiccans, and partial biceps injuries. MRI is not usually required in complete biceps tears with retraction or in the setting of traumatic fracture/dislocations where significant soft tissue injury can be assumed. Some have advocated the use of MR arthrogram to improve the sensitivity of collateral ligament injury diagnosis. Imaging can be performed safely with implanted metallic plates and screws, although scatter artifact limits image clarity.

Normal tendinous structures appear dark on T1- and T2-weighted images (Fig. 48-7A). Fluid and edema appear bright on the T2-weighted images, indicating soft tissue injury. Avascular bone appears dark on T1 images surrounded by the brighter signal of the normal cancellous bone. A fast spin echo, T2-weighted image with fat suppression is used to best image the collateral ligaments (Fig. 48-7B). Special positioning improves the image acquisition in patients with distal biceps injuries (Fig. 48-8).

ULTRASOUND

Ultrasound has been used to evaluate elbow tendons, ligaments, muscles, peripheral nerves, and joint structures. Advantages to ultrasound include accessibility, low cost, portability, and lack of contraindications (unlike MRI). In several specific applications, elbow ultrasound is the preferred imaging method, even over MRI. One such application is dynamic imaging of the elbow, where abnormalities may be present only with specific joint movements or

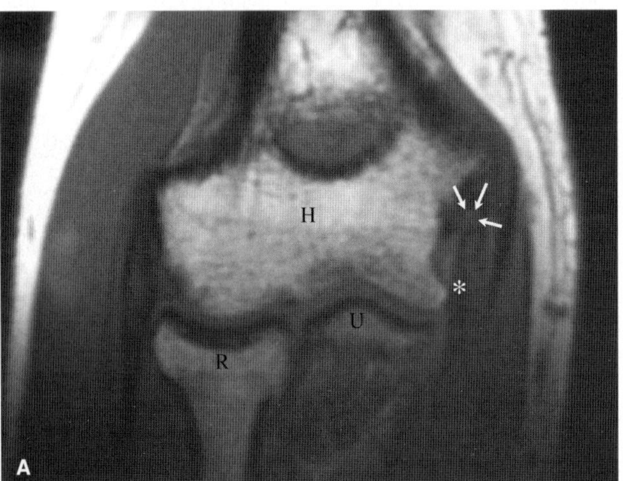

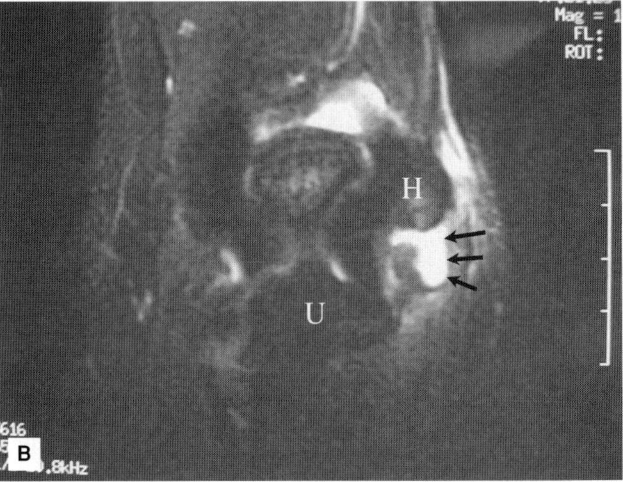

Figure 48-7 **A:** T1, spin echo, coronal image. Humerus (*H*), ulna (*U*), and radius (*R*). The low-signal, anterior bundle of the medial collateral ligament (MCL) (*asterisk*) is detached from its origin on the medial epicondyle; there is intermediate signal intensity (*white arrows*) seen at the site of the origin of the MCL indicating discontinuity. **B:** T2, fast spin echo with fat suppression, coronal image. Humerus (*H*), ulna (*U*). High-signal fluid (*arrows*) seen exiting through the tear of the origin of the MCL into surrounding soft tissues.

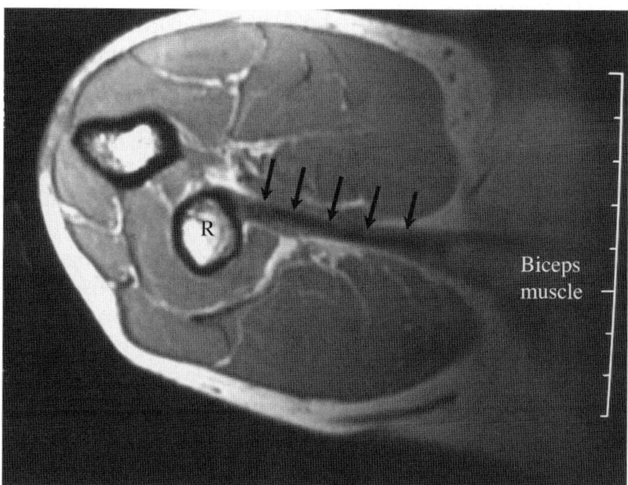

Figure 48-8 MRI of the distal biceps tendon (*arrows*) using the flexion, abduction, supination (FABS) view. Note that the entire length of the tendon is well visualized on one image, from the muscle belly (labeled) to the radius (*R*).

position. Examples include ulnar nerve dislocation and snapping triceps syndrome, which occurs with elbow flexion. An additional dynamic examination of the elbow under ultrasound observation is assessing injury to the anterior bundle of the ulnar collateral ligament with valgus stress applied to the elbow. Another advantage of ultrasound is evaluation of soft tissues superficial to metal hardware free of artifact. Peripheral nerves can also be efficiently evaluated with ultrasound, such as evaluation for the radial nerve injury after plate fixation of a humeral diaphyseal fracture.

CLINICAL SCENARIOS

Trauma

Imaging of the traumatized elbow usually starts with plain radiographs. Additional radiographic images should be included as indicated for specific pathology (Table 48-1). Evidence of associated fracture should be sought in all cases of elbow dislocation, as this affects treatment and prognosis. Thin-cut CT with multiplanar reconstructions are especially helpful in the evaluation of coronoid and capitellum fractures, as well as intracapsular distal humerus fractures. The CT images often demonstrate more significant pathology than suspected on plain films. Three-dimensional reconstructions with digital subtraction of uninvolved bony structures allow excellent visualization of complex intra-articular pathology. MR imaging provides excellent soft tissue definition, but is rarely indicated in high-energy trauma. Certain soft tissue injury patterns are common, such as lateral ulnar collateral ligament injury associated with radial head and coronoid fracture, and should be anticipated. MRI has increased utility in the evaluation of musculotendinous and ligamentous trauma, such as acute throwing injuries and biceps tendon pathology. Special imaging protocols have been developed to improve diagnostic accuracy.

TABLE 48-1 RECOMMENDED STUDIES I: TRAUMA

Radial head fracture or capitellum fracture	AP and lateral x-ray views External oblique view Radial head view Forearm rotation views CT with 2D or 3D reconstructions Consider ipsilateral wrist x-ray views if suspect Essex-Lopresti lesion
Coronoid fracture	AP and lateral x-ray views Internal oblique view 3D CT scan with digital removal of the humerus
Simple elbow dislocation	AP and lateral x-ray views
Complex fracture-dislocation	AP and lateral x-ray views Trauma series (AP forearm and humerus) CT scan with 2D or 3D reconstructions
Distal biceps injury	MRI with FABS protocol Ultrasound

AP, anteroposterior; CT, computed tomography; 2D, two-dimensional; 3D, three-dimensional; MRI, magnetic resonance imaging; FABS, flexion, abduction, supination.

Instability

Symptoms of instability may be acute or chronic. In the case of acute instability, the above trauma recommendations apply. Chronic instability is largely a clinical diagnosis. MRI is less sensitive in delineating attenuated ligamentous structures unless there is a superimposed acute on chronic injury. Gravity stress radiographs may confirm the diagnosis of valgus instability. In cases of posttraumatic chronic instability, CT images may clarify the competence of key structures such as the anterior and medial coronoid and radial head. Evaluation of the joint with real-time fluoroscopy before surgical procedures can be invaluable in clarification of instability patterns Examination of the awake patient to determine patterns of instability can be unreliable. It is highly recommended that all patients with a question of instability undergo a fluoroscopic examination after general anesthesia but prior to sterile surgical preparation of the patient.

Stiffness

Elbow stiffness may be related to soft tissue contracture, bony block, or most commonly, both causes. Plain films demonstrate bone causes such as heterotopic ossification (HO), loose bodies, or joint incongruity. CT scanning provides three-dimensional visualization of the bony abnormality and can be helpful in preoperative planning. Certain patterns of heterotopic bone formation are common. Posttraumatic HO typically occurs in the anterior lateral aspect of the joint. In cases of neuromuscular or burn HO, the posterior medial joint is most commonly involved. The ulnar nerve may be completely encased in bone;

TABLE 48-2 RECOMMENDED STUDIES II: NONTRAUMA

Osteochondritis dissecans or avascular necrosis in adults	AP and lateral x-ray views: late changes MRI: early changes
Elbow instability	Medial stress view Axial olecranon view MRI with or without gadolinium Fluoroscopy (EUA)
Heterotopic Bone	AP and lateral x-ray views Internal and external oblique views CT with 2D reconstructions
Suspected Loose bodies	AP and lateral x-ray views CT arthrogram or MRI arthrogram
Ulnar nerve pathology	Cubital tunnel view Ultrasound—instability
Snapping triceps	Ultrasound
Arthritis	AP and lateral x-ray views Rarely CT scan

AP, anteroposterior; MRI, magnetic resonance imaging; EUA, examination under anesthesia; CT, computed tomography; 2D, two-dimensional.

nevertheless, surprisingly, it almost always functions normally. CT images may clarify whether the ankylosis is complete or incomplete; in the latter case removal is simplified. MRI is of limited value in cases of soft tissue contracture and is not recommended.

The Painful Elbow

There are many causes for the painful elbow, and imaging is a useful adjunct in diagnosis (Table 48-2). The traumatized elbow is discussed above. In young athletes, osteochondritis dissecans (OCD) and apophysitis should be considered. These may be seen on plain x-ray films (contralateral images should be obtained), but MRI may be needed in early or subtle presentations. MRI or bone scan will demonstrate stress fractures, not seen on plain x-ray views. In cases of painful catching or locking, with or without limitation of motion, the author uses CT arthrogram to evaluate for loose bodies if the plain films are inconclusive. If the CT is positive, loose body removal is recommended; if negative, a symptomatic plica may be the cause of the symptoms. Throwers and other overhead athletes with medial elbow pain rarely exhibit gross instability. A medial stress view may show widening of the medial joint. An axial olecranon view may show posterior medial osteophytes associated with valgus extension overload syndrome. Finally, MRI may demonstrate medial collateral ligament (MCL) pathology or flexor pronator mass inflammation. Ulnar nerve instability may cause medial-sided pain. This is well evaluated by ultrasound. Ultrasound is also useful for demonstrating the snapping triceps syndrome, owing to the dynamic nature of the image acquisition. Additional imaging is rarely indicated in clinical cases of medial or lateral epicondylitis. Plain films may show periosteal reaction at the involved epicondyle. MRI adds little to the diagnosis or treatment of this condition. Avascular necrosis of the distal humerus is occasionally seen in patients on high-dose steroids, with alcoholism, or other lipid metabolism disorders. This may be seen on plain films, but often late in the course. MRI will demonstrate low-signal intensity of avascular bone on T1 images before changes can be detected on plain radiographs. Osteoarthrosis and inflammatory arthropathies are typically well visualized on plain x-ray films. CT is occasionally helpful to determine the extent of joint space involvement. Anterior cubital fossa pain, especially with resisted flexion and supination, may indicate a partial biceps injury. MR imaging can identify partial biceps injury or associated pathology. Ultrasound can provide similar information, often at lower cost, but the results are more operator dependent.

CONCLUSION

There are more options than ever before to provide high-resolution images of the bone and soft tissue anatomy of the elbow. Plain radiographs remain the appropriate initial choice in the diagnosis of many conditions and may indicate the need for confirmatory studies. MR imaging is most useful for the imaging of the soft tissues, whereas CT best defines the bony anatomy. Fluoroscopy and ultrasound provide motion images in real time, improving the diagnosis of dynamic conditions such as snapping triceps and instability patterns. All of these studies provide invaluable information to supplement, rather than replace, a careful history and physical examination for the diagnosis of complex elbow problems.

SUGGESTED READINGS

Berquist TH. Diagnostic imaging of the elbow. In: Money BF, ed. *The Elbow and Its Disorders*. 3rd ed. Philadelphia: WB Saunders; 2000;84–101.

Giuffre BM, Moss MJ. Optimal positioning for MRI of the distal biceps brachii tendon: flexed abducted supinated view. *AJR Am J Roentgenol*. 2004;182:944–946.

Haapamaki VV, Kiuru MJ, Koskinen SK. Multi detector computed tomography diagnosis of adult elbow fractures. *Acta Radiol*. 2004;45(1):65–70.

Hak DJ, Gautsch TL. A review of radiographic lines and angles used in orthopedics. *J Orthop*. 1995;Aug:590–601.

Jacobson JA. Musculoskeletal ultrasound and MRI: which do I choose? *Semin Musculoskelet Radio*. 2005:9:135–149.

Jacobson JA, van Holsbeeck MT. Musculoskeletal ultrasonography. Orthop Clin North Am. 1998;29:135–167.

Long B. The elbow. In: Long B, Rafert J, eds. *Orthopedic Radiography*. Philadelphia: WB Saunders; 1995;115–156.

Lowden C, Garvin G, King GJW. Imaging of the elbow following trauma. *Hand Clin Elbow Trauma*. 2004;20:353–361.

Potter HG, Sofka CM. Imaging. In: Altchek DW, Andrews JR, eds. *The Athlete's Elbow*. Philadelphia: Lippincott Williams & Wilkins; 2001;59–80.

CHRONIC MEDIAL INSTABILITY OF THE ELBOW

MAURICIO LARGACHA

In recent years there has been an increase in participation in sports that involve increased stress on the elbow. Much of the attention on the medial pathology around the elbow used to be related to throwing; presently, there are other sports that strain the medial structures, causing chronic medial instability. The process of better understanding the mechanics and pathophysiology of the elbow has increased our knowledge and treatment of chronic medial instability.

PATHOGENESIS

Etiology

Overhead and throwing athletic activities, such as baseball pitching, javelin throwing, tennis, throwing in football, and also floor gymnastics, expose elbows repetitively to valgus stress forces.

Anatomy and Biomechanics

In valgus stress to the elbow, with the elbow in flexion, the congruous osseous anatomy is the primary restraint. With lesser elbow flexion, between 20 and 120 degrees, the medial soft tissue restraints adopt a primary role in medial stability. In that arc of motion, the radial head is the secondary restrain on valgus stress.

The medial ligament complex is formed by three distinct structures that reinforce the capsule and form the medial collateral ligament (MCL) (Fig. 49-1). The anterior bundle of the MCL is the most important portion of the complex; it originates from the anteroinferior surface of the medial epicondyle and ends at the sublime tubercle of the ulna. Recent evidence suggests a two-band structure for the anterior bundle: the anterior band, which functions between 30 and 90 degrees of flexion (with 70 degrees being the position of greatest contribution to stability) and the posterior band, which is stressed most when flexion reaches 120 degrees. The posterior bundle of the MCL originates from the epicondyle and ends in the medial margin of the semilunar notch. It plays a secondary role in valgus stability. The transverse bundle originates from the medial olecranon and ends in the medial coronoid process and also plays a minor role in valgus stability.

Pathophysiology

Chronic MCL injury results from overuse activities such as throwing. With repetitive movements that produce valgus stress moments, the medial soft tissue structures are subjected to combined tension and bending stresses. An extension moment may also be present, producing internal shear stresses on the deep fibers of the MCL. This process is often a component of a multiple-compartment involvement (Table 49-1) that affects both the anterior and posterior compartment of the elbow. This can be best understood as a result of valgus extension overload syndrome.

During the mechanics of throwing, a rapid flexion-to-extension motion is accompanied by valgus stress moments. These combined forces produce medial tension forces of 300 N and external compression forces of 900 N. The repetitive nature of throwing puts the medial structures at risk of suffering chronic microtrauma, with partial or full rupture of the structures through chronically stressed ligaments.

Although infrequent, ulnar neuropathy may occur. With extreme positions of flexion, wrist extension, and shoulder abduction, the pressures in the ulnar tunnel increase up to six times. Additional pathology such as osteophytes, calcification of the MCL, and inflammation of the MCL can contribute to compression. Posteromedial osteophyte formation at the olecranon usually occurs in the latter stages of disease. With combined extension and valgus, early contact between the olecranon and the fossa is produced, resulting in posteromedial impingement. As a result of compression

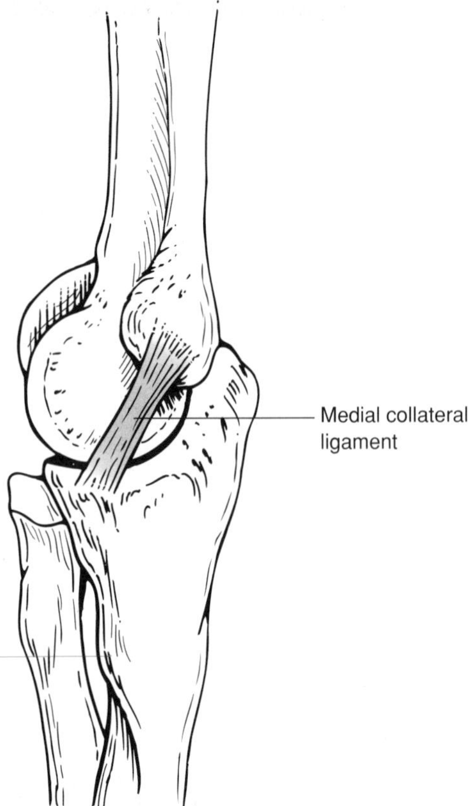

Figure 49-1 Medial collateral ligament.

forces across the radiocapitellar compartment, degenerative changes can be found beginning with chondromalacia of the capitellum to complete bone degeneration. In young athletes, osteochondritis dissecans may occur.

DIAGNOSIS

History

As with all chronic injuries of the upper extremity that involve overuse activities related to repetitive motion in sports, the history is essential. The examiner should investigate about the events that initiate the pain and if the evolution was acute in onset or chronic. In chronic medial elbow instability, pain is usually indistinct around the medial side with a slow progression over the season. Typically athletes complain about their inability to throw with the same power and speed before the onset of the injury, accompanied by pain in the late acceleration phase. On occasion a sudden dramatic pop may be felt by the patient when the medial collateral ligament ruptures.

TABLE 49-1 SPECTRUM OF INVOLVEMENT

- Medial side
  - Medial collateral ligament (MCL) rupture
  - Ulnar nerve compression
  - Medial-side osteophytes
- Lateral side
  - Chondromalacia of the radial head or capitellum
  - Osteochondritis dissecans
- Posterior compartment
  - Posteromedial osteophyte formation at the olecranon
  - Changes in the olecranon fossa shape and depth

Physical Examination

During examination, a complete arc of motion should be recorded with the forehand in supination for extension and flexion. If degenerative changes are present in the posterior compartment, pain may result at full extension during testing

With the elbow in 30 degrees of flexion, the surgeon can palpate the MCL through its normal course distal to the epicondyle. A valgus stress can also be applied to the elbow to examine for medial joint opening. Ulnar nerve palpation should also be done posterior to the course of the MCL to examine for tenderness or a possible Tinel sign.

Special Maneuvers

Moving Valgus Stress Test. The examiner must put the arm in 90 degrees of abduction and external rotation and,

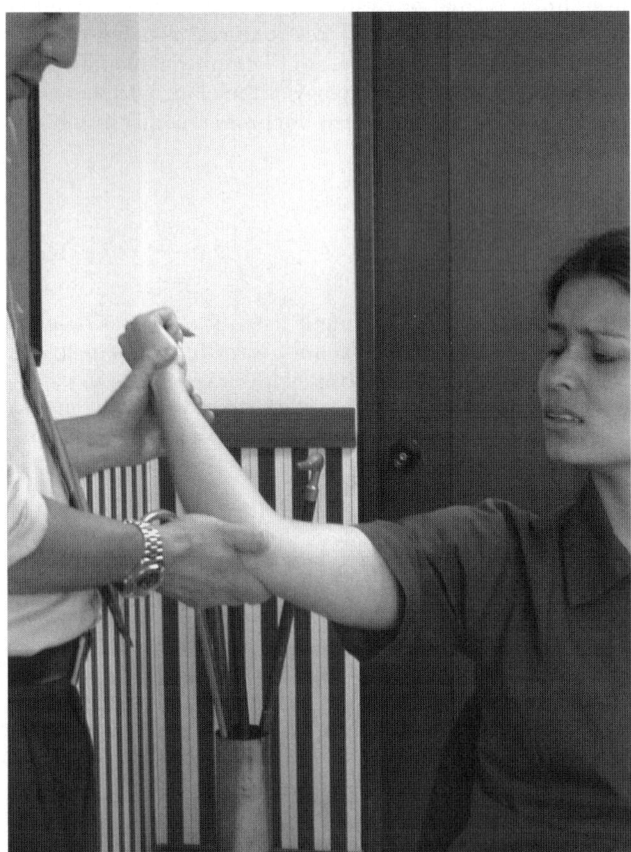

Figure 49-2 Moving valgus stress test. The examiner must put the arm in 90 degrees of abduction and external rotation, and, while applying a valgus stress, the arm is extended from a flexed position.

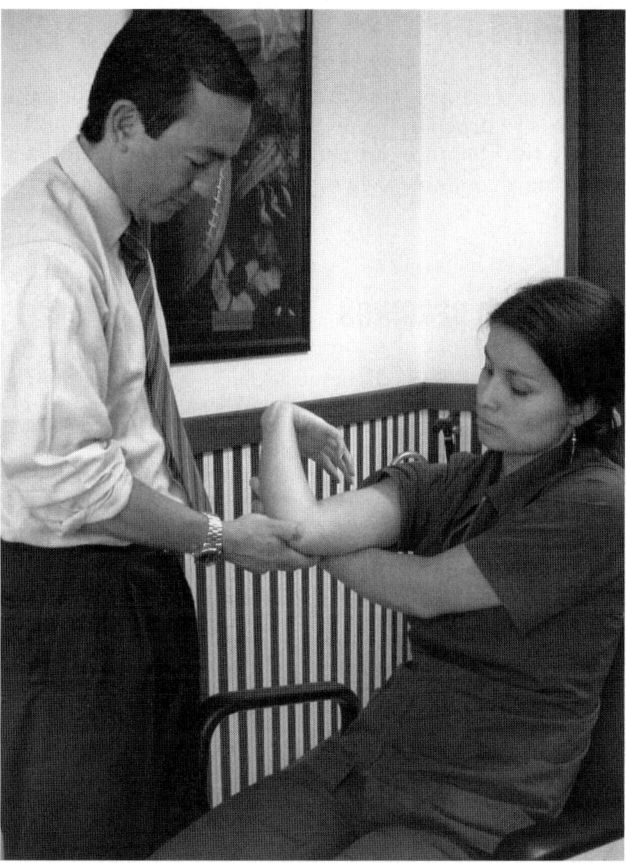

Figure 49-3 Milking maneuver. The affected elbow is flexed >90 degrees and the other hand grasps the thumb under the injured arm, exerting a valgus stress.

while the examiner applies a valgus stress, the arm is extended from a flexed position (Fig. 49-2). Pain is reproduced at about 70 degrees of flexion. Pain should be similar to the one produced by sports activities.

Milking Maneuver. The affected elbow is flexed >90 degrees and the other hand grasps the thumb under the injured arm, exerting a valgus stress (Fig. 49-3). The examiner palpates the MCL for pain.

Images

To make the diagnosis of chronic medial elbow instability, the history and physical exam are most important. Additional imaging studies can give further information to help confirm the diagnosis. Standard radiographic evaluation is routinely done, searching for calcification of the MCL. Degenerative changes may also be found, especially loose bodies and posteromedial osteophytes of the olecranon.

The use of radiographic evaluation with valgus stress under anesthesia may be helpful. However, it is important to remember that medial joint opening with stress radiographs can also be found in the asymptomatic thrower. Thus, a careful correlation with the clinical examination should be performed.

MRI imaging can be helpful, especially in the high-demand overhead athlete with suspected medial instability in whom clinical evaluation suggests chronic medial elbow instability. The use of intra-articular gadolinium increases the positive results of MCL tears.

TREATMENT

Different treatment options are available for athletes with medial elbow instability. Initially, the management includes a nonoperative program of rest combined with anti-inflammatory medications A formal rehabilitation program should be initiated. This should be done with an emphasis on regaining motion, followed by a dynamic stabilization and strengthening process that might permit the return to sports activities. Rehabilitation may require ≤16 weeks. With a nonoperative treatment, only between 50% and 60% of the patients may return to their previous level of throwing.

Reconstruction of the ligament using a tendon graft is the technique of choice for those patients who fail conservative treatment. Direct repair of the ligament is not usually possible. Either autograft or allograft can be used. It is unclear in the literature if there is an advantage of one over the other. Ipsilateral palmaris or plantaris tendon has often been used for reconstruction. Many patients will have an inadequate palmaris, and for this reason, allograft hamstring tendons are often quite helpful.

Reconstruction may be done by either a medial incision or a posterior incision. A posterior incision will provide access to the medial side but will help protect the underlying cutaneous nerves to a greater extent. A muscle split of the flexor carpi ulnaris allows for good surgical exposure and lowers the morbidity produced by a detachment of the flexor/pronator group. Transposing the ulnar nerve routinely is often not necessary and can increase the morbidity of the procedure.

Two 3.2-mm drill holes are placed 1 cm apart from each other, with the first one located slightly anterior to the sublime tubercle of the ulna in the medial aspect of the coronoid. The principal humeral drill hole is located at the anatomic origin, and two additional holes are placed anterior in the lateral column. Next, the graft is passed initially through the distal holes and through the anatomic hole in the humerus (Fig. 49-4). The graft is then sutured on itself with multiple nonabsorbable sutures. The split in the flexor pronator muscles is closed. A posterior splint at 90 degrees of flexion is used to immobilize the elbow. After 10 to 14 days, sutures are removed and the rehabilitation process begun. After discontinuing the splint, active progressive ROM exercises are started in the shoulder and elbow. A brace can be used during rehabilitation to protect the elbow from valgus stress. After restoring full range of motion, a strengthening program is begun first with isometric exercises, followed by resistance exercises. Attention should be focused on the flexor pronator group, which provides dynamic stabilization on the medial side of the elbow.

Beginning at 3 to 4 months, throwing should be progressively increased until the seventh month, at which time

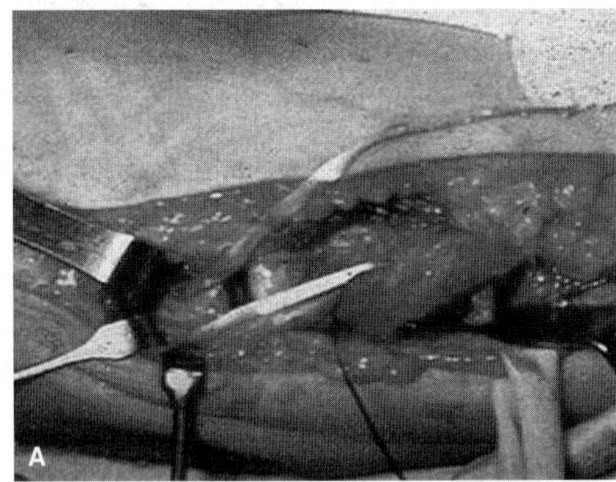

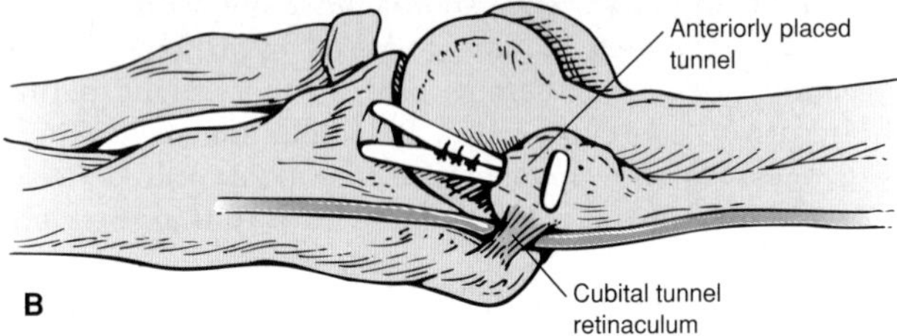

Figure 49-4 Tendon graft in place.

the athlete may throw at 50% of maximum velocity and can increase to 75% by the ninth month. Full rehabilitation of the athlete will take at least a year of treatment.

RESULTS

Studies suggest a good to excellent result occurs when the athlete is returned to the previous level of competition. Reports in the literature vary between 68% and 96% of athletes obtaining a good to excellent result after MCL reconstruction.

SUGGESTED READINGS

An KN, Morrey BF. Biomechanics of the elbow. In: Morrey BF, ed. *The Elbow and Its Disorders*. Philadelphia: WB Saunders; 1985:43–61.

Andrews JR, Timmerman LA. Outcome of elbow surgery in professional baseball players. *Am J Sports Med*. 1995;23:407–413.

Azar FM, Andrews JR, Wilk KE, et al. Operative treatment of ulnar collateral ligament injuries of the elbow in athletes. *Am J Sports Med*. 2000;28:16–23.

Conway JE, Jobe FW, Glousman RE, et al. Medial instability of the elbow in throwing athletes: treatment by repair or reconstruction of the ulnar collateral ligament. *J Bone Joint Surg Am*. 1992;74:67–83.

Jobe FW, Stark H, Lombardo SJ. Reconstruction of the ulnar collateral ligament in athletes. *J Bone Joint Surg Am*. 1986;68:1158–1163.

O'Driscoll SW, Lawton RL, Smith AM. The "moving valgus stress test" for medial collateral ligament tears of the elbow. *Am J Sports Med*. 2005;33:231–239.

Thompson WH, Jobe FW, Yocum LA, et al. Ulnar collateral ligament reconstruction in athletes: muscle splitting approach without transposition of the ulnar nerve. *J Shoulder Elbow Surg*. 2001;10:152–157.

CHRONIC POSTEROLATERAL ROTATORY INSTABILITY OF THE ELBOW

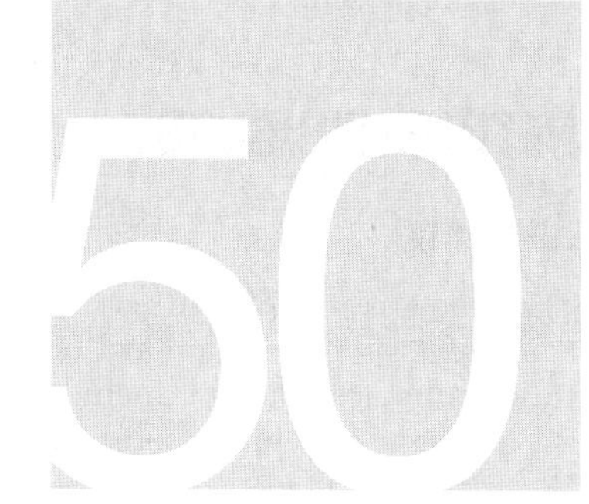

FELIX H. SAVOIE III
MELISSA A. YADAO
LARRY D. FIELD
J. RANDALL RAMSEY

In 1991, O'Driscoll introduced the term *posterolateral rotatory instability* (PLRI) to describe elbow instability caused by injury to the radial ulnohumeral ligament (RUHL) or lateral ulnar collateral ligament (LUCL). Since then the functional anatomy of the lateral collateral ligament complex has been closely examined, and the diagnosis and treatment of this condition have evolved with good results.

PATHOGENESIS

Etiology

The cause of PLRI may be traumatic or overuse. Traumatic injuries that produce subluxation events may result in PLRI. A fall onto a rotated forearm or a twisting event, such as a drill locking into an object and sending a supination force into the forearm or elbow, are typical mechanisms of injury. Unfortunately, surgical approaches to the lateral side of the elbow may also result in damage to the RUHL complex. Lateral epicondylitis surgery that involves the posterior/distal aspect of the epicondyle and radial head approaches for excision, replacement, or trauma may be associated with the development of PLRI.

Overuse conditions of the elbow have been reported by Cohen and Hastings to also result in PLRI. Repetitive use of the elbow when associated with a long-standing inflammatory response and weakness of the extensor musculature may result in stretching or disruption of the RUHL complex.

Epidemiology

O'Driscoll's original report described a group of patients who presented with symptoms of valgus instability after trauma but did not show typical clinical findings of a deficient medial collateral ligament complex. In this group, the radial head and lateral ulna rotated and subluxated posteriorly when the elbow was forced into valgus from a supinated and extended position. He attributed this instability to the incompetence of posterolateral structures, specifically the radial ulnohumeral ligament. Although these patients had responded poorly to the standard treatment for valgus instability, they did well after plication or reconstruction of this ligament. O'Driscoll named this condition posterolateral rotatory instability and developed the posterolateral rotatory instability test or pivot shift test to assist in diagnosis.

However, posterolateral rotatory instability is not really a new problem. In 1966 Osborne and Cotterill reported a group of patients with posterior subluxations of the radial head. Three of the 30 patients had normal exams. These authors felt that laxity in the posterolateral capsule caused this problem and successfully treated their patients with plication or repair of the lateral ligament complex.

In 1975, Symeonides et al. and Hassman et al. separately reported cases of recurrent elbow dislocations that were difficult to treat. One of the Hassman et al. patients clinically had a stable ulnohumeral joint despite a history of multiple dislocations. Other case reports described posttraumatic subluxations of the elbow that could be reproduced with maneuvers similar to the pivot shift test. The patients complained of locking and snapping of the elbow. Stress radiographs showed typical findings of PLRI: widening of the ulnohumeral joint space and posterior subluxation of the radial head.

These cases probably represent examples of what is now recognized as PLRI. The clinician should read the literature carefully as some reports of dislocations of the ulnohumeral joint or proximal radioulnar joint may indeed be misdiagnosed.

PATHOPHYSIOLOGY

Anatomy

The elbow is one of the most inherently stable joints because of its bony articulations and soft tissue stabilizers. The three bony articulations include the radiocapitellar joint, the proximal radioulnar joint, and the ulnohumeral joint. With trochlea cradled by the olecranon posterior and the coronoid anterior, the ulnohumeral joint provides the primary static restraint to varus/valgus, anterior/posterior, and rotatory motion at the elbow. The radiocapitellar joint is an important secondary stabilizer, accepting up to 60% axial loads when the elbow is extended.

The medial and lateral ligament complexes are the major static soft tissue stabilizers of the elbow. Three major components make up the medial or ulnar ligament complex (MCL): the anterior medial bundle, the posterior medial bundle, and the transverse oblique bundle. Although the proximal fibers have been described as distinct structures, distally they resemble more the ligaments of the shoulder as capsular thickenings.The medial ligament complex protects the elbow against valgus stress with the forearm in pronation.Biomechanical studies have shown that only the anterior and posterior bundles play important roles in elbow stability.

The lateral or radial ligament complex is made up of four components: the radial ulnohumeral ligament (RUHL) or lateral ulnar collateral ligament (LUCL), the radial collateral ligament (RCL), the annular ligament, and the accessory lateral collateral ligament (Fig. 50-1). Unlike the medial structures, these individual ligaments are often difficult to differentiate proximally where they originate as a broad band from the lateral epicondyle deep to the extensor wad. Distally, the fibers either remain as a single broad band or split into two bands, with the RCL constituting the more anterior band and the RUHL the posterior band. The annular ligament sweeps over the radial head and is thought to be a stabilizer of the proximal radioulnar joint. The RCL primarily restrains varus stress.

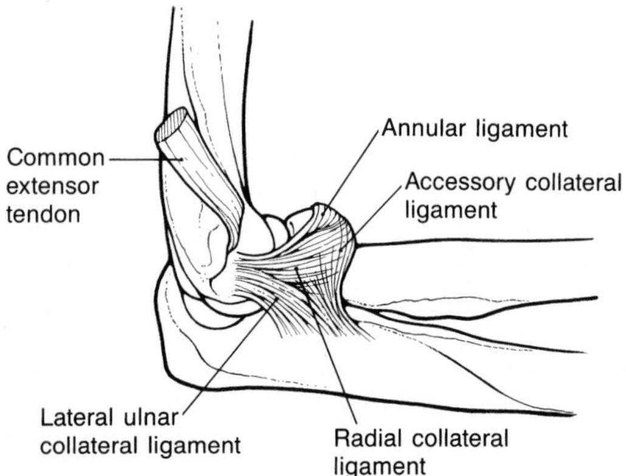

Figure 50-1 Anatomy of the lateral ligamentous complex of the elbow. Lateral ulnar collateral ligament = radial ulnohumeral ligament.

O'Driscoll has shown the RUHL to play a key role in PLRI. This ligament originates from the posterior inferior aspect of the lateral epicondyle and inserts on the supinator crest of the ulna. The RUHL is often difficult to distinguish proximally and is more easily identified at its distal insertion. Positioning the arm in varus and supination may help differentiate this structure from the RCL.

Other soft tissue structures of the elbow such as the capsule and musculature act as important dynamic stabilizers of the elbow. The capsule augments the strength of both the medial and lateral ligaments. With the elbow extended, the anterior capsule acts as a powerful restraint against varus and valgus stresses. Surgical techniques to restore stability incorporate the capsule with ligament plication. The anconeus and extensor wad are important dynamic restraints laterally whereas the flexor-pronator mass strengthens stability medially.

Injury Patterns

Anatomic studies by O'Driscoll and associates have shown that deficiencies of the RUHL and laxity of the lateral capsule allow the proximal radioulnar joint to rotate and the radial head to sublux posteriorly when stressed, leading to PLRI. In patients with this instability, the radial head subluxates, and on rare occasions, can dislocate posteriorly depending on the position of the elbow. With the forearm supinated and slightly flexed, valgus stress applied to the elbow causes rotation of the ulnohumeral joint, compression of the radiocapitellar joint, and posterior subluxation of the radial head. Extreme supination of the forearm stresses the posterolateral structures whereas flexing the elbow releases the olecranon tip from the olecranon fossa, allowing rotation of the ulnohumeral joint.

The proximal radioulnar joint must remain intact for PLRI to occur. During posterolateral rotation, the proximal forearm rotates as a unit so that the coronoid passes under the trochlea as the radial head moves posterior. This explains why hyperflexion or extensor results in reduction of the instability. In O'Driscoll's anatomic studies, the annular ligament was intact in all specimens. The integrity of this joint distinguishes PLRI from other instabilities such as recurrent dislocations of the radial head and elbow where disruption of this joint was thought necessary for dislocation to occur.

Recent biomechanical studies have attempted to define the functional anatomy of the entire lateral collateral ligament complex and its relation to PLRI. Cohen has shown that injury to the RUHL alone was not sufficient to cause instability. The entire lateral ligament complex as well as the lateral musculature played significant roles. Similarly, Dunning et al. demonstrated that the RUHL and the RCL needed to be cut before PLRI occurred. On the other hand, Seki et al. and Olsen et al. found that transection of either the RUHL or the RCL created this instability.

Although there is still much disagreement over the exact roles of the lateral ligament complex, most consider PLRI to be the first phase of elbow instability that can develop into frank dislocation. As proposed by Morrey and O'Driscoll individually, the mechanism leading to an unstable elbow is a progressive disruption of the ring of soft tissue stabilizers beginning laterally and sweeping medially. The first injured structure is the RUHL, resulting in PLRI that can reduce spontaneously. Further injury tears anterior and posterior capsules, resulting in ulnohumeral subluxations. Complete dislocation occurs when the medial structures are disrupted, although the anterior band of the medial collateral ligament may be only minimally injured.

Classification

There is no specific classification system for PLRI.

DIAGNOSIS

History and Physical Examination

Clinical Features

The patient with PLRI often presents with vague complaining of lateral elbow pain. The differential diagnosis of PLRI includes lateral epicondylitis, radial tunnel syndrome, valgus instability, and pure proximal radial head dislocation. Standard valgus/varus instability tests are often normal. Valgus instability should be tested with the forearm supinated and pronated. With valgus loads, pronation of the forearm tests the medial collateral ligamentous complex, whereas supination stresses posterolateral structures, in particular the RUHL.

Several provocative tests, including the posterolateral rotatory instability test or pivot shift test developed by O'Driscoll, can help make the diagnosis. The pivot shift test for the elbow resembles the pivot shift test for the anterior cruciate ligament (ACL)–deficient knee. With the patient supine, the arm is raised overhead, stabilizing the humerus to prevent external rotation. With the forearm fully supinated and the elbow extended, a valgus-supination force is applied to the elbow while slowing flexing it from an extended position. As a result, the ulnohumeral joint rotates and the radiohumeral joint subluxes posteriorly, sometimes even dislocating (Fig. 50-2A). Dimpling of the skin may be seen proximal to the subluxing radial head. As the elbow is flexed >40 degrees, the clinician may hear or feel the radiohumeral joint suddenly reduce.

This test is not easy to perform on the awake patient. Feelings of pain or apprehension are considered a positive result in such patients in the absence of instability. We prefer to perform the pivot shift test with the patient positioned prone. Resting the arm over the edge of the table stabilizes the humerus, allowing the examiner to more easily palpate the radiohumeral joint during the examination (Fig. 50-2B, C).

Two other provocative maneuvers designed by Regan simulate the pivot shift test. The first requires the patient to push up from a prone or wall position with the forearms maximally pronated so that the thumbs are turned toward each other. The test is repeated with forearms maximally supinated. The patient with PLRI will not want to allow the elbow to fully flex, describing a felling of pain and/or instability. Another test requires a patient to push up out of a chair using the armrests. With palms facing inward, essentially placing them in supination, pushing up will produce similar symptoms of pain.

Most patients will describe a history of trauma. Although elbow dislocation is the inciting event in 75% of patients younger than 20 years of age, varus extension stress without true dislocation is more likely the initiating event in older patients. PLRI can also occur secondary to repetitive stresses on the elbow. Some patients who present with lateral epicondylitis may also have PLRI. Repetitive motion may produce laxity in the lateral ligamentous complex, leading to secondary lateral epicondylitis. Previous surgery to the lateral side of the elbow can cause iatrogenic instability. PLRI has also been reported following radial head excision.

Most patients complain of pain, weakness to grip, and occasionally giving way of the elbow. As the instability may overstress the lateral musculature, lateral epicondylitis symptoms are common. The subluxation events may produce swelling in the posterolateral capsule and enlarged plica with resulting secondary plica syndrome. True dislocations tend to be rare. Rather, patients describe the elbow slipping in and out of the joint in certain positions but especially when the arm is supinated and slightly flexed.

Radiologic Features

Standard anteroposterior (AP) and lateral radiographs of the elbow should be obtained but are often normal. Bony avulsions following ligament injury can be identified. On lateral views, typical PLRI radiographic findings include widening of the ulnohumeral joint space with posterior subluxation of the radial head. These are best illustrated with radiographic or fluoroscopic stress views while performing the pivot shift test with the patient under anesthesia (Fig. 50-3A, B). Associated changes include degenerative changes on the capitellum and spur formation on the lateral aspect of the olecranon.

Currently MRI plays a limited role. Although the RUHL and any such injuries can be identified on MRI using special sequencing, this study requires experience in elbow MRI by both the radiologist and MRI technician.MR arthrograms may prove more useful, especially in posttraumatic cases.

Exam under Anesthesia and Arthroscopy

In difficult cases an exam under anesthesia with fluoroscopy may be valuable in making the diagnosis. Diagnostic arthroscopy can also demonstrate PLRI in a patient in whom instability is suspected. The pivot shift test should be performed while viewing from the anteromedial portal. The radial head will rotate and translate posterior if PLRI is present; with a competent ligament, the radial head will rotate but not translate (Fig. 50-4A, B). In addition, while viewing from the posterolateral portal, we have found the arthroscope can be easily driven through the lateral gutter and into the lateral aspect of the ulnohumeral joint if instability is present. We have described this as the "elbow drive through" sign, resembling the drive through sign in shoulder instability (Fig. 50-4C).

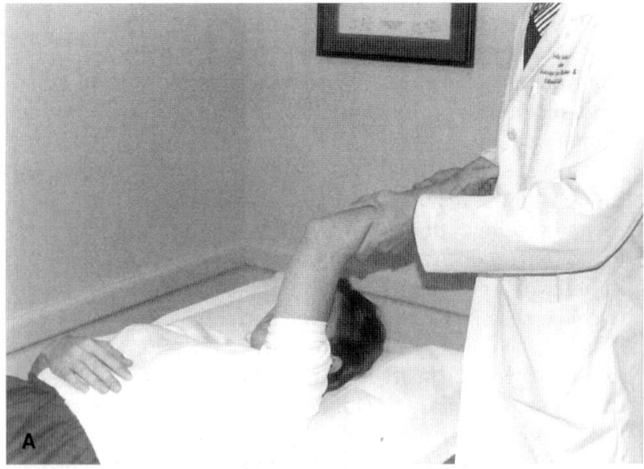

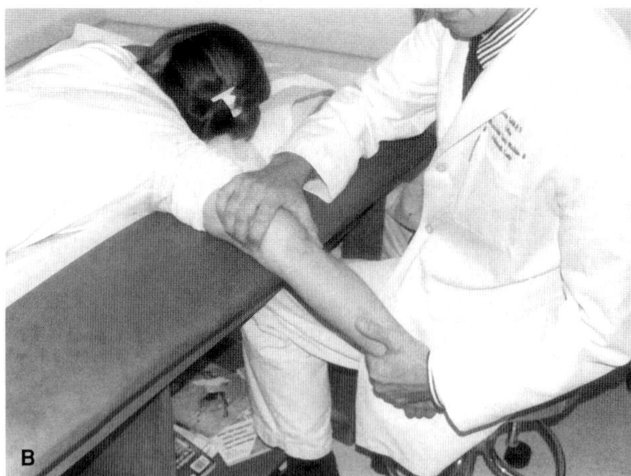

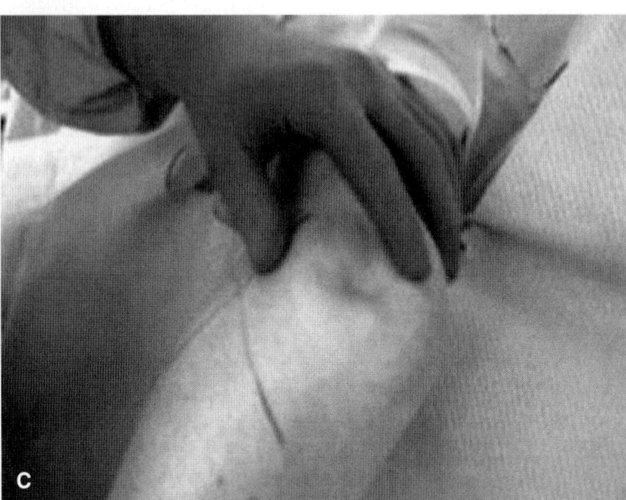

Figure 50-2 The posterolateral rotatory instability (PLRI) test or pivot shift test. The test is performed by applying a valgus stress to the elbow with the humerus stabilized and the forearm maximally supinated. Symptoms occur as the arm is brought from full extension into slight flexion. **A:** Performing the test in the supine position maximally externally rotates the arm and allows the examiner to use both hands to manipulate the elbow. **B:** Performing the test with the patient prone stabilizes the humerus and frees one hand to more easily palpate the radiohumeral joint. **C:** Exam under anesthesia demonstrates the subluxation of severe PLRI.

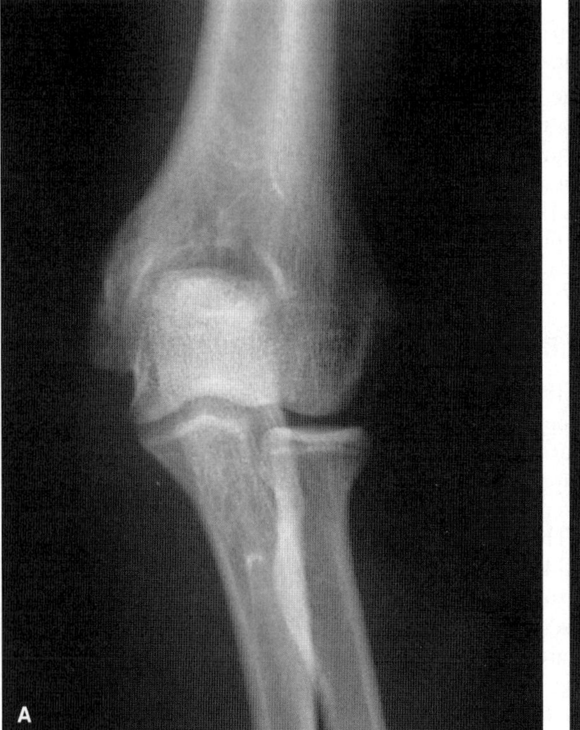

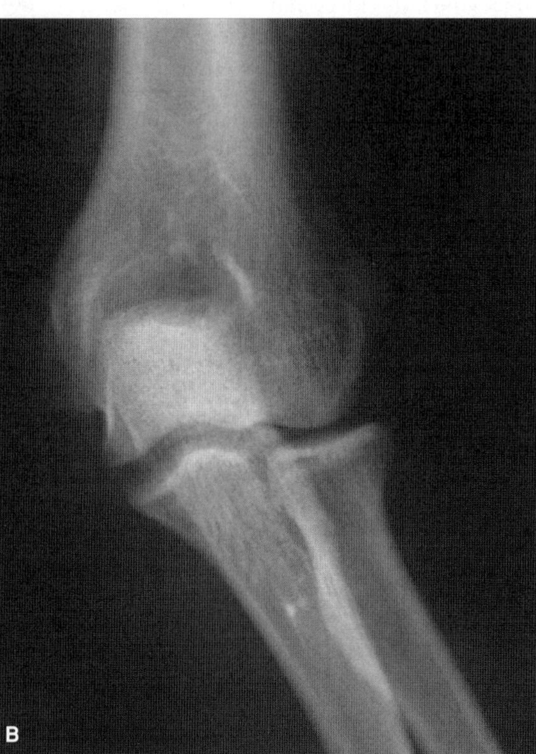

Figure 50-3 Neutral (**A**) and stress (**B**) views of the elbow demonstrate widening of the ulnohumeral joint and posterior subluxation of the radial head.

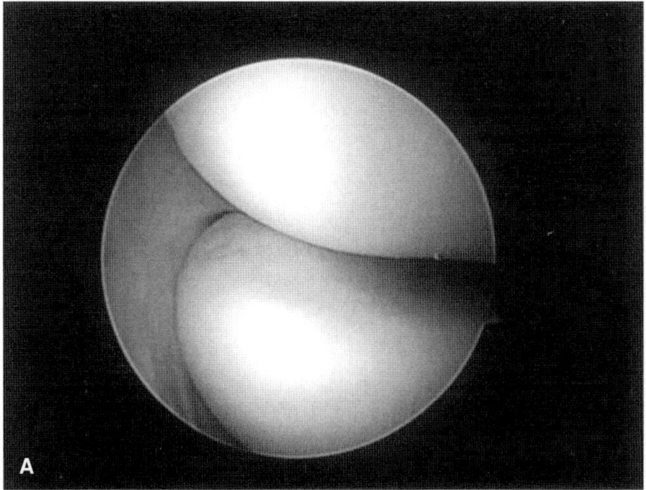

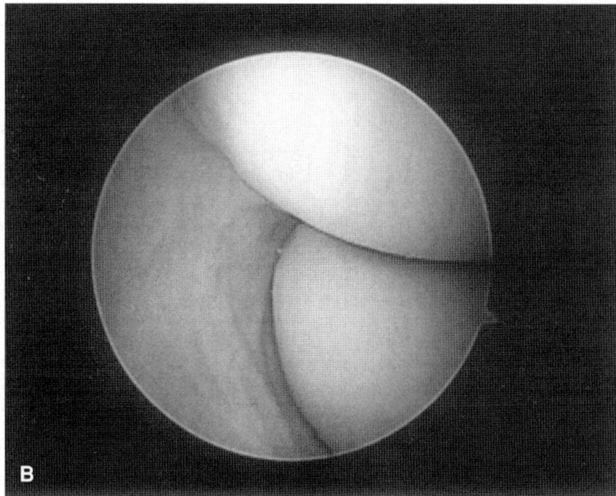

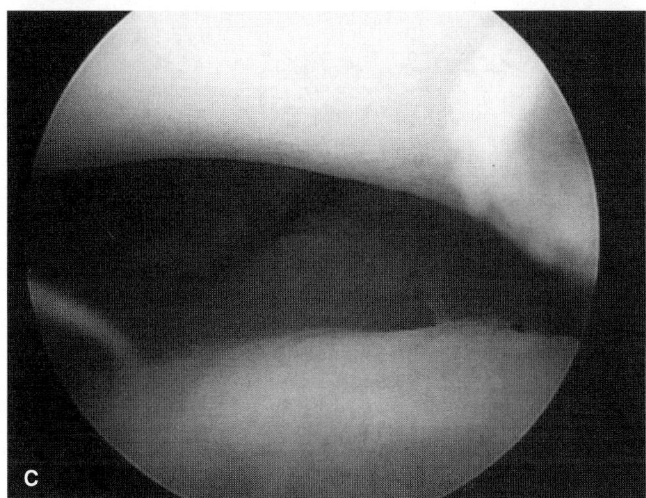

Figure 50-4 Arthroscopic findings of PLRI. **A:** The view from the anteromedial portal shows the normal position of the radial head with the forearm in pronation. **B:** During the PLRI or pivot shift test, the radial head can be seen to sublux posteriorly. In a stable elbow, the radial head would rotate but not translate posteriorly. **C:** Drive through sign.

SURGICAL INDICATIONS/ CONTRAINDICATIONS

The most difficult aspect of the management of posterolateral instability is often making the correct diagnosis. Once that is made, appropriate treatment measures may be taken.

Nonoperative Treatment

Nonoperative management of PLRI is focused on eliminating the secondary, pain-producing pathology; often a simple elbow sleeve will provide sensory feedback and stabilize the elbow enough to significantly reduce subluxation events. NSAIDs in pill and cream form may help with the swelling and inflammation of the extensors, muscles, and plica. Physiotherapy to include pain control modalities, tissue massage, extensor muscle strengthening, and biofeedback exercises to control subluxation may be helpful as well (Fig. 50-5).

Operative Treatment

The only indication for operative management is pain and functional impairment in the affected elbow not relieved by nonoperative management. Radiographic or MRI evidence alone is not a sufficient indication. Contraindications may include an uncooperative patient, psychiatric disorders, grade II or worse arthritis, or surgical inexperience with the reconstructive techniques and anatomic variations associated with this instability.

Posterolateral instability may be managed by open plication/repair, open graft reconstruction, or arthroscopic plication/repair. The specific technique used depends more on the surgeon's preference, experience, and the number of previous surgeries rather than any specific guidelines.

Open Technique

Open Repair. O'Driscoll originally described an open technique to plicate, repair, and reconstruct the RUHL. With the patient supine, the elbow is entered through a modified Kocher approach, exposing the entire lateral ligament complex from the lateral epicondyle to the supinator crest. The pivot shift test is performed to identify laxity in the lateral capsule and insufficiencies of the RUHL. An attenuated or detached ligament can be repaired by reattaching the ligament through bone to the posterior inferior lateral epicondyle. The ligament can be advanced or imbricated as needed. The loose capsule is

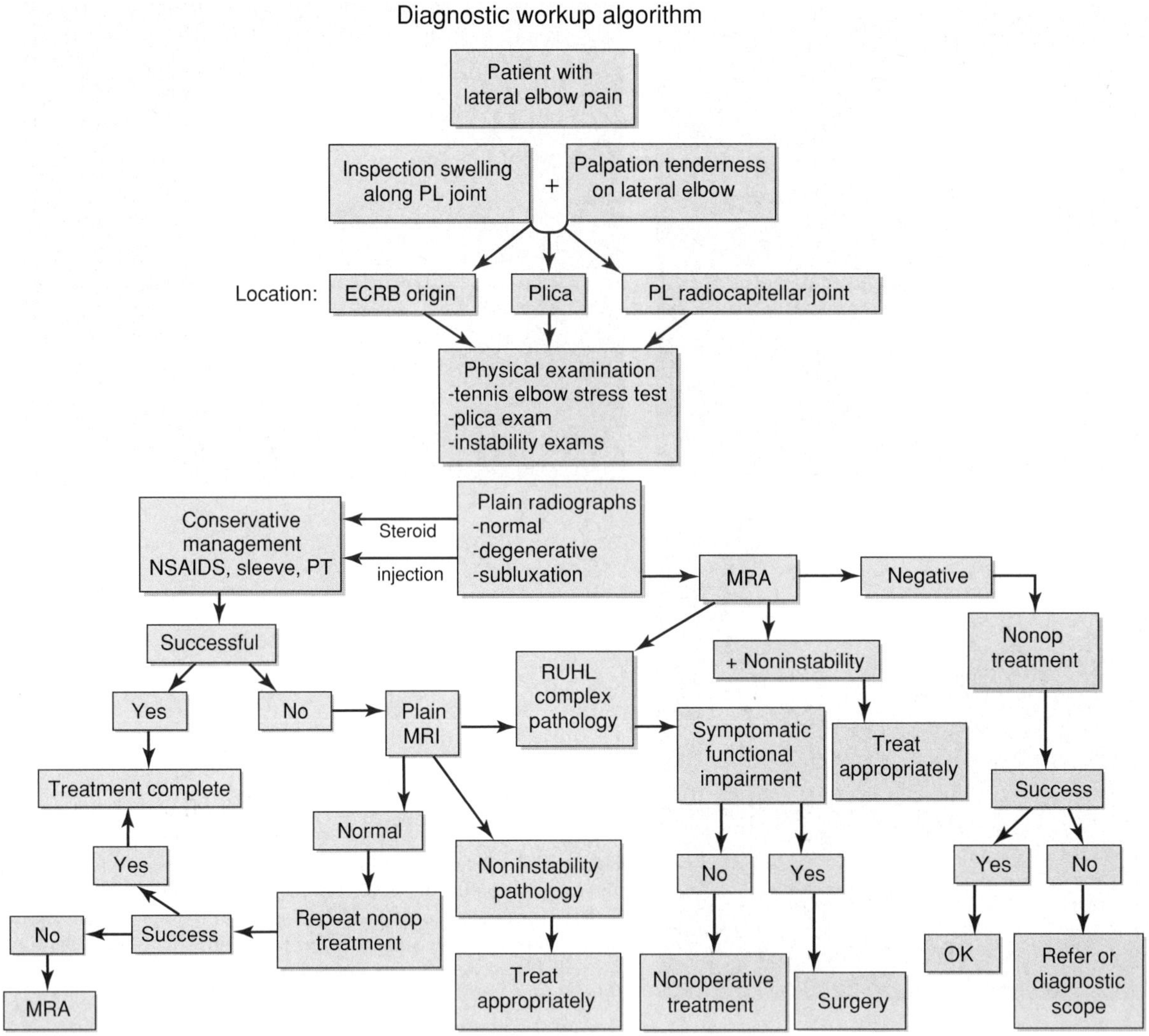

Figure 50-5 Diagnostic workup algorithm. PL, posterolateral; ECRB, extensor carpi radialis brevis; NSAIDs, nonsteroidal anti-inflammatory drugs; PT, physiotherapy; MRA, magnetic resonance arthrogram; MRI, magnetic resonance imaging; RUHL, radial ulnohumeral ligament.

plicated with sutures tied following completion of the repair (Fig. 50-6A). One simple technique for doing this is to place double-sutured anchors at the origin of the RUHL on the condyle. One set of sutures can be used to plicate the ligament and repair it to the epicondyle while the second is used to repair any associated damage to the extensor muscle.

Open Reconstruction. Reconstruction with tendon autograft or allograft may be necessary should the ligament tissue be of poor quality owing to extensive trauma, multiple previous surgeries, or excessive injections. In this technique an open posterolateral extensile approach is used. The anconeus is retracted and any residual ligament or capsule split longitudinally. The anatomic origin and insertion sites are identified and then tested using a suture while ranging the elbow. We normally drill our tunnel into the insertion site or the supinated crest of the ulna first using a Beath pin. This pin is then overreamed with a 5.5- or 6-mm reamer unicortically. The midportion of the graft is then pulled into the tunnel until it contacts the ulnar cortex, and the graft is fixed into the ulnar tunnel using an interference screw. The isometric point on the humerus is then retested, and the proximal end of the graft is passed into the tunnel and fixed using either a docking technique, Endobutton, or interference screw. The elbow is positioned in 40-degree flexion and the forearm fully pronated (Fig. 50-6B).

The palmaris graft is the most commonly used autograft. The semitendinosus is the most common allograft. Single or double limbs of the graft can be passed through the isometric origin of the lateral epicondyle. However, a recent study by King et al. has shown no biomechanical differences between single- or double-strand grafts.

Arthroscopic Repair and Plication

Arthroscopic techniques have recently been developed to plicate or repair the RUHL. As mentioned earlier, PLRI can be diagnosed by a posterior subluxing radial head during a pivot shift test or by seeing a drive through sign. While

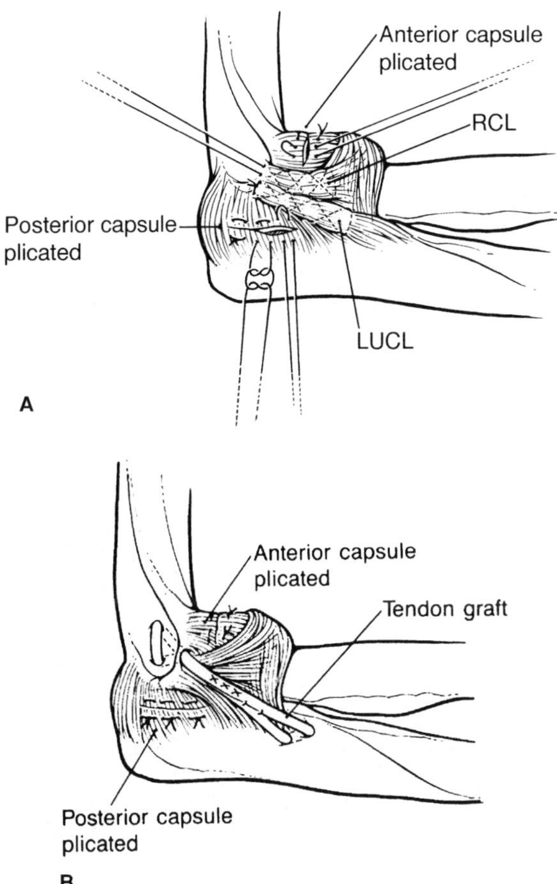

Figure 50-6 Open lateral reconstruction for PLRI as described by O'Driscoll. **A:** Repair of the radial ulnohumeral ligament by imbricating the ligament and reattaching it to its insertion point on the lateral epicondyle. The redundant posterolateral capsule is also plicated. **B:** Reconstruction of the ligament with a free tendon graft. It is essential to place the ligament in its correct anatomic position on the humeral epicondyle and supinator crest of the ulna. The posterolateral capsule is also plicated. RCL, radial collateral ligament; LUCL, lateral ulnar collateral ligament.

viewing through the posterolateral portal, the surgeon passes an absorbable suture into the joint through a spinal needle placed into the joint directly adjacent to the lateral aspect of the proximal ulna at the level of the supinator crest (Fig. 50-7A). The first two sutures pierce the annular ligament. The suture is retrieved adjacent to the posterior inferior aspect of the lateral epicondyle, near the normal origin site of the RUHL. Four to seven sutures can be passed, starting distal to proximal. The two ends of each suture are brought out together through a lateral incision and are tied separately in the same order. By pulling the sutures prior to tying, one should see the lateral structures tighten and the lateral gutter space collapse (Fig. 50-7B–D).

If a humeral avulsion is found, the repair can be augmented with a suture anchor. Through an additional portal, the anchor is placed at the isometric point onto the posterior aspect of the lateral epicondyle. One limb is passed into the joint, lassoing all the plication sutures before being retrieved near the ulna. The plication sutures are then tied, closing the lateral gutter and plication the entire lateral ligament complex. The suture from the anchor is then passed subcutaneously back over the tied sutures to the anchor portal; tying this suture then pulls the entire plicated ligament complex back toward the humerus, essentially reattaching the entire ligament complex to the lateral epicondyle.

Postoperative Management

Postoperative rehabilitation is similar following either technique. Patients are immediately immobilized in a splint with the elbow flexed to 70 to 90 degrees with the arm in full pronation. After 1 to 2 weeks, limited flexion of 45 to 90 degrees is initiated with the elbow protected in a double-hinged elbow brace. Full range of motion in the brace is allowed at 3 weeks. Full painless range of motion should be achieved by 6 weeks, following which wrist and elbow strengthening exercises in the brace are started. At 10 to 12 weeks, the brace can be removed once the patient can perform all strengthening exercises in the brace painfree.

RESULTS AND OUTCOME

Few results following surgical management of PLRI are described in the literature. In O'Driscoll's first paper, four of five patients were followed for 15 to 30 months. None had any recurrence of instability, and all achieved full range of motion. In a follow-up study by Nestor et al. on 11 patients, 3 patients underwent repair whereas 7 underwent ligament reconstruction with palmaris graft. Stability was achieved in ten patients with seven having an excellent functional result.

On reviewing his series of patients, O'Driscoll has found 90% satisfaction with no subluxations if the radial head is intact and no degenerative articular changes are present. Patient satisfaction decreases to 67% to 75% in the face of radial head excision or arthritis. Mild flexion contracture (10 degrees) is accepted as it protects against instability. Recurrent laxity or redislocation has been reported but usually occurs after reinjury involving significant stress.

We have retrospectively reviewed 54 patients with an average follow-up of 41 months (range 12 to 103 months) who underwent operative management of PLRI at our institution. Diagnostic arthroscopy confirmed PLRI in all patients. Thirty-seven patients were treated with open techniques: 34 had ligament repair and 3 had reconstruction with tendon graft. Seventeen patients were treated with arthroscopy: 11 had ligament plication alone whereas 6 required an anchor to augment the repair.

Twenty-five percent of patients had a previous history of lateral epicondyle release. Indications for open rather than arthroscopic repair included having concurrent procedures such as lateral epicondyle release, open extensor mass avulsion repairs, and release of the posterior interosseous nerve.

Overall Andrew-Carson scores improved significantly for all repairs from 145 to 180 ($p < 0.0001$). Subjective scores improved from 57 to 85 ($p < 0.0001$) and objective scores

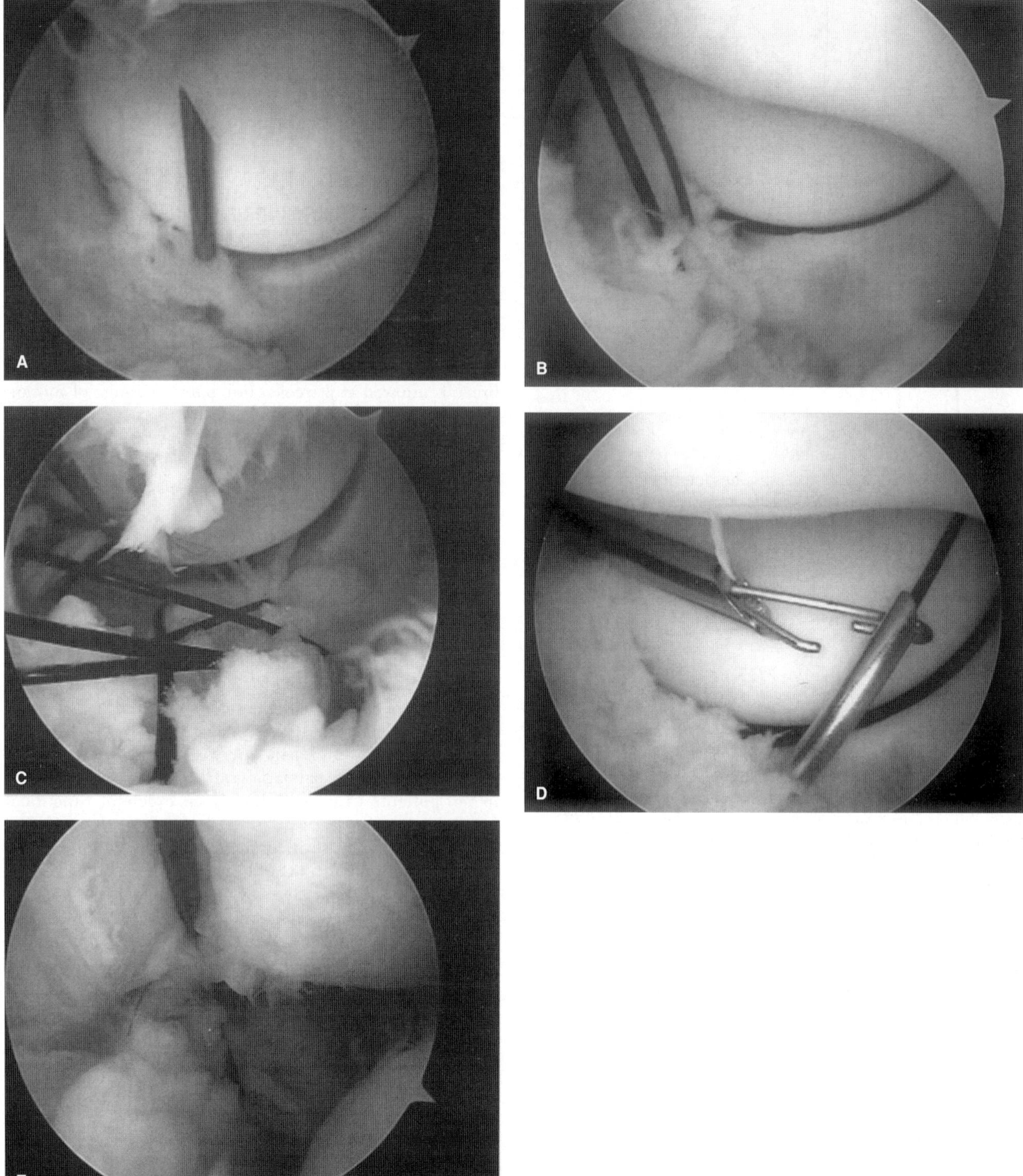

Figure 50-7 Arthroscopic reconstruction of posterolateral instability is accomplished by passing plication sutures through the ulnar side of the ligament with a spinal needle (**A**), retrieving them through the humeral side (**B**). These sutures are then retrieved out the soft spot portal and tied, closing the lateral ligament complex (**C**). This complex may be repaired to the humerus by passing a stitch around the plicated sutures (**D**) and tying the entire complex to the humerus.

from 88 to 95 ($p = 0.008$). Open repairs improved from 146 to 176 ($p = 0.0001$) and arthroscopic repairs from 144 to 182 ($p < 0.001$). Overall, open and arthroscopic techniques were shown to be equally effective (unpublished data).

CONCLUSION

Posterolateral rotatory instability should be considered in a patient who complains of vague elbow pain and giving way with a history of an elbow dislocation or previous lateral elbow surgery. Although the topic is currently debated, the radial ulnohumeral ligament does play an important role in this instability. Future investigations will help determine the exact role of the lateral collateral ligament complex in the unstable elbow. Indeed, PLRI is part of a continuum of injury from instability to frank dislocation.

The diagnosis of PLRI can be difficult as the provocative tests are challenging to perform and radiographic studies are not helpful. Early recognition following acute trauma and attention to detail during open elbow procedures provide the best prevention of PLRI. Diagnostic arthroscopy is an excellent tool to demonstrate this instability. Although arthroscopic plication and repair have shown to be as effective as open techniques, the clinician should be prepared for open reconstruction if needed.

SUGGESTED READINGS

Abe M, Ishizu T, Morikawa J. Posterolateral rotatory instability of the elbow after post-traumatic cubitus varus. *J Shoulder Elbow Surg*. 1997;6:405–409.

An KN, Morrey BF. Biomechanics of the elbow. In: Morrey BF, ed. *The Elbow and Its Disorders*. 3rd ed. Philadelphia: WB Saunders; 2000:43–60.

Burgess RC, Sprague HH. Post-traumatic posterior radial head subluxation. Two case reports. *Clin Orthop*. 1984;186:192–194.

Cohen MS, Hastings H II. Acute elbow dislocation: evaluation and management. *J Am Acad Orthop Surg*. 1998;6:15–33.

Cohen MS, Hastings H II. Rotatory instability of the elbow: The anatomy and role of the lateral stabilizers. *J Bone Joint Surg Am*. 1997;79:225–233.

Dunning CE, Zarzour ZDS, Patterson SD, et al. Ligamentous stabilizers against posterolateral rotatory instability of the elbow. *J Bone Joint Surg*. 2001;83A:1823–1828.

Eygendaal D, Verdegaal SHM, Obermann WR, et al. Posterolateral dislocation of the elbow joint: relationship to medial instability. *J Bone Joint Surg Am*. 2000;82:555–560.

Guerra JJ, Timmerman LA. Clinical anatomy, histology, and pathomechanics of the elbow in sports. *Operative Techniques Sports Med*. 1996;4:69–76.

Hassman GC, Brunn F, Neer CS II. Recurrent dislocation of the elbow. *J Bone Joint Surg Am*. 1975;57:1080–1084.

King GJW, Dunning CE, Zarzour DS, et al. Single-strand reconstruction of the lateral ulnar collateral ligament restores varus and posterolateral instability of the elbow. *J Shoulder Elbow Surg*. 2002;11:60–64.

Morrey BF. Acute and chronic instability of the elbow. *J Am Acad Orthop Surg*. 1996;4:117–128.

Morrey BF. Anatomy of the elbow joint. In: Morrey BF, ed. *The Elbow and Its Disorders*. 3rd ed. Philadelphia: WB Saunders; 2000:13–42.

Morrey BF, An KN. Articular and ligamentous contributions to the stability of the elbow joint. *Am J Sports Med*. 1983;11:315–319.

Morrey BF, An KN. Functional anatomy of the ligaments of the elbow. *Clin Orthop*. 1985;201:84–90.

Nestor BJ, O'Driscoll SW, Morrey BF. Ligamentous reconstruction for posterolateral rotatory instability of the elbow. *J Bone Joint Surg Am*. 1992;74:1235–1241.

O'Driscoll SW. Elbow dislocations. In: Morrey BF, ed. *The Elbow and Its Disorders*. 3rd ed. Philadelphia: WB Saunders; 2000:409–420.

O'Driscoll SW, Bell DF, Morrey BF. Posterolateral rotatory instability of the elbow. *J Bone Joint Surg Am*. 1991;73:440–446.

O'Driscoll SW, Jupiter JB, King GJW, et al. The unstable elbow. In: Sin FH, ed. *Instructional Course Lectures 50*. Rosemont, IL: American Academy of Orthopaedic Surgeons; 2001:89–100.

O'Driscoll SW, Morrey BF, Korinek S, et al. Elbow subluxation and dislocation: a spectrum of instability. *Clin Orthop*. 1992;280:186–197.

Olsen BS, Sojbjerg JO, Neilsen KK, et al. Posterolateral elbow joint instability: The basic kinematics. *J Shoulder Elbow Surg*. 1998;7:19–29.

Osborne G, Cotterill P. Recurrent dislocation of the elbow. *J Bone Joint Surg Br*. 1966:48:340–346.

Potter HG, Weiland AJ, Schatz JA, et al. Posterolateral rotatory instability of the elbow: usefulness of MR imaging in diagnosis. *Radiology*. 1997;204:185–189.

Rohrbough JT, Altchek DW, Hyman J, et al. Medial collateral ligament reconstruction of the elbow using the docking technique. *Am J Sports Med*. 2002;30:541–548.

Seki A, Olsen BS, Jensen SL, et al. Functional anatomy of the lateral collateral ligament complex of the elbow: configuration of Y and its role. *J Shoulder Elbow Surg*. 2002;11:53–59.

Smith JP III, Savoie FH III, Field LD. Posterolateral rotatory lateral instability of the elbow. *Clin Orthop*. 2001;20:47–58.

Symeonides PP, Paschaloglou C, Stavrou Z, et al. Recurrent dislocation of the elbow: report of three cases. *J Bone Joint Surg Am*. 1975;57:1084–1086.

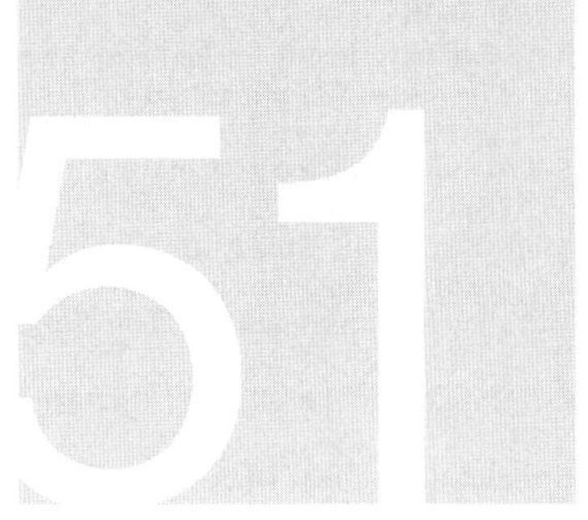

TREATMENT OF ACUTE ELBOW DISLOCATIONS

MICHAEL A. KUHN
HERVEY L. KIMBALL
GLEN ROSS

PATHOGENESIS

Etiology

Once poorly defined, the mechanism of elbow dislocation is now better understood. Traditional teaching stated that the mechanism of injury was hyperextension. A fall on the outstretched hand is the most common cause. The elbow experiences an axial compressive force during flexion as the body approaches the ground. The body rotates internally, with the forearm rotating externally to the trunk. This results in a supination moment at the elbow. At that point, the mechanical axis of the extremity is medial to the elbow, resulting in a valgus moment. O'Driscoll and Morrey suggest that an extension varus stress disrupts the lateral ligament complex first. If this dissipates the force, then a perched dislocation is the result. Continued force causes forearm rotation tearing the capsule, resulting in a complete dislocation. This has been described as the "ring of instability" progressing from disruption of the lateral ulnar collateral ligament (LUCL) to the capsule, and finally injury to the medial ulnar collateral ligament (MUCL). With a slightly flexed elbow, a tear in the medial collateral ligament complex occurs and the elbow dislocates.

While the tensile forces around the elbow result in ligamentous disruption, substantial compressive and shear forces occur on the articular surface. This can cause fractures of the proximal radius. Dislocations treated by open procedures have documented chondral injuries to the capitellum and trochlear surfaces at higher rates than previously believed. Understanding the mechanism of injury is important for appreciating classification, interpreting radiographs, formulating a treatment plan, anticipating complications, and guiding follow-up care.

Epidemiology

The elbow is the most commonly dislocated major joint in the pediatric age group and the second most common in the adult population. It is estimated that 6 of every 100,000 individuals will sustain an elbow dislocation during their lifetime. Elbow dislocations constitute 10% to 25% of all injuries to the elbow. More than one half of dislocations involve the nondominant extremity. It has been suggested that there is a protective instinct using the dominant side to protect from a fall. The mean age of an individual sustaining this injury is 30 years. There is a male predominance with 2 to 2.5 that of females with similar ratios in children.

Approximately 40% of elbow dislocations occur during sports. Gymnastics, wrestling, basketball, and football are commonly involved. Approximately 40% of dislocations have a poorly defined causes.

Pathophysiology

The injury progresses as a circle of tissue disruption from lateral to medial and can be broken into three stages. Stage 1 involves disruption of the ulnar component of the lateral collateral ligament. This results in posterolateral rotatory subluxation of the elbow, which reduces spontaneously. With continued force, disruption occurs anteriorly and posteriorly allowing for an incomplete posterolateral dislocation. This is a perched dislocation. Stage 3 has two parts. In stage 3A, all soft tissues are disrupted including the posterior part of the medial collateral ligament. The anterior band of the medial collateral ligament remains intact. This allows for posterior dislocation by the previously described posterolateral rotatory mechanism. In stage 3B, the entire medial collateral complex is disrupted. Varus, valgus, and rotatory instability are present. Surgical experience suggests that the medial collateral complex is disrupted in nearly 100% of elbow dislocations. Violation of the anterior bundle of the medial collateral ligament is considered the essential lesion. Disruption proximally from the humerus is most common. Dislocation is the final of three sequential stages of elbow instability, resulting from posterolateral ulnohumeral rotatory subluxation, with soft tissue disruption occurring from lateral to medial.

Classification

Traditional classification divides elbow dislocations into posterior, anterior, and divergent. Anterior dislocations are uncommon, occurring in only 1% to 2% of incidents. Anterior dislocations are usually seen in younger individuals. Posterior dislocations are divided based on the final relationship between the humerus and olecranon into posterior, posterolateral, posteromedial, and pure lateral dislocations. Posterolateral is most common, followed by lateral, and least commonly, posteromedial. A divergent dislocation is a rare injury associated with high-energy trauma. Displacement of the radius from the ulna occurs, resulting in disruption of the interosseous membrane, annular ligament, and distal radioulnar joint capsule.

Morrey proposed a simple classification distinguishing between a perched and complete dislocation. A medial or lateral resting position of the complete dislocation makes little difference with regard to treatment or prognosis. A perched dislocation is one in which the elbow is actually subluxated but the coronoid appears to impinge on the trochlea. In this type, the ligaments are less severely injured, and rehabilitation can be more rapid and recovery more complete.

DIAGNOSIS

Evaluation

Prior to any reduction, assessment of neurovascular status is mandatory. Anteroposterior and lateral radiographs should be obtained if possible. Evaluation of associated injuries should be reserved until reduction has been obtained. Computerized tomography and magnetic resonance imaging are often of limited value. These are reserved if adequate radiographs cannot be obtained, and can be used for later reconstructive planning.

Associated Injuries

Associated injuries with elbow dislocation are common. Radial head and neck fractures occur in 5% to 10% of elbow dislocations. Avulsion fractures of the medial or the lateral epicondyles occur in approximately 12% of the cases, and coronoid fractures occur in 10% of dislocations. The incidence of associated fractures in children is high, approaching 50%. With open physes, a medial epicondyle avulsion is the most common associated injury. Incarceration of the fragment can occur. Although prereduction and postreduction radiographs reveal periarticular fractures in 12% to 60% of dislocations, operative findings have revealed unrecognized osteochondral injuries in nearly 100% of acute elbow dislocations. The vast majority of these injuries are small fractures not requiring operative intervention.

Neurovascular injuries are rare, but can be potentially devastating. There are multiple case reports of brachial artery injuries with posterior dislocation. Although it may not be necessary to explore the brachial artery routinely if a radial pulse is present, it is accepted that disruption of the brachial artery should be treated with ligation and vein grafting. Median nerve entrapment has been reported with relocation of a dislocated elbow. The median nerve may be displaced posteriorly through a space created by avulsion of the medial epicondyle or the common flexor origin. This can result in a tension of the median nerve across the margin of the epicondylar flare and may "notch" the bone, producing a late radiographic sign known as the Matev sign.

With a dislocated elbow, extensive soft tissue swelling commonly occurs. Intact structures including the forearm fascia, the biceps tendon, and the lacertus fibrosis may exert a constricting effect resulting in increased compartment pressures. Compartment syndrome is possible and should be considered. Careful observation is required, and differentiation from neurologic stretch injuries is necessary.

TREATMENT

Nonsurgical Treatment

An expeditious atraumatic reduction is the goal. This is often best accomplished with conscious sedation or general anesthesia with adequate muscle relaxation. Muscle relaxation is the key to joint reduction. Care is taken to avoid multiple reduction attempts. A prone traction and countertraction maneuver is often successful (Fig. 51-1). Reduction is usually achieved by extending the elbow with countertraction on the arm and a thumb used to manipulate the coronoid clearing the trochlea. Perched dislocation can be treated with intra-articular analgesia and sedation whereas

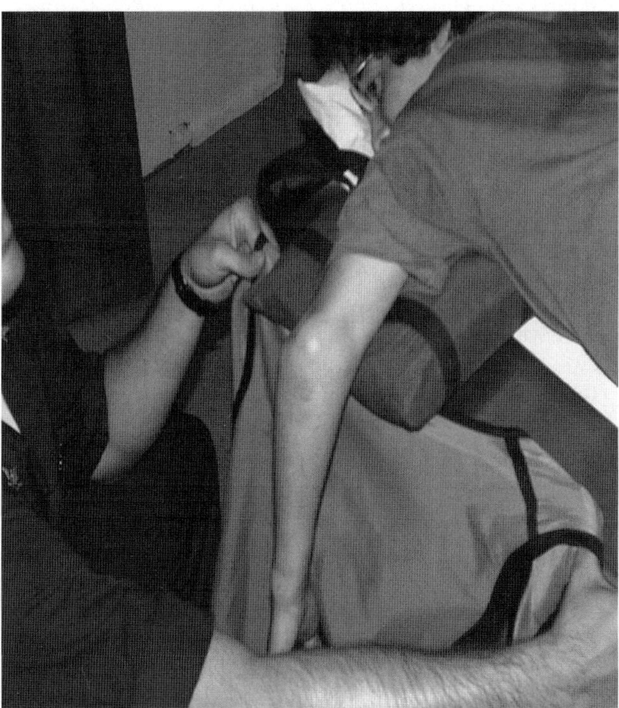

Figure 51-1 Prone position for traction/countertraction elbow relocation.

a complete dislocation may require general anesthesia and a muscle relaxant. Uncommonly, a dislocation occurs that is irreducible by closed reduction. This is most frequently associated with fractures. When a dislocation is irreducible, the radial head has been shown to be trapped in the soft tissues of the forearm or can buttonhole through the forearm fascia. These require surgical intervention. Surgical repair of ligaments without associated fractures in the acute dislocation has not been shown to improve return to activity or function.

Following reduction, instability is best assessed with the patient under anesthesia or an anesthetized elbow. The quality of joint reduction provides a clue to postreduction stability. Palpating a reduction "clunk" is a favorable sign of joint stability. The elbow is examined for valgus, varus, and posterolateral rotatory instability. Both varus and valgus instability are performed with the elbow in full extension and flexion up to 30 degrees. Most dislocated elbows are unstable to a valgus stress. This is best tested with the forearm in pronation to lock the lateral side. It is important to evaluate the tendency for redislocation occurring in extension, which can signify a potentially unstable joint. Posterolateral rotatory instability is diagnosed by the lateral pivot shift test. A positive test is manifested by a clunk that is heard and felt when the ulna and radius reduce on the humerus.

Postreduction radiographs should be obtained to confirm a concentric reduction. Anteroposterior and lateral views should be obtained. Widening of the joint space may indicate entrapped osteochondral fragments, which must be removed surgically. Posterolateral rotatory instability may also present as a nonconcentric reduction.

The wrist and shoulder should be examined to rule out concomitant injuries, which occur in 10% to 15% of cases. The distal radioulnar joint and interosseous membrane should be evaluated for tenderness and instability to rule out injury.

Surgical Treatment

All complete elbow dislocations without large periarticular fractures result in medial and lateral ligament ruptures. Rarely is surgical treatment necessary in the acute setting. Josefsson et al. evaluated 31 acute elbow dislocations without concomitant fractures. Under anesthesia nine were unstable with full extension. They surgically explored all 31 elbows, finding ruptures of the medial and lateral ligaments. The tendency of elbows to dislocate correlated with the degree of muscular injury to the flexor-pronator and extensor origins on the humerus. They concluded that muscular flexor and extensor origins represent secondary stabilizers of the elbow. If they are intact, they provide adequate stability to allow ligamentous healing after elbow dislocation. Prospective studies have failed to show improvement of early collateral ligament repair over early motion after a simple elbow dislocation.

Acute surgical intervention is indicated in few incidents. An open elbow dislocation and acute compartment syndrome require urgent intervention. Postreduction instability requiring 50 to 60 degrees of flexion to remain stable may require intervention. Elbow dislocations with unstable fractures require surgical stabilization. The unstable elbow will redislocate even with a well-fitting cast or splint (Fig. 51-2). If this occurs, rigid external fixation with pins in the humerus and ulna are required to maintain a stable concentric reduction. Dynamic external fixation may be used allowing motion in the stable range of motion.

Rehabilitation

The results of treatment of a simple closed elbow dislocation are not universally successful. Most authors recommend a period of immobilization lasting from 3 to 10 days. Restoration of full range of motion, especially extension, is not reliably achieved. Nonimmobilization and early rapid motion under supervision has been shown to achieve range of motion within 5 degrees of extension of the contralateral elbow with an excellent functional outcome.

Patients with persistent loss of motion by 6 to 8 weeks postinjury require additional intervention. If by 6 to 8 weeks full motion has not been obtained, patient-adjusted static flexion and extension splints are used to facilitate regaining motion. Rehabilitation should be closely supervised.

Results

Melhoff et al. reviewed the long-term sequelae of simple dislocations. Sixty-five percent reported loss of motion especially in extension. They found a direct correlation with the period of immobilization. Immobilization >3 weeks resulted in a high incidence of contractures. Uncomplicated dislocations generally have very satisfactory results. Excellent results with full range of motion, normal strength, absent pain, and good stability may be expected in 50% of patients. Good results, defined as <15 degrees of motion loss, minimal discomfort, and normal stability, may be expected in one third of patients. Fair or poor results are generally associated with complications and severe injuries and occur in 15% of cases.

Most patients note continued improvement up to 6 months and rarely up to 18 months. Limitations in extension are the most common problem. Recurrent instability has not been commonly reported, but symptoms have been noted in ≤ 35 percent of cases. Even long after healing, approximately 50% of patients followed up long term complain of discomfort or residual symptoms attributed to their elbow after a dislocation. This is predominately reported during heavy loading of the affected extremity. Approximately 60% of patients reported that their elbow did not feel as "good" as the contralateral elbow. Mechanical testing reveals a 15% average loss of elbow strength.

Complications

Neurologic problems occur in $\leq 20\%$ of dislocations. Symptoms range from transient paresthesia to a rare permanent ulnar palsy. Median nerve involvement is less common. Stretching and distortion of the anterior structures may result in spasm, intimal damage, thrombosis, or rupture of the brachial artery. Because dislocation involves disruption of collateral circulation, the forearm can be placed at risk.

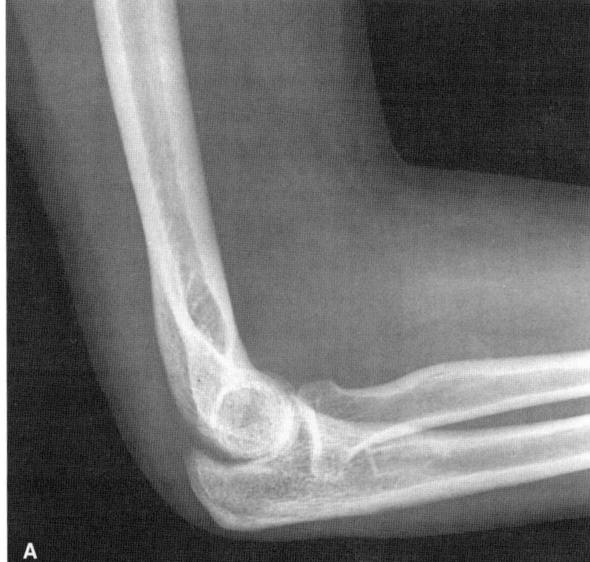

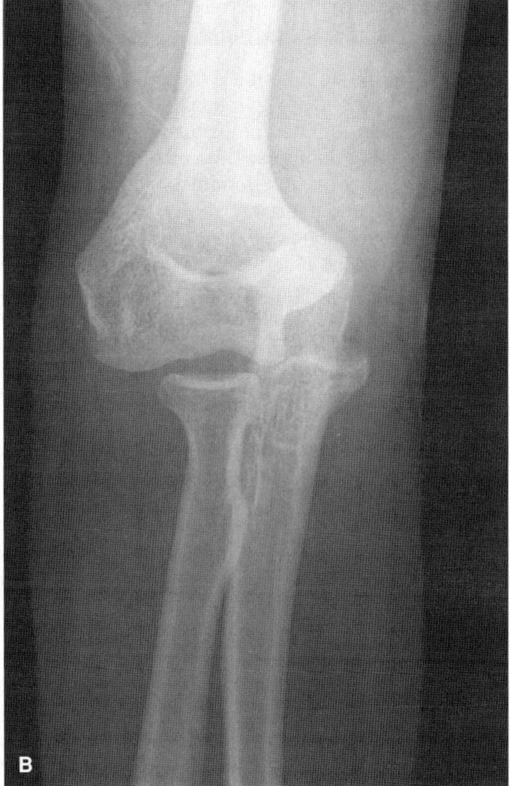

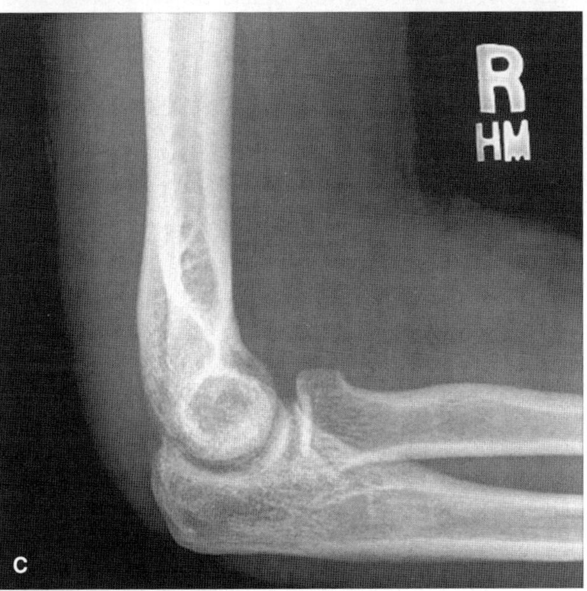

Figure 51-2 Patient with recurrent instability and dislocated 2 weeks after closed reduction. **A:** The redislocation was not initially recognized with only a lateral radiograph. The joint is not congruent. **B:** Orthogonal anteroposterior (AP) view shows the clear dislocation. **C:** Lateral radiograph obtained after open repair of medial and lateral ligaments with a congruent, stable joint.

Ischemic myositis, myonecrosis, impaired vascularity, or claudication may result.

Compartment syndrome can result from intramuscular bleeding and edema formation within the flexor compartment of the forearm. Pain with passive finger and wrist extension out of proportion to the injury raises clinical suspicion. Compartment pressures are obtained when the diagnosis is in doubt, and arteriography is obtained if arterial injury is suspected.

Posttraumatic stiffness is much more common than instability after elbow dislocation. Limitation of extension is common with frequent loss of 10 to 15 degrees of terminal extension. Bracing and therapy are not generally useful after 1 year. If there is sufficient limitation of 30 degrees or more, capsulolysis may be considered. The anterior capsule can be released via an open or arthroscopic approach.

Heterotopic bone formation occurs at three primary locations following dislocations. Ossification in the lateral and medial collateral ligaments occurs most frequently (reported in approximately 75% of cases) but seldom causes impairment. Ossification occurs in the anterior capsule above the coronoid process. True ectopic ossification that limits motion is rare, occurring in <5% of cases. Motion-limiting ossification excision is delayed until reactive bone has matured, generally at 1 year.

Elbow dislocations with radial head fractures can be associated with distal radioulnar instability. This is a variant of the Essex-Lopresti injury. The combined injury makes radial head reconstruction important for both elbow stability and axial stability of the forearm. If the radial head is not reconstructible, a metal prosthesis or allograft radial head will provide axial support to the radius and improve valgus stability of the elbow. Temporary pin fixation of the distal radioulnar joint in a neutral position may be added to resist the tendency of proximal radial migration.

TABLE 51-1 ELBOW DISLOCATION PROTOCOL

Daily measurements	Before treatment: (1) Measure arm circumference 3 inches above and 3 inches below the medial epicondyle; (2) measure elbow range of motion. After treatment: Measure elbow range of motion
Treatment day 1	Begin with neuromuscular electrical stimulation under cold water for 20 minutes. Immediately after the treatment, place the athlete supine on a table. Use a 6-inch latex compression wrap to apply compression from distal to proximal (metacarpophalangeal joints to the top of the shoulder). The injured extremity should be elevated above the heart. Maintain compression for 60 seconds on, then 60 seconds off, for a total treatment time of 30 minutes. Unwrap the bandage rapidly (the patient will feel the blood rush to the hand). On release of the wrap, instruct the athlete to open and close the hand rapidly while simultaneously working on flexion and extension of the elbow. This must be a painfree *active* exercise, not passive. After treatment, use a doubled 3-inch rubberized stockinette from the metacarpophalangeal joints to the top of the shoulder to secure two 5-inch oval foam pads to the elbow. Place the pads over the condyles, with the sleeve maintaining their position to provide gentle compression. The sleeve should be removed only for treatment. The entire procedure should be comfortable for the patient.
Treatment day 2	Repeat day 1 modalities. Replace the pads and sleeve. Also, instruct the patient to add a bounce/catch/squeeze exercise using a tennis ball, incorporating biceps flexion/extension and wrist pronation/supination through a painfree range of motion. This can be accomplished during short, intermittent breaks throughout the day.
Treatment days 3 and 4	Repeat day 1 modalities. On completion, instruct the patient in using the injured extremity in the swimming pool. Breast stroke for 30 to 45 minutes is recommended. If available, begin use of an upper body exerciser (UBE) (Cybex, Ronkonkoma, New York). Adjust the UBE handgrip length to accommodate for the injury and the tolerable range of elbow motion. After exercise, ice the elbow for 20 minutes and replace the pads and sleeves for compression.
Treatment days 5 to 7	Repeat day 1 modalities. Continue with the compression wrap routine until swelling is reduced to within 1 cm of the contralateral elbow. At that time, begin isokinetic exercises, focusing on wrist flexion/extension/pronation/supination and biceps/triceps strengthening. After exercise, ice the elbow for 20 minutes and replace the pads and sleeve for elbow compression until edema is completely eliminated.

Author's Preferred Treatment

Diagnosis of acute elbow dislocation is usually straightforward, and careful evaluation of radiographs should allow classification of a complex or simple dislocation. Most injuries will be simple, without significant associated fracture. A rapid but complete neurovascular assessment is documented.

Reduction is carried out expeditiously. On-field reduction may be performed under select conditions if indicated. This will involve an obvious dislocation and an experienced provider at the injury site. Most patients will require transportation to an acute care facility for radiographic evaluation.

Ease of reduction is generally inversely proportional to the degree of muscle spasm present. Analgesia may be provided with conscious monitored sedation, or regional or general anesthesia. The prone position with an assistant controlling the proximal humerus for traction/countertraction has been helpful. The forearm is supinated, and with pressure on the proximal olecranon, a successful reduction can usually be achieved. The stability of the reduction is assessed with range of motion, and the patient is temporarily placed in a sling for postreduction x-ray films.

Most reductions will be stable. We have found for this group, an aggressive early range of motion (ROM) protocol, emphasizing *active* motion, has been helpful for maximizing final range of motion and minimizing extension loss (Table 51-1). Rarely, an elbow dislocation without fracture will be grossly unstable following reduction. In this circumstance, an early MRI, followed by exploration and repair of the medial collateral ligament, flexor-pronator tendon, and lateral ulnar collateral ligament can restore stability. Our experience has been that early range of motion is critical to ensuring a successful outcome.

SUGGESTED READINGS

Cohen MS, Hastings HH. Acute elbow dislocation: evaluation and management. *J Am Acad Ortho Surg*. 1998;6:15–23.

Josefsson PO, Gentz CF, Johnell O, et al. Surgical versus non-surgical treatment of ligamentous injuries following dislocation of the elbow joint. *J Bone Joint Surg Am*. 1987;69:605–608.

Matev I. A radiological sign of entrapment of the median nerve in the elbow joint after posterior dislocation: a report of two cases. *J Bone Joint Surg*. 1976;58B:353.

Melhoff T. The elbow dislocation revisited: pathoanatomy, stabilizing structures, and keys to rehabilitation. In: *Current Concepts of Elbow Surgery, A Comprehensive Review*. Rosemont, IL: American Academy of Orthopaedic Surgeons; 1992.

Melhoff TL, Noble PC, Bennett JB, et al. Simple dislocation of the elbow in the adult: results after closed treatment. *J Bone Joint Surg Am*. 1988;70:244–249.

Mezera K, Hotchkiss RN. Fractures and dislocations of the elbow. In: Rockwood CA Jr, Green DP, Bucholz RW, et al. *Fractures in Adults*. 5th ed. Philadelphia: Lippincott, Williams & Wilkins; 2001:921–934.

O' Driscoll SW, Morrey BF. Elbow dislocation and subluxation: a Spectrum of instability. *Clin Orthop*. 1992;280:186–197.

O'Driscoll SW. Elbow dislocations. In: Morey B, ed. *The Elbow and Its Disorders*. 3rd ed. Philadelphia: WB Saunders; 2000;409–420.

Ross G, McDevitt ER, Chronister R, et al. Treatment of simple elbow dislocation using an immediate motion protocol. *Am J Sports Med*. 1999;27:308–311.

BICEPS TENDON INJURIES

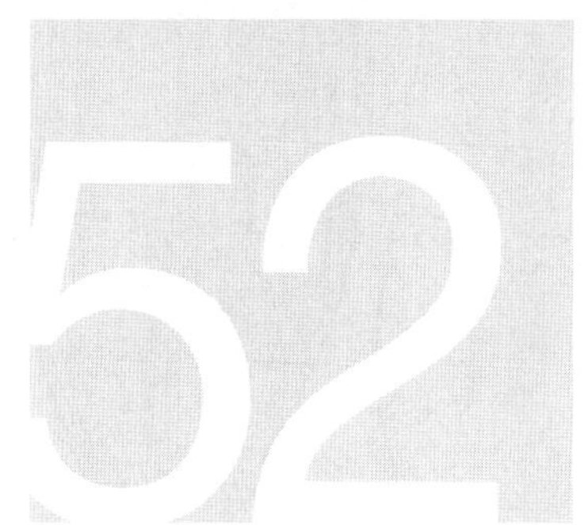

EDWARD W. KELLY

Injury to the biceps tendon encompasses a spectrum from insidious partial tears, complete traumatic tears, to chronic neglected ruptures. Nonoperative treatment was commonly advocated in the past and still plays a role in the elderly or inactive patient. Many surgeons now recognize that early surgical reattachment of the torn tendon to the radial tuberosity will restore function and prevent deformity.

PATHOGENESIS

Etiology

Chevallier proposed that complete biceps tears occur in two stages; the first is the partial tear, which can be insidious in onset, followed by a complete disruption of the remaining tendon with a sudden traumatic event. Davis and Yassine in 1956 presented two cases, one a partial and one a complete rupture of the distal biceps tendon, which illustrated the degenerative changes that occur in the tendon. In both cases, spurring had occurred at the bicipital tuberosity, which acted as a knife to separate the tendon with supination and pronation. In each case, the disruption occurred in the lateral aspect of the tendon first and progressed medially (Fig. 52-1). The tendon avulsion almost always occurs at the insertion site, and at the time of surgery, the torn tendon end is bulbous and frayed, confirming the degenerative process of this injury.

Epidemiology

The ruptures tend to occur in active, middle-aged men, whereas women rarely present with this injury. In a review of >100 cases of distal biceps injuries surgically repaired at the Mayo Clinic, only one patient was a woman, and her tear was only partial. Distal biceps injuries were once considered uncommon, mostly based on a report by Gilcrest in 1925 in which he stated that only 3 of 100 patients with biceps tendon injuries that he reviewed were at the distal insertion. Currently, greater recognition of this condition has led to more diagnoses.

Classification

Distal biceps tears can be classified into partial or complete tears. Complete tears can be further divided into acute (<10 days from injury), subacute (11 to 21 days), or delayed/chronic (>21 days). The subclassification of the complete tear is important when considering surgical management of the torn tendon. On average, if the patient is operated on ≤10 days of the injury, the retracted tendon is easily identifiable, the tract to the tuberosity is intact, and the tendon can be reapproximated to the tuberosity without significant dissection. If >10 but <21 days have passed since the injury at the time of surgical repair, the scarring makes the surgery more difficult and increases the risk of complications, but the tendon can usually be reapproximated to the tuberosity. At ≥21 days postinjury, primary repair becomes more difficult and a graft may be necessary to restore length.

DIAGNOSIS

Physical Examination and History

Clinical Features

Complete distal biceps tears are most often associated with a sudden traumatic event of forced extension against an actively flexing elbow. Patients present with ecchymosis, pain, swelling, weakness, and a palpable defect of the biceps tendon. The ecchymosis is fairly characteristic, extending along the entire medial aspect of the arm and forearm. The deformity of the retracted biceps is also characteristic with the tendon stump retracted proximally and the Popeye-shaped muscle belly retracted into the upper arm. Initially the patients may complain of pain, but this often subsides by the time they present to the orthopaedist. The patients will be tender in the antecubital fossa and have pain with

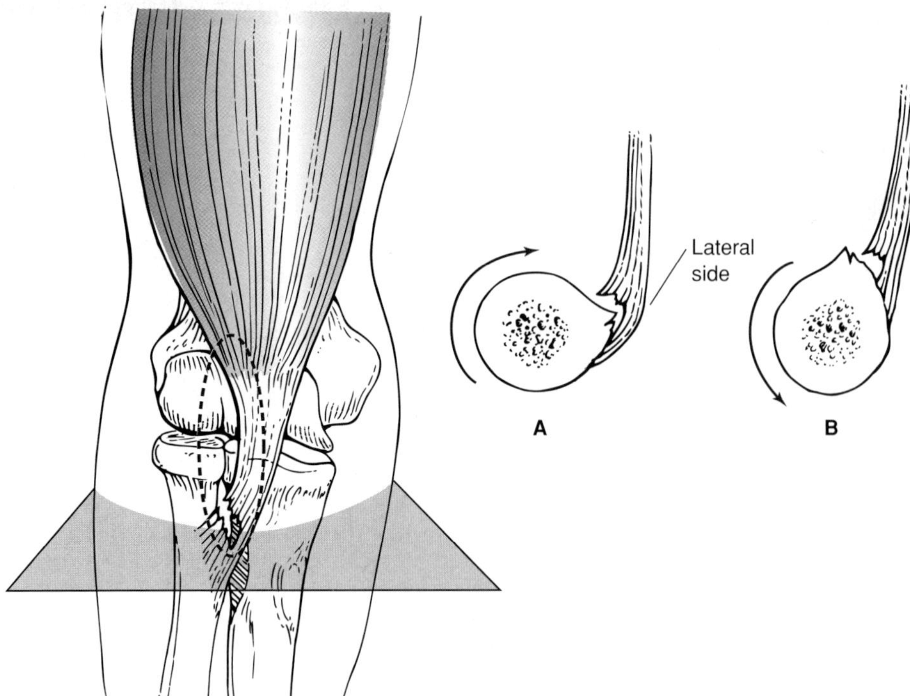

Figure 52-1 The degenerative tear occurs on the deep side of the tendon. **Left:** drawing demonstrating the appearance of the lesion at surgery, in which the *dotted line* represents the enlarged bicipital bursa. **Right:** A cross section of the area of the arm indicated by the *straight line* in the left figure. When the arm is pronated (**A**), the sharp margin of the tuberosity impinges on the tendon; when the arm is supinated (**B**), the tendon is pulled free. (Reprinted from Davis WM, Yassine Z. An etiological factor in tear of the distal tendon of the biceps brachii: report of two cases. *J Bone Joint Surg* A. 1956;39:1365–1368, with permission.)

resisted supination and flexion as well as mild to moderate weakness with these resisted motions. In some cases, the lacertus fibrosis may remain intact, making it difficult to palpate the tendon defect. In thin individuals, the diagnosis can be confirmed by comparing the motion of the bicep muscle belly with the elbow flexed 90 degrees while the forearm is passively rotated. While moving the forearm from supination to pronation, the biceps muscle belly should move distally with an intact tendon. In addition, as the examiner grips a patient's right injured forearm with the right arm, he or she should be able to grip the arm above the elbow and place the left thumb under an intact biceps tendon.

In more chronic cases, the ecchymosis and swelling will no longer be apparent; however, the muscle belly will remain retracted and may be atrophic. The retracted tendon is often scarred, fibrosed, and not palpable, and the patient remains weak in flexion and supination. These patients complain more of a "cramping" and weakness rather than a sharp pain with activity.

Unlike the often dramatic and well-characterized presentation of complete distal biceps tendon ruptures, patients with partial tears often fail to describe an acute traumatic event, describing an insidious onset to their symptoms. The tendon is intact anteriorly but tender to palpation. In addition, the bicipital tuberosity is also tender when palpated with the forearm in full pronation. The patients tend to have weakness with resisted supination and flexion but not as marked as with complete tears. A local cortisone and anesthetic injection from a posterior approach to the radial tuberosity may be both therapeutic and diagnostic in these cases. This should be done with the arm in full pronation, aiming the needle at the level of the tuberosity, just between the radius and ulna. The patients should be warned that temporary posterior interosseous nerve palsy may result as the anesthetic diffuses through the surrounding tissues.

Radiographic Features

In acute disruptions, plain radiographs are most often normal; however, they may occasionally demonstrate osteophytic spurring at the level of the radial tuberosity. Although occasionally helpful in the patient with a questionable diagnosis, MRI is often unnecessary. In partial tears, however, MRI evaluation is very helpful is assisting in the diagnosis of these cases. The presence of increased intratendinous signal intensity and abnormal tendon diameter along with fluid around the tendon can confirm the diagnosis (Fig. 52-2).

TREATMENT

Surgical Indications/Contraindications

Nonoperative treatment of acute, complete distal biceps tears may provide acceptable results in older or more sedentary individuals. The resulting weakness, pain, and deformity, however, have lead many surgeons to recommend surgical reattachment of the avulsed tendon to the tuberosity. The issue of surgical approach, however, has been controversial.

The significant anterior exposure initially required to reattach the biceps to the radial tuberosity was associated with several complications including radial and median nerve palsies. In an attempt to avoid such complications, Boyd and Anderson advocated a two-incision technique. They were able to limit the anterior dissection by exposing the radial tuberosity through a second posterior incision. Although this technique was thought to decrease the

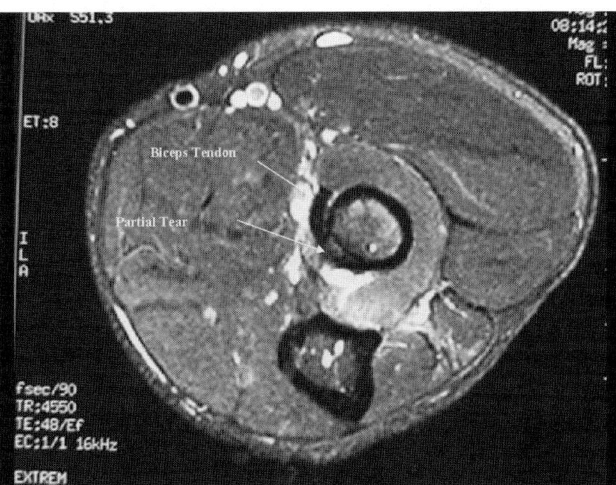

Figure 52-2 Axial MRI image from a patient with a partial distal biceps tendon tear demonstrating increased signal intensity at the tendon insertion site coinciding with the site of the tendon tear on the radial surface of the tendon. (Reprinted from Kelly EW, Steinmann SP, O'Driscoll SW. Surgical treatment of partial distal biceps tendon ruptures through a single posterior incision. *J Shoulder Elbow Surg*. 2003;12:456–461, with permission.)

potential of nerve injury associated with an anterior approach, it was perceived to increase the likelihood of radioulnar synostosis.

There have been reports of heterotopic bone formation occurring with the anterior approach and nerve injury occurring with the two-incision approach. Firm evidence is lacking attributing either excess bone formation or nerve injury with either surgical technique.

Surgical Technique

Regardless of whether the surgeon plans on using only a single anterior or a two-incision approach, the patient is placed supine on the operating table with the arm out on a hand table. The arm is then prepped and draped from the wrist to the axilla and a sterile tourniquet is used. The first important task is to milk the muscle belly distally prior to applying the tourniquet (Fig. 52-3A). This maneuver pushes the tendon down toward the antecubital fossa where is can easily be retrieved through the anterior incision.

Mini Two-Incision Technique

When using the two-incision technique, a 3-cm transverse incision is made in the antecubital crease along the flexion lines (Fig. 52-3A). The incision is centered over the bicipital tract just medial to the midline. The lateral antebrachial cutaneous nerve lies just to the lateral aspect of the incision but does not need to be exposed. Just deep to the subcutaneous tissues lies the fascia of the bicipital tunnel, which can be incised with scissors longitudinally. In the acute setting, hemorrhagic fluid is frequently encountered, indicating the correct plane. Blunt digital dissection can now be used to identify the radial tuberosity distally in the tunnel, and proximally to identify the tendon. The tendon may be grasped with an Allis clamp and then pulled out the anterior incision. The bulbous end is then debrided back just a few millimeters and the tendon prepared with a running locking Krackow stitch using a strong nonabsorbable no. 2 suture. This is done twice to provide four strands of suture (Fig. 52-3B).

The bicipital tuberosity of the radius is then palpated from the anterior incision by following the bicipital tunnel. A blunt, curved hemostat is carefully inserted into the space previously occupied by the biceps tendon. The instrument slips past the tuberosity between the radius and ulna and is advanced below the radius past the ulna while pronating the forearm so that its tip may be palpated on the dorsal aspect of the proximal forearm (Fig. 52-4). A second, 4-cm-long incision is made over the instrument, which should be 1 cm anterolateral to the subcutaneous border of the ulna. The tuberosity is exposed by a muscle-splitting incision. The ulna is never exposed. The supinator fascia is identified after splitting through the common extensor muscles. Fibers are then split to expose the bicipital tuberosity, taking care to keep the forearm in maximal pronation to protect the posterior interosseous nerve. Small Hohmann retractors are carefully placed underneath the supinator on the radius. A small round (4 to 5 mm) high-speed burr is used to excavate a trough 1.5 cm long and 5 mm wide in the radial tuberosity. The trough is taken into the medullary canal of the radius. Two or three drill holes are then placed 7 to 8 mm apart and ≥7 mm from the edge of the excavation using a small drill bit or 0.062 K-wire (Fig. 52-5). Copious irrigation is used to remove bone dust at each stage during preparation of the cavity and the suture holes. The sharp leading edge of the radial bone trough should be smoothed off to prevent irritation of the tendon with supination and pronation.

Once the trough is created, the surgeon passes the four strands of suture through the anterior incision and out the posterior incision, taking care to be aware of the tendon's orientation in the tunnel. The strands of suture are then threaded through the bone trough and out the drill holes, one at each of the proximal and distal holes and two out the middle hole (if using three drill holes). A Hewson suture passer is helpful for this step. The tendon is pulled into the bone trough by supinating the forearm and pulling on the sutures. The sutures are tied over the bone bridges. The wound is carefully lavaged and the wound closed in layers. The patient is placed in a posterior plaster splint overnight for comfort.

Single Anterior Incision

If an anterior-only approach is used, the distal portion of a Henry, S-shaped incision is performed with the transverse aspect similar to that described above for the mini two-incision procedure, but with the lateral edge curving distally. The lateral antebrachial cutaneous nerve is identified in the lateral aspect of the incision and protected. The brachioradialis is retracted laterally and the pronator is retracted medially, exposing the radial tuberosity with the forearm in supination. The posterior interosseous nerve is at risk in this exposure but can be kept out of the surgical field by supinating the forearm. The radial tuberosity is debrided of any remaining soft tissue but is not decorticated. Two suture anchors are then placed in the most medial aspect of the radial tuberosity. The tendon is identified and prepared

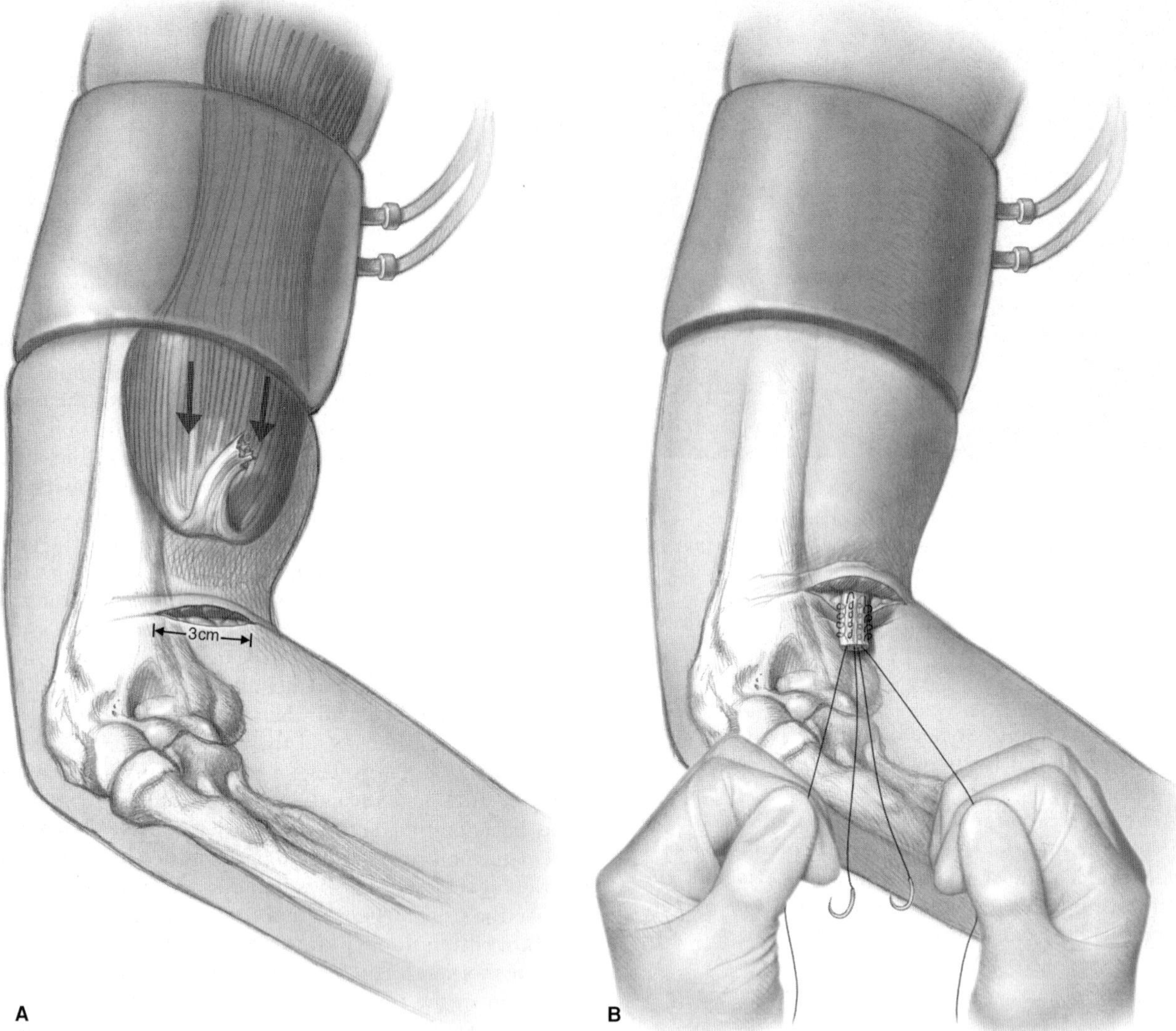

Figure 52-3 **A:** The tendon stump is milked distally with the tourniquet applied and then expressed through the anterior incision. **B:** Two running, locking stitches are placed in the tendon stump providing four strands of suture to tie to the radius. (Reprinted from Kelly EW, O'Driscoll SW. Mini-incision for acute distal biceps repair. *Techniques Shoulder Elbow Surg*. 2002;3[2]:57–62, with permission.)

as noted above up to the point of placing sutures. One limb of each of the two sutures is then placed in Krackow fashion up the medial or lateral edge of the tendon. The two sutures are then tied to each other proximally. The two free suture ends at the anchors are then tied to each other pulling the tendon to the tuberosity with the arm in full supination and 90 degrees of elbow flexion. The wound is closed in layers and the patient placed in a posterior rigid splint for 7 to 10 days. If using an interference screw, the exposure is the same while the tuberosity is drilled and the screw inserted per the manufacturer's instructions.

Subacute and Chronic Tears

If the tendon has been torn for >14 days, but <30 days, it is often quite retracted and it is difficult to get the tendon back to the radius without flexing the elbow. If the tendon can be reapproximated with the elbow flexed <90 degrees, a primary repair may be performed with the confidence that the muscle belly will relax within a few days once tension has been restored. Often, however, in the chronic setting, the tendon itself is very atrophic or so scarred that primary repair is not an option. In this situation, a tendon graft is the best option to restore length and contour. The biceps is first exposed through a larger, Henry type of anterior incision taking the smaller transverse incision as described above and carrying it out laterally, then curving proximally as far as necessary to expose the muscle. Care is taken to identify and protect the lateral antebrachial cutaneous nerve. Different types of tendon grafts have been described including semitendinosus, brachioradialis autografts, and Achilles tendon allografts. The latter are ideally suited for chronic biceps reconstructions. The graft has excellent mechanical and physical properties. The aponeurotic portion of the graft is wide and long enough to permit secure suturing to the host biceps muscle, while the distal part of the allograft can be easily trimmed to the appropriate length.

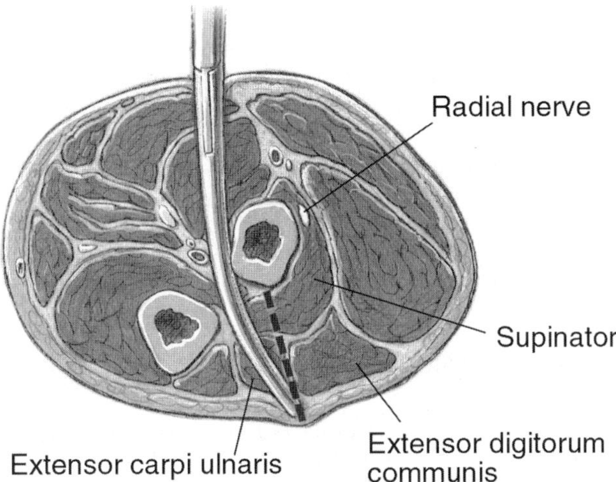

Figure 52-4 A large blunt curved hemostat is placed through the anterior incision, down the tunnel of the biceps tendon, and between the radius and ulna to identify the site for the posterior incision. (Reprinted from Kelly EW, O'Driscoll SW. Mini-incision for acute distal biceps repair. *Techniques Shoulder Elbow Surg.* 2002;3[2]:57–62, with permission.)

The wide expansive portion of the Achilles allograft tendon is attached to the biceps muscle belly and tendon stump with multiple no. 2 nonabsorbable sutures (Fig.52-6). The tendon insertion end is then passed through the bicipital tunnel and out through the posterior incision as described above for the primary repair. The distal end of the allograft can then be trimmed back to create the proper length for tensioning prior to inserting the distal tendon end into the prepared bone trough at the bicipital tuberosity. The sutures are to be tied with the elbow in 60 to 90 degrees of flexion and full pronation. Once the tendon is trimmed to the appropriate length, it is prepared as described for the primary repair above with two no. 2 nonabsorbable sutures in a Krackow fashion providing four suture stands. The repair is then completed as described above using the two-incision technique.

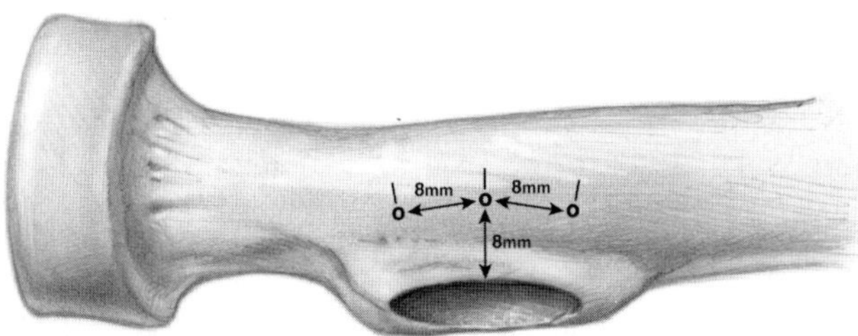

Figure 52-5 Illustration of the proximal radius describing the position of the holes placed to pass the suture and tie over the bone bridge. The holes should be 7 to 10 mm from the trough edge and 7 to 8 mm apart, creating a very stable bone bridge over which to tie the suture. (Reprinted from Kelly EW, O'Driscoll SW. Mini-incision for acute distal biceps repair. *Techniques Shoulder Elbow Surg.* 2002;3[2]:57–62, with permission.)

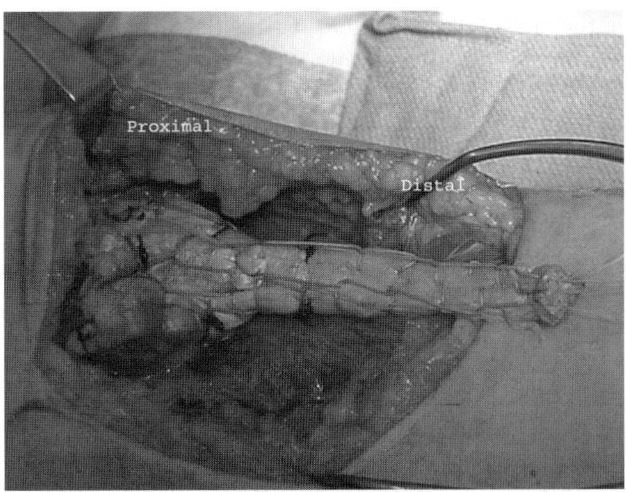

Figure 52-6 The aponeurosis of the Achilles allograft is secured proximally to the muscle belly and remaining tendon stump of the biceps while distally it is prepared with two running, locking sutures to secure the allograft to the radius.

Partial Tears

For partial repairs that require surgery, the entire repair can be accomplished through a single posterior incision avoiding any anterior dissection. The radial tuberosity is located by palpating the lateral forearm in full pronation, or by measuring down from the olecranon on the lateral preoperative x-ray view. A 4-cm incision is then made centered over the radial tuberosity, 1 cm anterolateral to the subcutaneous border of the ulna. The fascia of the extensor digitorum communis is identified and split longitudinally in line with the skin incision, avoiding the subcutaneous border of the ulna. With the forearm fully pronated to protect the posterior interosseous nerve, the supinator fascia is identified and split longitudinally over the radial tuberosity, exposing the underlying biceps tendon at its insertion on the radius. As the partial tear and pathology occurs on the undersurface of the tendon, which is not exposed, the tendon in the wound often appears normal.

To expose the tendon and explore the pathology, the tendon needs to be pulled out of the wound and probed. To accomplish this, a stay suture is placed in the most proximal portion of the biceps that is visible in the wound and the tendon pulled down and out of the wound. This same maneuver is repeated two or three times with the elbow flexed, each time placing a new stay suture more proximal in the tendon to pull more tendon out of the wound. With 2 to 3 cm of biceps tendon pulled out through the posterior wound, the undersurface of the tendon can be inspected and probed to reveal the defect in the undersurface of the tendon. Once the pathology has been confirmed, the remaining portion of the intact tendon can be detached while the tendon is held securely with the stay sutures to prevent retraction into the wound. The degenerative and frayed end of the tendon is sharply debrided, cutting back a few millimeters into healthier tendon. The tendon is then made to retract between the radius and ulna by extending the elbow while the stay sutures permit it to be brought back posteriorly after preparation of the bicipital tuberosity. The trough in the radial tuberosity is created and the tendon prepared and secured to the radius as described above in the two-incision technique.

Results and Outcome

The results for primary repair of avulsed distal biceps tendon in the acute or subacute setting (<30 days) are uniformly excellent. Numerous reports, regardless of the technique used, have demonstrated return of function, contour, and strength by 6 months. The results from partial repairs are similar but much less commonly reported. Pain relief can be achieved in 90% of patients with the posterior-only incision. The results from chronic repairs using a tendon graft are also limited in number but similarly acceptable with 90% of patients satisfied and few complaints of pain. The restoration of objective strength, however, has not been well documented.

Postoperative Management

Having full confidence in the strength of a repair using a bone trough and transosseous sutures, immobilization of the elbow can be limited to only the first night and rehabilitation of the tendon can be started the day after surgery in the setting of acute, chronic, or partial repairs. The patients are instructed to begin gravity-assisted extension exercises with active-assisted and passive flexion the day they are removed from the postoperative dressing. The sling is worn for comfort the first 6 weeks to prevent a constant gravitational pull on the tendon. As their initial postoperative pain subsides, they are instructed to "use no more force than would be required to lift a glass of water or a telephone receiver" for 6 weeks, then to "use common sense" and avoid heavy force (e.g., getting a window unstuck, and so on) until 3 months. From 3 to 6 months postoperatively, they are simply advised to avoid violent force such as occurs in contact sports but can work against unlimited resistance. They can begin a self-directed strengthening program with light weights. Formal physical therapy is rarely indicated. Unlimited activities are permitted after 6 months in all patients.

SUGGESTED READINGS

Boyd HB, Anderson LD. A method for reinsertion of the distal biceps brachii tendon. *J Bone Joint Surg*. 1961;43A:1041–1043.

Chevallier CH. Sur un cas de desinsertion au tendons bicipital in terieur. *Mem. Acad Chir*. 1953;79:137.

Davis WM, Yassine Z. An etiological factor in tear of the distal tendon of the biceps brachii: report of two cases. *J Bone Joint Surg*, 1956;39A:1365–1368.

Failla JM, Amadio PC, Morrey BF, et al. Proximal radioulnar synostosis after repair of distal biceps brachii rupture by the two-incision technique. Report of four cases. *Clin Orthop*. 1990;253:133–136.

Gilcrest EL. Rupture of muscle and tendons. *JAMA* 1925;84:1819.

Kelly EW, Morrey BF, O'Driscoll SW. Complications of distal biceps tendon repairs. *J Bone Joint Surg*. 2001;82-A:1575–1581.

Kelly EW, Steinmann S, O'Driscoll SW. Surgical treatment of partial distal biceps tendon ruptures through a single posterior incision. *J Shoulder Elbow Surg*. 2003;12:456–461.

Le Huec JC, Moinard M, Liquois F, et al. Distal rupture of the tendon of biceps brachii. Evaluation by MRI and the results of repair. *J Bone Joint Surg*. 1996;78B:767–770.

Morrey BF. Distal biceps tendon rupture. In: Morrey BF, ed. *The Elbow*. 2nd ed. New York: Raven Press; 2002:173–191.

Morrey BF. Tendon injuries about the elbow. In: Morrey BF, ed. *The Elbow and Its Disorders*. 3rd ed. Philadelphia: WB Saunders; 2000:468–479.

LATERAL EPICONDYLITIS

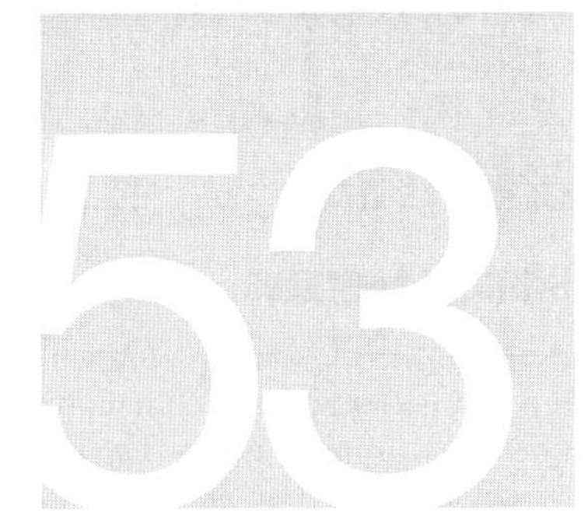

KEVIN J. RENFREE

ETIOLOGY

The cause of lateral epicondylitis is poorly understood, although most likely a symptom of overuse microtrauma (a small tear) to the common wrist extensor tendon origin, usually the extensor carpi radialis brevis (ECRB). A commonly used term, *epicondylitis* inaccurately implies an inflammatory process. Numerous pathologic studies have confirmed vascular proliferation and focal hyaline degeneration in surgical specimens, most likely as a result of disrupted healing response, with fibrosis and granulation tissue forming rather than normal tendon. Nirschl has also used the term "angio-fibroblastic tendinosis" to describe the pathologic changes. This process leads to progressive shortening of the tendon, which may increase the chance of reinjury. Other authors have postulated that it may be a degenerative process with vascular compromise and hypoxia, similar to that found in rotator cuff pathology. A possible link to fluoroquinolone ingestion has also been proposed. Excessive eccentric loading may be a factor in the etiology of tendinopathy, as fewer muscle fibers are recruited to perform the work, which increases the stress load on each, resulting in an elevated risk for injury.

EPIDEMIOLOGY

Lateral epicondylitis is a common complaint, with an annual incidence between 1% and 3% in the general population. In one study, which attempted to identify industries at high risk for work related disorders of the neck, back, and upper extremity, epicondylitis was found to be the only one in which claims increased over a near-10-year period. Most likely the process is a cumulative one, resulting from the use of heavy hand-held tools or a combination of vigorous work, abnormal posture of hands and arms, and repetition. It is also very common in the dominant extremity of a typically average recreational athlete involved in racquet sports who may have a faulty single-handed backhand ground stroke. The commonly used term "tennis elbow" is unfortunately misleading, though, as only a small percentage (5% to 10%) of patients afflicted with this disorder play at all.

PATHOPHYSIOLOGY

The specific areas of elbow abnormality include the extensor carpi radialis brevis–extensor digitorum communis (EDC) complex laterally. Pathologic specimens of patients operated on for this condition have not revealed any evidence of acute or chronic inflammation, although in vitro analysis of painful tendons has revealed the presence of interleukin-1 and cytokines. This molecular inflammation cascade could be a source of pain and dysfunction. One study in which catheters were inserted into tendons with tendinosis showed no prostaglandin E2, a component of inflammation. Higher levels of glutamate, a potent pain modulator in the central nervous system, were found, though, which may also be a source of pain in tendinosis. Although it is debatable whether radial nerve entrapment (analogous to carpal tunnel syndrome) causes the forearm discomfort seen in many cases of lateral epicondylitis, decompression of the posterior interosseous nerve may also be necessary to relieve the forearm pain and tenderness associated with lateral epicondylitis.

As mentioned, the cause of pain in lateral epicondylitis is poorly understood. Magnetic resonance images in patients with lateral epicondylitis have demonstrated thickening with separation of the ECRB tendon from the radial collateral ligament and abnormal signal change on the T1-weighted sequences. There were no associations between pathological signal intensity within the ECRB tendon on T1- and T2-weighted sequences, however, and the degree of self-reported pain. In one arthroscopic study, 31.3% of patients were noted to have a type I lesion, characterized as fraying of the undersurface of the ECRB; 31.3% had a type II lesion noted by linear tears within the ECRB; and 37.5% had a type III lesion, consisting of a partial or complete avulsion of the ECRB origin. Therefore, an overuse injury resulting in progressive disruption of the tendinous origin of the ECRB may produce an excessive inflammatory response during the healing process leading to pain and possible swelling and compression of the posterior interosseous nerve. If overuse of the tendon leads to the pain that patients experience, rest should decrease symptoms. Unfortunately, injections of the muscle with botulinum toxin, providing temporary paralysis of the painful common extensor origin, showed no benefit over placebo.

DIAGNOSIS

Clinical Features

Patients with lateral epicondylitis typically are adults who report insidious onset of symptoms with no clear recollection of a traumatic event. The pain is localized to the lateral aspect of the elbow and proximal forearm. It is typically aggravated with activities such as lifting an object with the arm extended away from the body and the forearm in a pronated position. Tenderness along the lateral aspect of the elbow is present. Although rest pain is unusual, patients often experience pain and stiffness in the morning while initially attempting to mobilize their elbow and wrist with their daily activities. Secondary stiffness of the elbow and wrist is uncommon, and if present, should prompt suspicion for an underlying articular disorder. Furthermore, any mechanical symptoms such as catching, locking, popping, or giving way may indicate an internal derangement of the elbow joint. Lateral epicondylitis is rare in patients in their teenage years or younger and should prompt a more aggressive workup.

Physical Examination and History

Overlying changes in skin color or temperature are not typically seen. Although swelling may be seen in a thin individual, it is uncommon. Tenderness is typically present about 1 cm anterior and distal to the lateral epicondyle, which is easily palpated in most patients. Although patients may also experience tenderness in the proximal forearm musculature, this may also indicate a coexisting radial tunnel syndrome, particularly if the tenderness is in the area of the radial tuberosity. Elbow motion is typically full, smooth, and painless, although some patients with severe epicondylitis may experience lateral elbow pain in full extension. If pain is present with passive forearm rotation, combined with elbow flexion and valgus stress, a radiocapitellar plica may be the cause. Elbow stability should be assessed with a posterolateral pivot shift maneuver while the patient is in a supine position. A careful neurologic exam should be performed, although it is unusual to find any deficits, even in a patient in whom radial tunnel syndrome is suspected. Pain in terminal extension with a bounce maneuver, especially in a throwing athlete, might be related to impingement from an olecranon spur. A common finding in tennis elbow is pain in the region of the lateral epicondyle during resisted extension of the middle finger (the Maudsley test). This may be owing to disease in the EDC muscle rather than compression of the radial nerve or disease within the ECRB. A positive chair test may be identified if pain is exacerbated when the patient lifts a chair with the affected arm in extension. If unilateral symptoms are present, diminished grip strength compared with the opposite side is often found, most likely is a reflection of painful wrist extension.

Radiographic Features

The role of radiographs in the clinical evaluation of lateral epicondylitis is unclear. In one study, standard anteroposterior, lateral, and radiocapitellar views of the elbow in patients with a diagnosis of lateral epicondylitis demonstrated calcification along the lateral epicondyle in 7%. In only two of the 294 sets of films did the radiographs alter management. The author concluded that obtaining radiographs as an initial step in the evaluation of patients with lateral epicondylitis is not necessary. Certainly in patients who present with atypical symptoms such as night pain and mechanical abnormalities, radiographs are recommended.

Although the use of ultrasound has been described for the diagnosis of tennis elbow, magnetic resonance imaging (MRI) is a more sensitive modality to diagnose and evaluate treatment response, although rarely necessary in my opinion. MRI of epicondylitis demonstrates tendon thickening with increased T1 and T2 signal, but these findings may be seen in a small minority of asymptomatic individuals. Tears of the extensor origin may be identified, and anconeus edema, previously demonstrated on MRI in epicondylitis, is rarely found. Increased marrow T2 signal within the involved epicondyle is occasionally seen. Abnormalities of the lateral collateral ligament complex and areas of osteochondritis dissecans, which can also produce lateral elbow pain, may also be identified with MR imaging. CT scan and isotope bone scan may be helpful in distinguishing lateral epicondylitis from bony tumors such as osteoid osteoma.

TREATMENT

Surgical Indications/Contraindications

A poor prognosis for spontaneous recovery may be related to manual work and high baseline pain. If modifications to reduce physical demands during recovery cannot be realized, than operative treatment may eventually be necessary. One concept that is important to make the patient understand, however, is that (assuming all other diagnostic possibilities have been excluded) lateral epicondylitis is a condition in which pain may secondarily effect function. The surgical solutions proposed to correct it, therefore, are elective with very focused goals. If patients can live with their pain, or modify their activities in such a way as to make their symptoms tolerable, then surgery may not be advisable.

Nonoperative Options

The primary goal of nonsurgical treatment is to encourage healing of the abnormal tissue that produces pain. Most successful nonsurgical treatment programs center on the concept of an adequate, progressive rehabilitative resistance exercise program. Nonetheless, many modalities have been described in an attempt to hasten or improve the healing process. Unfortunately, many of these interventions have been advocated on the merit of insufficient evidence, contradicting results, insufficient power, short-term follow-up, or a low number of studies per intervention. They may, therefore, not actually produce results superior to rest alone, which can be expected to result in improvement in 80% to 85% of patients. Although rest is important with respect to avoiding symptom-provoking activities, complete rest is ill advised as muscle atrophy may begin within 6 days of complete disuse.

As mentioned, physical therapy is probably the most commonly used nonoperative treatment modality. In one systematic review of many studies on various modalities (laser therapy, electrotherapy, exercises, mobilization techniques, and ultrasound), weak evidence for efficacy was found only for ultrasound. Other studies have failed to demonstrate any additional benefit of including phonophoresis with a topical corticosteroid to ultrasound. With strengthening, eccentric contraction should be emphasized. Eccentric strengthening may help to heal tendinopathies by stimulating mechanoreceptors and tenocytes to produce collagen. Animal experiments have shown that eccentric loading improves tendon collagen alignment and simulates formation of collagen cross-linkage to improve tensile strength. In addition, tendon cells respond to an eccentric mechanical load by up-regulation of gene expression for synthesis of collagen proteins. One large Dutch randomized, controlled study found that, after 12 months, the success rate in the physiotherapy group (91%) was significantly higher than an injection group (69%), but only slightly higher than in a "wait-and-see" group (83%).

Brace treatment might be useful as initial therapy. Overload of the wrist extensors, which is considered to be a major pathogenic factor in lateral epicondylitis, has been shown to be reduced by braces. Forearm/hand splints are not more effective than elbow bands as a treatment for lateral epicondylitis, and currently no definitive conclusions can be drawn concerning the effectiveness of orthotic devices for lateral epicondylitis.

Most authors recommend treatment with nonsteroidal anti-inflammatory medications (NSAIDS), despite the growing evidence that the condition is noninflammatory. Nonetheless, these medications may be helpful in decreasing the level of pain, at least in the short term, but must be weighed against the risks of gastrointestinal adverse effects. There is also evidence that topical NSAIDS are similarly effective in the short term, and without the gastrointestinal risks. These compounds can typically be produced at many pharmacies or apothecary shops. A direct comparison between topical and oral NSAID has not been made, though. Some authors have expressed concern, however, as NSAIDS may inhibit the inflammatory response necessary for tissue repair. One study demonstrated that when NSAIDS were compared with placebo, tendon strength was reduced at 28 days.

Despite the fact that most evidence points to corticosteroid injections providing only short-term relief at best, lateral epicondylitis is the most common extra-articular use for corticosteroid injections by orthopedic surgeons. A meta-analysis review found superior short-term effects of corticosteroid injections for lateral epicondylitis, but it was not possible to draw firm conclusions on the effectiveness of injections owing to the lack of high-quality studies. No beneficial effects were found for intermediate or long-term follow-up. Other authors have reported on the use of an injection of autologous blood, felt to possibly provide the necessary cellular and humoral mediators to induce a healing cascade, with a reported 80% success rate. A double-blind, randomized, controlled trial comparing injections of botulinum toxin type A with those of a placebo (normal saline solution) in the treatment of chronic tennis elbow failed to find a significant difference between the two groups. Acupuncture also may provide improved pain relief in the short term when compared with placebo, but no clear long-term benefit has been demonstrated.

Numerous investigators have recommended extracorporeal shock wave therapy as an alternative treatment for chronic lateral epicondylitis of the elbow. The mechanism of action of shockwave therapy is not fully understood but may stimulate the healing process of damaged tendons and encourage revascularization, release of local growth factors, and the recruitment of appropriate stem cells to the area. Although some studies comparing low-dose or low-energy shockwave therapy with sham treatment demonstrated improvement in pain scores, most other studies have failed to demonstrate a clear benefit of this treatment modality.

Patient Selection

Studies on the natural history and surgical management of lateral epicondylitis have shown that surgical intervention is necessary in only 5% to 10% of patients. Only those patients with persistent or recurrent local pain and muscle weakness, nonresponsive to conservative measures for at least 6 months, should be considered for surgery. Symptoms of radial tunnel syndrome can resemble those of tennis elbow and result from compression of the radial nerve by the free edge of the supinator muscle or closely related structures in the vicinity of the elbow joint. It can be difficult to objectively differentiate these two disorders, and they may often occur simultaneously. Radial tunnel syndrome should be strongly considered in patients who have failed to respond to previous extensor release or debridement. Differential diagnostic injections can be helpful in distinguishing these two problems or confirming the presence of both. The first injection is given at the point of maximal tenderness, near the lateral epicondyle typically 1 cm anterior and 1 cm proximal with 3 to 4 mL of 1% plain lidocaine. After 5 to 10 minutes have elapsed, the patient is re-examined, and if pain is eliminated with provocative maneuvers (resisted wrist extension). and tenderness over the radial tuberosity region is diminished, then a diagnosis of lateral epicondylitis alone is appropriate. If, however, pain and tenderness persists, an injection is given toward the radial tuberosity with the forearm in supination with a long 25- or 27-gauge needle (Fig. 53-1). Once the needle strikes bone, it is redirected anteriorly and 10 mL of 1% plain lidocaine (a reasonable volume of local anesthetic is important) is injected. After 10 minutes, the patient is re-examined and if a posterior interosseous nerve palsy has been produced and pain is relieved, a posterior interosseous nerve decompression is included in the surgical plan. If pain persists following both injections, suspicion is raised for intra-articular pathology such as degeneration of the orbicular ligament or a redundant synovial fold, in which case a confirmatory intra-articular injection can be

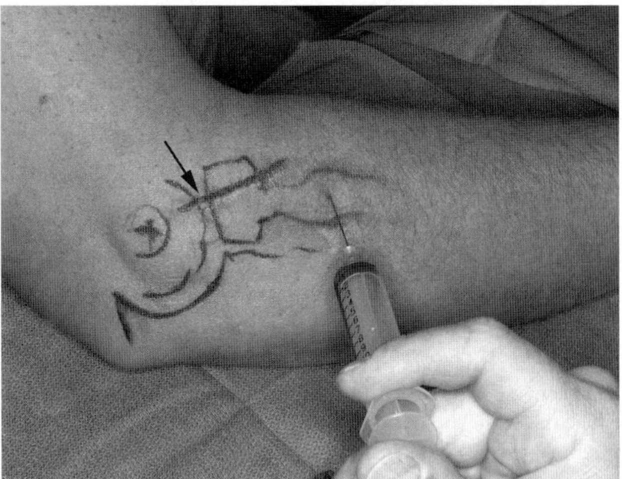

Figure 53-1 With the forearm in supination, a fine gauge (1.5 in.) needle is directed anterior to the radial tuberosity in this patient with persistent pain after a previous open release of the extensor origin (surgical scar marked with indelible pen depicted by *solid black arrow*) suspected of having radial tunnel syndrome.

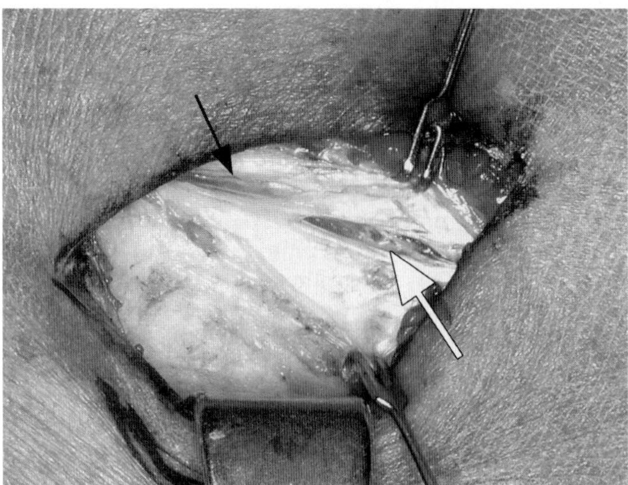

Figure 53-2 Intraoperative photograph of a patient with refractory epicondylitis. *Solid black arrow* depicts area of tendon degeneration; *open arrow* depicts longitudinal rent in extensor carpi radialis brevis (ECRB) tendon.

performed. This is particularly helpful in patients who have failed previous surgery for lateral epicondylitis.

My personal preference is an open procedure, in which case the patient is placed in the supine position with an arm board. If there is any suspicion of instability or intra-articular pathology, an examination under anesthesia is included, as well as a possible arthroscopy. The presence of a palmaris longus is confirmed, or alternate graft choices are discussed with the patient in advance

Surgical Techniques

Percutaneous release can be done in an office setting and has a significant advantage of cost savings. Local anesthetic is injected at the point of origin of the ECRB. An 11 blade is then used to release the extensor origin from the epicondyle. The goal is to achieve about a 1-cm distal muscle slide to a new resting length. Immediate motion is allowed in a soft dressing. A more popular technique involves excising the abnormal tissue through an open incision, which I prefer to perform under a Bier block anesthetic. A longitudinal split is made between extensor carpi radialis longus (ECRL) and EDC tendons. After elevating the origin of the ECRL, the grayish-yellow pathologic tissue in the origin of the ECRB has a distinct fish-flesh appearance and consistency in contrast to the normal glistening longitudinal tendinous tissue (Fig. 53-2). It is excised in an elliptical fashion, with care taken to avoid injury to the underlying lateral collateral ligament. The underlying lateral epicondyle is then excoriated with a curette, and a small drill is used to create some channels for bleeding to promote scar and healing. One randomized double-blind comparative prospective trial has shown, however, that drilling conferred no benefit and actually caused more pain, stiffness, and wound bleeding than not drilling.

If the joint capsule is violated, I prefer to repair it with absorbable sutures to prevent a synovial cutaneous fistula from developing postoperatively (Fig. 53-3). The defect in the extensor tendon is then reapproximated. A soft, compressive dressing is applied and immediate gentle range of motion is encouraged. Alternatively, complete release of the extensor mechanism, debridement of abnormal tissue, with reattachment of the extensor origin back to lateral epicondyle out through drill holes can be performed. A V-Y lengthening, or slide, of the common extensor origin has also been described with good results. One must limit lifting and activities for 6 weeks following these latter two procedures to prevent detachment of the extensor origin in the postoperative period. In patients with persistent pain requiring revision surgery, or in whom a synovial cutaneous fistula has developed after a previous release, a wider debridement of the extensor origin may be performed with coverage using a vascularized rotational pedicle flap of the anconeus muscle.

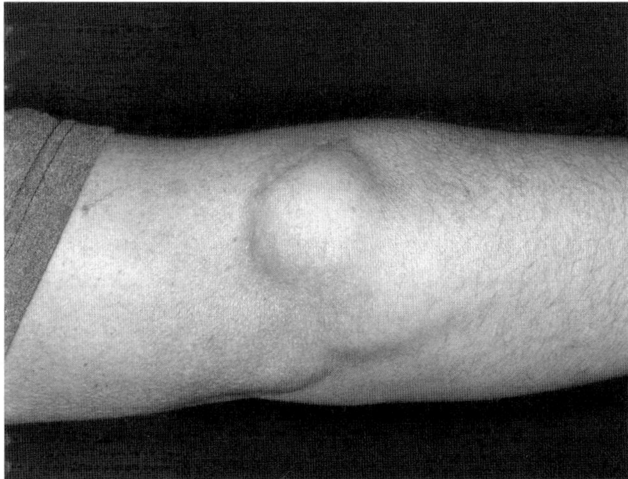

Figure 53-3 Patient with a persistent subcutaneous synovial fluid collection after extensor origin debridement and arthrotomy, in whom the joint capsule was not repaired.

Arthroscopic release of the ECRB origin has also become a popular technique. This is accomplished using proximal medial and proximal lateral portals. It has an added advantage of addressing any intra-articular pathology, which has been reported in 19% to 70% of patients. Baker et al. have classified the arthroscopic appearance of these lesions as follows: type 1, a normal-appearing undersurface of the capsule; type 2, a horizontal rent in the capsule; or type 3, complete rupture of the capsule with exposure of the ECRB tendon. The capsule is removed to allow visualization of the origin of the extensor muscles and tendon. The debridement is then performed from proximal to distal and is complete when all visible abnormal tissue is excised, exposing muscle fibers with a healthy appearance. Elbow stability is not compromised as long as resection does not extend posteriorly to an intra-articular line bisecting the radial head. Contraindications to arthroscopic debridement include significant calcific tendonitis, previous ulnar nerve transposition since visualization must be from the medial side (proximal-medial portal), and significant ankylosis, which may lead to inadequate joint distention and an increased risk of vascular injury because of inadequate displacement from the portal site from incomplete distention. Denervation (Wilhelm technique) has also been reported as an effective method for relieving pain, and is accomplished blindly by detachment of certain muscles, as well as simultaneous indirect decompression of the posterior interosseous nerve.

Surgical Complications

Posterolateral instability may result from inadvertent release of the lateral collateral ligament, as this structure is confluent with the origins of the ECRB and EDC. When performing a percutaneous release, the surgeon should keep a thumb over the posterolateral aspect of the radiocapitellar joint to avoid extension of the scalpel. If a posterior interosseous nerve decompression is performed, direct injury or neurapraxia, particularly involving branches to the EDC, is possible. One must keep in mind during an arthroscopic release that cadaveric studies have demonstrated varying courses of the lateral and posterior antebrachial nerves, which place these superficial sensory nerves at risk during portal placement. The radial nerve is also about an average of 5 mm from the proximal lateral portal. Painful neuromas of the posterior antebrachial nerve have also been reported after open releases and can be treated with neuroma resection and implantation of the nerve proximally into the brachioradialis muscle. Synovial cutaneous fistulas can result if the capsule has been violated to a significant degree and not repaired sufficiently. Heterotopic ossification after lateral epicondylectomy, although rare, has also been reported.

Results and Outcome

As mentioned previously, most studies on lateral elbow pain are limited by methodologic weaknesses in selection and definition of the study population, length of follow-up, and analysis of prognostic factors. Outcome scores, such as proposed by Roles and Maudsley or DASH (Disabilities of the Arm, Shoulder, and Hand), are not routinely used, and even objective data such as grip-strength measurements with an extended elbow are seldom reported. Systematic reviews of interventions have confirmed that there is a surprising lack of published controlled trials of surgery for lateral elbow pain. Without a control group, it is very hard to draw any conclusions about the effectiveness of a given modality of treatment, since the natural history of the syndrome is uncertain.

Of the published studies, pain relief following open debridement or releases ranges from 78% to 97%, 91% to 96% after percutaneous releases, and 85% to 90% after denervation. Reported rates involving return to work average about 5 weeks following open, 9 to 21 days for percutaneous, and 6 to 15 days after arthroscopic releases. When reported, grip-strength improvements range from 30% to 100%, with a good result considered >90% compared with the uninvolved side. One prospective, randomized, controlled trial comparing formal open release with percutaneous tenotomy showed significant improvements in patient satisfaction, time to return to work, the DASH score, and sporting activities in the percutaneous group. In another retrospective comparison, 69% of open cases and 72% of arthroscopic cases had good or excellent outcomes. Patients treated with arthroscopic release returned to work earlier than patients treated with open release did, and they required less postoperative therapy. Poorer results have been reported in patients seeking compensation.

SUGGESTED READINGS

Almquist EE, Necking L, Bach AW. Epicondylar resection with anconeus muscle transfer for chronic lateral epicondylitis. *J Hand Surg (Am)*. 1998;23:723–731.

Baker CL Jr, Murphy KP, Gottlob CA, et al. Arthroscopic classification and treatment of lateral epicondylitis: two-year clinical results. *J Shoulder Elbow Surg*. 2000;9:475–482.

Boyer MI, Hastings H. Lateral tennis elbow: "Is there any science out there?". *J Shoulder Elbow Surg*. 1999;8:481–491.

Dunkow PD, Jatti M, Muddu BN. A comparison of open and percutaneous techniques in the surgical treatment of tennis elbow. *J Bone Joint Surg Br*. 2004;86:701–704.

Haahr JP, Andersen JH. Prognostic factors in lateral epicondylitis: a randomized trial with one-year follow-up in 266 new cases treated with minimal occupational intervention or the usual approach in general practice. *Rheumatology (Oxford)*. 2003;42:1216–1225.

Hayton MJ, Santini AJ, Hughes PJ, et al. Botulinum toxin injection in the treatment of tennis elbow. A double-blind, randomized, controlled, pilot study. *J Bone Joint Surg Am*. 2005;87:503–507.

Labelle H, Guibert R, Joncas J, et al. Lack of scientific evidence for the treatment of lateral epicondylitis of the elbow. An attempted meta-analysis. *J Bone Joint Surgery Br*. 1992;74:646–651.

Nirschl RP, Ashman ES. Tennis elbow tendonitis (epicondylitis). *Instructional Course Lectures*. 2004;53:587–598.

Pomerance J. Radiographic analysis of lateral epicondylitis. *J Shoulder Elbow Surg*. 2002;11:156–157.

Verhaar J, Walenkamp G, Kester A, et al. Lateral extensor release for tennis elbow. A prospective long-term follow-up study. *J Bone Joint Surg Am*. 1993;75:1034–1043.

Wilhelm A. Tennis elbow: treatment of resistant cases by denervation. *J Hand Surg (Br)*. 1996;21:523–533.

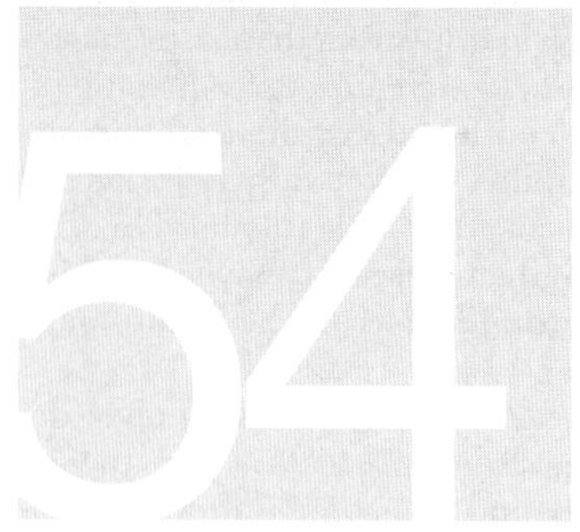

MEDIAL EPICONDYLITIS

SCOTT DUNCAN

Medial epicondylitis is a confusing and poorly understood condition. It is frequently referred to as "golfer's elbow." There have been few studies with proper design methodology or power to scientifically delineate definitive treatment requirements. Medial epicondylitis is perhaps the most common cause of medial elbow pain. The term *epicondylitis* is really a misnomer because there is minimal histologic evidence of inflammatory disease. It most likely is a tendinosis, i.e., a degenerative condition of the tendon. This tendinosis appears to be a failure of tendon healing in the face of continual microtrauma. The diagnosis can be difficult and may be found in conjunction with ulnar neuropathy at the elbow.

PATHOGENESIS

Etiology

The etiology of medial epicondylitis suggests that there is a repetitive overuse or stressing of the flexor pronator mass musculature resulting in microtrauma. Degenerative changes involving the musculotendinous unit of the medial epicondyle appear to be brought about by a chronic repetitive concentric and eccentric loading of the flexor pronator musculature. These repetitive eccentric and concentric contractions load the muscle and tendon, causing microtrauma. These microtears fail to heal and can build up over time. The degenerative changes are usually seen in the pronator teres as well as the flexor carpi radialis muscles. A single traumatic event such as a direct blow or sudden-overload eccentric contraction can result in the development of epicondylitis; however, the repetitive overuse theory is usually attributed as the main cause. Activities that require repetitive forearm pronation as well as wrist flexion have been associated with causing medial epicondylitis.

Medial epicondylitis has been related to sports such as golf, tennis, baseball, racquetball, bowling, football, archery, javelin throwing, and weight lifting. However, this is not just an athletic-type injury; some occupations require significant physical activity. For example, butchers, carpenters, and plumbers are at potential risk because of the repetitive forearm pronation and wrist flexion involved with their occupations. It is thought that overload from extrinsic valgus stresses and intrinsic muscular contractions can predispose the flexor pronator mass musculature to injury and accumulative microdegenerative trauma involving the pronator teres, flexor carpi radialis, and occasionally the flexor carpi ulnaris. Most commonly what is seen is a microtear in the interface between the pronator teres and the flexor carpi radialis origins with subsequent development of fibrotic granulation tissue.

Epidemiology

Medial epicondylar tendinosis occurs much less frequently than its lateral counterpart, lateral epicondylitis. The predominant age groups affected are fourth and fifth decades although almost any age group can potentially be affected. However, it has not been described in children. Male and female prevalence appears to be equal in most studies. Other studies have suggested a 2:1 male-to-female ratio. Approximately 75% of patients are usually symptomatic in their dominant extremity. Approximately 30% of patients describe the pain being associated with an acute injury. Most patients, roughly 70% of cases, describe a much more insidious onset of their symptoms. Almost half of all cases will have some ulnar nerve symptoms associated with them. Other conditions commonly seen in patients with medial epicondylitis include an approximately 30% rate of prior history of lateral epicondylitis, a 25% rate of history of carpal tunnel syndrome, and a 20% rate of prior rotator cuff tendinosis. In younger patients other causes of epicondylar pain should be ruled out prior to considering this degenerative condition more commonly seen in middle-aged adults. Other literature has suggested no predilection for the dominant hand or between genders.

Pathophysiology

Early descriptions of medial and lateral epicondylitis were posed and postulated in inflammatory conditions that involved bursa, periosteum, synovium, and ligaments. The recent literature has discounted these theories, and the histologic analysis of Nirschl and Pettrone has demonstrated normal collagen and architecture disrupted by fibroblastic immature vascular response as well as an incomplete reparative process. Importantly, there is a lack of acute and chronic inflammatory cellular architecture. In the very early stages of medial epicondylitis, there may be some inflammatory or synovitis-type patterns present. However, more definitively in the later stages there is evidence of microtearing with tendon degeneration, with or without calcification, and failure to complete a neovascular healing response. The pathologic tissue appears grossly friable and has a gray to tannish color.

Nirschl and Pettrone have coined the term "angiofibroblastic hyperplasia" to describe such structural changes. Nirschl has described four stages of epicondylar tendinosis. In stage one there is generalized inflammation that can recede. In stage two the injury is noted to have pathologic tissue changes of the angiofibroblastic type. Stage three is noted to have degeneration that results in structural failure. Finally, stage four can include components of stages two and three but is also accompanied by marked fibrosis or calcifications. The exact pathophysiology of medial epicondylitis has not yet been established. It is agreed that the injury results from microtearing of the tendon origin at the epicondyle with failure of the usual reparative processes to mount a response. The subsequent tendon tearing and degeneration changes the usual musculotendinous biomechanics of the elbow, resulting in the pain and dysfunction seen clinically.

Classification

Gable and Morrey have described a classification for medial epicondylitis based on the presence and severity of concomitant ulnar neuropathy at the elbow. In their classification system, type 1A includes patients without any associated ulnar nerve symptoms. Type 1B has mild ulnar nerve signs or symptoms. In the type 2 medial epicondylitis patient, there are moderate or severe ulnar nerve symptoms with objective deficits noted on the physical exam as well as denervation noted on electromyography.

DIAGNOSIS

History and Physical Examination

Clinical Features

A patient who presents with medial epicondylitis can come from various situations. Some are from the workplace and have an environment that is consistent with repetitive activity. Others relate it to being problematic with their athletic endeavors. When obtaining the history, it is useful to divide patients based on the manner of onset, provocative activities, localization of pain, and severity of discomfort. Other specific characteristics to specifically ask about include onset of pain with the date, time, and activity being performed. For example, a golfer may recall a missed hit striking the ground with the club that resulted in a sudden deceleration, or the tennis player or racquetball player may remember a specific extra-hard hit or serve that resulted in pain about the medial aspect of the elbow. Is the patient able to localize the pain with one specific finger to the medial epicondylar region or is he or she vague in where the symptoms are located? Are symptoms better with rest and reproduced with certain provocative activities? Do they have other areas of significant pain about the upper extremity or neck or is it again specifically localized to the medial epicondylar region? Is worker's compensation or other potential secondary gain involved? Do they describe numbness and tingling in an anatomic or in a nonanatomic distribution?

The textbook case of medial epicondylitis should be mechanically based in that the pain is exacerbated or reproduced by the stress and strain of the wrist flexors and forearm pronators on the medial side. Otherwise other conditions need to be considered (Table 54-1). The most important injuries to exclude when evaluating a patient with medial epicondylitis involve, again, the amount of ulnar nerve involvement and any type of injury to the medial collateral ligament. In overhead throwing athletes, this can be a challenging differential. One technique for trying to differentiate medial tendon injury from medial collateral ligament insufficiency is by placing a valgus force to a slightly flexed elbow with the wrist in volar flexion and the forearm pronated. This test usually does not elicit pain or demonstrate laxity if the diagnosis is medial epicondylitis only. Other considerations to think about are lower cervical radiculopathies involving C7 through T1 that may cause radiating pain along the medial aspect of the upper extremity.

Ideally the physical exam should be done with the patient relaxed and sitting. The patient frequently is able to help identify the tenderest spot. Classic findings consist of exquisite and repeatable localization of medial epicondylar tenderness with palpation. Some patients may have maximal tenderness just distal to the epicondylar region in the proximal flexor pronator mass. The medial pain can be exacerbated with resisted pronation and flexion of the wrist. The usual physical exam shows some tenderness over the anterior aspect of the medial epicondyle. More than 90% of patients will have pain with resisted pronation and more than 70% pain with resisted wrist flexion. Wrist and elbow range of motion are typically normal. Local injection of lidocaine or Marcaine results in near complete obliteration of the discomfort.

Of course the ulnar nerve needs to be evaluated including the Tinel sign over the ulnar nerve in the region of the elbow, an elbow flexion test, ulnar nerve compression test, and

TABLE 54-1 MEDIAL ELBOW PAIN DIFFERENTIAL DIAGNOSIS

Medial epicondylitis
Medial collateral ligament tear/attenuation
Flexor pronator mass muscle injury
Pronator teres syndrome
Ulnar trochlear arthritis/synovitis
Intra-articular loose body
Snapping triceps
Ulnar nerve compression/subluxation
Cervical radiculopathy

TABLE 54-2 ULNAR NERVE TRANSPOSITION INDICATIONS IN PATIENTS WITH MEDIAL EPICONDYLITIS

Sensory or motor loss
Positive elbow flexion test
Neurapraxia with valgus stress
Subluxating ulnar nerve
Cubital tunnel scarring
Marked cubital valgus

checking the ulnar nerve for subluxation about the medial epicondyle (Table 54-2) Distally, function of the ulnar nerve needs to be assessed with two-point discrimination in intrinsic strength and dorsal cutaneous nerve status. Other things to check for include the cervical spine to rule out a radiculopathy. The skin about the elbow should be inspected. Palpation about the biceps insertion, brachialis, and lacertus needs to be performed. The triceps insertion and olecranon should also be palpated. Kurvers and Verhaar have noted that in their patient series, approximately 20% of patients with medial epicondylitis for >12 months had flexion contractors ranging from 10 to 25 degrees. Furthermore, 15% of their patient population had decreased active supination range of motion by 5 to 15 degrees. Occasionally local swelling and warmth may be present.

Radiographic Features

The radiographs of elbows affected with medial epicondylitis are usually normal. Approximately 20% to 25% of patients, however, may have some soft tissue calcification in the proximity of the medial epicondyle. Other patients, especially throwing athletes, may have ulnar-sided traction spurs and medial collateral ligament calcifications. Radiographs are also useful to rule out associated conditions such as osteoarthritis as well as medial instability with valgus stress views (if medial instability is suspected). An MRI arthrogram can be helpful in differentiating medial collateral ligament injury from medial epicondylitis. Other findings potentially seen on radiographs are loose bodies, radiocapitellar and ulnar trochlear arthritis, olecranon or coronoid impingement. In trying to differentiate calcification to the medial tendon from the medial collateral ligament, it should be noted that the calcifications in the medial tendon are usually relatively superficial whereas those in the medial collateral ligament are deep to the flexor pronator mass.

Other Studies

Electrodiagnostic evaluation of the ulnar nerve is useful in cases where ulnar neuropathy is suspected clinically. This can be used to document the severity of axonal changes. This can also be used to show nerve conduction slowing in an absolute or relative fashion compared with other nerves or the other side. The author's preference is to obtain electrodiagnostic studies with nerve conduction velocities as well as electromyographic analysis. Surgical outcome can be compromised by failing to address the ulnar neuropathy (Table 54-2). In obtaining the MRI, make sure that the facility to be used has the appropriate coils and imaging protocols as well as technical knowledge to adequately evaluate the elbow; otherwise the study will be for naught.

DIAGNOSTIC WORKUP

Algorithm

The reader is referred to Figure 54-1 for the work-through algorithm in evaluating the patient and proceeding with study intervention and treatment options.

Anatomy

The anatomy of the medial epicondyle consists of the flexor pronator origin; this is at the anterior medial epicondyle. The pronator teres originates in part from the superior interior medial epicondyle; however, its main origin is from an intramuscular tendon otherwise known as the medial conjoint tendon. In going from the radial to ulnar aspect of the forearm, the musculature includes the pronator teres, the flexor carpi radialis, the palmaris longus, the flexor digitorum superficialis, and the flexor carpi ulnaris. The pronator teres and flexor carpi radialis tendon and muscles are most afflicted with the alteration of stretching and acceleration during throwing and swinging.

The critical lesion of medial epicondylitis comes from the medial conjoint tendon and its associated pronator teres and flexor carpi radialis origins. The medial conjoint tendon serves as the landmark for the surgical excision of the pathology as well as a way to identify and avoid the anterior oblique ligament. Medial conjoint tendon arises from the anterior inferior epicondyle with an oblique parasagittal orientation that traverses approximately 12 cm into the proximal forearm. Any surgical dissection and elevation off the medial epicondyle posterior to the medial conjoint tendon will violate the anterior oblique ligament of the medial collateral ligament.

Professional throwing athletes can develop hypertrophy of the flexor pronator mass resulting in a flexion contracture. Frequently 50% of these individuals will have some type of flexion contracture and 30% will have an increased valgus angle compared with their contralateral extremity. Of note, though, is that these features have never been correlated with the recurrence of medial epicondylitis. The ulnar nerve transverses posteromedially about the medial epicondyle. Also, the medial antebrachial cutaneous nerve passes in this zone. Occasionally the triceps can snap over the medial epicondyle causing pain that is not related to medial epicondylitis, and this is known as a snapping triceps syndrome.

TREATMENT

Nonoperative Options

Nonoperative treatment works for most cases of medial epicondylitis. The purpose of this nonsurgical care is to relieve pain and allow sufficient rehabilitation so that the

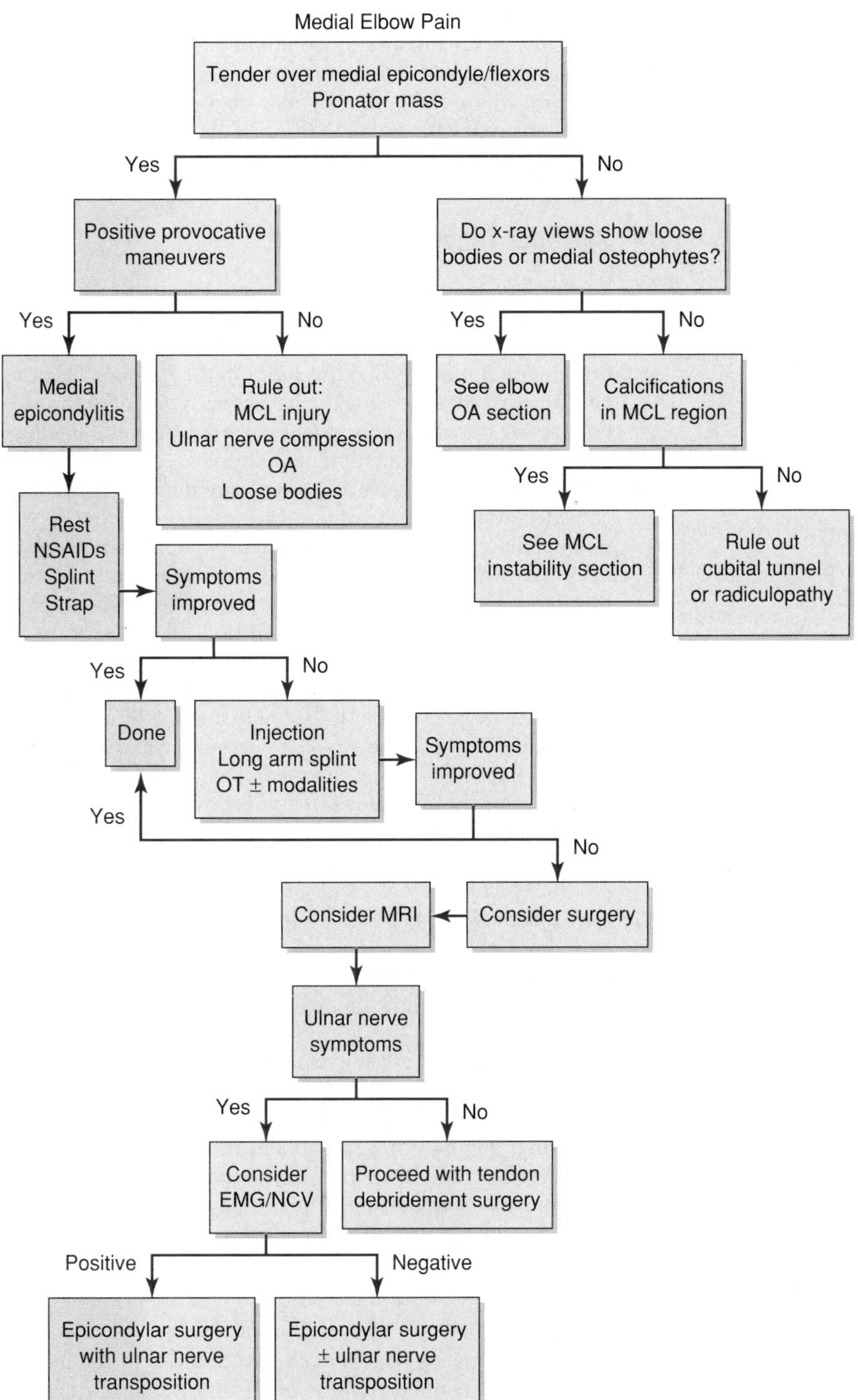

Figure 54-1 Algorithm for patient evaluation and treatment. MCL, medial collateral ligament OA; osteoarthritis; NSAIDs, nonsteroidal anti-inflammatory drugs; MRI, magnetic resonance imaging; EMG/NCV, electromyogram/nerve conduction velocity.

patient can return to the previous activities. Current literature suggests that roughly 5% to 15% of patients suffer recurring episodes of medial epicondylitis. However, this may represent incomplete rehabilitation or premature termination of the rehabilitative program. The initial nonoperative treatment usually consists of rest, ice, nonsteroid anti-inflammatories, local modalities, splinting, and cortisone injections. The author's preference for cortisone injection consists of a water-soluble corticosteroid mixed with 2 mL of half percent plain bupivacaine.

The injection can be both therapeutic and diagnostic. The bupivacaine should substantially reduce the pain and this should last for several hours. If the patient does not notice any relief from the symptoms or minimal relief from the symptoms, then it is unlikely the diagnosis is epicondylitis, assuming the injection was placed in the proper location.

Most cases of medial epicondylitis do benefit from the initial injection, and this can last several months. However, repeat injections tend to have a decreasing benefit. When performing an injection about the medial aspect of the elbow for medial epicondylitis, care needs to be taken to make sure the ulnar nerve is palpated and that the needle is directed away from the cubital tunnel. I prefer to do the injection with the elbow extended and the thumb of my nondominant hand over the cubital tunnel.

A commercial wrist splint can help a patient whose pain is of sudden onset and severe. Usually a cock-up wrist splint resting the wrist at approximately 10 degrees of extension is adequate. In combination with the previously mentioned items, a 2-week course of oral nonsteroid anti-inflammatories may also be helpful. A medial counterforce brace can also be helpful for some patients, and the pad of the brace needs to be anteromedial on the flexor pronator mass but not medial or posterior medial over the ulnar nerve. If ulnar nerve symptoms are exacerbated, the brace should be discontinued.

If symptoms are improved at 6 to 8 weeks, a conditioning program can be initiated. This part of the rehabilitation starts with wrist flexor and forearm pronator stretching and progressive isometric exercises. Provocative activities, however, need to be avoided until predisease strength is restored. Eccentric and concentric resistive exercises are added once the flexibility, strength, and endurance of the patient have improved adequately to tolerate the program. Success rates of this combined approach range between 70% and 90%. The use of modalities such as ultrasound and iontophoresis may help some patients with their symptoms. However, there is no strong evidence in the literature to support widespread use of one modality over another, and no studies have shown modalities to provide prolonged long-term benefit.

Surgical Indications

If after one or two injections that provided temporary relief of the patient's symptoms the patient finds recurrence of the symptoms inhibiting function of daily activities, then these patients can be considered for surgical intervention. Patients with continued minor or intermittent symptoms whose hobbies such as tennis or golf are bothered but are not incapacitated in their activities of daily living are marginal candidates for surgery. Contraindications to surgery would be those patients who medically could not tolerate the surgery. The other candidate obviously would be those patients who received no benefit, even temporary, from an injection and are not able to demonstrate or localize the pain to the medial epicondyle.

Patients need to understand that not everyone benefits from surgery and it is rare for anyone to achieve 100% improvement. Certainly strenuous or provocative activities that brought the symptoms on before can still bring the symptoms on postoperatively. A rough rule to give patients in counseling them about surgery is that 80% of patients see 80% improvement in their symptoms. The author prefers to try a minimum of 6 months of nonoperative treatment prior to considering surgical intervention. Some authors recommend MRI or MRI arthrogram as part of the preoperative planning to rule out any concomitant pathology, to evaluate the condition of the tendons prior to surgery, and to help focus on where the pathology may be present. However, by no means is MRI mandated; this is a diagnosis that is made clinically and not by imaging studies.

Surgical Technique

Various procedures have been described such as percutaneous epicondylar release and epicondylectomy; however, the standard surgical treatment at this time consists of debridement of the degenerative nidus in the tendon. This can be summarized as excising the pathologic portion of the tendon, trying to enhance local vascularity to promote healing, performing stout reattachment of any elevated tissues to the medial epicondyle, repairing any tissue defects, and surgically decompressing the ulnar nerve and reconstructing the ulnar collateral ligament if needed. Nirschl and Pettrone have performed a debridement of abnormal tendon tissue through a longitudinal split of the medial tendon complex. The diseased tendon can be identified and excised in an elliptical fashion. The tendon origin is not disrupted.

Vangsness and Jobe described a technique that provided a greater exposure of the flexor origin and facilitated a complete debridement. They used a curvilinear incision at the medial elbow centered at the medial epicondyle. The interval between the pronator teres and flexor carpi radialis is then identified. The medial tendon is incised along the interval in the common flexor origin and is reflected directly off the epicondyle with sharp dissection. The medial collateral ligament is exposed but not disturbed. Any diseased and abnormal tissue is sharply excised, and the epicondyle is prepared with a rongeur to remove fibrous tissue. Small holes can be drilled in the medial epicondyle that create a vascular bed. Care needs to be taken to avoid entrapping any soft tissue around the drill. The common flexor origin is then reattached to the bleeding bone surface with interrupted stitches. Morrey describes his type 1A cases as requiring epicondylar debridement only, whereas type 1B cases require debridement with or without cubital tunnel decompression or transposition. Finally, his type 2 cases receive debridement with submuscular transposition of the ulnar nerve.

Technique

A 5-cm oblique incision is made just anterior to the medial epicondyle. I usually apply a sterile tourniquet and use an arm board. The medial antebrachial cutaneous nerve and its branches are identified. The incision may be easily enlarged if ulnar nerve transposition is to be considered. The common flexor pronator origin is found along with the ulnar nerve, which is protected. Usually an incision to the pronator teres and flexor carpi radialis interval is developed longitudinally (Fig. 54-2). This exposes the medial conjoint tendon. Again, care must be taken along the posterior aspect of the medial conjoint tendon because that is where the anterior oblique ligament lies. The degenerative tissue is then debrided with a rongeur as seen in Figure 54-3. The flexor pronator fascia is then repaired back to the retained rim

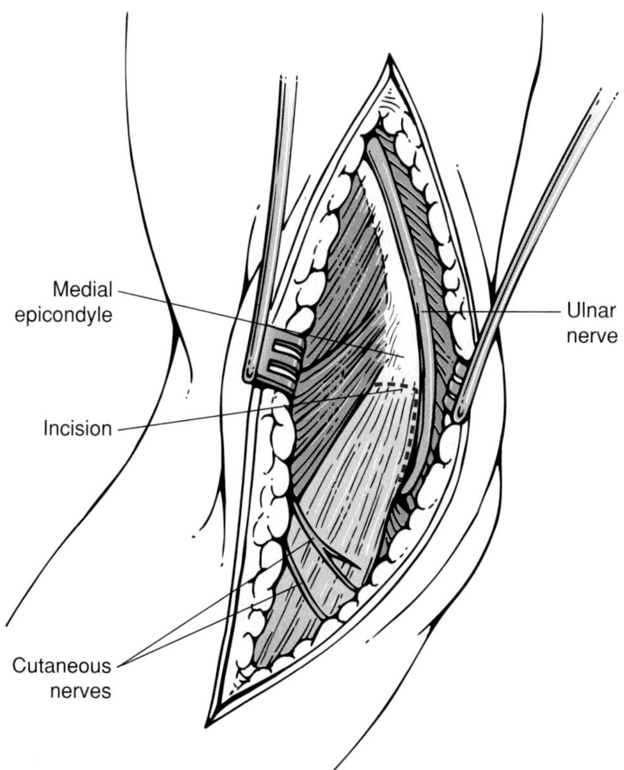

Figure 54-2 Anatomy and exposure of the medial epicondyle. Note the medial conjoint tendon, anterior oblique ligament, and medial antebrachial cutaneous nerve branches.

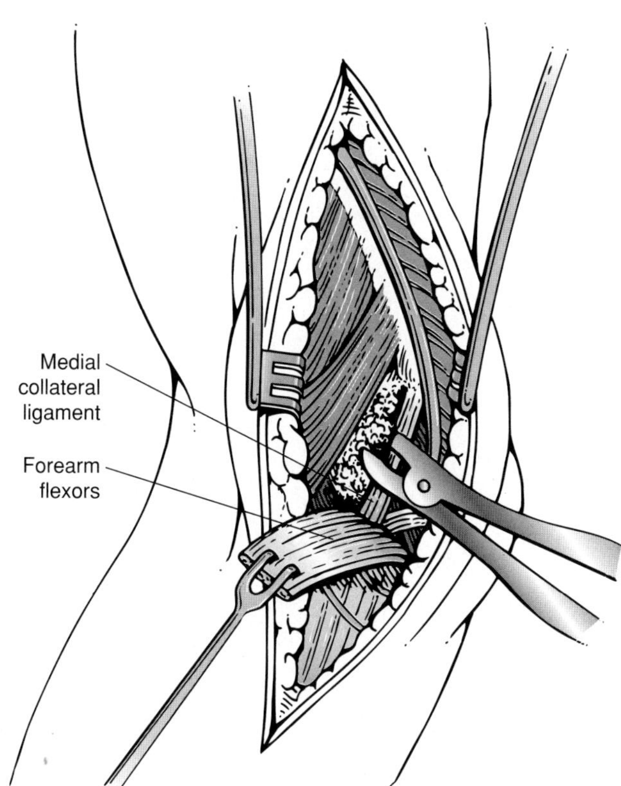

Figure 54-3 Note reflection of forearm flexors and debridement of degenerative tissue with a rongeur.

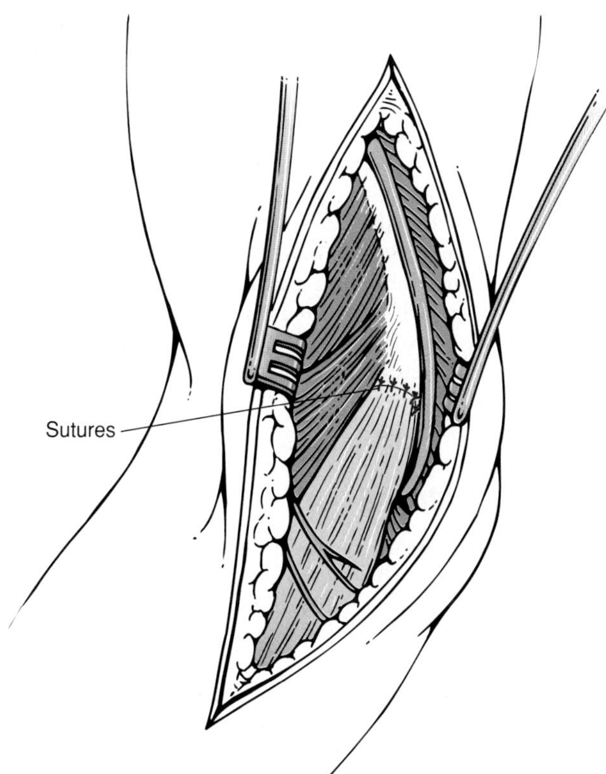

Figure 54-4 The common flexor tendon is then reattached with interrupted sutures, creating a secure closure.

of fascia at its original position or in a slightly lengthened position but not by more than >1 cm. The flexor pronator origin can be reattached to the bleeding bony surface with either interrupted sutures or through drill holes or with the attached adjacent flexor pronator origin (Fig. 54-4).

Rehabilitation

The patient is then placed in a posterior plaster splint that is applied to the elbow and wrist with the elbow at 90 degrees of flexion and the forearm in neutral rotation. At approximately 10 days postoperatively, the splint is removed and any skin sutures are removed. At this point gentle passive and active nonresistive range of motion exercises are begun for the hand, wrist, and elbow. Gentle isometric exercises are usually begun at 3 to 4 weeks postoperatively. Finally at 6 weeks, more aggressive resistant wrist flexion and forearm pronation are begun. Finally the progressive strengthening program is initiated. A gradual careful return is encouraged. Total body and extremity conditioning is encouraged throughout the entire rehabilitative process. The average return for most patients to their regular activities is 3 to 6 months postoperatively. However, in some series this has been anywhere in the range from 3 to 24 months.

Complications

Potential complications associated with this surgery include injury to branches of the medial antebrachial cutaneous nerve with subsequent neuromas around the incision site. Other complications involve injury to the ulnar nerve. Ulnar neuritis after surgery is not uncommon for a short period of time. Scarring along the cubital tunnel can lead to ulnar nerve symptoms developing postoperatively. Medial collateral ligament injury can destabilize the elbow and result in new symptoms that were not present preoperatively. Excessive release and debridement of flexor fascia without careful repair can lead to permanent flexor weakness. After surgery hematoma formation can result, causing discomfort. Patients should be warned about numbness around the incision area as well as potential numbness in the forearm. The other potential complication of course relates to failure to obtain improvement in the patient's preoperative symptoms.

Results and Outcome

Surgical results appear to correlate with the class of medial epicondylitis. Types 1A and 1B have roughly ≥90% good or excellent results as reported in two studies and have slightly lower rates in another two studies. Two thirds of patients can take ≤6 months to obtain the good to excellent level, whereas the remaining third may take up to ≤2 years. Type 2 with its associated ulnar nerve neuropathy has a poorer prognosis. The results of type 2 medial epicondylitis are related to the failure of the ulnar neuropathy to respond to the surgical treatment. Cubital tunnel release alone as treatment for type 2 medial epicondylitis has been shown to be suboptimal. Vangness and Jobe have reported the results of their surgical intervention with 86% of patients having no limitation in use of the elbow. In their study, isokinetic and grip-strength testing revealed no significant functional loss. Gabel and Morrey have reported similar success rates after surgical treatment of medial epicondylitis, but again found ulnar neuropathy to be correlated with a poor prognosis. Using Nirschl debridement technique Ollivierre et al. analyzed 50 cases of intractable medial epicondylitis and found partial or complete pain relief in all patients. Yet, one quarter of these patients were not able to return to painfree participation after surgery.

Summary

Medial epicondylitis will continue to remain an enigmatic and problematic disease until surgeons have a better understanding of the failure of the reparative mechanisms by which this degenerative condition occurs. Nonoperative management remains the mainstay of treatment, but surgical intervention is warranted in those patients who fail nonoperative treatment and can no longer tolerate the effect of their symptoms on their activities of daily living. Most patients will have improvement in their symptoms after surgery.

SUGGESTED READINGS

Chen FS, Rokito AS, Jobe FW. Medial elbow problems in the overhead-throwing athlete. *J Am Acad Orthop Surg.* 2001;9:99–113.

Ciccotti MC, Schwartz MA, Ciccotti MG. Diagnosis and treatment of medial epicondylitis of the elbow. *Clin Sports Med.* 2004;23:693–705.

Gabel GT, Morrey BF. Operative treatment of medial epicondylitis. Influence of concomitant ulnar neuropathy at the elbow. *J Bone Joint Surg Am.* 1995;77:1065–1069.

Hotchkiss RN. Epicondylitis—lateral and medial. A problem-oriented approach. *Hand Clin.* 2000;16:505–508.

Jobe FW, Ciccotti MG. Lateral and medial epicondylitis of the elbow. *J Am Acad Orthop Surg.* 1994;2:1–8.

Kurvers H, Verhaar J. The results of operative treatment of medial epicondylitis. *J Bone Joint Surg Am.* 1995;77:1374–1379.

Nirschl RP, Pettrone FA. Tennis elbow: the surgical treatment of lateral epicondylitis. *J Bone Joint Surg Am.* 1979;61:832–839.

Ollivierre CO, Nirschl RP, Pettrone FA. Resection and repair for medial tennis elbow. A prospective analysis. *Am J Sports Med.* 1995;23(2):214–221.

Stahl S, Kaufman T: The efficacy of an injection of steroids for medial epicondylitis. A prospective study of sixty elbows. *J Bone Joint Surg Am.* 1997;79:1648.

Vangsness C, Jobe FW. Surgical technique of medial epicondylitis: results in 35 elbows. *J Bone Joint Surg Br.* 1991;73:409–411.

RADIAL HEAD FRACTURES

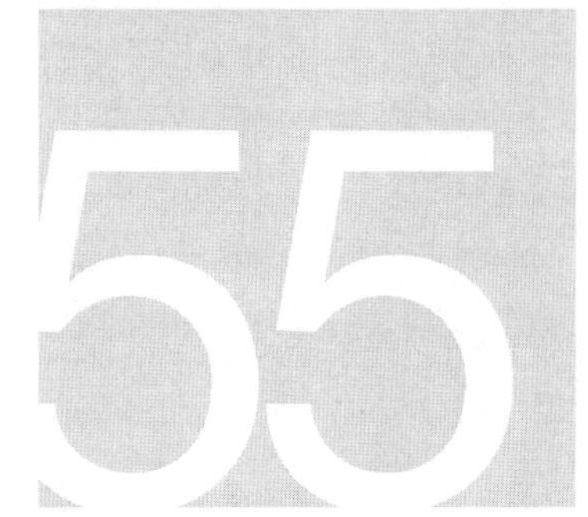

MICHAEL W. HARTMAN
SCOTT P. STEINMANN

Radial head fractures represent the most common fracture of the elbow in the adult population, accounting for 1.7% to 5.4% of all adult fractures. Approximately 85% of these fractures occur in young, active individuals ranging in age from 20 to 60 years old. Radial head fractures may occur in isolation or may be part of a more extensive traumatic elbow injury. An estimated 20% of all acute elbow injuries have an associated radial head fracture (Fig. 55-1). In elbow dislocations, a radial head fracture is commonly associated with other traumatic pathologies including medial collateral ligament (MCL) rupture, olecranon fracture, and/or coronoid fracture. Therefore, in the setting of trauma, the elbow must be carefully evaluated to rule out associated ligamentous and bony pathology.

Radial head fractures usually result from a fall onto the outstretched hand with the elbow slightly flexed and the forearm in a pronated position. Biomechanical studies have demonstrated that the greatest amount of force is transmitted from the wrist to the radial head when the elbow and forearm are oriented in this position. During a fall, the body rotates internally on the elbow; the weight of the body contributes an axial load to the radius; and a valgus moment is applied to the elbow since the hand becomes laterally displaced from the body. The resultant combination of axial, valgus, and external rotatory loading mechanisms forces the anterolateral margin of the radial head to come into contact with the capitellum, resulting in a fracture of the radial head and/or capitellum.

SURGICAL INDICATIONS AND OTHER OPTIONS

The modified Mason classification is useful in predicting the surgical management of radial head fractures. Type I fractures include nondisplaced or minimally displaced fractures of the head and neck, fractures with intra-articular displacement of <2 mm, or marginal lip fractures. There should be no mechanical block to forearm rotation; however, rotation may be limited by acute pain and swelling. The mainstay of treatment of type I fractures involves nonoperative measures that encourage early elbow and forearm range of motion. In the acute setting, the elbow hemarthrosis should be aspirated and injected with local anesthetic to allow a better assessment of forearm rotation, improve patient discomfort, and encourage earlier range of motion. The patient is placed into a sling for comfort and instructed to begin active and passive range of motion as tolerated within 7 days. Protected weight bearing of the upper extremity for a period of 6 weeks is encouraged to prevent fracture displacement. Serial x-ray views are obtained on a weekly basis to assess for fracture displacement. Open reduction internal fixation (ORIF) is indicated if the fracture displacement subsequently occurs. Good to excellent results are expected in most type 1 fractures managed nonoperatively with a program of early elbow and forearm range of motion.

Type II fractures include displaced (>2 mm) fractures of the radial head or neck without severe comminution. These fractures may have mechanical block to motion or be incongruous. Nonoperative management of type II fractures should be considered only if elbow stability is not dependent on fracture fixation and no significant block to elbow motion is present. In the absence of comminution, these fractures are usually amenable to ORIF (Fig. 55-2). Recent data suggest that ORIF should be reserved for minimally comminuted fractures with three or fewer articular fragments.[1] These data also suggest that fracture-dislocations of the elbow or forearm managed with ORIF result in less optimal results, especially with regard to forearm rotation. Other surgical options for type II fractures include fragment excision, head excision, or radial head replacement arthroplasty. Fragment excision alone may be indicated when a fracture fragment blocks forearm rotation but is too small, comminuted, or osteoporotic to adequately gain fixation (Fig. 55-3). The fracture fragment should not involve the lesser sigmoid notch or involve more than one third of the circumference of the head's articular surface. Most elbow surgeons discourage fragment excision because of the possibility of subsequent radial head subluxation.

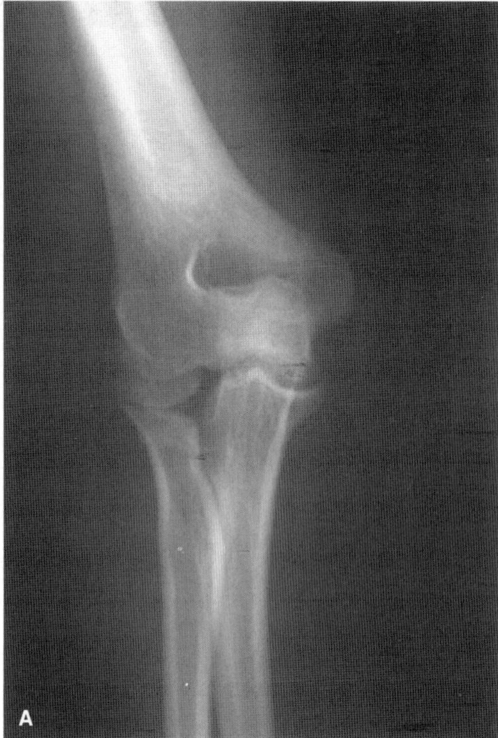

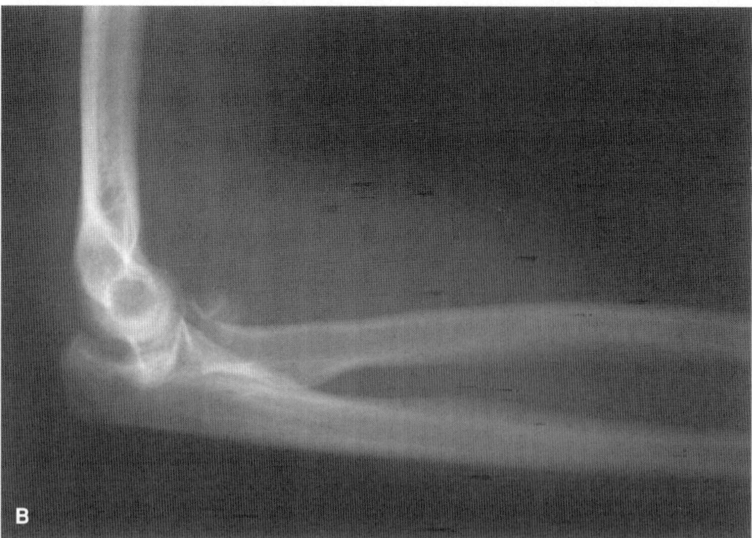

Figure 55-1 Type III radial head fracture. **A:** Anteroposterior view. **B:** Lateral view.

Type III fractures include severely comminuted radial head or neck fractures that are deemed unreconstructable based on radiographic and/or intraoperative appearance. Surgical options include radial head excision with or without radial head replacement arthroplasty. Prosthetic head replacement is indicated under associated conditions of instability such as complex elbow instability, Essex-Lopresti lesion, Monteggia lesion with instability, or a fracture of a major portion of the coronoid (Fig. 55-4).

Radial head excision alone may be indicated in elderly, low-demand patients without ligamentous instability. Numerous series report good to excellent results in terms of pain relief and elbow range of motion after head excision alone. The potential disadvantages of head excision include decreased grip strength, weak forearm rotation, and radial shortening with resultant wrist pain. Altered load transfer at the elbow joint may also lead to the development of early ulnar trochlear arthrosis and elbow pain. When compared with head excision, results of metal prosthetic radial head replacement demonstrate similar range of motion, better clinical scores, less proximal radial migration, and decreased elbow arthritis (Fig. 55-5).

SURGICAL TECHNIQUES

Preoperative planning is essential in the surgical management of radial head fractures. A full selection of internal fixation and reconstructive options should be available at the surgeon's disposal. Options for internal fixation include various combinations of threaded K-wires, screws, and plates. The ultimate goal of these hardware devices is to obtain rigid fixation and hence, allow early postoperative range of motion. The surgeon should be prepared to replace the radial head if indicated, preferably with a metallic prosthesis. The patient is positioned supine on the operating table and general or regional anesthesia is administered. A sandbag is placed under the ipsilateral scapula to facilitate positioning of the upper extremity across the chest. Prophylactic antibiotics are administered 30 minutes prior to making the incision. An examination under anesthesia is performed prior to prepping and draping the involved extremity. Examination under anesthesia is absolutely essential in evaluating elbow and forearm stability and range of motion prior to proceeding. A skin incision is centered laterally over the lateral epicondyle and extended distally over the radial head and neck. Alternatively, a posterior elbow incision just lateral to the tip of the olecranon may be used in complex injuries in which access to the radial head, coronoid, medial collateral ligament, and/or lateral collateral ligament may be required (Fig. 55-6). Full-thickness flaps are developed down to the level of the fascia.

The classic approach to the radial head uses the Kocher interval between the anconeus and extensor carpi ulnaris. This approach is disadvantageous for two reasons. First, the approach tends to expose the radial head too posteriorly, making internal fixation of the commonly fractured anterolateral head difficult, if not impossible. Second, iatrogenic injury to the lateral ulnar collateral ligament is difficult to avoid and may lead to posterolateral rotatory instability. An alternative approach that splits the extensor digitorum communis is the preferred approach. This approach is more anterior and hence avoids disruption of the posterolateral

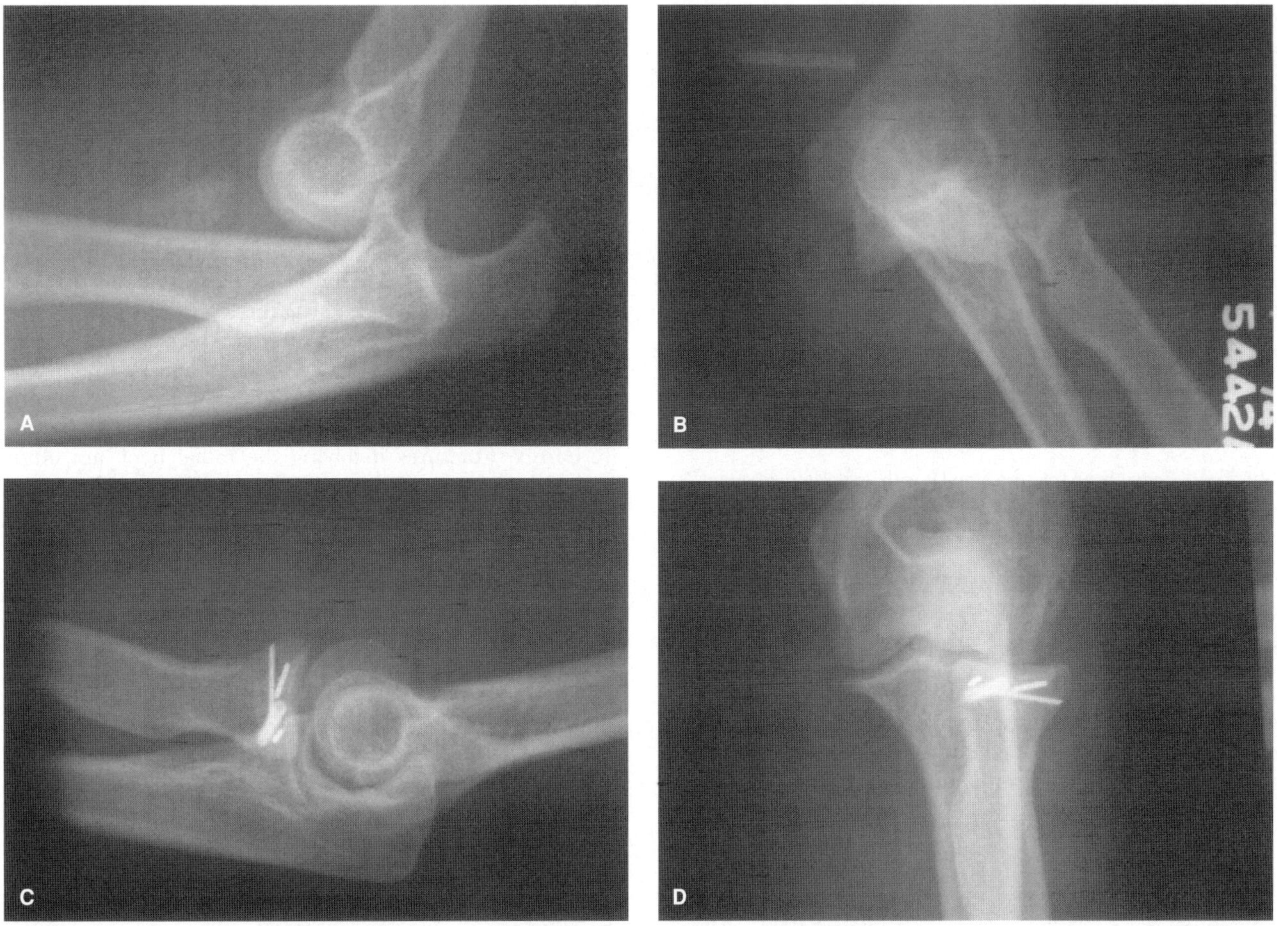

Figure 55-2 **A:** Lateral radiograph of fracture dislocation of elbow type II fracture radial head. **B:** Anteroposterior radiograph type II fracture radial head. **C:** Postoperative view: pin and screw fixation of radial head fracture (lateral view). **D:** Postoperative view: pin and screw fixation of radial head fracture (anteroposterior view).

collateral ligamentous complex (Fig. 55-7). The lateral epicondyle is identified, and the elbow capsule is elevated subperiosteally off its anterior aspect. Anterior capsular elevation is continued distally to the level of the capitellum and elbow joint taking care to avoid the collateral ligamentous complex posteriorly. Dissection next proceeds through the annular ligament exposing the radial head. If the fracture involves only the radial head, minimal distal (1 to 2 cm) dissection is usually necessary. If the radial neck is involved, further distal exposure is required. The forearm is fully pronated and the posterior portion of the extensor digitorum communis is divided. To avoid placing the posterior interosseous nerve at risk, distal dissection should not proceed more than two fingerbreadths from the radial head. If the location of the posterior interosseous nerve is in doubt, definitive identification of the nerve may be required.

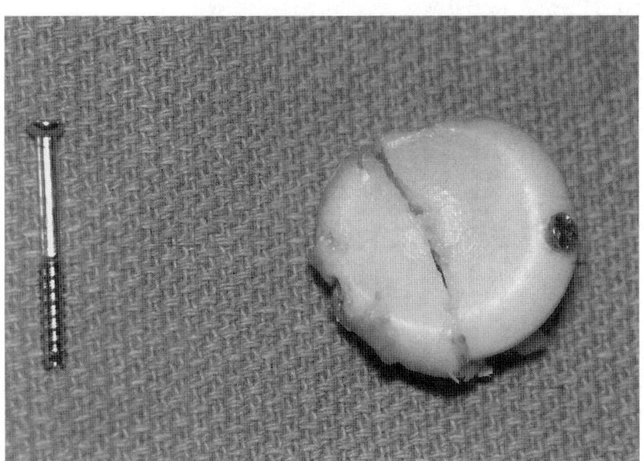

Figure 55-3 Attempted screw fixation of radial head fracture.

Once sufficient exposure is obtained, the character of the fracture is thoroughly assessed. The capitellum is also visually assessed for the presence of an associated chondral injury or osteochondral fracture. The decision to proceed with fragment excision, head excision, ORIF, or radial head replacement arthroplasty can be made at this point. At the time of closure, the annular ligament and the posterolateral collateral ligament complex (if disrupted) are repaired. The fascial layer over the common extensor group is closed to augment lateral elbow stability. Elbow and forearm range of motion and stability are carefully assessed and recorded.

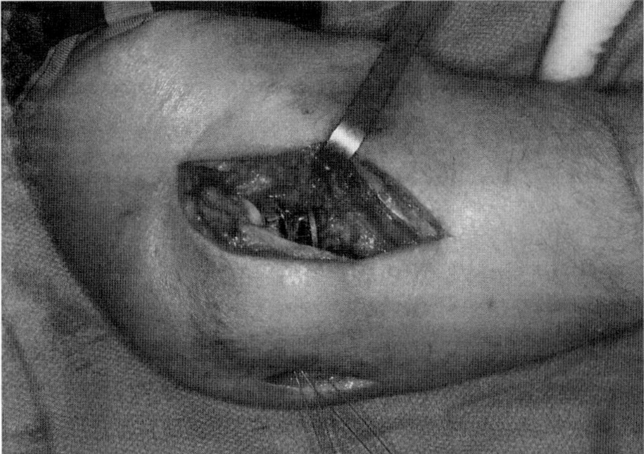

Figure 55-4 Radial head fracture type III with associated coronoid fracture. The radial head was replaced with a prosthesis and the coronoid fracture repaired with suture (second smaller, posterior incision).

Open Reduction Internal Fixation

The concept of an anatomic "safe zone" must be understood when attempting hardware placement into the radial head. Hardware may be placed into this zone without causing impingement of the proximal radioulnar joint. The safe zone is defined by a 110-degree arc centered anterolaterally over the equator of the radial head with the forearm in neutral rotation. Alternatively, one may identify the safe zone as a 90-degree arc defined by the right angle from the radial styloid to the Lister tubercle. Surface anatomy can also help to identify the proper location for hardware placement.

Once the fracture has been reduced, K-wires may be used for provisional fixation. K-wires should be absolutely avoided for definitive fixation given their tendency for migration postoperatively. For fractures that do not involve the radial neck, definitive fixation is typically obtained by using small screws (sizes 1.5, 2.0, or 2.7 mm) and 3.0-mm cannulated screws. Screws should be countersunk beneath the articular surface but not protrude through the opposite cortex. Fractures involving the radial neck are often impacted and require bone grafting to elevate the radial head. These fractures may be amenable to screw and/or plate fixation. One technique that has been successful in the authors' experience avoids the inherent problems associated with plate fixation for impacted neck fractures. In this technique, the radial head is first elevated to its anatomic position and temporarily secured using threaded K-wires. Screws are then placed obliquely from the radial head proximally to the opposite cortex of the radial neck distally. This arrangement may be likened to a bar stool in which the seat (the radial head) is supported by the eccentrically

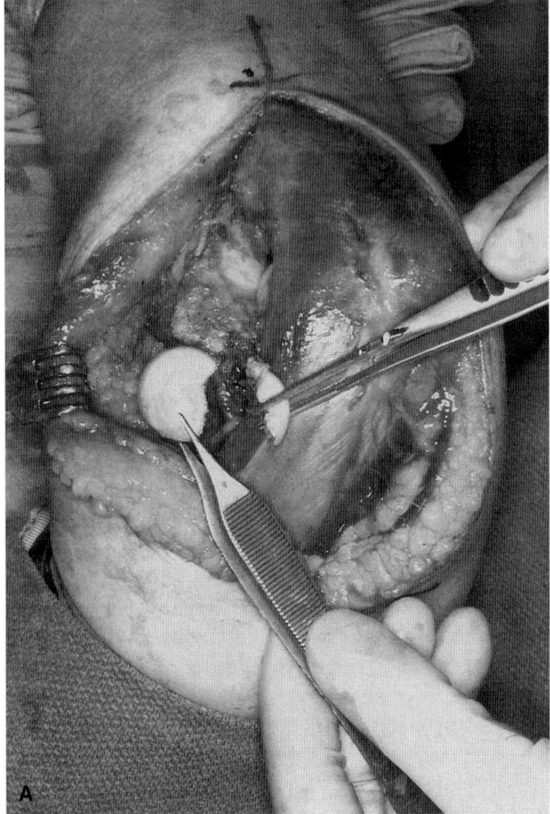

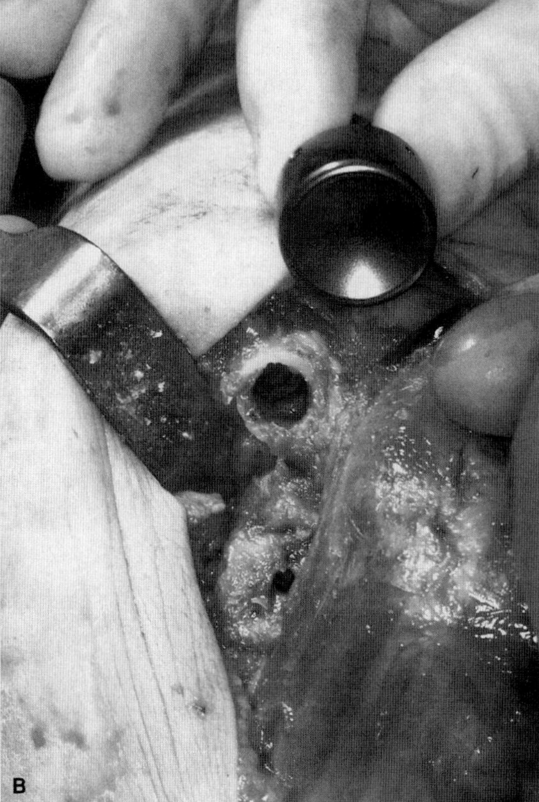

Figure 55-5 **A:** Type III radial head fracture. Attempt at open reduction internal fixation was unsuccessful. **B:** Radial neck has been prepared for implantation of radial head prosthesis.

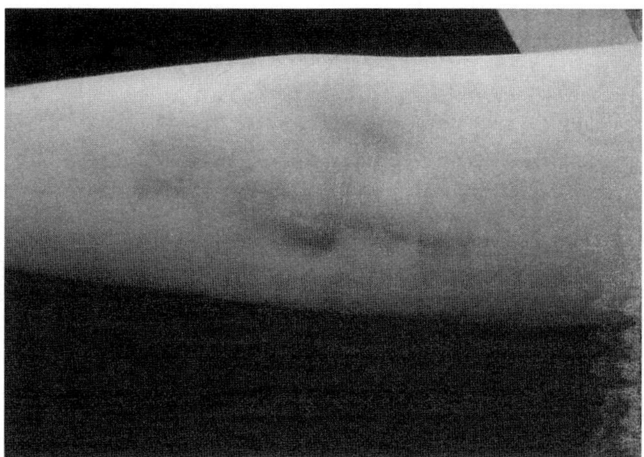

Figure 55-6 Postoperative photograph of posterior incision for radial head fracture. This is the standard approach used by the authors because of the pleasing cosmetic result.

arranged legs (the screws). The resultant bony defect in the radial neck secondary to impaction is filled with autogenous bone graft or bone graft substitute. This technique has several advantages over plate fixation for radial neck fractures. First, screws are less bulky than plates and may decrease annular ligament impingement. Second, placement of screws generally requires less dissection and periosteal stripping, which may lessen the amount of blood supply disruption to the neck and decrease risk of injury to the posterior interosseous nerve. These advantages should theoretically result in decreased postoperative stiffness, painful hardware, heterotopic ossification, proximal radioulnar synostosis, and nonunion rates. If plate fixation is chosen, lowprofile plates are necessary given the close proximity of the annular ligament and paucity of overlying soft tissues. Minicondylar L-plates, T-plates, and fixed-angled blade plates are all available for radial head and neck fixation.

There are few studies comparing internal fixation devices. A recent biomechanical study compared the average stiffness of several radial neck fracture plate fixation constructs axially loaded in compression.[2] The study demonstrated statistically greater stiffness with a 2.7-mm T-plate modified with a fixed-angle blade when compared with a 2.0-mm T-plate and 2.0mm fixed-angle blade. The investigators also noted increased proximal screw hole toggle when a fixed-angle device was not used. Contouring of the plate to the radius was observed to be the most important factor affecting overall construct stiffness. In another biomechanical study, investigators found no statistically significant difference in fixation stiffness when a low-profile blade plate and 3.0-mm cannulated screws were compared, but both constructs were statistically stiffer when compared with a 2.7-mm T-plate.[3]

Radial Head Replacement Arthroplasty

For all practical purposes, metal radial head prostheses have replaced silicone radial heads as the implant of choice in radial head replacement arthroplasty. When compared with metal radial heads, silicone implants are associated with worse clinical scores, increased elbow arthritis, and increased radial shortening. Furthermore, silicone implants are associated with increased failure secondary to fracture, fragmentation, and production of silicone synovitis. Both monoblock and modular radial head prostheses are now available. Anthropometric studies of cadaver proximal radii demonstrate that the head is inconsistently elliptical in shape, the head is variably offset from the axis of the neck, and the head diameter correlates poorly with the diameter of the medullary canal of the neck.[4] These findings may support the use of modular implants that allow improved sizing options that more closely approximate the anatomy of the proximal radius.

The radial head is approached in the manner previously described. The annular ligament is incised transversely to expose the radial head. The appropriate radial head resection guide is used to determine proper alignment and resection level. The neck should be osteotomized proximal to the bicipital tuberosity. The medullary canal of the proximal

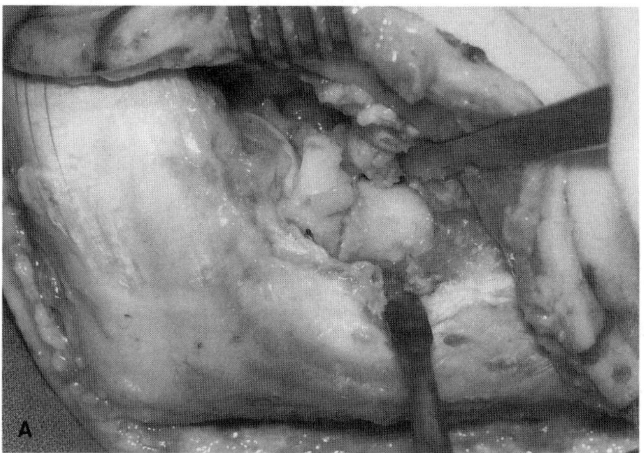

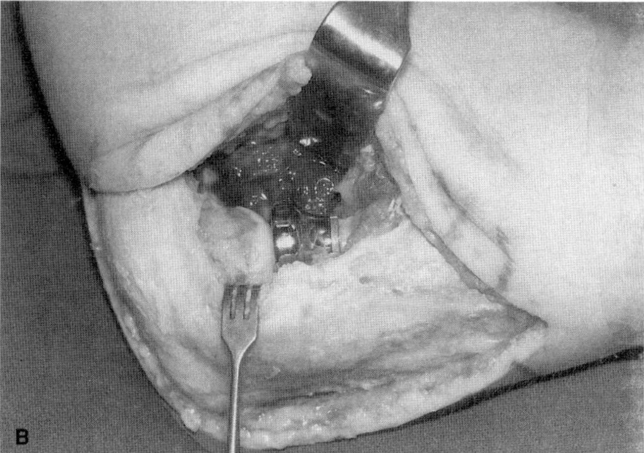

Figure 55-7 **A:** Type III fracture. Severe comminution noted at surgery. Surgical approach involved posterior skin incision with split of the extensor digitorum communis (EDC) tendon origin to gain exposure. **B:** Radial head prosthesis. Note metallic head centered on capitellum.

radius is then prepared with a starter awl, burrs, and broaches to accept the implant. Exposure may be improved by applying varus stress and placing the forearm in supination. Serial sized broaches are used until a snug fit is obtained in the canal at the appropriate depth. The appropriate-sized trial stem is inserted, ensuring that the collar of the prosthesis is flush with the resected neck. In modular designs, the trial head is secured to the trial stem, and the elbow and forearm are placed through a full arc of motion. Tracking as well as the relationship between the prosthesis and the capitellum are carefully assessed. Once acceptable alignment and tracking are determined, the trial components are removed and the final prosthesis is inserted. The stem may be press-fit or cemented in place depending on the design and stability of the stem in the medullary canal. The head is inserted over the taper of the stem and secured using an impactor. Final assessment of motion and stability of the elbow and forearm is performed.

CONCLUSION

Radial head and neck fractures are common injuries that require a thorough understanding of elbow anatomy and biomechanics for proper management. The goals of current management are aimed at restoring the normal anatomic and biomechanical relationships of the elbow in an effort to prevent the development of elbow stiffness, instability, and arthritis. Preservation of the radial head should be attempted in fractures that are amenable to internal fixation. Severely comminuted fractures that are not salvageable should be managed with radial head replacement. Regardless of the type of fracture and chosen method of management, a program of early range of motion should be incorporated.

REFERENCES

1. Ring D, Quintero J, Jupiter J. Open reduction and internal fixation of fractures of the radial head. *J Bone Joint Surg Am*. 2002;84:1811–1815.
2. Patterson J, Jones C, Glisson R, et al. Stiffness of simulated radial neck fractures fixed with 4 different devices. *J Shoulder Elbow Surg*. 2001;10:57–61.
3. Griffin J, Rath D, Chess D, et al. *Internal fixation of radial neck fractures: in-vitro biomechanical analysis. Transactions of the 44th Annual Meeting, Orthopaedic Research Society*. 1998;23: 73 1.
4. King G, Zarzour Z, Patterson S, et al. An anthropometric study of the radial head: implications in the design of a prosthesis. *J Arthroplasty*. 2001;16(1):112–116.

SUGGESTED READINGS

Boyer M, Galatz L, Borrelli J Jr, et al. Intraarticular fractures of the upper extremity: new concepts in surgical treatment. *Instr Course Lect*. 2003;52:591–605.

Furry KL, Clinkscales CM. Comminuted fractures of the radial head. Arthroplasty versus internal fixation. *Clin Orthop Rel Res*. 1998;353:40–52.

Hotchkiss R. Displaced fractures of the radial head: internal fixation or excision? *J Am Acad Ortho Surg*. 1997;5:l–l0.

King GJ. Management of comminuted radial head fractures with replacement arthroplasty. *Hand Clin*. 2004;20(4):429–441.

Morrey BF. Radial head fractures. In: Money BF, ed. *The Elbow*. 2nd ed. Philadelphia: Lippincott Williams & Wilkins; 2002:83–102.

Morrey BF. Radial head prosthetic replacement. In: Money BF, ed. *Joint Replacement Arthroplasty*. 3rd ed. Philadelphia: Churchill Livingstone; 2003:294–302.

O'Driscoll S, Jupiter J, Cohen M, et al. Difficult elbow fractures: pearls and pitfalls. *Instr Course Lect*. 2003;52:113–134.

Parasa R, Maffulli N. Surgical management of radial head fractures. *J R Coll Surg Edinb*. 2001;46:76–85.

Van Glabbeek R, Van Riet R, Verstreken J. Current concepts in the treatment of radial head fractures in the adult a clinical and biomechanical approach. *Acta Orthop Belg*. 2001;67: 430–441.

FRACTURES OF THE OLECRANON

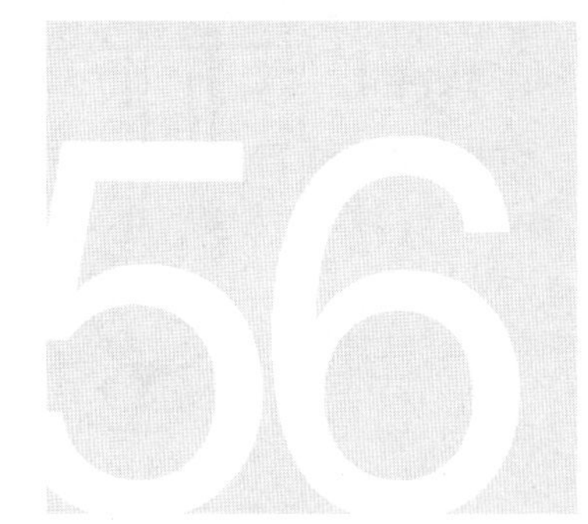

JULIE E. ADAMS
SCOTT P. STEINMANN

The subcutaneous location of the olecranon makes it vulnerable to injury, and fractures are not uncommon following low-energy trauma. Fractures of the olecranon are generally amenable to treatment and usually have a favorable prognosis.

PATHOGENESIS

Epidemiology, Etiology, and Pathophysiology

Isolated fractures of the olecranon constitute approximately 10% of fractures about the elbow, with an estimated incidence of 1.08 per 10,000 person-years. Most olecranon fractures follow low-energy trauma such as a fall from a height of <2 meters, a direct blow to the elbow, or from forced hyperextension. A fall on a partially flexed elbow may generate an avulsion fracture of the olecranon from the pull of the triceps. Amis and Miller investigated variable-impact mechanisms and the resultant fracture patterns in a cadaveric model. Whereas radial head and coronoid fractures tended to occur with forearm impacts with the elbow in ≤80 degrees of flexion, olecranon fractures followed direct blows at 90 degrees of flexion, and injuries occurring with the elbow in >110 degrees of flexion tended to result in distal humerus fractures. The olecranon and coronoid process constitute the semilunar or greater sigmoid notch of the ulna, which articulates with the trochlea. The constraints of this articulation confer stability to the elbow joint and facilitate anterior-posterior motion. A transverse "bare area" devoid of cartilage is found at the midpoint between the coronoid and the tip of the olecranon. An appreciation of this anatomic structure is necessary to avoid inadvertently discarding structurally significant portions of the olecranon when reconstructing the fractured olecranon. The ossification center of the olecranon generally appears by 9 to 10 years of age and fuses to the proximal ulna by age 14 years. Persistence of the physis into adulthood may occur and can be confused with a fracture; clues to this condition include its commonly bilateral nature and often familial tendency. In addition, patella cubiti, an accessory ossicle embedded in the distal triceps, may be present and likewise be mistaken for a fracture.

Classification of Olecranon Fractures

Morrey classified olecranon fractures according to criteria regarding stability, comminution, and displacement (Fig. 56-1). The Mayo Classification thus divides olecranon fractures into three types, provides a basis for a rational treatment algorithm by fracture type and subtype, and conveys prognostic value.

Mayo Type I

Mayo type I fractures are undisplaced fractures characterized by displacement of <2 mm with separation remaining <2 mm with flexion of the elbow to 90 degrees or with extension against gravity. Patients with these fractures are able to actively extend the elbow against gravity. Type I fractures may be further subdivided into type IA, noncomminuted fractures, and type IB, comminuted fractures. Since these fractures are nondisplaced by definition, the degree of comminution is not practically significant, and types IA and IB may essentially be regarded as and treated as the same lesion.

Mayo Type II

Mayo type II fractures are the most common type. These fractures, which are stable fractures with >3 mm of displacement, may be noncomminuted (type IIA) or comminuted (type IIB). Because the collateral ligaments are intact, the forearm is stable relative to the humerus.

Mayo Type III

Mayo type III fractures are unstable, displaced fractures and represent fracture-dislocations. Like types I and II, type III

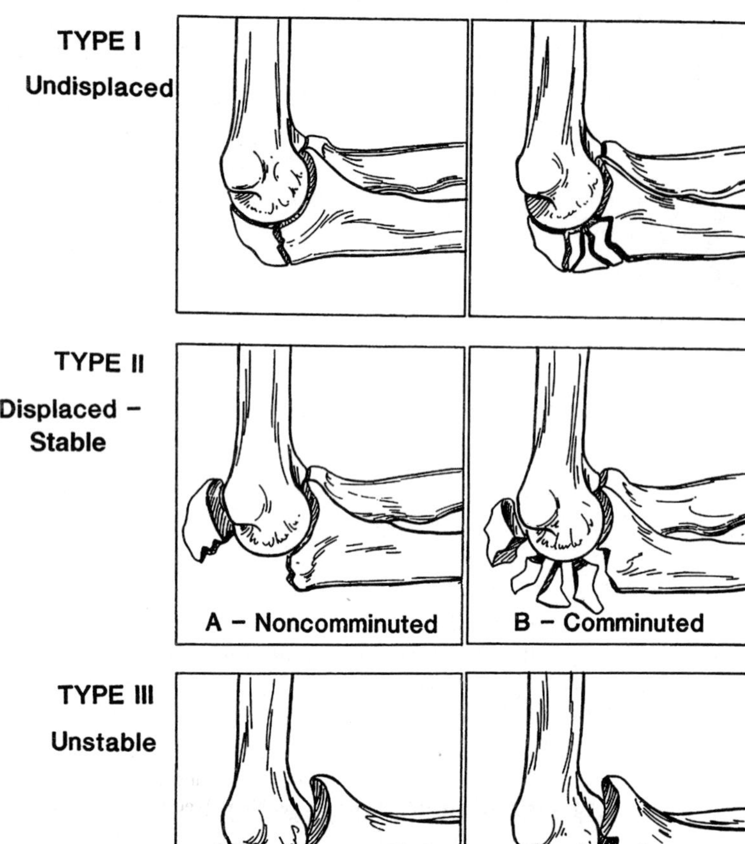

Figure 56-1 Mayo Classification of olecranon fractures. Type I fractures are nondisplaced noncomminuted (IA) or comminuted (IB) fractures. Type II fractures are stable displaced fractures and may be noncomminuted (IIA) or comminuted (IIB). Type III fractures are unstable, displaced fractures and may be noncomminuted (IIIA) or comminuted (IIIB). (From Cabenela ME, Morrey BF. Fractures of the olecranon. In: Morrey BF, ed. *The Elbow and Its Disorders*. Philadelphia: WB Saunders; 2000, with permission.)

fractures may be subclassified into noncomminuted (IIIA) or comminuted (IIIB) types.

Avulsion-Type Fractures

Avulsion-type fractures do not fit into the Mayo Classification categories well but are common in the elderly and may result from forces generated by the triceps. In general, little comminution is present.

Complex Olecranon Fracture-Dislocations

Olecranon fractures associated with subluxation of the radial head and or the coronoid process are typically multifragmentary, complex injuries that may be adequately described by the Mayo Classification scheme. Anterior fracture dislocations are often referred to as transolecranon fracture-dislocations, as the mechanism of injury appears to involve anterior displacement of the forearm resulting in the trochlea being driven through the olecranon process. The radial head is displaced anteriorly. This injury, unlike the Bado type I Monteggia fracture, is characterized by instability of the ulnohumeral joint with a preserved radioulnar relationship. Posterior fracture dislocations of the olecranon are more similar to type II Monteggia fractures, with posterior dislocation of the radial head, an apex posterior fracture of the ulna, and similar implications for the stability and function of both the ulnohumeral joint as well as the forearm. These fractures may be considered a variant of the posterior Monteggia lesion. Both posterior and anterior variants are commonly associated with basal fractures of the coronoid. In anterior olecranon fracture dislocations, reduction of the olecranon and coronoid fracture fragments results in restoration of stability with little implications for forearm dysfunction. Posterior olecranon fracture dislocations, in contrast, have important implications with elbow instability and forearm dysfunction common despite fracture reduction.

DIAGNOSIS

Physical Examination and History

Clinical Features

Because the olecranon is subcutaneous, the fracture may often be felt as palpable crepitation. With the exception of some avulsion-type fractures of the olecranon, the fracture

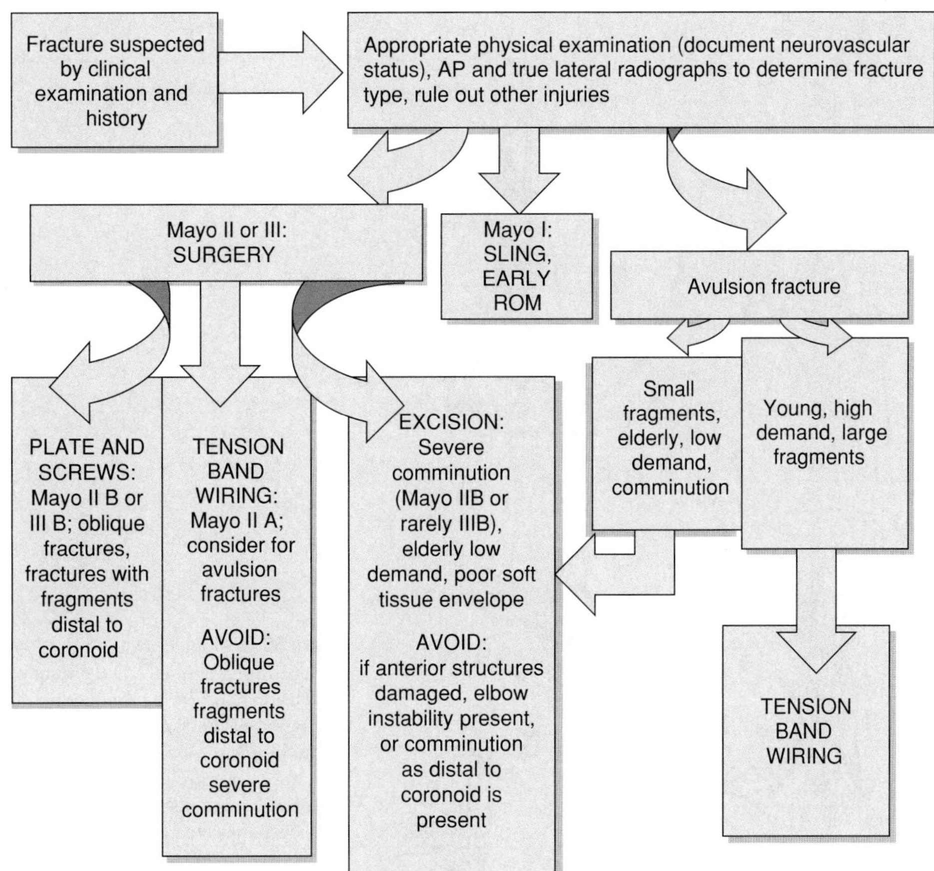

Figure 56-2 Flow chart representing the evaluation and decision-making processes involved in the workup and treatment of olecranon fractures.

by nature is intra-articular, so hemarthrosis is frequently present in conjunction with olecranon fracture. Although this sign may be obfuscated by pain caused by the injury, inability to actively extend the elbow against gravity may be an important indication of triceps discontinuity. Because of the proximity of the ulnar nerve, the first and each subsequent examination should document the status of the ulnar nerve.

Radiologic Features

Anteroposterior and true lateral radiographs should be obtained to aid in diagnosis and treatment considerations. The true lateral film should be examined to determine the extent and nature of the fracture pattern and to evaluate for the presence of other lesions such as a radial head fracture or dislocation, or distal humerus or coronoid fractures. A radiocapitellar view may be helpful to assess concomitant pathology.

Diagnostic Workup Algorithm

Figure 56-2 presents a diagnostic workup algorithm.

TREATMENT

Surgical Indications/Contraindications and Postoperative Management

For Mayo type I fractures, conservative nonoperative management is preferred. The patient is placed in sling immobilization for comfort with early active gentle range of motion exercises commencing no later than 7 to 10 days postinjury. Close follow-up (weekly) with radiographs is essential to rule out displacement and need for alternative treatment. Restrictions on active resisted elbow extension and weight bearing should be maintained for 6 to 8 weeks with gradual increases in these activities as tolerated. Rarely, in select patients, type I fractures may benefit from open reduction and internal fixation to allow immediate motion and stability. Some type I fractures may be treated with immobilization in a long arm cast at 90 degrees of flexion for 3 to 4 weeks. Thereafter, protected range of motion with avoidance of flexion >90 degrees until radiographic evidence of bony healing occurs, usually at 6 to 8 weeks, is recommended. Range of motion exercises may be commenced at an earlier time point in select patients, such as the elderly, in whom stiffness occurs more frequently.

Displaced fractures (Mayo types II and III) are best treated surgically with either excision or open reduction and internal fixation. Goals of surgical management include restoring the articular congruity and stability of the elbow, maintaining extension power, and providing stable anatomic fixation such that early range of motion is possible, thereby lessening the risk of postoperative stiffness. Options include tension band wiring, intramedullary screw placement, plate-and-screw constructs, bioabsorbable pins, or excision. Tension band wiring using standard AO technique is generally accepted and widely used as treatment for most olecranon fracture patterns amenable to this fixation technique

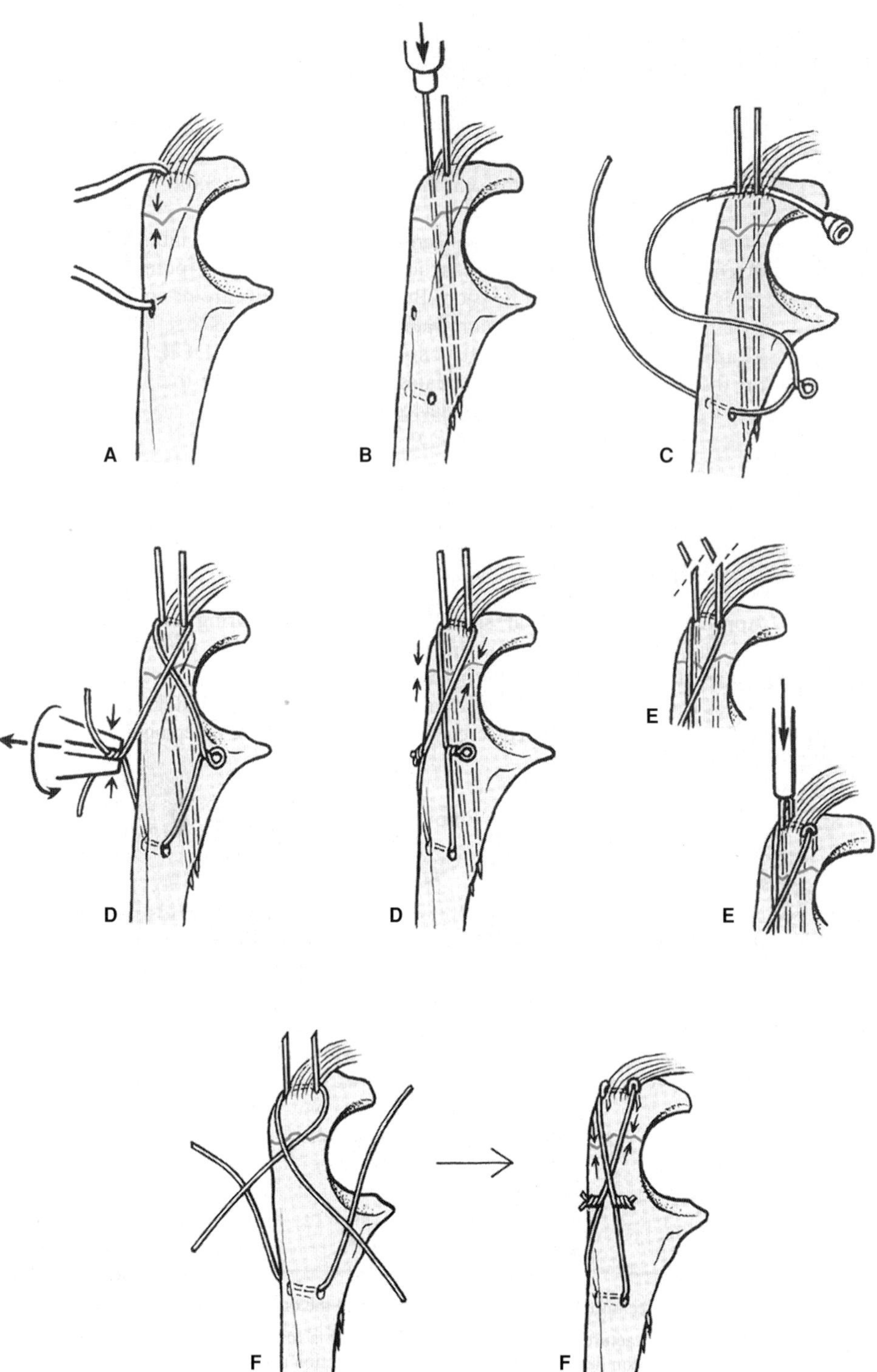

Figure 56-3 Line drawing demonstrating optimal AO technique for tension band wiring. Reduction of the fracture is performed with pointed forceps (**A**), and parallel Kirschner wires are driven obliquely from proximal to distal until the volar cortex is penetrated (**B**). A 2.5-mm drill is used to create a transverse hole distally to accept the tension wire (**B**). The 1.0- or 1.2-mm wire with a prefabricated loop is introduced under the triceps and the two K-wires, then through the transverse hole (**C**). As an alternative, two separate wires may be used (**C**). The wires are grasped at the base and twisted together and the twists laid down flat on the bony surfaces (**D′** and **F′**). Subsequently, the K-wires are pulled back slightly, cut obliquely, and bent into hooks. The hooks are then impacted into bone over the tension band (**E**, **E′**, and **F′**). (From Heim U. Forearm and hand/mini-implants. In: Muller ME, et al., eds. *Manual of Internal Fixation: Techniques Recommended by the AO-ASIF Group*. 3rd ed. New York: Springer-Verlag; 1991, with permission.)

(Fig. 56-3). Tension band wiring converts tensile forces across the fracture to compressive forces that, with motion, exert compression across the fracture site. It may be favored over plate-and-screw fixation due to requirements for less soft tissue dissection and less periosteal stripping. However, this fixation technique may have technical challenges and be associated with undesirable postoperative sequelae. Because of the subcutaneous nature and location of the elbow, prominent hardware may be problematic, with many patients in one series reporting hardware-related pain (24%) and functional difficulties (32%) relieved by hardware removal. Hardware removal rates are ≤81% in some series. Nevertheless, ≤97% good to excellent results have been widely reported with use of tension band wiring using proper technique. However, for fractures with fragments distal to the coronoid, plate-and-screw osteosynthesis is preferred, as these more distal fragments are usually not adequately fixed by tension band wiring. Likewise, more comminuted

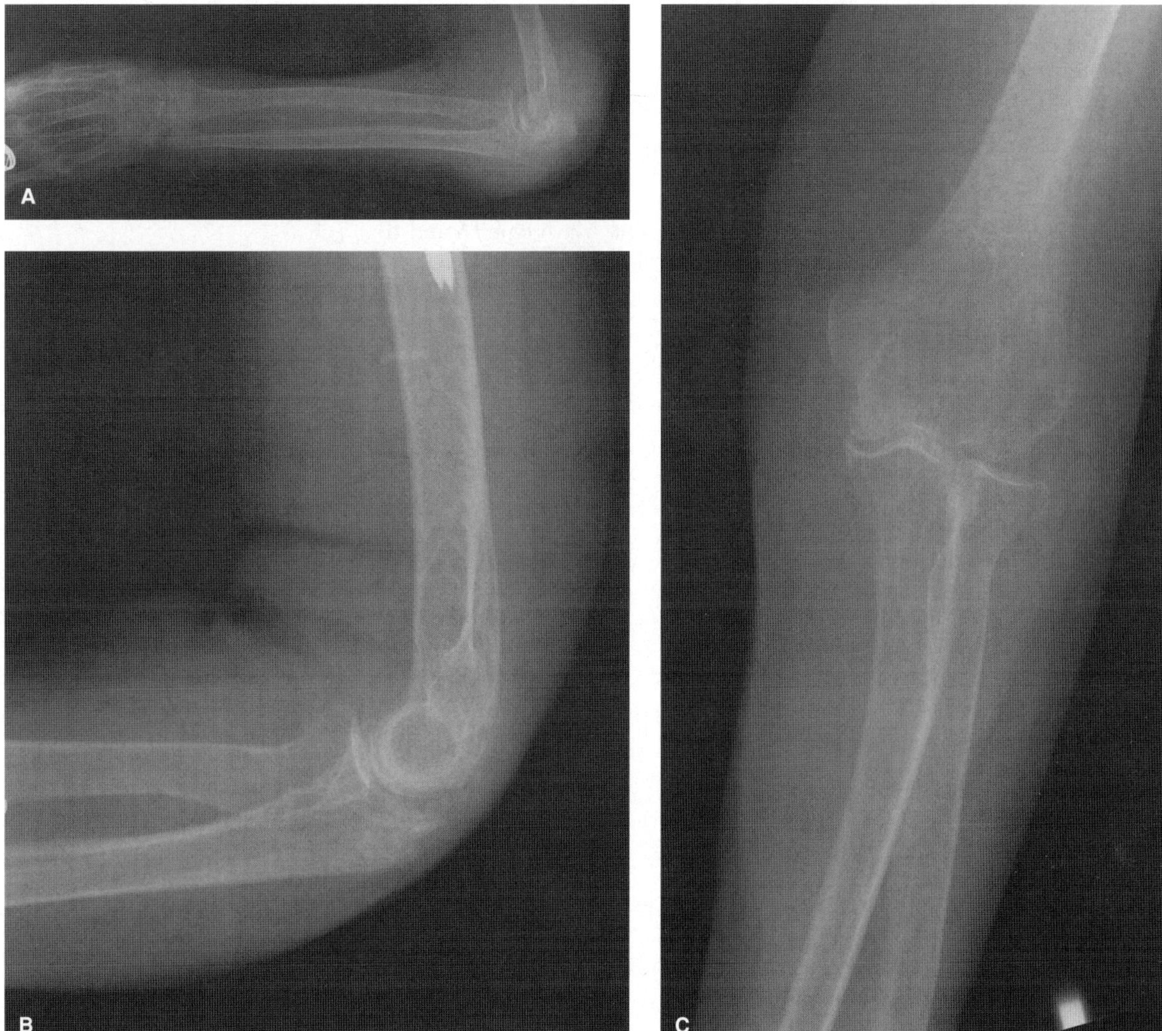

Figure 56-4 This 84-year-old right hand–dominant woman experienced a syncopal episode and fell down the stairs at home. She sustained concomitant fractures of the left proximal humerus, left distal radius, left ulnar styloid, and a fracture of the left olecranon (A) treated with excision of the proximal fragment (B and C). At 6 months postoperatively, she was painfree and her range of motion in the flexion extension arc was from 20 to 135 degrees; pronation was to 70 degrees and supination was to 70 degrees.

fractures or oblique patterns are best treated with plate-and-screw fixation to optimize stability. In the authors' experience, plate-and-screw osteosynthesis provides the optimal fixation stability with minimal complications.

Excision of fracture fragments with advancement and reinsertion of the triceps is preferred for elderly, low-demand patients (Fig. 56-4A,B), for nonunions, in those with poor soft tissue viability, for avulsion-type extra-articular fractures, and in cases with severe comminution as in Mayo type IIB, or rarely, type IIIB fractures (Fig. 56-4). Disadvantages of excision include subsequent risks of triceps weakness, instability, stiffness, and a theoretical risk for increased arthrosis. Biomechanical studies suggest that decreased extension strength may be minimized with reattaching the triceps at a more posterior site. McKeever and Buck determined that one may excise ≤80% of the olecranon without sacrificing stability if the coronoid and anterior soft tissues are intact. If anterior damage is present or if comminution extends as far distally as the coronoid process, instability is a sequela if too much proximal ulna is excised. In addition, An et al. noted increasing instability of the elbow with olecranon excision. However, satisfactory clinical outcomes (Fig. 56-4A,B) have been described for treatment of olecranon fracture by excision when used in appropriate patient populations. The nature of the procedure, in which hardware is absent, may lead to decreased local complications and need for subsequent procedures relative to other surgical treatment options. Despite documented satisfactory outcomes with excision, some speculate that excision may lead to development of arthrosis. Biomechanical studies document increased forces across the ulnohumeral joint following excision relative to fixation with tension band wiring, suggesting that abnormal joint forces that may predispose to arthrosis may follow excision.

Intramedullary screw or nail fixation is generally not recommended because of their less reliable fixation stability in vivo. In addition, potentially problematic with intramedullary nailing are fracture malreduction secondary to off-axis placement of the nail, possible damage to the triceps muscle or the ulnar nerve during locking-screw placement, and the effect of cyclical loading as well as union rate.

Bioabsorbable fixation may be desirable because of the potential to avoid future operations for hardware removal. Satisfactory outcomes in a few patients have been noted; however, further clinical experience is needed to determine the role that bioabsorbable fixation techniques will assume in the future.

Plate-and-screw constructs are preferred by the authors for most fractures and are necessary to treat all oblique fractures, fractures with extensive comminution, and fractures with fragments distal to the coronoid.

Mayo type IIA fractures are usually adequately treated with tension band wiring. Intramedullary fixation has also been described for selected patients, although reported outcomes have been variable and biomechanical data is less supportive of this technique.

Type IIB fractures are treated according to the age and activity level of the patient. In patients younger than 60 years of age, anatomic reduction of fracture fragments followed by plate-and-screw fixation is the treatment of choice. Care should be taken to avoid shortening the articular groove of the ulna between the olecranon process and the coronoid process, as doing so may lead to early arthritis. In older patients, or when comminution is severe, excision of proximal fragments with advancement and reinsertion of the triceps tendon may be preferred.

Mayo type III fractures, displaced unstable fractures, represent the most difficult treatment challenge of all olecranon fractures and are associated with the highest complication rates and least satisfactory outcomes. Type III fractures are associated with a high incidence of concomitant pathology, such as ligamentous trauma or bony injuries of the radial head or coronoid or distal humerus; these should be addressed at the time of olecranon fixation. Type III olecranon fractures typically require plate fixation and ligamentous reconstruction. One may consider application of a hinge fixator if stability is not restored.

Noncomminuted (IIIA) fractures may be treated with a plate-and-screw construct and anatomic reduction. Comminuted (type IIIB) fractures may likewise be treated with plate osteosynthesis or very rarely be treated with excision of fracture fragments, although instability is likely.

Olecranon fracture dislocations require special considerations for treatment. Because of inherent instability of these fracture patterns, they are best treated with plate-and-screw osteosynthesis. Contoured plates are preferred; one-third tubular plates lack the stiffness necessary to withstand early range of motion and have been associated with early loosening or fatigue fractures. If a concomitant anteromedial coronoid fracture fragment is present, it should be fixed to optimize stability of the elbow. The integrity of the lateral collateral ligament (LCL) and the anteromedial coronoid are important factors in stability of the fracture.

When comminution is extensive, a skeletal distractor or temporary external fixation device may be helpful to facilitate reduction; after satisfactory reduction is obtained, definitive fracture fixation using plate and screws with or without augmentation with tension band wiring is usually possible. If extensive comminution is present such that plate and screw fixation does not provide sufficient fracture stability, augmentation with tension band wiring through the triceps insertion may facilitate stable fixation.

- Mayo type IA and IB:
  - Undisplaced (<2 mm) fractures with no comminution (IA) or with comminution (IIB).
  - Sling immobilization, early active range of motion, close follow-up.
- Mayo type II A:
  - Stable fractures with >3 mm displacement, no comminution.
  - Tension band wiring usually adequate. Consider plate-and-screw constructs if fracture lines are distal to coronoid; consider excision in low-demand patients or when small fragments are present.
- Mayo type II B:
  - Stable fractures with >3 mm displacement; comminution is present.
  - Plate-and-screw constructs preferred, especially in patients <60 years old.
  - Consider excision in low demand patients or those older than age 60 years, fractures with extensive comminution, or when small fragments are present.
- Mayo type III A:
  - Unstable, displaced fracture-dislocations. No comminution is present.
  - Plate-and-screw constructs preferred.
- Mayo type III B:
  - Unstable, displaced fracture-dislocations. Comminution is present.
  - Plate-and-screw constructs preferred.
- Avulsion fractures
  - Tension band wiring or excision may be used.

Surgical Technique

A dorsal midline longitudinal incision curving over the olecranon is recommended to avoid placing the incision over the subcutaneous bone. Medial and or lateral flaps may be raised to access other bone or ligamentous structures; alternatively, concomitant radial head or coronoid fractures may be treated through the window created by the olecranon fracture.

Excision may be performed by sharp dissection of fracture fragments from the triceps aponeurosis, and longitudinal drill holes made through the proximal ulna to secure the triceps tendon down to bone (Fig. 56-4).

Tension band wiring may be performed using the standard AO technique (Figs. 56-3 and 56-5). Bone reduction clamps are used to reduce the fracture. A superficial drill hole in the distal fragment may be useful to give a traction site for the jaws of the bone reduction forceps. Following reduction, two parallel 1.6-mm K-wires are introduced from the posterior aspect of the olecranon aiming anteriorly and obliquely just through the anterior cortex. A 2.5-mm hole is

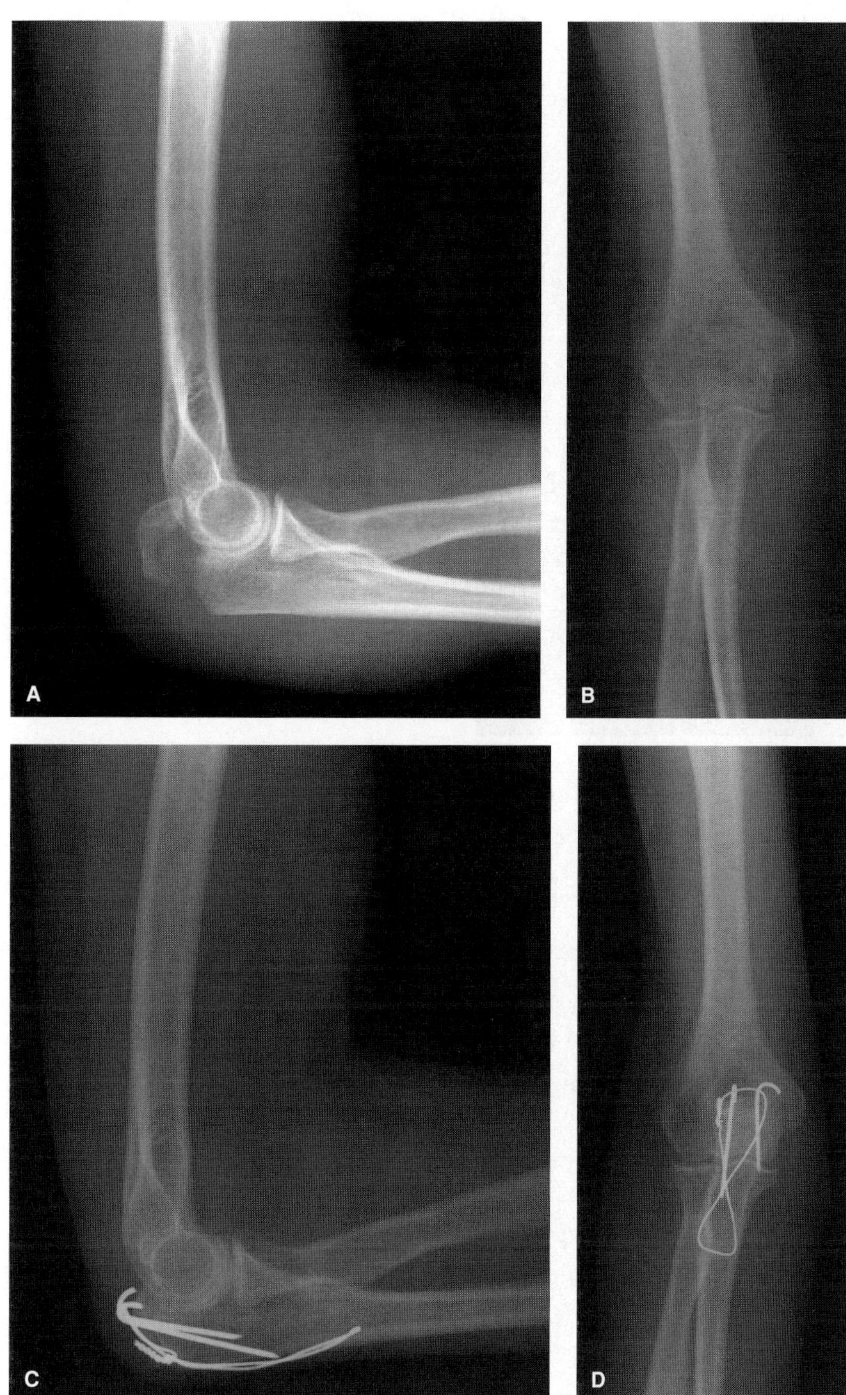

Figure 56-5 This 60-year-old nurse practitioner fell while running and sustained a type IIA olecranon fracture (**A** and **B**). She underwent open reduction and internal fixation with tension band wiring (**C** and **D**). Subsequently, at latest follow-up she had range of motion from 10 to 100 degrees in the flexion/extension arc. She complained of prominent hardware and underwent hardware removal at 20 months after her fracture fixation.

drilled transversely in the distal fragment for placement of a 1.0-mm or 1.2-mm cerclage wire with a prefabricated loop; alternatively, two cerclage wires may be used. The wire is then routed under the triceps tendon and K-wires to create a figure-of-8 construct. Tensioning is performed symmetrically on each side. The K-wires are pulled back slightly, cut and bent, and finally the bend ends are impacted into bone.

Plate osteosynthesis is likewise performed using standard AO technique (Fig. 56-6). The plate may be applied over part of the triceps insertion without muscle or periosteal elevation to optimize bone healing, or the triceps may be split longitudinally and mobilized. If a concomitant anteromedial coronoid fracture fragment is present, it should be fixed to optimize stability of the elbow. When comminution is extensive, a skeletal distractor or temporary external fixation device may be helpful to facilitate reduction; after satisfactory reduction is obtained, definitive fracture fixation using plate and screws with or without augmentation with tension band wiring is usually possible. If extensive comminution is present such that plate-and-screw fixation does not provide sufficient fracture stability, augmentation with tension band wiring through the triceps insertion may facilitate

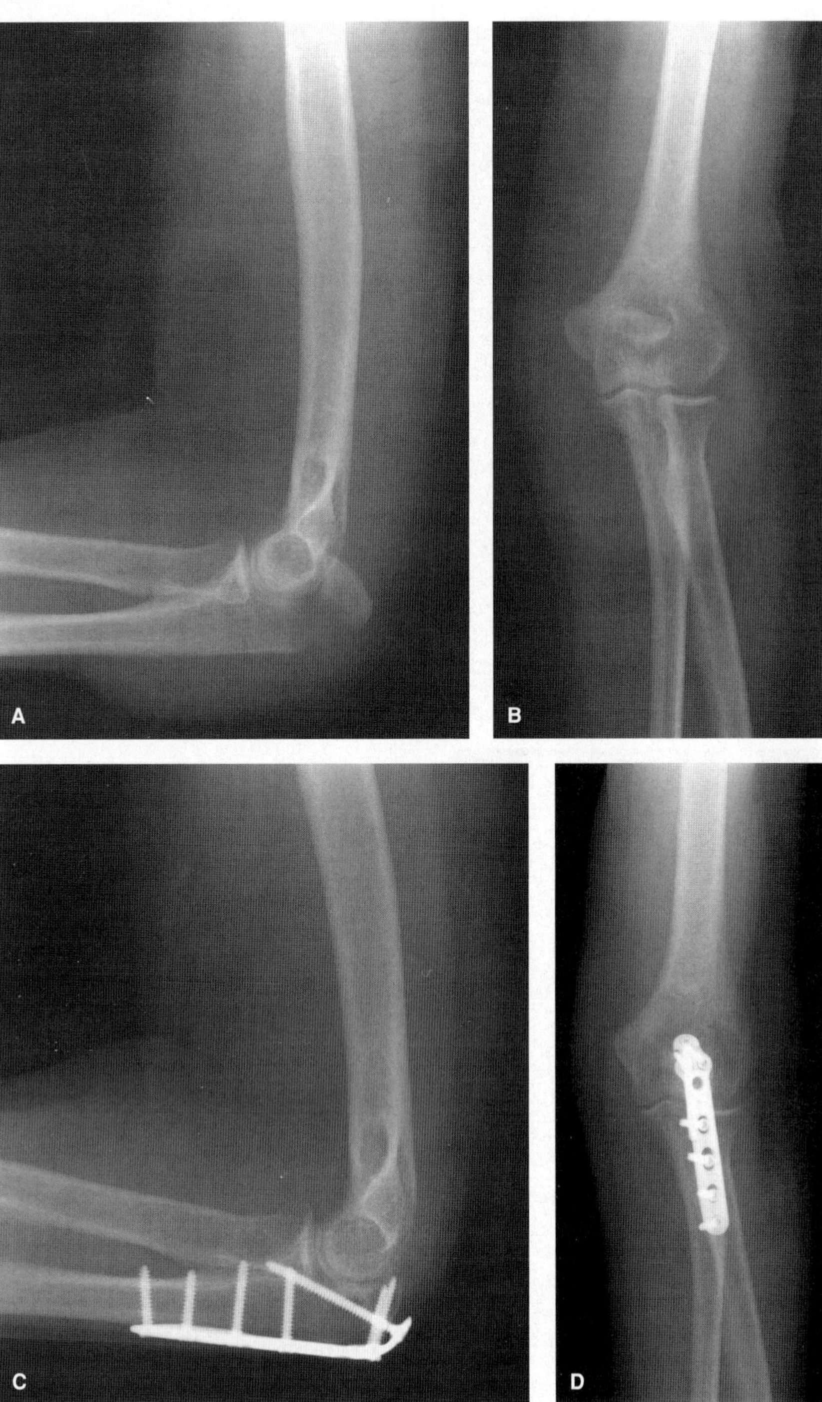

Figure 56-6 This 66-year-old right hand–dominant retired laboratory technician slipped on the ice and fell, sustaining a direct blow to her left elbow and this Mayo type IIA fracture of the olecranon (**A** and **B**). She underwent plate-and-screw osteosynthesis (**C** and **D**). At 18 months postoperatively, she was painfree and her range of motion was 0 to 140 degrees, with supination to 70 degrees and pronation to 80 degrees.

stable fixation. Restoration of the olecranon and coronoid facets is key as the intervening segment, the transverse ridge of the olecranon, contributes little surface contact area to the articular interface.

The wound is then closed in the standard fashion and a posterior plaster dressing is applied in full extension. The arm should be elevated overnight and the initial dressing changed on the second day. Active and passive motion is then initiated. Alternatively, if for any reason the operative fixation was felt to be less than optimal, splinting may be continued for 3 to 4 weeks to allow for some bony healing. Protected use of the extremity is maintained with minimal weight bearing and no resistance greater than that of gravity for 6 weeks or until radiographic evidence of healing is seen.

Complications

Complications of olecranon fracture include nonunion or malunion, infection, loss of motion, ulnar nerve symptoms, arthrosis, and need for additional procedures, such as hardware removal. Loss of motion may be problematic, particularly a 10- to 15-degree extension lag. This appears to be related to immobilization. Radiographic evidence of degenerative changes in the ulnohumeral joint has been documented in 20% to 50% of patients ≤15 to 25 years following olecranon fracture, but is generally asymptomatic. Symptomatic hardware is the most frequent complication, requiring removal in 11.4% to 81% of patients. Hardware prominence is more common in tension band wiring relative to other fixation techniques, such as figure-of-8 wiring or plate-and-screw constructs. The risk of problematic hardware with tension band wiring is decreased if attention to proper AO technique is observed and wires are bent 180 degrees and impacted into bone with the triceps securely sutured over the wires.

Results and Outcomes

Outcomes following olecranon fracture are generally good to excellent, with most series noting satisfactory outcomes and restoration of normal or near-normal function in >95% of patients.

In conclusion, olecranon fractures are commonly seen in orthopedic practice and with appropriate treatment, generally have good to excellent outcomes with little adverse sequelae. Decreased range of motion, radiographic evidence of degenerative changes, and requirement for hardware removal are common but generally are not devastating complications, and may be obviated by attention to proper technique, anatomic reduction, and proper postoperative management.

SUGGESTED READINGS

Amis AA, Miller JH. The mechanisms of elbow fractures: an investigation using impact tests in vitro. *Injury*. 1995;26(3):163–168.

An KN, Morrey BF, Chao EY. The effect of partial removal of the proximal ulna on elbow restraint. *Clin Orthop*. 1986;209:270–279.

Bailey CS, MacDermid J, Patterson SD, Outcome of plate fixation of olecranon fractures. *J Orthop Trauma*. 2001;15:542–548.

Bostman OM. Metallic or absorbable fracture fixation devices. A cost minimization analysis. *Clin Orthop*. 1996;329:233–239.

Boyer MI, Galatz LM, Borrelli J, Jr, et al. Intra-articular fractures of the upper extremity: new concepts in surgical treatment. *Instr Course Lect*. 2003;52:591–605.

Bucholz RW, Heckman JD, eds. *Rockwood and Green's Fractures in Adults*. 5th ed. Philadelphia: Lippincott, Williams & Wilkins; 2001.

Cabenela ME, Morrey BF. Fractures of the olecranon. In: Morrey BF, ed. *The Elbow and Its Disorders*. Philadelphia: WB Saunders; 2000.

Colton CL. Fractures of the olecranon in adults: classification and management. *Injury*. 1973;5(2):121–129.

Compton R, Bucknell A. Resection arthroplasty for comminuted olecranon fractures. *Orthop Rev*. 1989;18(2):189–192.

Didonna ML, Fernandez JJ, Lim TH, et al. Partial olecranon excision: the relationship between triceps insertion site and extension strength of the elbow. *J Hand Surg Am*. 2003;28(1):117–122.

Doornberg JD, Ring JD, Jupiter JB. Effective treatment of fracture-dislocations of the olecranon requires a stable trochlear notch. *Clin Orthop*. 2004;429:292–300.

Estourgie RJ, Tinnemans JG. Treatment of grossly comminuted fractures of the olecranon by excision. *Neth J Surg*. 1982;34(3):127–129.

Evans MC, Graham HK. Olecranon fractures in children. Part 1: a clinical review; Part 2: a new classification and management algorithm. *J Pediatr Orthop*. 1999;19:559–569.

Fern ED, Brown JN. Olecranon advancement osteotomy in the management of severely comminuted olecranon fractures. *Injury*. 1993; 24(4):267–269.

Fyfe IS, Mossad MM, Holdsworth BJ. Methods of fixation of olecranon fractures. An experimental mechanical study. *J Bone Joint Surg Br*. 1985;67(3):367–372.

Gartsman GM, Sculco TP, Otis JC. Operative treatment of olecranon fractures. Excision or open reduction with internal fixation. *J Bone Joint Surg Am*. 1981;63:718–721.

Hak DJ, Golladay GJ. Olecranon fractures: treatment options. *J Am Acad Orthop Surg*, 2000;8(4):266–275.

Heim U. Forearm and hand/mini-implants. In: Muller ME, et al., eds. *Manual of Internal Fixation: Techniques Recommended by the AO-ASIF Group*. 3rd ed. New York: Springer-Verlag; 1991.

Helm RH, Hornby R, Miller SW. The complications of surgical treatment of displaced fractures of the olecranon. *Injury*. 1987;18(1):48–50.

Horne JG, Tanzer TL. Olecranon fractures: a review of 100 cases. *J Trauma*. 1981;21(6):469–472.

Horner SR, Sadosivan KK, Lipka JM, et al. Analysis of mechanical factors affecting fixation of olecranon fractures. *Orthopedics*. 1989;12:1469–1472.

Kamineni S, Hirahara H, Pomianowski S, et al. Partial posteromedial olecranon resection: a kinematic study. *J Bone Joint Surg Am*. 2003;85-A(6):1005–1011.

Karlsson MK, Hasserius R, Kailsson C, et al., Fractures of the olecranon: a 15- to 25-year followup of 73 patients. *Clin Orthop*. 2002;403:205–212.

Karlsson MK, Hasserius R, Besiakov J, et al. Comparison of tension-band and figure-of-eight wiring techniques for treatment of olecranon fractures. *J Shoulder Elbow Surg*. 2002;11(4): 377–382.

McKay PL, Katarincic JA. Fractures of the proximal ulna olecranon and coronoid fractures. *Hand Clin*. 2002;18(1):43–53.

McKeever FM, Buck RM. Fracture of the olecranon process of the ulna: treatment by excision of fragment and repair of triceps tendon. *JAMA*. 1947;135:1–5.

Moed BR, Ede DE, Brown TD. Fractures of the olecranon: an in vitro study of elbow joint stresses after tension-band wire fixation versus proximal fracture fragment excision. *J Trauma*. 2002;53:1088–1093.

Molloy S, Jasper LE, Elliott DS, et al. Biomechanical evaluation of intramedullary nail versus tension band fixation for transverse olecranon fractures. *J Orthop Trauma*. 2004;18(3): 170–174.

Morrey BF. Current concepts in the treatment of fractures of the radial head, the olecranon, and the coronoid. *Instr Course Lect*. 1995;44:175–185.

Morrey BF. Master techniques in orthopaedic surgery. In: Morrey BF, ed. *The Elbow*. 2nd ed. Philadelphia: Lippincott Williams & Wilkins; 2001.

Mullett JH, Shannon F, Noel J, et al. K-wire position in tension band wiring of the olecranon—a comparison of two techniques. *Injury*. 2000;31(6):427–431.

Nowinski RJ, Nork SE, Segina DN, et al. Comminuted fracture-dislocations of the elbow treated with an AO wrist fusion plate. *Clin Orthop Relat Res*. 2000;378:238–244.

O'Driscoll SW, Jupiter JB, Cohen MS, et al. Difficult elbow fractures: pearls and pitfalls. *Instr Course Lect*. 2003;52:113–134.

Ring D, Jupiter JB, Sanders RW, et al. Transolecranon fracture-dislocation of the elbow. *J Orthop Trauma*. 1997;11:545–550.

Rommens PM, Schneider RU, Reuter M. Functional results after operative treatment of olecranon fractures. *Acta Chir Belg*. 2004;104(2):191–197.

Wolfgang G, Burke F, Bush D, et al. Surgical treatment of displaced olecranon fractures by tension band wiring technique. *Clin Orthop*. 1987;224:192–204.

SURGICAL EXPOSURES OF THE ELBOW

JOAQUIN SANCHEZ-SOTELO

Adequate surgical exposure of the elbow joint is one of the most critical factors in achieving a successful outcome in both trauma and reconstruction. Elbow exposure is complicated by the need to identify and protect surrounding neurovascular structures, some of which are extremely close to the joint capsule. Various surgical exposures have been developed to mobilize the extensor mechanism or to allow access from the medial or lateral side of the joint while preserving the collateral ligaments; anterior exposures are seldom used for very specific indications (such as distal biceps tendon repair). The skin incision will be determined by the selected deep exposure as well as prior surgical skin incisions, but many elbow surgeons favor a universal posterior midline skin incision that allows almost circumferential exposure of the elbow joint. It is not the purpose of this chapter to discuss all the approaches to the elbow joint but rather to provide a summary of the approaches more commonly used by elbow surgeons at the present time.

SKIN

Posterior Midline Skin Incision

Many elbow surgeons favor the use of a posterior midline skin incision for many elbow procedures. It has several advantages: (i) medial and/or lateral skin flaps can be elevated on demand to provide access to virtually any deep exposure, (ii) the risk of neuromas is minimized, as the number and diameter of nerve fibers crossing the posterior aspect of the elbow are low compared to the medial or lateral side, and (iii) should future surgery be needed, the same skin incision can be used for almost any procedure. Exposures that involve mobilization of the extensor mechanism are performed through this incision. It is also extremely useful for the treatment of elbow fracture-dislocations, which may require sequential access to both the medial and lateral side of the joint depending on the pathology found.

Wound-related complications are relatively uncommon provided full-thickness fasciocutaneous flaps are elevated; seromas or hematomas do happen occasionally, but they seldom compromise the outcome. The posterior midline skin incision is placed slightly off the tip of the olecranon either medially or laterally to facilitate healing. When the elbow needs to be splinted, the splint can be placed anteriorly to avoid direct pressure on the wound, and the elbow can be immobilized in extension and kept elevated to decrease swelling and surgical wound tension, as well as seroma or hematoma accumulation underneath the skin flaps.

Lateral and Medial Skin Incisions

Lateral or medial incisions are useful when no need for a more extensile approach is anticipated (Table 57-1); they can be complicated occasionally by neuromas (from transected branches of the lateral or medial antebrachial cutaneous nerves), especially on the medial side, but these more limited skin incisions are associated with a lower rate of wound complications than the posterior midline skin incision.

LATERAL APPROACHES

The Köcher Approach

Classically, the lateral side of the elbow is exposed through the Köcher interval. This interval between the *anconeus* and the *extensor carpi ulnaris* is easily identified distally and developed proximally in line with the lateral epicondyle and humeral column. The underlying annular ligament, lateral collateral ligament complex, and elbow capsule are easily exposed. The Köcher approach can be used for radial head open reduction and internal fixation (ORIF) or replacement and is especially useful when the lateral collateral ligament complex is already injured, as in most fracture-dislocations; it represents the standard approach for reconstruction of the lateral collateral ligament (Fig. 57-1). Release of the lateral collateral complex off the lateral epicondyle through the Köcher interval allows great exposure of the subluxed or

TABLE 57-1 PROCEDURES COMMONLY PERFORMED THROUGH A LATERAL OR MEDIAL SKIN INCISION

Lateral Skin Incision	Medial Skin Incision
■ Radial head ORIF/ replacement ■ Contracture release through the lateral column procedure ■ Lateral collateral ligament reconstruction ■ Tennis elbow release/posterior interosseous nerve decompression	■ Coronoid ORIF/ reconstruction ■ Contracture release through the medial column procedure ■ Medial collateral ligament reconstruction ■ Medial epicondylitis release ■ Ulnar nerve decompression/ transposition

ORIF, open reduction and internal fixation.

dislocated joint. However, increased understanding of the role of the lateral collateral ligament complex and concerns about its residual laxity after detachment have prompted the use of alternative ligament-sparing deep exposures.

Common Extensor Group Split

One of the best exposures for internal fixation or replacement of the radial head is through a split in the *extensor carpi radialis brevis* (ECRB) in line with the Lister tubercle that is then continued proximally by detachment of the common extensor origin and anterior capsule off the lateral column. Incision of the annular ligament underneath the ECRB provides access to the radial head, and the supinator muscle can be elevated from proximal to distal if the radial neck needs to be exposed (Fig. 57-2). Care should be taken to protect the posterior interosseous nerve; placing the forearm in pronation displaces this nerve distally and allows safe exposure of at least 35 mm of proximal radius. A retractor placed around the neck may be used to lever the radial head and neck anteriorly for fixation or replacement.

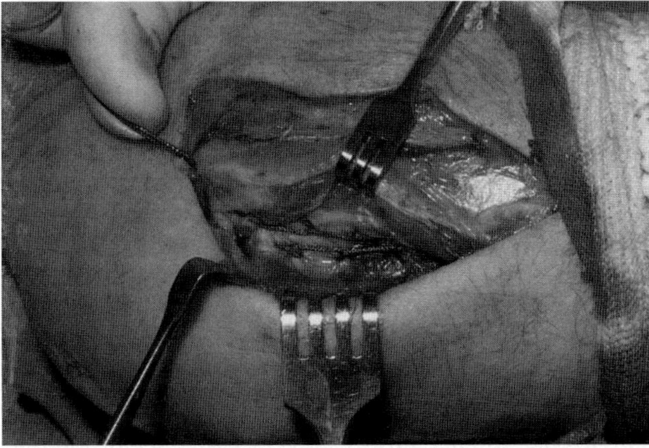

Figure 57-1 The Köcher approach uses the interval between anconeus and extensor carpi ulnaris. The interval is being used in this case to expose the lateral collateral ligament complex.

Lateral Column

The proximal aspect of this approach, through detachment of the extensor muscle group origin off the lateral column and distal split of the extensor group in line with the Lister tubercle, allows excellent exposure to the anterior compartment; the posterior compartment can be easily exposed from the lateral side by elevation of the triceps and anconeus off the lateral column. These two combined form the basis of the so-called lateral column procedure (Fig. 57-3).

MEDIAL APPROACHES

As noted above, the skin of the medial aspect of the elbow is richly innervated by multiple branches of the medial antebrachial cutaneous nerve. Incisions placed on this area have a high risk of neuroma formation, and some authors recommend identification and preservation of these branches when a medial skin incision is used. Alternatively, the medial aspect of the elbow may be exposed through a posterior midline skin incision by elevation of a medial skin flap.

Deep medial exposures vary depending on the procedure to be performed (Table 57-1). The medial side of the elbow joint is covered by the flexor-pronator group anteriorly and the triceps posteriorly. *Medial collateral ligament (MCL) reconstruction* used to be performed through detachment of the flexor-pronator group; currently, a muscle split is used for most MCL reconstructions, and detachment of the flexor-pronator group is reserved for submuscular transposition of the ulnar nerve, and may also be used for coronoid exposure and sometimes resection of heterotopic ossification.

Different approaches may be used for *coronoid exposure*. Coronoid plating and reconstruction require ample exposure. The author favors elevation of the flexor-pronator group off the subcutaneous border of the ulna from proximal to distal (Fig. 57-3). This exposure allows identification and preservation of the MCL which appears as a white collection of fibers as the fleshy flexor-pronator group is elevated; it does not require formal transposition of the ulnar nerve and limits the amount of muscle that needs to be detached from the distal humerus, providing good exposure to both the coronoid and the ulnar shaft.

The so-called *medial column procedure* provides access to both the anterior and the posterior compartments of the elbow and is used mainly for contracture release The principles of this approach are similar to those of the lateral column approach: preservation of the collateral ligament and ample access to the joint through a somewhat limited muscle dissection. The posterior compartment of the elbow is exposed by elevation of the triceps off the medial column. The anterior compartment is exposed by elevation of the pronator teres off the medial intermuscular septum and the anterior column; the exposure is extended distally

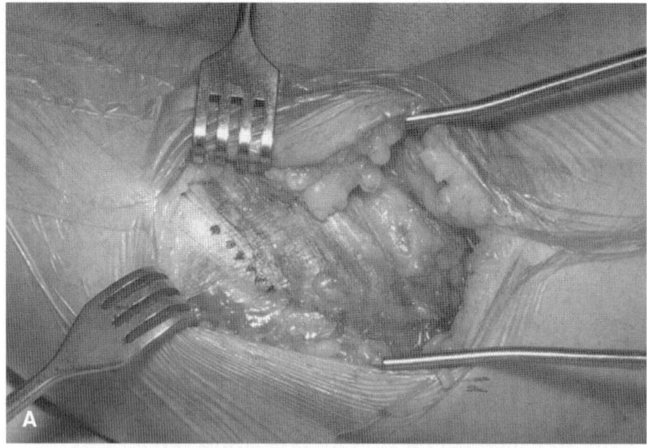

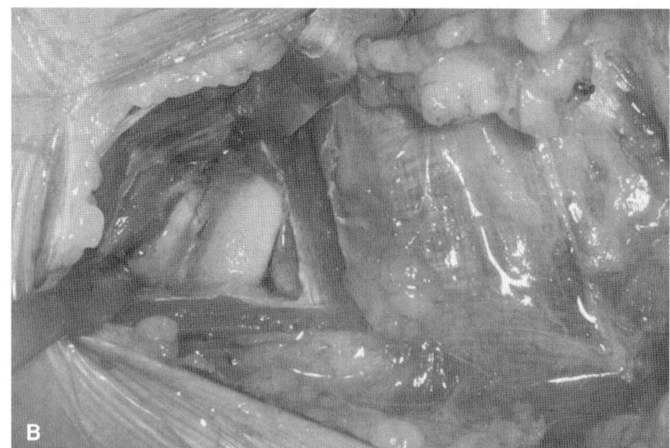

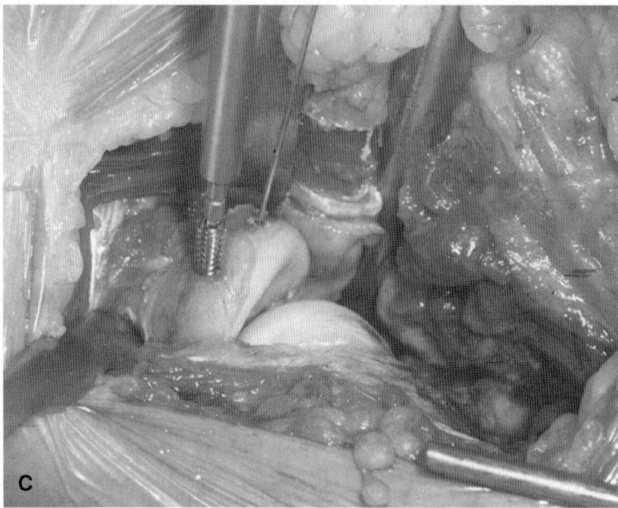

Figure 57-2 Radial head exposure through a muscle-splitting approach. **A:** The split in extensor carpi radialis brevis (ECRB) and proximal extension along the lateral column are marked in blue. **B:** The radial head is easily exposed through the split. **C:** Proximal extension of the approach along the column provides an excellent exposure for fixation or replacement.

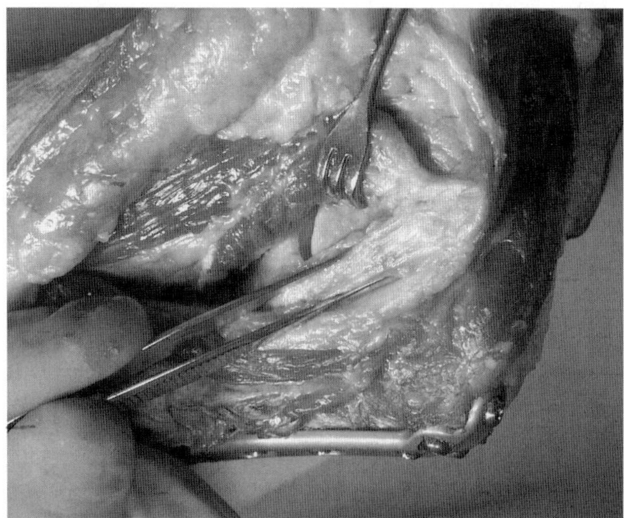

Figure 57-3 Coronoid fractures may be exposed medially by elevation of the flexor-pronator group from distal to proximal. The medial collateral ligament, deep to the muscle group, is pointed out by the forceps. The medial side of the trochlea and the coronoid lie just anterior to the ligament.

through a split in the raphe between the flexor and pronator components of the flexor-pronator group.

THE EXTENSOR MECHANISM

Internal fixation of most distal humerus fractures and reconstruction of the elbow joint with either a joint prosthesis or interposition arthroplasty often require mobilization of the extensor mechanism. Table 57-2 summarizes surgical approaches to mobilize the triceps with some of their advantages and disadvantages.

Working on Both Sides of the Triceps

This approach was originally described by Alonso-Llames for the treatment of children's supracondylar fractures and their sequelae. Access to the distal humerus working on both sides of the triceps is ideal, as it preserves the extensor mechanism intact. However, it provides limited exposure to the articular surface. It is used mainly for internal fixation of selected simple distal humerus fractures, elbow arthroplasty in the presence of distal humeral bone loss, and supracondylar osteotomies.

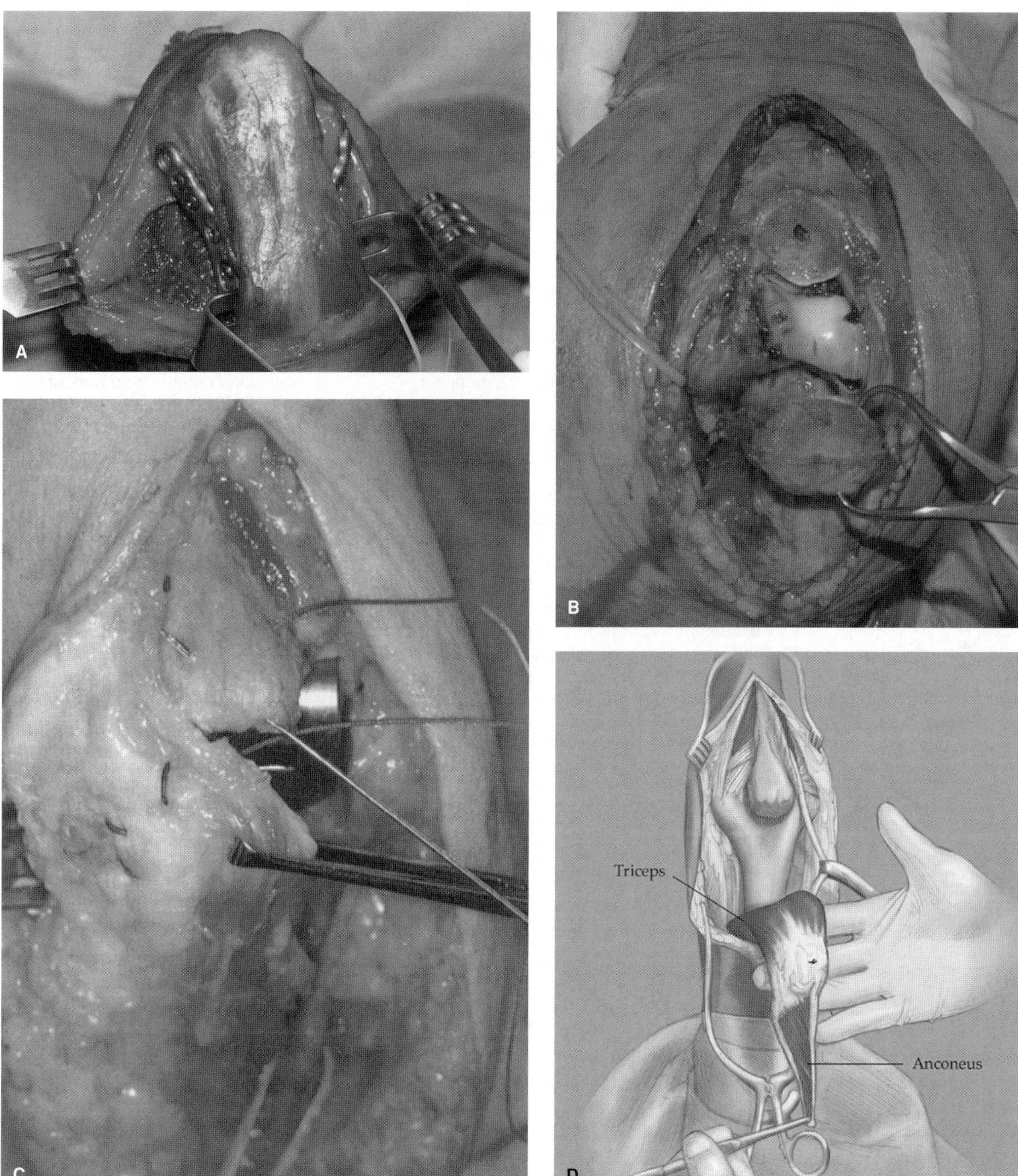

Figure 57-4 Some of the posterior exposures of the elbow joint. **A:** Paratricipital approach. **B:** Olecranon osteotomy. **C:** Bryan-Morrey triceps reflection. **D:** Triceps-reflecting anconeus pedicle (TRAP) approach.

Triceps-Reflection

The triceps can be detached off the olecranon and reflected in continuity with the anconeus, forearm fascia, and ulnar periosteum from either lateral to medial or medial to lateral (Fig. 57-4). Reflection from medial to lateral, the Bryan-Morrey approach, is more commonly used, especially for elbow arthroplasty. The Köcher interval may be identified and developed laterally and the approach extended by reflecting the triceps and anconeus from lateral to medial, the so-called Mayo modified extensile Köcher approach. Both approaches require secure reattachment of the extensor mechanism with nonabsorbable transosseous sutures and avoidance of extension against resistance for about 6 weeks.

TABLE 57-2 SURGICAL EXPOSURES TO MOBILIZE THE EXTENSOR MECHANISM

Approach	Advantages	Disadvantages
Paratricipital/bilaterotricipital (Alonso-Llames) approach	■ Avoids interruption of the extensor mechanism (less morbidity and potential for complications) ■ No postoperative protection of the extensor mechanism needed ■ Decreased surgical time	■ Limited exposure of the articular surface
Triceps reflection approaches ■ Bryan-Morrey (medial to lateral) ■ Mayo modified extensile Köcher (lateral to medial)	■ Avoid complications related to the olecranon osteotomy ■ Preserve anconeus muscle vascularity and continuity with the triceps ■ Prevent proximal migration of the extensor mechanism ■ Provide excellent exposure	■ Failure to heal or lateral/medial subluxation of the extensor mechanism may cause weakness ■ Continuity may be difficult to maintain in rheumatoid patients with poor tissues ■ Exposure may be limited for complex intra-articular fractures (AO/OTA C3)
Triceps split	■ Avoids complications related to olecranon osteotomy ■ Keeps the extensor mechanism centralized ■ Provides excellent exposure for arthroplasty ■ May be associated with less postoperative weakness ■ The triceps turn down allows distal slide of the triceps tongue to facilitate elbow flexion	■ Greater soft-tissue disruption ■ Risk of radial nerve injury with proximal split extension ■ Exposure may be limited for complex intra-articular fractures (AO/OTA C3)[19]
Olecranon osteotomy	■ Provides excellent exposure ■ Limits the amount of soft tissue dissection ■ Offers the potential of bone-to-bone healing	■ Nonunion ■ Intra-articular adhesions ■ Need for hardware removal (local discomfort) ■ Limits the ability to convert intraoperatively to total elbow arthroplasty ■ The proximal ulna cannot be used as a template to judge reduction or motion
Triceps-reflecting anconeus pedicle (TRAP)	■ Provides excellent exposure ■ Avoids the complications of olecranon osteotomy ■ Preserves anconeus muscle vascularity and continuity with the triceps ■ Keeps the extensor mechanism centralized	■ Extensive soft tissue disruption ■ Increases surgical time ■ Substantial gravity-induced pedicle swelling may compromise closure ■ Some patients complain of residual weakness

(AO/OTA C3)[19].

Olecranon Osteotomy

This approach provides excellent exposure to the elbow joint, especially for the management of complex distal humerus fractures. There are some controversies regarding the ideal osteotomy configuration and fixation technique. Currently, most authors favor a chevron-shaped osteotomy initiated with a saw and completed with an osteotome to create additional microinterdigitation at the osteotomy site and avoid inadvertent damage to the articular cartilage. The osteotomy should be centered at the bare area of the olecranon (Fig. 57-4).

Plate fixation provides excellent stability, but it seems to increase the rate of wound complications. Tension band wiring using either a large-fragment partially threaded cancellous screw or two Kirschner wires is commonly used. When screw fixation is selected, drilling and tapping should be completed before performing the osteotomy, and screw length should be enough to provide cortical engagement while avoiding mediolateral translation of the osteotomized fragment with introduction of a long straight screw in the bowed ulnar canal. When Kirschner wires are used, wire placement through the anterior ulnar cortex may decrease the risk of postoperative migration. The main complications of olecranon osteotomy are nonunion and hardware-related complications.

Triceps Split

The triceps can be split in the midline to expose the distal part of the humerus. The split may be extended distally by elevation of medial and lateral subperiosteal flaps off the ulna. This approach is recommended by some mainly for elbow arthroplasty. It maintains the extensor mechanism centralized, but the attachment of the medial half of the triceps is often thin, which may compromise the quality of the repair.

The Triceps-Reflecting Anconeus Pedicle Approach

The triceps-reflecting anconeus pedicle (TRAP) approach was developed for internal fixation of complex distal humerus fractures to avoid the disadvantages of olecranon osteotomy while providing improved exposure over triceps-reflection approaches. It basically involves complete detachment of the triceps and anconeus off the proximal ulna by combining the Bryan-Morrey and the extensile Köcher approaches (Fig. 57-4). The joint can be exposed by elbow hyperextension, and the ulna is kept intact to be used as a template for reconstruction of the distal humerus articular surface or in case conversion to elbow replacement becomes necessary. It may lead to weakness in terminal extension.

ANTERIOR APPROACHES

Anterior approaches to the elbow have very specific indications. Some authors recommend an anterior approach for contracture release, but access to the posterior compartment is required for most contracted elbows, which makes this approach somewhat unappealing. Currently, the anterior aspect of the elbow is exposed most commonly for repair of distal biceps tendon injuries. Either a small anterior incision used to retrieve the tendon is then combined with a second incision in the proximal aspect of the dorsal forearm, or a single larger anterior approach is used for both tendon retrieval and reattachment. Care should be taken to protect the median and radial nerves as well as the brachial artery. Care should also be taken to avoid crossing the elbow flexion crease at a right angle to decrease the chance of skin contracture limiting elbow extension. Moisture accumulated in the elbow flexion crease when the joint is immobilized in some flexion may increase the risk of wound-related complications after any anterior approach.

SUGGESTED READINGS

Aldridge JM III, Atkins TA, Gunneson EE, et al. Anterior release of the elbow for extension loss. *J Bone Joint Surg*. 2004;86A(9):1955–1960.

Alonso-Llames M. Bilaterotricipital approach to the elbow. Its application in the osteosynthesis of supracondylar fractures of the humerus in children. *Acta Orthop Scand*. 1972;43(6):479–490.

Bryan RS, Morrey BF. Extensive posterior exposure of the elbow. A triceps-sparing approach. *Clin Orthop*. 1982;166:188–192.

Diliberti T, Botte MJ, Abrams RA. Anatomical considerations regarding the posterior interosseous nerve during posterolateral approaches to the proximal part of the radius. *J Bone Joint Surg*. 2000;82A:809–813.

Dowdy PA, Bain GI, King GJ, et al. The midline posterior elbow incision. An anatomical appraisal. *J Bone Joint Surg*. 1995;77B:696–699.

Frankle MAMD. Triceps split technique for total elbow arthroplasty. *Techniques Shoulder Elbow Surg*. 2002;3(1):23–27.

Husband JB, Hastings H II. The lateral approach for operative release of post-traumatic contracture of the elbow. *J Bone Joint Surg*. 1990;72A:1353–1358.

Mansat P, Morrey BF. The column procedure: a limited lateral approach for extrinsic contracture of the elbow. *J Bone Joint Surg*. 1998;80A:1603–1615.

Morrey BF. Anatomy and surgical approaches. In: Morrey BF, ed. *Joint Replacement Arthroplasty*. Philadelphia: Churchill-Livingstone; 2003:269–285.

O'Driscoll SW. The triceps-reflecting anconeus pedicle (TRAP) approach for distal humeral fractures and nonunions. *Orthop Clin North Am*. 2000;31(1):91–101.

Ring D, Gulotta L, Chin K, et al. Olecranon osteotomy for exposure of fractures and nonunions of the distal humerus. *J Orthop Trauma*. 2004;18(7):446–449.

Schildhauer TA, Nork SE, Mills WJ, et al. Extensor mechanism-sparing paratricipital posterior approach to the distal humerus. *J Orthop Trauma*. 2003;17(5):374–378.

Wada T, Ishii S, Usui M, et al. The medial approach for operative release of post-traumatic contracture of the elbow. *J Bone Joint Surg*. 2000;82B:68–73.

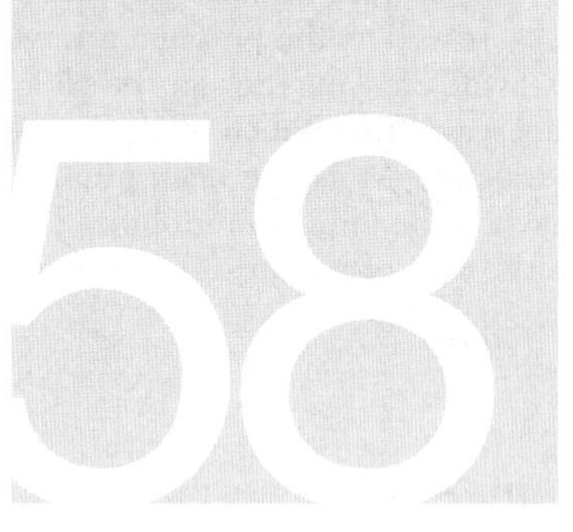

ELBOW ARTHROPLASTY: SURGICAL TECHNIQUE

RICK F. PAPANDREA

Total elbow arthroplasty has evolved into a reliable treatment for the appropriately selected patient. The advent of reliable devices in the 1980s allowed this joint to be replaced with outcomes similar to other joints. Not that total elbow arthroplasty is without its potential complications or problems. At least as important as in other joints, if not more important because of potential pitfalls, proper surgical technique is paramount for a successful arthroplasty.

IMPLANT TYPES

The type of implant used can dictate the surgical approach and various technical details; although much about total elbow arthroplasty surgical technique is not implant design specific. Current devices are most easily categorized as being either linked or unlinked. Constraint of the implant is important, but is not dependent on linkage. A linked implant is best thought of as a hinge, with the ulnar and humeral components coupled, or linked. Initial designs had no play or toggle between the components, and these devices failed quickly. Modern-design linked implants allow for angular and rotational play between the humeral and ulnar components. Unlinked components have no direct connection between the components. The amount of congruity or conformity between the articulating surfaces of the implants dictates the constraint of the device. A highly congruent articulation has more constraint than an articulation with little conformity. Thus, a linked or unlinked device can be either constrained or unconstrained. An unlinked device with little constraint has the highest risk of dislocation; particular attention has to be given to both pre-existing deformity and adequate soft tissue repair, especially the ligaments. A linked device cannot, by design, dislocate; but, attention to pre-existing deformity is just as important as when considering an unlinked design.

SURGICAL INDICATIONS AND CONTRAINDICATIONS

The disease-specific indications and contraindications will be discussed in the following chapters. General indications for a total elbow arthroplasty include a painful elbow joint that does not have less-extensive reconstructive options available. Adequate bone stock for reconstruction with the chosen prosthesis is necessary, and the surgeon should have familiarity with the technical limitations of the prosthesis considered for implantation. Bone deficit can be compensated for by some devices, but each device has limitations. Custom devices are rarely if ever needed. A functional elbow flexor is necessary. A competent extensor mechanism is considered important; but, a functional limb can be reconstructed without, if the patient is willing to accept a compromise. Gravity is then used for elbow extension, and overhead function with the involved limb is not possible. An adequate soft tissue envelope is necessary, especially with the higher risk of infection in total elbow arthroplasty. Understanding of and compliance with the restrictions inherent to any total elbow arthroplasty is a mandatory requisite for surgery. Longevity of newer implants has improved to parallel hip arthroplasty in rheumatoid patients. Failures have been noted in patients placing high demands on their reconstructed joint. Because of this, most surgeons have placed the permanent restriction on their patients of not lifting >10 pounds as a single, occasional event, and 1 to 2 pounds as a repetitive event.

Contraindications for total elbow arthroplasty include noncompliant patients, inadequate bone stock or soft tissue envelope, active or recent infection, or a dysfunctional elbow flexor.

SURGICAL APPROACH

As discussed in the preceding chapter, there are several approaches to the elbow, but a posterior incision allows for much freedom in the deeper exposure. Although a laterally based skin incision (and deeper exposure) has been used in elbow arthroplasty (especially some unlinked designs), it does have inherent limitations. This author routinely uses a universal posterior skin incision for elbow arthroplasty. Multiple approaches can be easily accomplished, and future revision surgery is not compromised by other skin incisions. Fewer problems with the cutaneous nerves are encountered when the incision is placed posteriorly. Many elbows requiring arthroplasty have pre-existing deformity, which can be challenging to correct. Laterally based approaches can make a challenging deformity nearly impossible to correct.

When planning the surgical approach to elbow arthroplasty, there are three structures that require consideration regardless of the implant used. These include the triceps, the ulnar nerve, and the collateral ligaments. The implant used may dictate certain needs, but each of these three factors must be considered in every elbow arthroplasty.

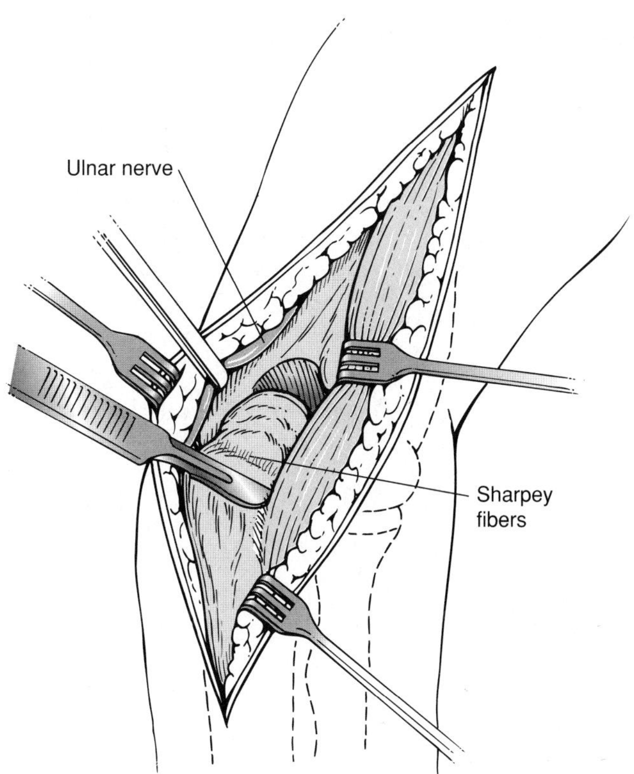

Figure 58-1 The Bryan-Morrey, or Mayo, approach reflects the triceps with the anconeus laterally. The distal extent continues to the extensor musculature and fascia of the forearm, which is kept in continuity with the triceps.

Triceps

Recent attention has focused on the potential complications with triceps reattachment after elbow arthroplasty. Postoperative weakness has been attributed to failure of the repair site of triceps to the olecranon. This has caused a scrutiny of current techniques and reconsideration of alternative methods to deal with the triceps. Most available implants for elbow arthroplasty recommend that the triceps be released or transected at some level. The ideal method of release is unknown. Although more challenging, implants can be placed through a medial and/or lateral deep exposure. The triceps can then be left alone. Visualization is more difficult and extreme care must be taken to ensure proper implant orientation.

One exception to the requirement for triceps release occurs when treating chronic nonunions with a linked prosthesis. As described by Morrey, these are readily approached by excising the distal humeral fragment(s). The epicondyles are, by default, excised, but this does not compromise the result. By excising the distal humerus, the triceps can be left attached to the olecranon and the components can be implanted through the gap from the resection. This has the advantage of allowing full triceps activity without the need to protect a repair. If surgical exposure is adequate from this approach, the risk of extensor weakness should be eliminated. The potential drawback of the approach is the limitation of exposure and the potential inability to correct significant deformity. A similar technique has also been described for routine elbow linked arthroplasty by Matsen.

When the triceps is dealt with directly, the tendon needs to be released from the olecranon is some fashion. Early techniques (Campbell/Van Gorder) involved leaving a tongue of triceps tendon attached to the olecranon, detaching the tendon proximally in a "V" fashion. This did allow for a V-Y lengthening if needed and also did not disturb the Sharpey fibers attachment of the triceps. This approach has been essentially abandoned for modern elbow arthroplasty, but as concern regarding the healing potential of the triceps to the olecranon is raised, it could once again be considered.

The Bryan-Morrey, or Mayo, approach to the triceps is a reflection of the triceps laterally off of the olecranon. The anconeus is kept in continuity with the triceps, and the whole sleeve of tissue, with the extensor fascia, is reflected laterally (Fig. 58-1).

The triceps is repaired to the olecranon using bone tunnels to pass sutures. This technique allows for complete separation of the olecranon from the triceps. If the reattachment does not heal completely, there will be at minimum triceps weakness and possibly complete extensor mechanism failure. The tissue distal to the Sharpey fibers can be quite atrophic, resulting in a defect of the sleeve of soft tissue. This approach can also be performed leaving a small wafer of bone on the triceps to allow for precise attachment back to the olecranon and also allow for bone-to-bone healing of the extensor mechanism. Unfortunately, in clinical practice, this addition did not bear out any advantage to the all–soft tissue approach.

Another approach to dealing with the triceps and allowing for the potential of bone-to-bone healing is the Gschwend approach (Fig. 58-2). This is a midline triceps splitting approach. As the distal dissection is undertaken, the split continues along the subcutaneous border of the

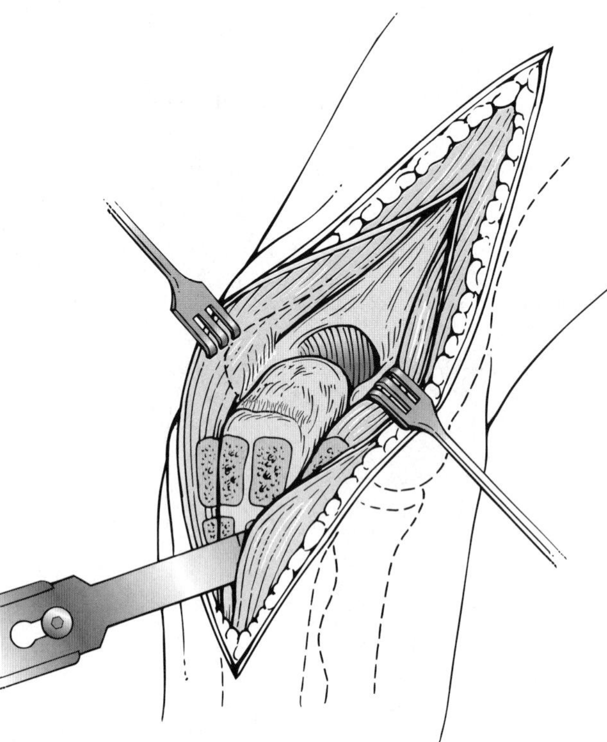

Figure 58-2 The Gschwend approach splits the triceps and continues distally, osteotomizing triceps attachment with bone from the olecranon.

ulna. As originally described, an osteotome is then used to remove the medial and lateral cortex of the ulna with the soft tissue attachments. The collateral ligaments can be left in situ, but releasing them allows for significantly more exposure. The split and the bone wafers are reattached through drill holes at closure. This approach can be done strictly as a soft tissue exposure by carrying the dissection along the medial and lateral ulna, forgoing any bone resection.

Ulnar Nerve

Prior to undertaking any elbow arthroplasty, the status of the ulnar nerve should be documented. If there has been previous surgery, attempts should be made to study the old operative records. In cases of old trauma or surgery, one should never assume the location of the ulnar nerve. It must be identified and protected throughout the procedure. The proximal medial triceps border is usually a reliable location to identify the nerve in an elbow with previous surgery.

Transposition of the nerve into a subcutaneous pocket is standard practice by many surgeons regularly performing elbow arthroplasty. The nerve can be safely removed from the primary surgical field and should not cause further difficulty in the future, should a revision be needed. Although there is always risk when transposing the ulnar nerve, the risk is far less than that incurred by leaving it in the cubital tunnel. A transposition was not originally described by Gschwend in his triceps splitting approach. At a minimum the nerve needs to be identified in this technique and can be readily transposed with little additional effort.

Collateral Ligaments

The lateral collateral ligament must be released to allow dislocation or subluxation of the elbow sufficient to allow for implantation of any total elbow device. Releasing the medial collateral ligament will allow for better correction of any pre-existing deformity and give better access. If the device implanted is linked, neither ligament needs to be repaired.

If an unlinked device is used, the lateral collateral must be repaired or reconstructed. Although a medial collateral ligament–deficient elbow may not dislocate in the native state, the increased instability will jeopardize an unlinked implant, and consideration should be given to repair or reconstruction.

BONE PREPARATION

Humerus

Each different elbow arthroplasty system has its own cutting blocks and guides. However, there are some general principles for humeral preparation. The posterior aspect of the capitellum is the origin for the anconeus. The muscle should be dissected off of this area to allow for complete exposure of the lateral column.

Care needs to be taken when cutting out the trochlea for the humeral component. Although consisting of cortical bone, the columns are narrow, and if notched or too generous a cut is made, the column may fracture, separating the epicondyle from the humerus. If this occurs, the most efficacious treatment is to excise the fractured fragment if a linked implant is being placed. The loss of the epicondyle and associated collateral will not have bearing on the outcome. Attempts at fixation of these small fragments have little to no net benefit. If the device is unlinked, this fracture will have significant bearing on the potential stability. Either the fragment has to be fixed or a linked device has to be used. If an unlinked device is used, fixation can be done with a tension band and wires, or if the fragment is large, a unicortical plate.

The humeral canal narrows to a point in the sagittal plane. Because of this, if the starting hole is not proximal enough, or attention is not paid to the opening, there may be remnant cortical bone tapering inward. This obscures the true diameter of the humeral canal, and more important, can cause the humeral instrumentation or implant to be pushed anterior or posterior. It is imperative to recognize this, and if the canal is not accepting the rasps or trials, to ensure that a sufficient amount of the distal humerus is removed to allow a straight approach up the medullary canal. If it is apparent that there is impeding bone, it is often easiest to remove with a rongeur.

Ulna

Most implants require that the tip of the olecranon is excised to allow for instrumentation of the medullary canal and implantation of the device. The attachment site for the triceps must be retained. Like the humerus, the opening to the medullary canal may not initially allow for correct broaching or rasping. This is especially true in patients with osteoarthritis and/or dense bone. When the subchondral bone is too dense, using a burr to open the canal will save time and prevent potential catastrophic fracture of the proximal ulna.

IMPLANTATION

Each total elbow arthroplasty device has a specific technique for implantation. However, some universal concepts are worthy of consideration.

Linked implants can often be implanted separately, then linked, or implanted all at once already linked. The advantage of implanting each component separately is the ability to focus technique on each side individually. The disadvantage is that of having to mix two separate batches of cement and the extra time it takes for the two sides to cure sequentially. The advantages of separate component implantation far outweigh the disadvantages for the surgeon with limited experience implanting total elbows. Linked implantation should be done only by surgeons with high-volume experience.

Humerus

The trefoil shape of the humerus, as well as the guides for most systems, help with proper rotational alignment. The anterior flange on many humeral components also aids in rotational alignment. The flange's main purpose is to resist posterior and rotationally directed forces on the humeral component. These stresses are significant and can lead to early failure if not neutralized. For this reason, the flange should be grafted if the technique calls for it. Evidence of the stress on the flange is noted postoperatively, when most of these grafts heal and many hypertrophy.

Ulna

Rotational alignment can be more difficult to account for in the ulnar component. Once the medullary canal is prepared, it is cylindrical, allowing for rotation of the component. Some devices account for this and have flanges or flat posterior aspects of the component. Even with these additions, if one is not careful, the rasps and trials (and eventually the final components) can be placed with rotation. This will cause undue stress on the coupling in a linked component and potential for dislocation in an unlinked device. There are two reliable methods to ensure proper rotational alignment of the ulnar component. As described by King, the flat spot on the dorsal ulna is almost perfectly perpendicular to the plane of the greater sigmoid notch. O'Driscoll has recently described the use of the radial head (or shaft if the head has been resected) to align the ulnar component. The ulnar component must be aligned so that the flexion axis of the device passes through the radial head (or shaft) center when viewing from end on.

Every effort should be made to balance the elbow while using the trial implants. This is especially true in elbows with significant pre-existing deformity. Unlinked devices have a high dislocation rate. Unbalanced devices that are

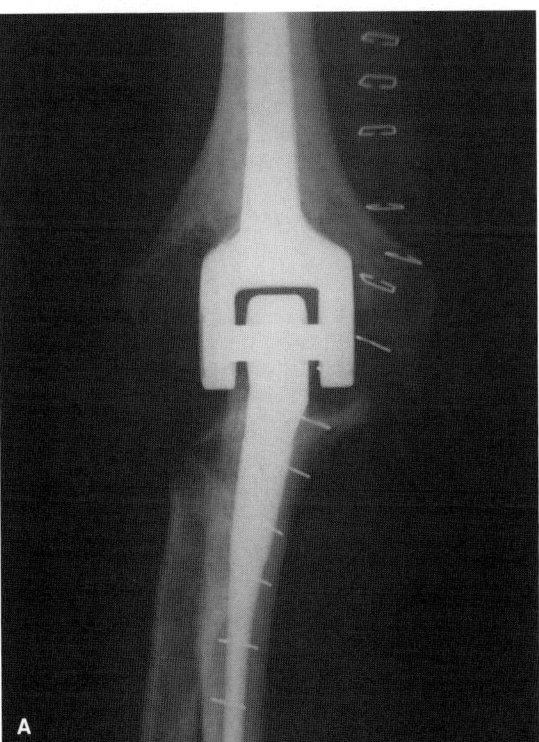

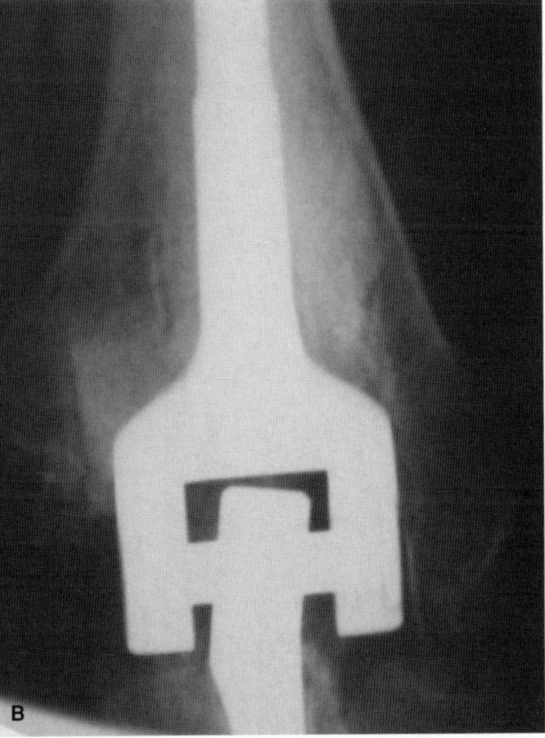

Figure 58-3 Plain radiographs of a balanced (A)and unbalanced (B) linked total elbow arthroplasty.

not linked are even more likely to dislocate. A linked device will not dislocate, but if unbalanced, will load the bearings more than will a balanced elbow (Fig. 58-3). This has been proposed as a cause of early failure.

CLOSURE

Details of the triceps repair depend on the type of approach that was used. Every effort should be made to reattach the triceps to its native location. Marking the area of the Sharpey fibers attachment with a suture can ensure later reattachment to the proper location. If the triceps was detached only as soft tissue, drill holes should be used for suture passage of no. 2 or no. 5 nonabsorbable sutures to secure the repair. One can usually pass straight needles directly through the ulna with a pin driver, obviating the need to drill, and then pass the sutures with another device.

If the ligaments were taken down, which is usually necessary for adequate exposure, they need not be repaired in the case of a linked device. If the device implanted is unlinked, stability must be restored or else the chance of dislocation is high. The ligaments should be repaired, or if this is not possible, reconstructed.

Seroma formation is not uncommon postoperatively, owing to the skin flaps created during dissection. To decrease the likelihood or severity of this, the subcutaneous tissue can be tacked down to the fascia to close this potential space. When doing this, the cutaneous nerves must be avoided to prevent neuromas.

Since most patients have trouble obtaining extension postoperatively, splinting in full extension is helpful. This allows a compressive bandage to be applied, and the elbow can then be elevated or hung in a stockinette to decrease swelling.

SUGGESTED READINGS

Bryan RS, Morrey BF. Extensive posterior exposure of the elbow. a triceps-sparing approach. *Clin Orthop*. 1982;166:188–192.

Duggal N, Dunning CE, Johnson JA, et al. The flat spot of the proximal ulna: a useful anatomic landmark in total elbow arthroplasty. *J Shoulder Elbow Surg*. 2004;13:206–207.

Gill DR, Morrey BF. The Coonrad-Morrey total elbow arthroplasty in patients who have rheumatoid arthritis. A ten to fifteen-year follow-up study. *J Bone Joint Surg Am*. 1988;80:1327–1335.

King GJ, Itoi E, Niebur GL, et al. Motion and laxity of the capitellocondylar total elbow prosthesis. *J Bone Joint Surg Am*. 1994;76:1000–1008.

Ring D, Kocher M, Koris M, et al. Revision of unstable capitellocondylar (unlinked) total elbow replacement. *J Bone Joint Surg Am*. 2005;87:1075–1079.

Schuind F, O'Driscoll S, Korinek S, et al. Loose-hinge total elbow arthroplasty. An experimental study of the effects of implant alignment on three-dimensional elbow kinematics. *J Arthroplasty*. 1995;10:670–678.

Wright TW, Hastings H. Total elbow arthroplasty failure due to overuse, C-ring failure, and/or bushing wear. *J Shoulder Elbow Surg*. 2005;14:65–72.

TOTAL ELBOW ARTHROPLASTY FOR RHEUMATOID ARTHRITIS

DAVID R. J. GILL

PATHOGENESIS

Etiology and Epidemiology

Rheumatoid arthritis (RA) is a chronic systemic inflammatory disorder in which the body's immune system mistakes articular cartilage for foreign (nonself) material. The exact cause for RA is unknown. Genetic susceptibility is recognized, including monozygotic HLA DR4, which has a 12% to 15% concordance rate. Women, especially postpartum and those breastfeeding, have an increased risk along with smokers.

In the United States approximately 2.1 million people are affected with rheumatoid arthritis, or approximately 1 per 300,000. It is generally believed that the ratio of women to men is between 2 to 1 and 3 to 1. It is rare in men younger than the age of 45 years; in this age group, the condition is predominately among women (6 to 1). The peak incidence is between the ages of 20 and 50 years, but it can affect both the young and the elderly. Its prevalence is lowered among black African and Chinese and among certain Indian tribes. It most commonly affects adults as a polyarticular disease where extra-articular features are uncommon.

PATHOPHYSIOLOGY

The pathologic changes of RA can be separated into the following three phases:

1. *Synovitis*—The synovial lining of the joint is congested and at times villous. Subsynovial infiltrates of lymphocytes and plasma cells are present. The effusion is cellular, and the capsule is thickened.
2. *Joint destruction*—Within the first 2 years, proteolytic enzymes and direct invasion of the pannus of granulation tissue destroys the articular surface. The joint margins are eroded by the same process. Tendon sheaves develop tenosynovitis, and this process causes invasion of the collagen bundles.
3. *Deformity*—Over time, joint destruction capitula thickening and distension along with tendon rupture leads to progressive instability and deformity.

CLASSIFICATION

The classification most commonly used is summarized in Table 59-1. This classification system is based on both the pathologic changes and the changing x-ray film appearances. This classification system can be used to guide the orthopaedist with regard to treatment options.

DIAGNOSIS

The diagnosis of RA in general requires four of the seven revised American Rheumatism Association (ARA) criteria in the last 6 months.

When focusing on the elbow, it is important in the history to focus on pain, associated stiffness, and/or instability. One should inquire about neurologic symptoms, especially that of the ulnar nerve, remembering that approximately 40% of rheumatoid arthritic patients with elbow pathology have either clinical or subclinical peripheral neuropathy or nerve compressions. Previous surgery to the elbow (radial head excision or replacement and/or interposition) has prognostic implications. A more general view of the patient including the joints above and below the elbow and cervical spine in mode and abilities and ambulation is important. The overall functional capacity, e.g., the ARA classification, may also be useful.

TABLE 59-1 CLASSIFICATION OF RHEUMATOID ARTHRITIS OF THE ELBOW

Pathology	Radiographic Appearance
Grade 1. Synovitis alone	Osteoporosis with normal joint space, effusion
Grade 2. Synovitis cartilage destruction	Joint space narrowing, periarticular erosions
Grade 3. Loss of cartilage, ligamentous redundancy, capsular stretching	Loss of joint space
Grade 4. Bone destruction, deformity	Instability, loss of joint congruity

Examination

The aim here is to carefully consider the elbow and then the patient as a whole.

1. *The integument*—the skin, especially posteriorly where the incision will be made. The muscles, the flexors of the elbow: What are their strengths, and what is their condition? Neurovascular considerations, particularly to the course of the ulnar nerve and its behavior in flexion.
2. *The joint*—the range of motion and both flexion and extension along with pronation/supination; its stability in reference to whether the joint is enlocated or whether it remains subluxed or flail.
3. *The patient*—particular reference to the joints above and below (wrist and shoulder), the cervical spine, and the patient's general ambulatory ability and if the affected elbow is used in ambulation in any way (cane, crutch, or wheelchair).

RADIOLOGIC FEATURES

The general radiographic changes are summarized in Table 59-2; specifically, one should examine the plain x-ray films to determine surgical requirements. Canal capacity length and alignment relative to the articulate surfaces are important. Any bone thinning, particularly cortical bone thinning, especially at points of entry of the prosthesis or at the tips of potential prosthetic replacement, needs to be noted (Fig. 59-1).

TABLE 59-2 SEVERITY OF RHEUMATOID ARTHRITIS OF THE ELBOW

Worsening disease ↓	Osteopenia Effusion Periarticular erosion Joint space narrowing Subluxation Bone destruction

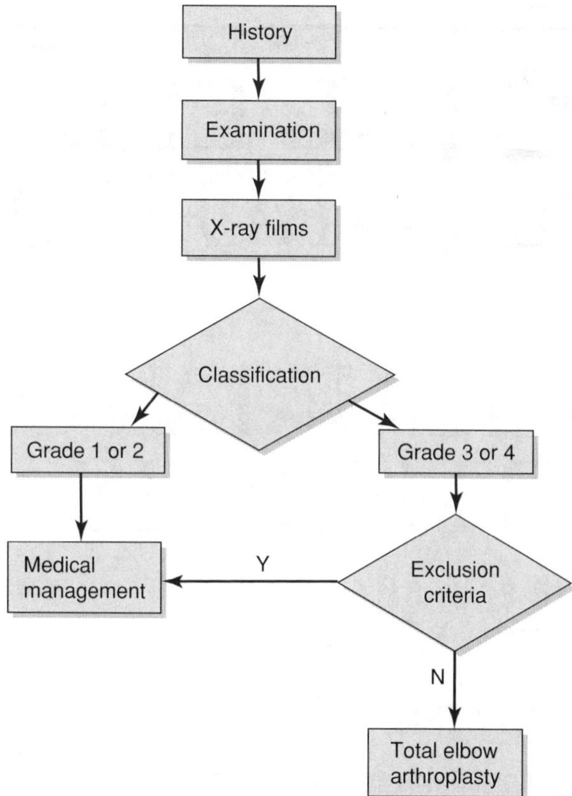

Figure 59-1 Diagnostic workup algorithm.

TREATMENT

Surgical Indications/Contraindications

The primary surgical indication is pain; the specific surgical goal is the relief of pain. Total elbow arthroplasty for rheumatoid arthritis should be considered in patients with grade 3 or 4 disease. The contraindications are bone or joint infection or an open wound about the elbow. Relative contraindications include the medical state of the patient specifically with regard to Parkinsonian or other neurologic disorders, particularly if the patient has a history of recurrent falls. The possibility that anaesthesia will place the patient at unnecessary risk must also be considered. The other relative risk is bone ankyloses. The technical demands of joint replacement at the elbow are such that the general orthopaedist should refer to those surgeons with high-volume experience in total elbow arthroplasty.

Surgical options relate to prosthetic choice. Both unconstrained and semiconstrained joint replacements are currently available. Traditionally, unconstrained joint replacement (with which there is no direct linkage between the humeral and ulnar components) has been considered for those patients with grade 3 disease where there is still primary ligamentous stability. Semiconstrained implants have a loose linkage between the humeral and ulnar components, allowing approximately 7 to 10 degrees of toggle at the articulation but at the same time maintaining the articulation's

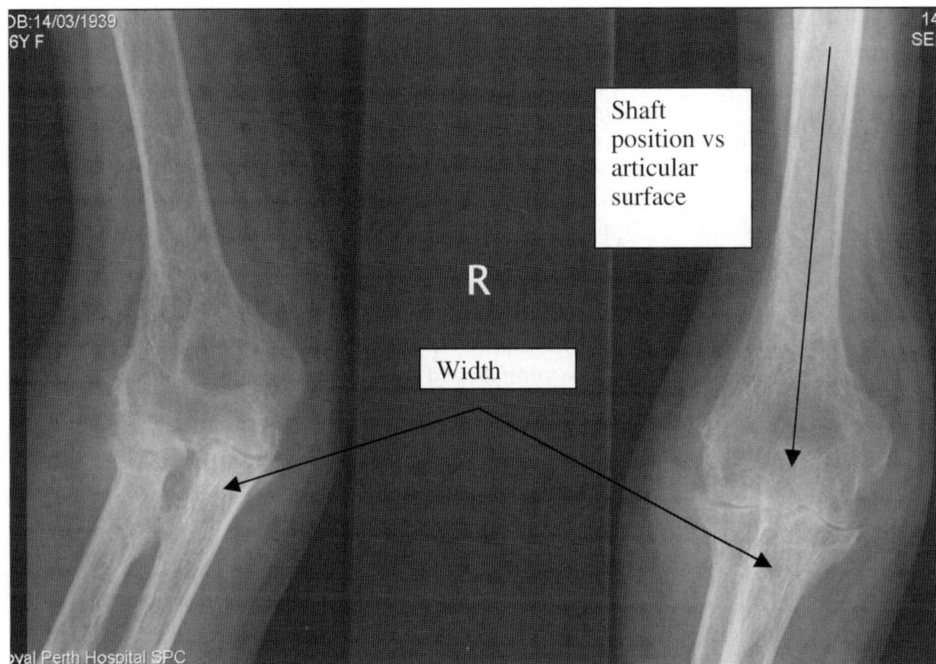

Figure 59-2 Anteroposterior radiograph of an elbow with rheumatoid arthritis.

stability. This type of prosthesis is the most commonly used and may be considered for both grade 3 and grade 4 patients.

Preoperative planning starts from the time of the history and examination, the orthopaedist having satisfied himself or herself that the patient is a surgical candidate and has no contraindications. The examination can specifically review those aspects important for the joint replacement itself—soft tissue coverage and the quality of the integument: There must be at least one flexor of antigravity power and preferably an extensor of similar power both for extension and to cover the prosthesis. Bone deficiency is covered both clinically and on the radiographs; the minimum requirement for a semiconstrained prosthesis is two tubes of bone (the humeral canal, the ulnar canal, and a grade 4 flexor). These are the minimum requirements for undertaking elbow replacement arthroplasty.

Templating prior to surgery, preferably during the clinic appointment, focuses the orthopaedist on any technical difficulties of implantation of the preferred implant. The size, the position of the humeral and ulnar cuts, and the relationship of the intramedullary canals to the articular surface are brought to the orthopedist's attention. Also of note is the curvature of the humerus on lateral view and therefore its relationship to the prosthesis being used and the narrowing on lateral view of the ulna beyond to the olecranon with specific reference to the stem of the prosthesis to be used (Figs. 59-2 and 59-3).

The specific surgical technique used for elbow replacement arthroplasty is covered in other chapters. Important steps to be focused on include the following:

- Exposure
- Ulnar nerve identification and transposition
- Dislocation
- Release of anterior humerus
- Accurate identification of the canals
- Bone cuts as per manufacturer requirements
- Trial components; Ensure soft tissue releases for balance of prosthesis
- Cement prosthesis (sequentially is recommended)
- Rearticulation

Complications

Approximately 10% of total elbow arthroplasty patients will experience some type of complication. Most of these are

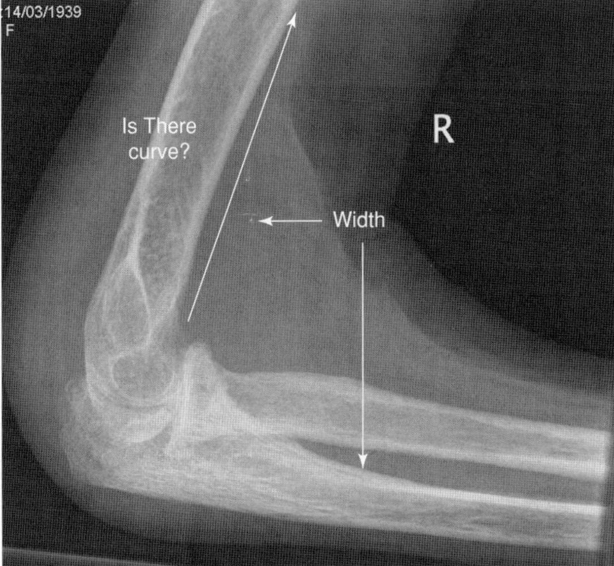

Figure 59-3 Lateral radiograph of an elbow with rheumatoid arthritis.

minor and permit easy recovery. Intraoperative bone fracture, either that of the condyles or perforation of the canals, can occur without careful preoperative planning. If there is canal perforation, more distant neurovascular structures such as the radial or median nerve are at risk. Early complications include wound-healing difficulties, bleeding, and joint stiffness. Temporary paresthesia, particularly of the ulnar nerve, is also recognized. Late complications that have been recognized and should be considered are loosening of the implant's bushing in those implants using bushings, triceps failure, and component fracture. Infection of total elbow arthroplasty in rheumatoid patients is said to be approximately 2%, which is slightly higher than that of standard lower extremity (hip and knee) joint replacement.

Results

The expected result for total elbow arthroplasty in patients with rheumatoid arthritis is a 100-degree arc motion generally from approximately 30 degrees of fixed flexion to 130 degrees of flexion. The patient should expect excellent relief of pain, which provides a high degree of satisfaction. When scored by a common elbow evaluation rating at 10 years, 85% of patients will have a good or excellent result. The survivor rate is approximately 92% at 10 years for this group of patients.

Postoperative Management

After surgery, the elbow is splinted straight with a commercial or plaster of Paris splint until the following day. This achieves a decrease in elbow joint volume and therefore reduces swelling. Thermal regulation that caused the joint may also be used to reduce the initial swelling. Typically, once the dressings are removed, simple dressings are applied to the wound, a compressive long arm stocking is applied, and unrestricted elbow motion can be commenced. Discharge of the patient from the hospital is dependent on overall recovery as semiconstrained implants are stable from the beginning and no specific postoperative splinting is required. If an unconstrained implant is chosen, the manufacturer's specific recommendations must be followed regarding postoperative splinting and protection.

Total elbow arthroplasty in patients with rheumatoid arthritis requires specific restrictions in use of the limb and can be summarized as follows: no more than 5 kg repeated lifting and no more than 10 kg in a single event.

SUGGESTED READINGS

Gill DRJ, Morrey BF. The Coonrad-Morrey total elbow arthroplasty in patients who have rheumatoid arthritis. A ten to fifteen-year follow-up study. *J Bone Joint Surg Am*. 1998;80:1327.

Gschwend N, Scheier NH, Baehler AR. Long-term results of the GSBIII elbow arthroplasty. *J Bone Joint Surg Br*. 1999;81:1005.

Hildebrand KA, Patterson SD, Regan WD, et al. The functional outcome of semiconstrained total elbow arthroplasty. *J Bone Joint Surg Am*. 2000;82:1379.

Morrey BF. *The Elbow and Its Disorders*. 3rd ed. WB Saunders; 2000.

Potter D, Claydon P, Stanley D. Total elbow replacement using the Kudo prosthesis. Clinical and radiological review with five- to seven-year follow-up. *J Bone Joint Surg Br*. 2003;85:354.

Sanchez-Sotelo J, O'Driscoll S, Morrey BF. Periprosthetic humeral fractures after total elbow arthroplasty: treatment with implant revision and strut allograft augmentation. *J Bone Joint Surg Am*. 2002;84:1642.

Van der Lugt JC, Geskus RB, Rozing PM. Primary Souter-Strathclyde total elbow prosthesis and rheumatoid arthritis. *J Bone Joint Surg Am*. 2004;86A:465.

TOTAL ELBOW ARTHROPLASTY FOR PRIMARY OSTEOARTHRITIS

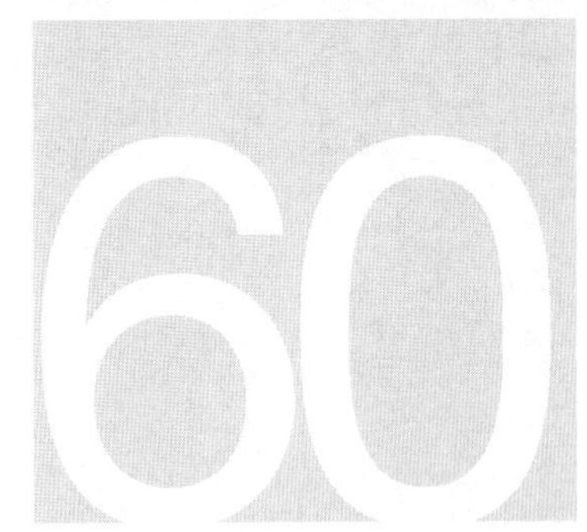

BASSEM ELHASSAN
SCOTT P. STEINMANN

DEFINITION

Degenerative primary arthritis of the elbow is an uncommon problem.[1] It occurs in less than 2% of the population and principally affects the dominant extremity in middle-age manual laborers. It has also been reported in people who require continuous use of a wheelchair or crutches, athletes, and in patients with a history of osteochondritis dissecans of the elbow. It has different pathologic changes than the age-related changes of the distal humerus and the radiohumeral joint.

Because of the younger age and increased activity levels of patients with primary osteoarthritis of the elbow, the treatment options are more limited and the role of total elbow arthroplasty is less defined in this population of patients.

PATHOLOGY

Histopathologic Changes in Elbow Osteoarthritis

The degenerative changes of the elbow joint are usually more advanced in the radiohumeral joint, where bare bone is often in wide contact and the capitellum appears to have been shaved obliquely (Fig. 60-1). This is owing to the high axial, shearing, and rotational stresses at this articulation, which result in marked erosion of the capitellum and callus hypertrophy formation in a skirtlike pattern on the radial neck.

The ulnohumeral joint is usually less involved in the beginning of the disease process and becomes more pronounced with more advanced disease. The central aspect of the ulnohumeral joint is characteristically spared. The anterior and posterior involvement of this joint is usually manifested by fibrosis of the anterior capsule in the form of cordlike band and hypertrophy of the olecranon.

Osteophyte growths are seen over the olecranon (especially medially), the coronoid process, and the coronoid fossa. These changes in the radiohumeral and ulnohumeral joints lead to the loss and fragmentation of the cartilaginous joint surfaces with distortion, cyst formation, and bone sclerosis. Kashiwagi noted that the early stage of the disease is characterized by small, round bony protuberances that progress into various shapes of osteophytes and bony sclerosis with more advanced cases.

Clinical Presentation

Despite considerable radiographic severity, many patients with osteoarthritis of the elbow report minimal symptoms. This is partly related to the fact that the elbow is a slight weight-bearing joint compared with the lower extremity joints.

Mechanical symptoms of locking and catching caused by intra-articular loose bodies, pain at the end points of the arc of motion (flexion or extension), and progressive loss of range of motion are characteristic manifestations of osteoarthritis of the elbow. In athletes who are required to hyperextend their elbows, pain can be significant and limits their performance.

With more progressive disease, the patients may have pain with forearm rotation and throughout the range of elbow motion. This could lead to disability in this patient population as well as in the older laborers who extensively use their upper extremity.

Medial joint pain in patients with advanced osteoarthritis of the elbow might be the first manifestation of ulnar neuropathy. It is reported that ≤20% of patients with primary osteoarthritis of the elbow have some degree of ulnar neuropathy. The proximity of the ulnar nerve to the arthritic posteromedial aspect of the ulnohumeral joint makes it susceptible to impingement. The expansion of the capsule as a result of synovitis and the presence of osteophytes in that area of the joint result in direct compression and ischemia of the ulnar nerve. Acute onset of

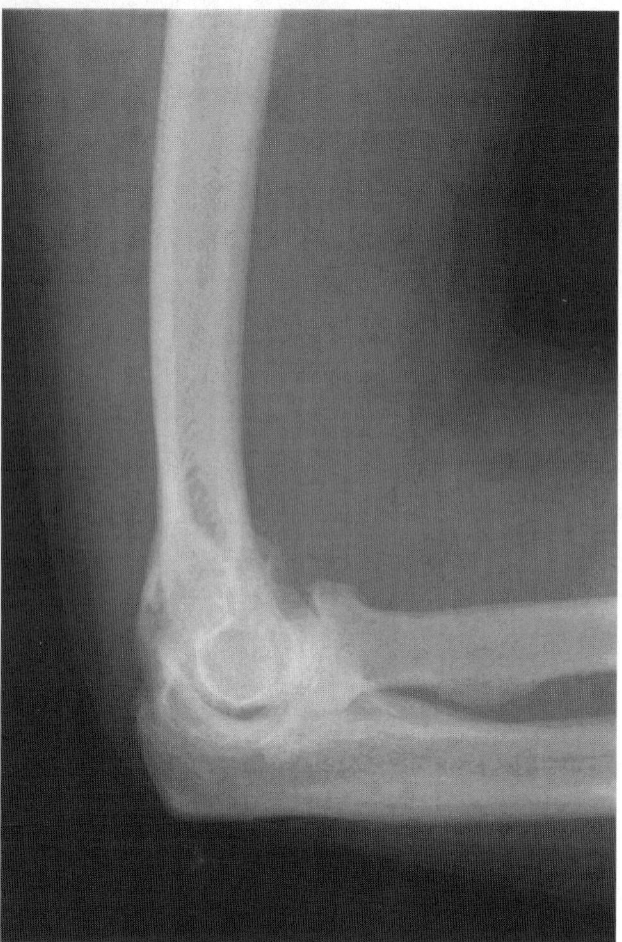

Figure 60-1 A lateral view of the right elbow, showing advanced osteoarthritis specifically involving the radiocapitellar joint. Notice the formation of osteophytes anteriorly and posteriorly.

cubital tunnel syndrome in patients with osteoarthritis of the elbow might be also the first manifestation of medial elbow ganglion.

IMAGING AND OTHER DIAGNOSTIC STUDIES

The characteristic radiographic features seen on the anteroposterior and lateral radiographs of the elbow include radiocapitellar narrowing, ossification, and osteophyte formation in the olecranon fossa in almost all patients with osteoarthritis of the elbow. Loose bodies and fluffy densities might be observed filling the coronoid and olecranon fossae (Fig. 60-2).

Computer tomography (CT) also helps in delineating the detailed structural anatomy of the articular surface of the elbow with an accurate determination of the locations of the osteophytes and loose bodies. When contemplating surgical treatment of the osteoarthritic elbow, a CT is quite helpful for determining which osteophytes need to be removed. Radiographs do not allow for accurate visualization of all osteophytes.

NONOPERATIVE MANAGEMENT

Because of the young age of the patients with primary osteoarthritis of the elbow, most of these patients tend to be active and involved in manual labor work, which will place a great demand on any kind of prosthetic replacement. All limited operative debridement options should be exhausted before contemplating elbow replacement in this group of patients.

Early in the course of the disease, treatment by nonsurgical measures should be followed. This consists of activity modification, physical therapy, anti-inflammatory medications, and possibly steroid injection. As in other joints arthritis, if there is no improvement with these symptomatic measures, operative management is warranted.

SURGICAL MANAGEMENT

Elbow arthroscopy is a good option for removal of intra-articular loose bodies and is effective in relieving the patient's mechanical symptoms of catching and locking. Elbow arthroscopy has proved quite effective in removing osteophytes and releasing tight areas of capsule in the arthritic elbow. Surgeons with significant experience in elbow arthroscopy can remove all restricted capsule and reach all areas of the anterior and posterior elbow joint and areas of impinging osteophytes. To release a similar amount of the elbow joint with an open approach would require a wide exposure.

TECHNIQUES

Kashiwagi popularized the open elbow decompression described by Outerbridge, which consisted of decompression of the ulnohumeral joint with resection of the coronoid and olecranon osteophytes and fenestration of the distal part of the humerus. A disadvantage of this technique is the difficulty in exposing and excising the osteophytes in the radial head fossa.

Savoie et al. reported good results with extensive arthroscopic debridement involving capsular release, fenestration of the distal part of the humerus, and removal of osteophytes. Also, Morrey reported good results with open ulnohumeral arthroplasty, a variation of the original technique in which a trephine is used to remove the osteophytes encroaching on the olecranon and coronoid fossae.

If the above options fail to relieve the patient symptoms, then total elbow arthroplasty (TEA) may cautiously be considered as the next alternative of treatment. Most studies in the literature reporting on total elbow arthroplasty involve large numbers of patients, mostly with rheumatoid arthritis or other inflammatory pathologies, but very few patients with primary osteoarthritis. This makes it difficult to make accurate conclusions on the value of this treatment option for this population of patients. There are few studies in the English literature reporting specifically on the

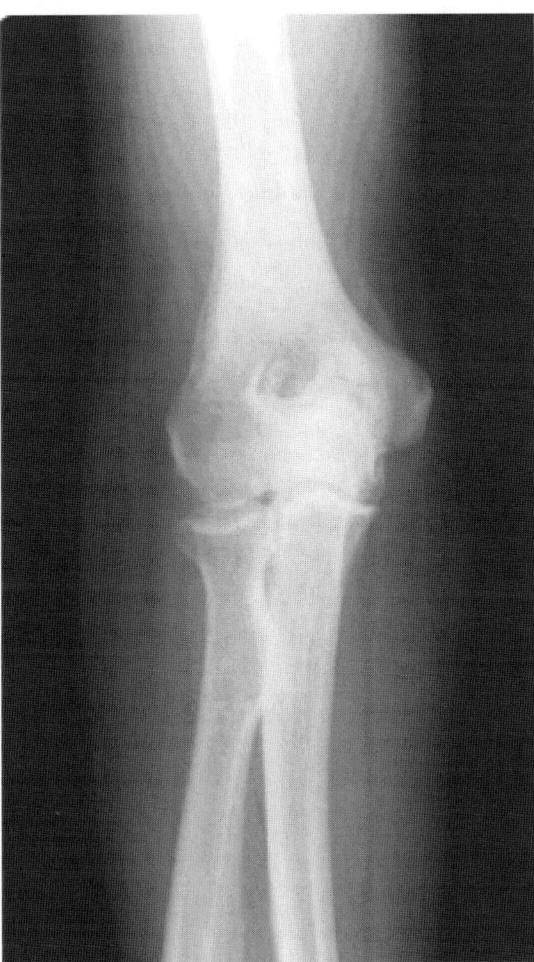
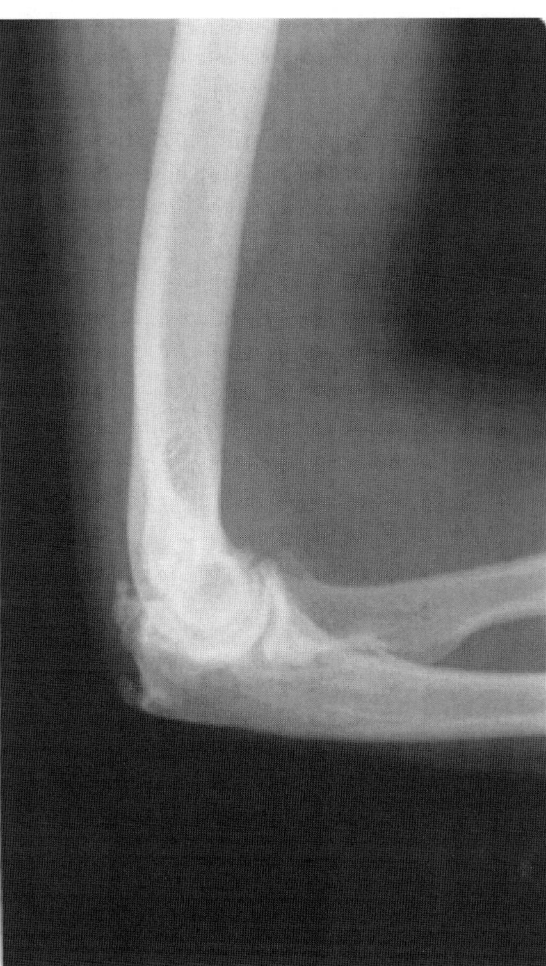

Figure 60-2 An anterior-posterior and lateral view of a right osteoarthritic elbow showing narrowing of the joint line and subchondral sclerosis, with formation of osteophytes in the coronoid, capitellar, and olecranon fossae.

outcome and complications of TEA as a treatment option for patients with primary osteoarthritis of the elbow.

Kozak et al. reported on the Mayo clinic experience. Over a 13-year period, only 5 out of 493 patients (<1%) who underwent TEA had the procedure performed for primary osteoarthritis of the elbow. The Coonrad-Morrey prosthesis (Zimmer, Warsaw, IN) cemented semiconstrained prosthesis was used in three patients, and the Pritchard elbow-resurfacing system (ERS) (De Puy, Warsaw, IN) cemented unconstrained prosthesis was used in the other two patients. The average age of the patients was 67 years, and a follow-up ranged from 37 to 121 months. Two minor and four major complications were reported in four elbows, two of which required revision. This rate of complications according to the authors is much higher than the rate of complication reported in TEA performed for other reasons in the same institution during the same period of time, including revision TEA, posttraumatic arthritis, nonunion of distal humerus, and rheumatoid arthritis.

Espag et al. reported on 11 Souter-Strathclyde cemented unlinked primary total elbow arthroplasties in 10 patients with osteoarthritis of the elbow. The diagnosis was primary osteoarthritis of the elbow in nine patients and posttraumatic osteoarthritis in two patients. The average age of the patients was 66 years, with a mean follow-up of 68 months. Only one patient required revision after 97 months for ulnar component loosening. All patients reported good symptomatic relief of pain and a significant increase in range of motion, and all patients considered the procedure to be successful.

The authors compared these results with the result of Souter-Strathclyde total elbow arthroplasty used in patients with rheumatoid arthritis. The revision rate in their series (9%) performed for ulnar component loosening compares favorably with the revision rate with the rheumatoid patients (5% to 21%), in which the main indications for revision included dislocation and perioperative fracture. The authors attributed the decrease in the incidence of perioperative and postoperative fracture to the good amount of bone stock in patients with primary osteoarthritis of the elbow that makes the risk of fracture very minimal.

As evident from this review, the outcome studies of TEA in patients with primary osteoarthritis of the elbow are very limited. The above-mentioned studies included small numbers of patients, and no final recommendation could be drawn at this time.

It is hoped that a greater understanding of elbow anatomy and kinematics will lead to advances in prosthetic design and surgical technique. The newer anatomic unlinked implants may improve the outcome of elbow replacement in younger patients. More outcome studies are needed on these implants or any other modern implants before openly recommending elbow replacement in younger active patients with primary osteoarthritis of the elbow.

SUGGESTED READINGS

Antuna SA, Morrey BF, Adams RA, et al. Ulnohumeral arthroplasty for primary degenerative arthritis of the elbow: long-term outcome and complications. *J Bone Joint Surg*. 2002;84A:2168–2173.

Bullough PG. *Atlas of Orthopedic Pathology*. 2nd ed. New York: Gower Medical Publishing; 1992;10:4–10.

Doherty M, Preston B. Primary osteoarthritis of the elbow. *Ann Rheum Dis*. 1989;48:743–747.

Espag MP, Black DL, Clark DI, et al. Early results of the Souter-Strathclyde unlinked total elbow arthroplasty in patients with osteoarthritis. *J Bone Joint Surg*. 2003;85B:351–353.

Ewald FC. Total elbow replacement. *Orthop Clin North Am*. 1975;3:685–696.

Goodfellow JW, Bullough PG. The pattern of aging of the articular cartilage of the elbow joint. *J Bone Joint Surg*. 1967;49B:175–181.

Gramstad GD, King GJ, O'Driscoll SW, et al. Elbow arthroplasty using a convertible implant. *Tech Hand Up Extrem Surg*. 2005;9(3): 153–163.

Kashiwagi D. Intra-articular changes of the osteoarthritis of the elbow. *Orthop Clin North Am*. 1995;26:691–706.

Kashiwagi D. Osteoarthritis of the elbow joint: intra-articular changes and the special operative procedure, Outerbridge-Kashiwagi method (O-K method). In: Kashiwagi D, ed. *Elbow Joint*. Amsterdam: Elsevier Science; 1985:177–188.

Kato H, Hirayama T, Minami A, et al. Cubital tunnel syndrome associated with medial elbow ganglia and osteoarthritis of the elbow. *J Bone Joint Surg*. 2002;84A:1413–1419.

Kellgren JH, Lawrence JS. Radiological assessment of osteoarthrosis. *Ann Rheum Dis*. 1957;16:494–501.

King GJW, Adams RA, Morrey BF. Total elbow arthroplasty: revision with use of a non-custom semiconstrained prosthesis. *J Bone Joint Surg*. 1997;79A:394–398.

Kozak TK, Adams RA, Morrey BF. Total elbow arthroplasty in primary osteoarthritis of the elbow. *J Arthroplasty*. 1998;13:837–842.

Kraay MJ, Figgie MP, Inglis AE, et al. Primary semiconstrained total elbow arthroplasty. *J Bone Joint Surg*. 1994:76B:636–640.

London JT. Kinematics of the elbow. *J Bone Joint Surg*. 1981;63A: 529–535.

Meachim G. Age changes in articular cartilage. *Clin Orthop*. 1969;64:33–44.

Mintz G, Fraga A. Severe osteoarthritis of the elbow in foundry workers. *Arch Environ Health*. 1973;27:78–80.

Morrey BF, Adams RA, Bryan RS. Total replacement for post-traumatic arthritis of the elbow. *J Bone Joint Surg*. 1991;73B:607–612.

Morrey BF, Adams RA. Semiconstrained elbow replacement arthroplasty for distal humeral non-union. *J Bone Joint Surg*. 1995;77B:67–72.

Morrey BF, Bryan RS, Dobyns JH, et al. Total elbow arthroplasty. *J Bone Joint Surg*. 1981;81A:80–84.

Morrey BF. Primary degenerative arthritis of the elbow. *J Bone Joint Surg*. 1992;74B:409–413.

O'Driscoll SW. Arthroscopic treatment for osteoarthritis of the elbow. *Orthop Clin North Am*. 1995;26:691–706.

O'Driscoll SW. Elbow arthritis: treatment options. *J Am Acad Orthop Surg*. 1993;1:106–116.

Ogilvie-Harris DJ, Schemitsch E. Arthroscopy of the elbow for removal of loose bodies. *Arthroscopy*. 1993;9:5–8.

Oka Y. Debridement for osteoarthritis of the elbow in athletes. *Int Orthop*. 1999;23:91–94.

Ortner DJ. Description and classification of degenerative bone changes in the distal joint surfaces of the humerus. *Am J Phys Anthop*. 1968;28:139–155.

Rozing P. Souter-Strathclyde total elbow arthroplasty. *J Bone Joint Surg*. 2000;82B:1129–1134.

Savoie FH 3rd, Nunley PD, Field LD. Arthroscopic management of the arthritic elbow: indications, technique, and results. *J Shoulder Elbow Surg*. 1999;8:214–219.

Stanley D. Prevalence and etiology of symptomatic elbow osteoarthritis. *J Shoulder Elbow Surg*. 1994;3:386–389.

Trail IA, Nuttal D, Stanley JK. Survivorship and radiological analysis of the standard Souter-Strathclyde total elbow arthroplasty. *J Bone Joint Surg*. 1999;81B:80–84.

Tsuge K, Mizuseki T. Debridement arthroplasty for advanced primary osteoarthritis of the elbow. Results of a new technique used for 29 elbows. *J Bone Joint Surg*. 1994;76B:641–646.

Wadworth TG. Osteoarthritis. In Wadworth TG, ed. *The Elbow*. Edinburgh: Churchill Livingstone; 1982;292–293.

ELBOW ARTHROPLASTY: REVISION

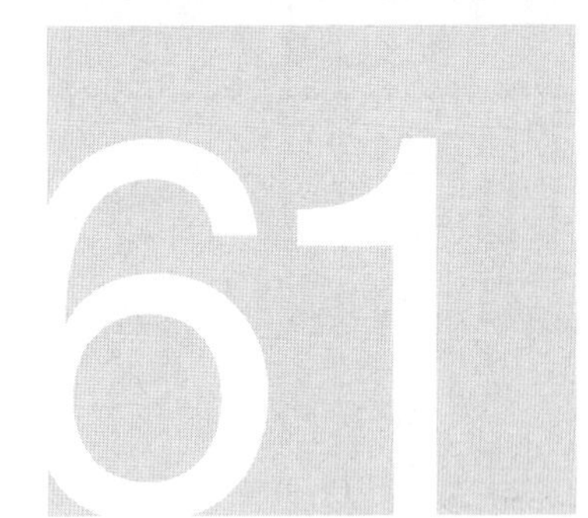

PIERRE MANSAT

EPIDEMIOLOGY

A meta-analysis of 22 publications reviewing 838 total elbow arthroplasties (TEAs) was published in 1996. With an average follow-up of 5 years, the complication rate was 43% with a revision rate of 18%. Main complications were the following: aseptic loosening (radiographic 17.2% and clinical 6.4%), infection (8.1%), ulnar nerve involvement (10.4%), instability (7% to 19%), and periprosthetic fracture (3.2%). The French Orthopedic and Traumatology Society reviewing 370 TEAs found a complication rate of 27% with a revision rate of 17%. In this chapter, several specific features of the presentation are discussed and surgical options available to deal with failed TEAs are presented.

ASSESSMENT

Failed elbow arthroplasty can be caused by sepsis, device failure, instability, periprosthetic fracture, and loosening. Assessment to exclude the possibility of sepsis is the most important consideration prior to any revision procedure, but especially in those with early unexplained or unanticipated failure. Analysis of the sedimentation rate and C-reactive protein are regularly performed along with aspiration of the joint if there is any question of sepsis. Based on the plain radiograph to analyze bone quality, the appropriate preoperative plan is formulated. Surgery is not performed if radiolucent lines are not painful. In such cases, the patient is followed on a regular basis. Stiffness, scarring, and contracture of the soft tissue and prior evidence of sepsis and status of the ulnar nerve must also be noted.

PRESENTATION—TREATMENT OPTIONS

Device Failure

Wear of the polyethylene in TEA has been the most common mode of material failure. Although often contributing to component loosening owing to polyethylene debris, mechanical symptoms may develop because of metal-on-metal articulation or dislocation of the component. Fracture of the metal components has been reported but is now less common owing to improvements in implant design and materials. Isolated bushing exchange is a successful procedure if there is no osteolysis compromising component fixation.

Instability

Instability is typically seen with unlinked resurfacing types of TEA. Although usually occurring in the early postoperative period as a frank dislocation, this also can present more insidiously as weakness, giving way, clunking, or other mechanical symptoms. Instability can be caused by ligament insufficiency, malpositioning of the components, or uneven wear of the polyethylene. Examination under fluoroscopy may show the cause of instability and allow the diagnosis to be made. Splinting for a few weeks may help restore stability, but if the elbow remains unstable after a period of splinting, a surgical procedure may be indicated. Attempts to salvage an unlinked TEA that is unstable can be unpredictable. One can attempt at least one soft tissue procedure before undertaking removal of a well-cemented unlinked prosthesis. Attention should be paid to maintaining or restoring an adequate lateral collateral ligament complex by firmly reattaching it to the lateral epicondyle with use of sutures through drill holes in bone or by reconstructing the ligament with a tendon graft. Elbows with malpositioned components do not respond to conservative treatment or ligament reconstruction. Revision of the component positioning or conversion to a semiconstrained implant is usually required.

Periprosthetic Fracture

Fractures in proximity to TEA can occur at the time of implant insertion, as a consequence of neglected component loosening with bone loss, or as a result of a traumatic

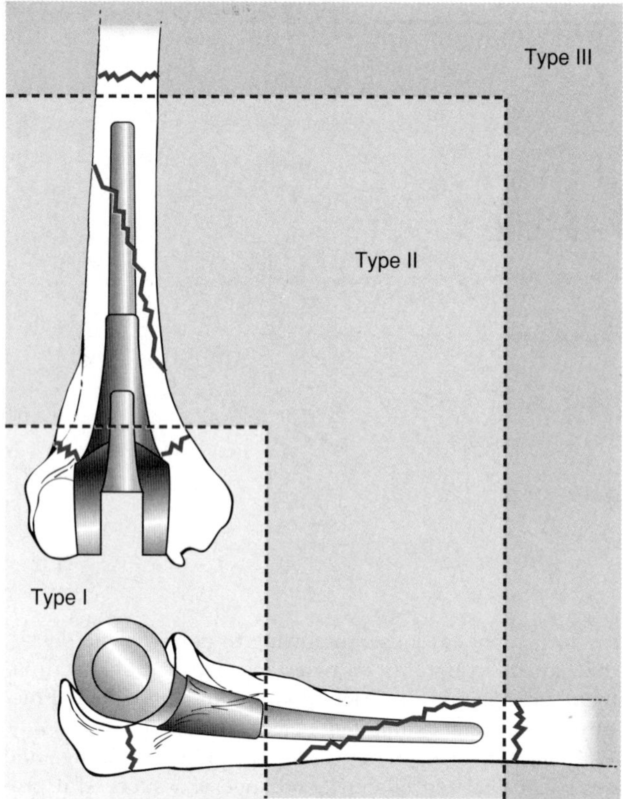

gure 61-1 Mayo Classification of periprosthetic elbow fractures. Type I: metaphyseal; type II: involves stem; type III: beyond stem.

event. Mayo has proposed to classify these fractures as type I—metaphyseal; type II—stem involvement; type III—proximal or distal to the stem tip (Fig. 61-1).

Humeral periprosthetic fractures that occur in the periarticular segment (type I) usually do not require surgical treatment if a linked prosthesis has been used. In unlinked prostheses, fixation of the fragment is necessary to preserve implant stability. Fractures that involve the olecranon, however, should be fixed in all patients since this will restore triceps function. Proximal or distal to the stem (type III), cerclage wire or plate and screw fixation may be required to stabilize the fracture (Fig. 61-2). Fractures around the stem of the prosthesis (type II) almost always require revision surgery because the implant is often loose. A longer revision stem should be used to bypass the fracture, with cortical strut allograft around the fracture.

Implant Loosening

Loosening of the implant is the most frequent cause of long-term implant failure. A loose implant can be associated with bone resorption, cortical thinning, and ballooning of the humerus or ulna. Revision options are predicated on the quality of bone and presence of a periprosthetic fracture. A salvage procedure such as arthrodesis is rarely indicated. Arthrodesis requires a sufficient amount of bone present. Resection arthroplasty is indicated in the presence of a septic prosthesis. A stable resection arthroplasty can provide a relatively comfortable joint. Not all patients after resection arthroplasty will desire a reimplantation procedure. A revision procedure with reimplantation can be performed when infection has been eradicated.

TECHNIQUE OF REVISION ARTHROPLASTY

Implant Selection

The most important consideration is whether adequate fixation can be obtained with another stemmed implant given the amount and quality of the intact cement mantle. If bone

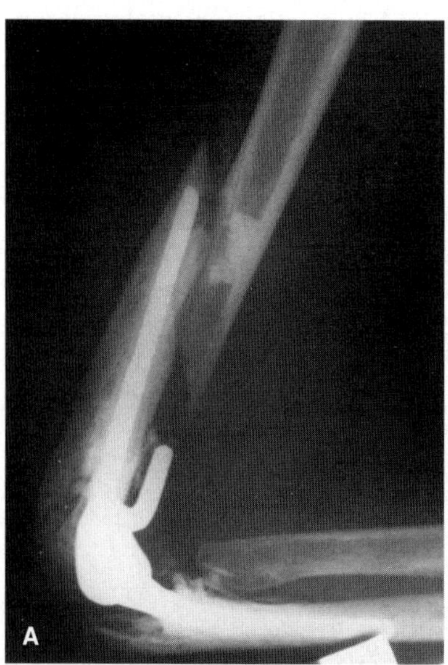

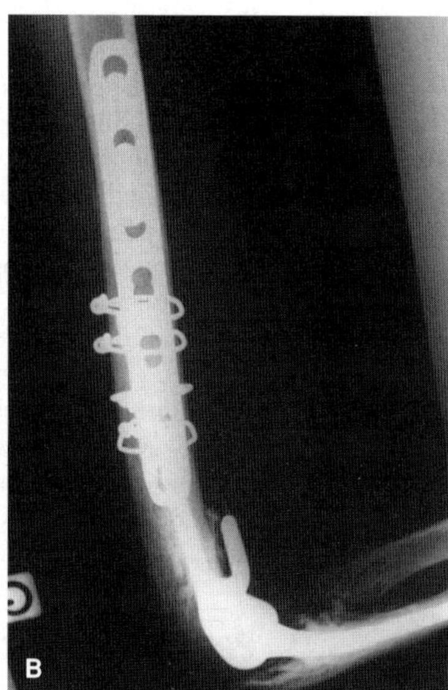

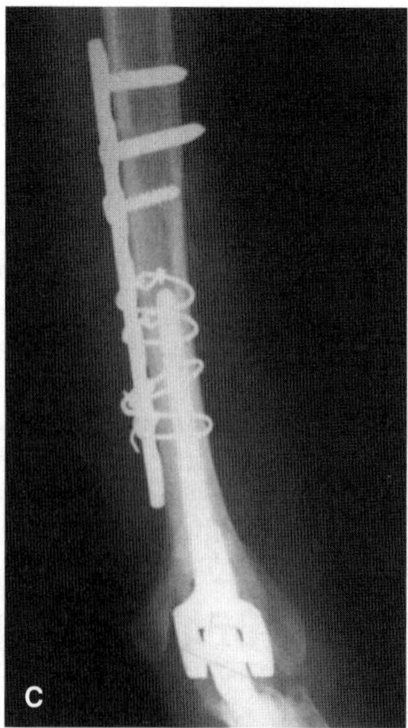

Figure 61-2 Periprosthetic type III fracture at the stem of the humeral component; the implant is well fixed (**A**). Osteosynthesis with plate and screw and cerclage wire (**B, C**).

stock remains, a nonconstrained implant can be used. However, most of the time a semiconstrained implant is preferred. Long-stem devices should be available. For humeral revisions, a 15- or 20-cm-long humeral stem is often needed. Long-stemmed ulnar components should also be available.

Surgical Technique

Preparation for iliac crest bone should be routine. A sterile tourniquet is often used. The lateral decubitus position is preferred by some surgeons to allow wide exposure of the humerus and radial nerve if necessary. The use of a posterior midline elbow incision is preferred, but use of a previous skin incision is recommended. The technical features of all revision options must address the preservation of the triceps, identifying and protecting all neurovascular structures, and protection of the cortical bone. If the distal humeral columns are deficient, a triceps-preserving approach should be considered. If the olecranon process is fractured, a trans-olecranon approach is used for revision of the elbow arthroplasty and repaired with tension band wire technique at the end of the procedure. Proximally, the radial nerve is always identified, at least by palpation. The ulna is extensively exposed in a subcutaneous fashion as distally as necessary to have adequate exposure and to avoid violation of the ulnar cortex. Extensive synovectomy is always necessary; tissue samples are sent for pathology and culture.

Extraction of the components is straightforward in cases of aseptic loosening but more problematic if they are firmly fixed. If the implant design is tapered, the component sometimes can be extracted by grasping the articulating surface and tapping on the prosthesis in a retrograde direction. Removing as much cement as possible allows the device to be removed more easily. Fracture or further bone loss from aggressive attempts at cement removal should be avoided. A cortical window around the stem or at the tip of the prosthesis should be considered to avoid intraoperative fracture caused by more aggressive attempts to remove the components. It should be fixed with cerclage wire at the end of the procedure before cement injection. Once the prosthesis is removed, cement that is firmly adherent should be left in place unless it interferes with placement of the new components (Fig. 61-3). Powered cement removal instruments should be used with caution. Ultrasonic cement removal devices can be particularly useful.

The implant chosen for revision should have stems of adequate length to bypass cortical defects or fractures and have sufficient constraint to provide adequate joint stability (Fig. 61-4). Modern cement technique is used with cement restrictors and pressurized gun. Antibiotic cement should be routinely used. Caution should be exercised in patients with cortical perforations or fractures to ensure that cement does not damage adjacent neurovascular structures.

Closure is done with steps to ensure triceps function and the arm placed in extension with a splint to avoid tension or pressure on the wound. The arm is elevated for 48 hours. Gentle active motion can then be initiated. If the bone is fractured or if a bone graft has been used, protection in a cast brace or splint for several weeks may be undertaken. No formal therapy is prescribed, but activities of daily living are encouraged.

SPECIFIC REVISION OPTIONS

Osseous Enhancement Options

If the process is associated with bone resorption, osteolysis, or a periprosthetic fracture, an impaction or strut grafting augmentation procedure is indicated.

Impaction Grafting

Impaction grafting is designed for two specific purposes, to restore bone stock and to enhance the bone/cement interface. At least 2 to 3 cm stem depth into intact bone in addition to the augmentation fixators is needed. The

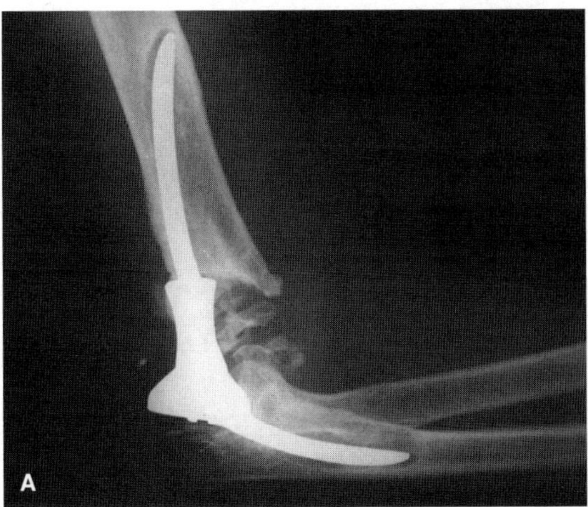

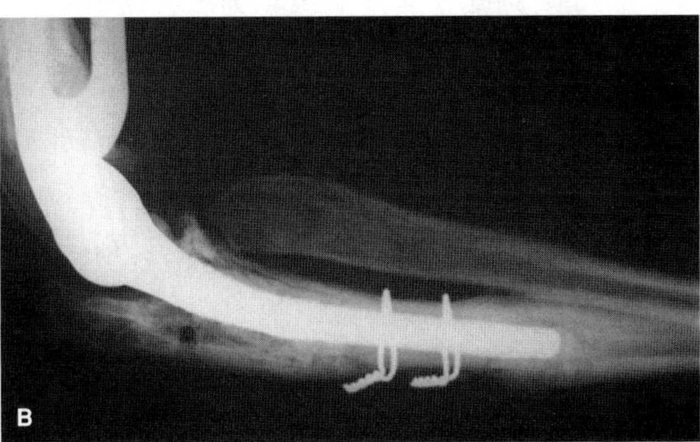

Figure 61-3 Revision of a loose constrained implant (**A**). A long-stem semiconstrained implant has been used to bypass the area of loosening (**B**).

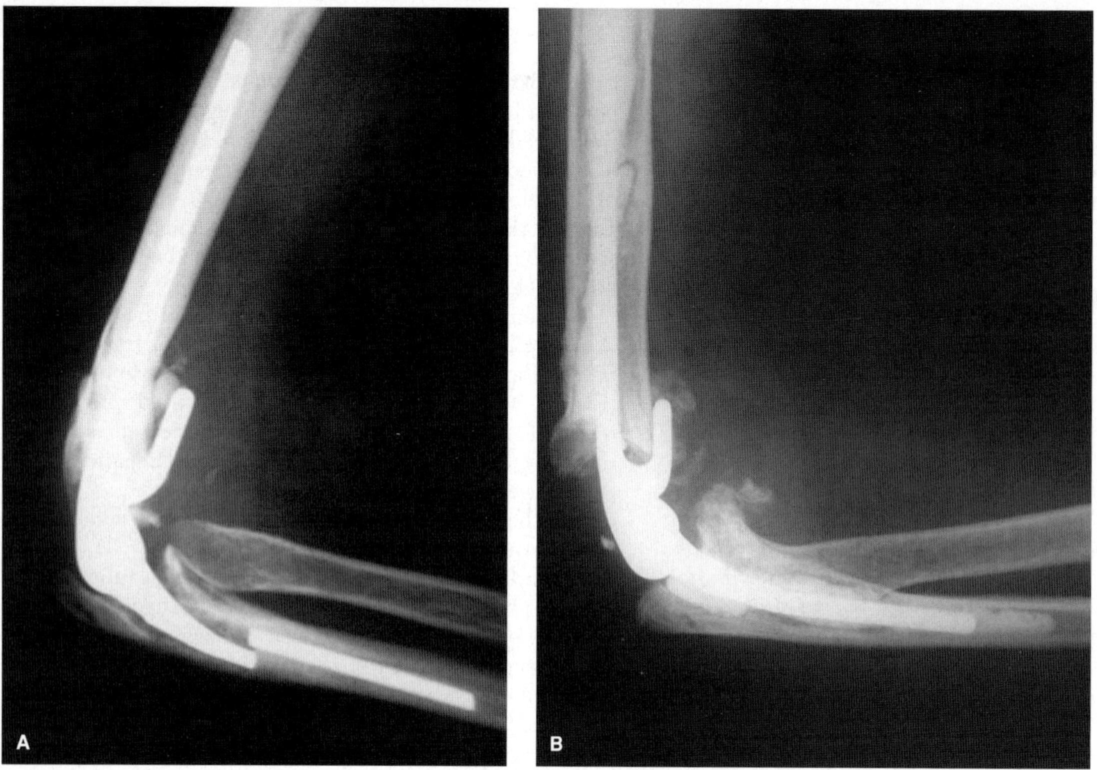

Figure 61-4 Ulna fenestration has been made to remove a fractured well-fixed ulnar component (**A**). Cerclage wire has been used to fix the cortical window before cementing a new ulnar component (**B**).

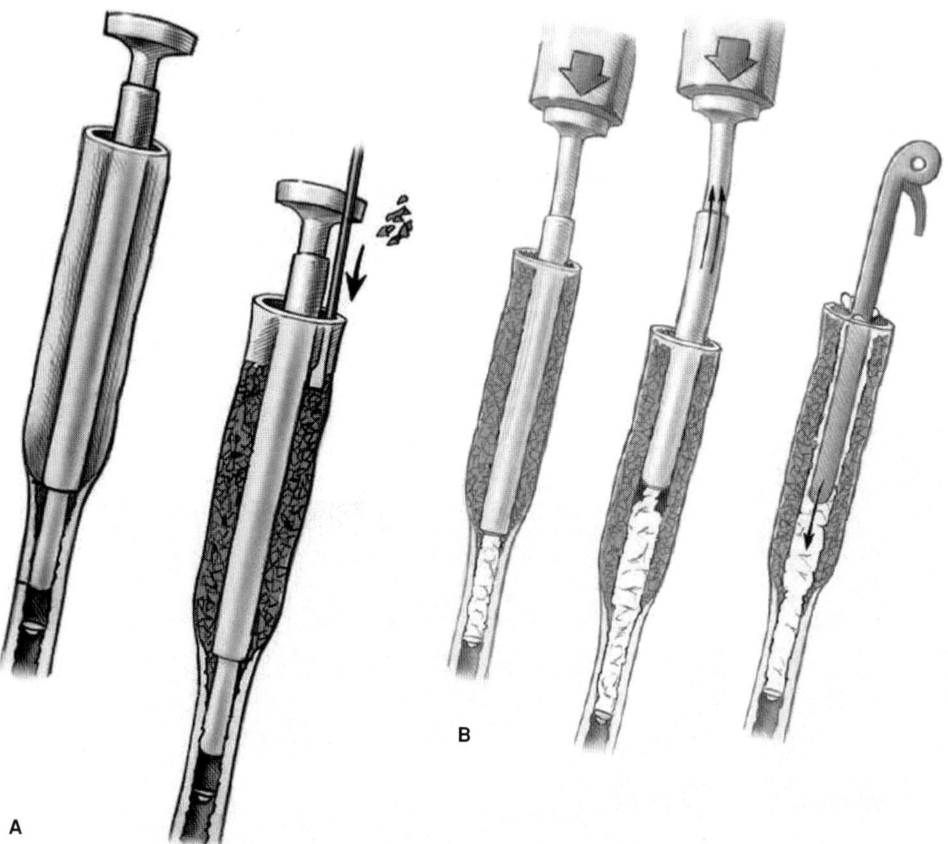

Figure 61-5 A double tube is used and allograft bone is packed around the outer tube (**A**); The cement is injected through the smaller tube, which is slowly withdrawn to the level of the outer tube; then both tubes are withdrawn simultaneously while injecting cement into the void created by the larger tube (**B**).

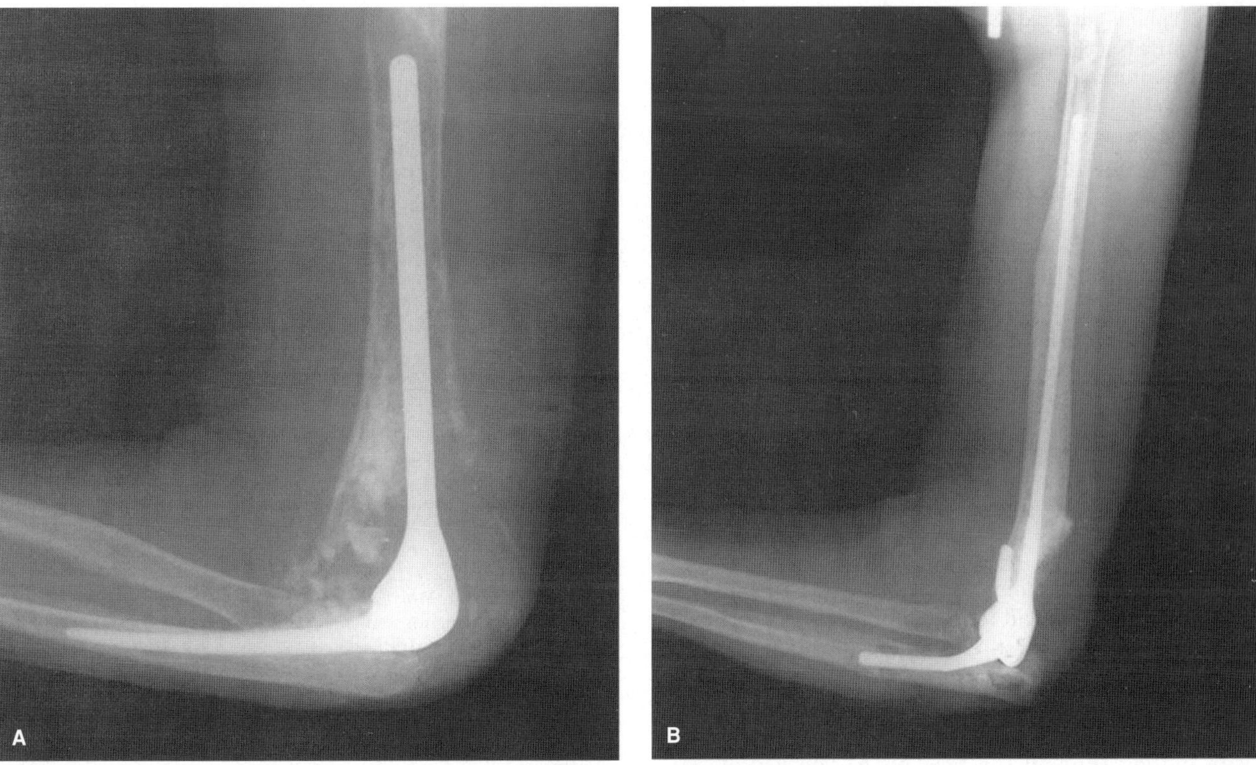

Figure 61-6 Marked osteolysis (A) effectively treated with impaction grafting at 6 years (B).

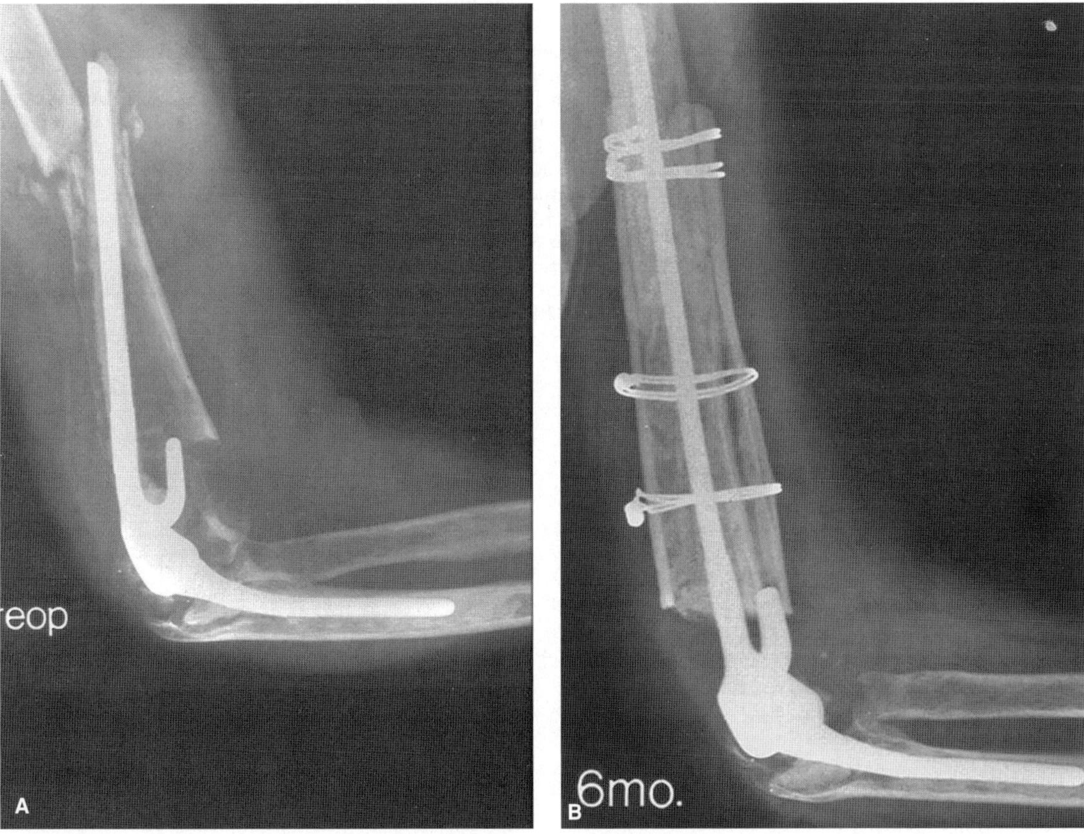

Figure 61-7 Patient with severe bone loss and fracture after failed Coonrad/Morrey implant (A). At 2 years, the struts have incorporated with a successful clinical and radiographic outcome (B).

medullary canal is plugged with a silastic device. A double-tube apparatus is assembled. The nozzle of tubing used for femoral cementation is cut to the length that corresponds to the extent of the lytic process. The elbow cement injector tube is then inserted within the femoral tube, extending distally into normal host bone. Cancellous bone graft or graft substitute is tightly packed around the outer tube. The cement is then mixed in the canister of the smaller elbow injector system and inserted on the nozzle in situ. It is injected through the nozzle while withdrawing to the level of the outer tube. At this point both inner and outer tubes are simultaneously withdrawn while injecting cement into the void created by the larger tube. The implant is carefully inserted to the desired length (Fig. 61-5). This technique may be used for both the humerus and ulna, as an adjunct in the re-establishment of bone stock (Fig. 61-6).

Strut Graft

This technique is especially useful for types II and III periprosthetic fractures and for distal humeral or proximal ulnar bone loss. The most effective application to the humerus is that of an anterior strut that transverses the osteolysis or fracture and captures the flange anteriorly. A posterior strut is used to enhance stability and to prevent the wire cutting through the host bone. The use of an extended flange, anterior strut graft, and 2 cm of shortening allows management of distal humeral deficiencies of ≤ 7 cm (Fig. 61-7).

Allograft-Prosthetic Composite (APC) Reconstruction

When bone loss is significant, either a custom implant, a component reconstruction with strut graft, or an allograft-prosthesis composite (APC) are options. In this last option, the prosthesis is fitted and cemented to the allograft. When that has hardened, the prosthesis is cemented in the host. The difficulty of obtaining interface union between the host and allograft bones has limited the use of this strategy.

CONCLUSION

Revision elbow arthroplasty is a challenging procedure. An evolution in prosthetic components and varied surgical options has allowed the surgeon to deal with different presentations of TEA failure. Although the complication rate is higher than in primary TEA, the frequency of problems continues to decrease as experience with revision surgery increases.

SUGGESTED READINGS

Augereau B, Mansat P. Total Elbow Arthroplasty [in French]. *Rev Chir Orthop*. 2005;91(suppl 5):2S31–2S96.

Gschwend N, Simmen BR, Matejovsky Z. Late complications in elbow arthroplasty. *J Shoulder Elbow Surg*. 1996;5:86–96.

Kamineni S, Morrey BF. Proximal ulnar reconstruction with strut allograft in revision total elbow arthroplasty. *J Bone Joint Surg Am*. 2004;86:1223–1229.

King GJ, Adams RA, Morrey BF. Total elbow arthroplasty: revision with use of a non-custom semiconstrained prosthesis. *J Bone Joint Surg Am*. 1997;79:394–400.

Lee BP, Adams RA, Morrey BF. Polyethylene wear after total elbow arthroplasty. *J Bone Joint Surg Am*. 2005;87:1080–1087.

Loebenberg MI, Morrey BF, O'Driscoll SW. Impaction grafting in revision total elbow arthroplasty. *J Bone Joint Surg Am*. 2005;87:99–106.

Mansat P, Adams RA, Morrey BF. Allograft-prosthesis composite for revision of catastrophic failure of total elbow arthroplasty. *J Bone Joint Surg Am*. 2004;86:724–735.

Morrey BF. Complications of elbow replacement surgery. In: Morrey BF, ed. *The Elbow and Its Disorders*. 3rd ed. WB Saunders; 2000: 667–677.

O'Driscoll SW, Morrey BF. Periprosthetic fractures about the elbow. *Orthop Clin North Am*. 1999;30:319–325.

Redfern DRM, Dunkley AB, Trail IA, et al. Revision total elbow replacement using the Souter-Strathclyde prosthesis. *J Bone Joint Surg Br*. 2001;83:635–639.

Ring D, Kocher M, Koris M, et al. Revision of unstable capitellocondylar (unlinked) total elbow replacement. *J Bone Joint Surg Am*. 2005;87:1075–1079.

Sanchez-Sotelo J, O'Driscoll SW, Morrey BF. Periprosthetic humeral fracture after total elbow arthroplasty treatment with implant revision and strut allograft augmentation. *J Bone Joint Surg Am*. 2002;8:1642–1650.

NONPROSTHETIC TREATMENT OF ELBOW ARTHRITIS

KENNETH J. FABER
SCOTT P. STEINMANN

INFLAMMATORY ARTHRITIS

Rheumatoid arthritis (RA) is a chronic, systemic inflammatory disease that affects synovial joints. The prevalence is approximately 1.0% of adults, and the disease is associated with significant morbidity and mortality. The treatment of RA has changed significantly over the past decade. In addition to new medications that have improved the treatment of inflammatory arthritis, advancements in elbow arthroscopy have resulted in the introduction of new surgical techniques.

Pathogenesis

The exact cause of RA remains unknown. One proposed mechanism involves the interaction between an unknown exogenous antigen and the host immune system that precipitates a response that recruits and activates monocytes and macrophages. The activated monocytes and macrophages release proinflammatory cytokines such as tumor necrosis factor-α (TNF-α) and interleukin-1 (IL-1) into the joint. The cytokines mediate joint destruction by activating chondrocytes and fibroblasts that release metalloproteinases and collagenases capable of cartilage and bone destruction. A second proposed pathway for joint destruction is through deregulation of B lymphocytes that subsequently produce rheumatoid factor and autoantibodies and promote the formation of destructive immune complexes.

Diagnosis

History and Physical Examination

Clinical Features. Joint destruction is acknowledged to occur early in the disease process, and $\leq$60% of patients will have radiographic evidence of erosions by 2 years. Intra-articular symptoms associated with RA can be clustered into three groups: (a) pain, (b) restricted motion, and (c) instability. Extra-articular symptoms secondary to joint synovitis include local nerve compression, tenosynovitis, and tendon rupture.

Pain as a consequence of persistent inflammation is a common feature of RA. A secondary fibrotic reaction can occur in response to the inflammation and results in decreased elbow flexion and extension. If the radiocapitellar articulation is affected, forearm rotation can be restricted. As the disease progresses, cartilage destruction, bone loss, and ligament incompetence can result in joint instability.

Radiographic Features. The radiographic features of rheumatoid arthritis have been classified by Larsen[1] and subsequently modified by Morrey[2] (Table 62-1; Figs. 62-2–62-5).

Treatment

Pharmacotherapy

Conventional pharmacotherapy for the treatment for RA includes nonsteroidal anti-inflammatory medications and disease-modifying antirheumatic drugs (DMARDs) such as methotrexate, prednisone, sulfasalazine, and gold. Combination therapy with these agents has been shown to decrease disease activity and reduce radiographic progression of bone erosions. In most patients, this form of treatment is adequate.

Newer therapies take advantage of the improved understanding of the alteration in the immune system that contributes to the development of RA.[3] For example, leflunomide (Arava) inhibits the synthesis of pyrimidine by activated T lymphocytes, thereby hindering the

TABLE 62-1 CLASSIFICATION

Stage	Description	Pathology	Imaging
I	Normal architecture, osteoporosis	Synovitis present	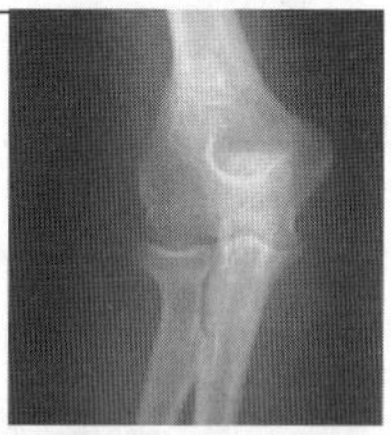
II	Joint space narrowing, intact joint architecture	Synovitis persists	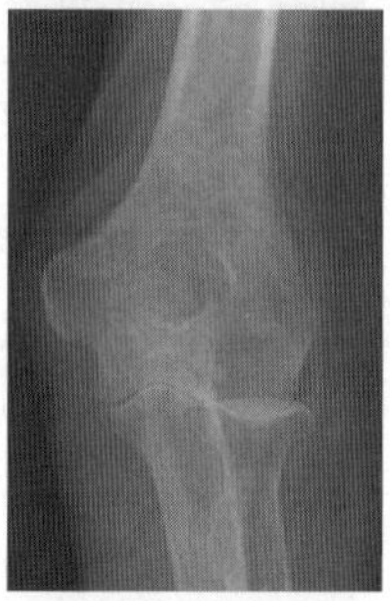
III	Alteration of joint architecture	Variable synovitis	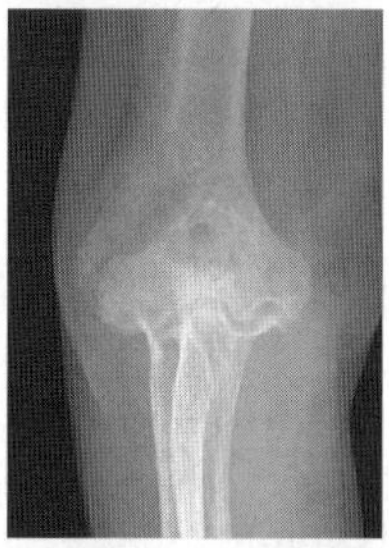
IV	Gross joint destruction	Minimal synovitis	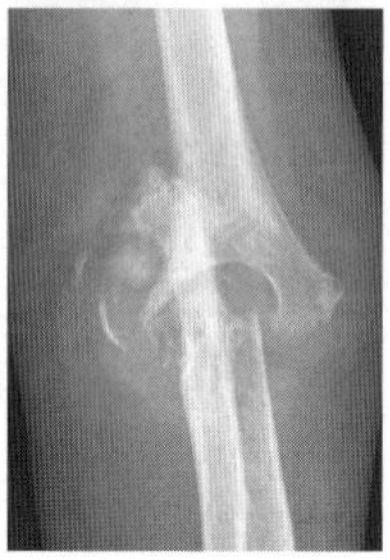

(From Larsen A. Radiological grading of rheumatoid arthritis. An interobserver study. *Scand J Rheumatol*. 1973;2[3]:136–138. Modified in Morrey BF, Adams RA. Semiconstrained arthroplasty for the treatment of rheumatoid arthritis of the elbow. *J Bone Joint Surg Am*. 1992;74:479–490, with permission.)

T lymphocytes' ability to initiate an inflammatory response. Etanercept (Enbrel), infliximab (Remicade), and adalimumab (Humira) all exploit strategies to bind the inflammatory cytokine TNF-α. Anakinra (Kineret) is an IL-1 receptor antagonist that competes with IL-1 and blocks the production of metalloproteinases that have been shown to destroy cartilage and create bone erosions. Each of these medications has demonstrated efficacy according to the definition of improvement in rheumatoid arthritis guidelines described by the American College of Rheumatology.[4]

Surgical Indications/Contraindications

The indications for surgical intervention include the failure of an appropriately supervised course of pharmacotherapy, symptoms of sufficient severity to justify the risks of surgery, and satisfactory general health to permit the safe performance of a surgical procedure. Ensuring satisfactory general health may require the assistance of rheumatologists, anesthesiologists, and general internists. In general, synovectomy is considered in patients with stage I or II disease and in select cases of stage III disease in young individuals. More advanced disease, manifested by joint destruction and mechanical instability, is likely to benefit most from total elbow arthroplasty (Fig. 62-1).

Open Synovectomy. The standard treatment of early rheumatoid arthritis involves radial head excision and synovectomy. This procedure is usually performed through

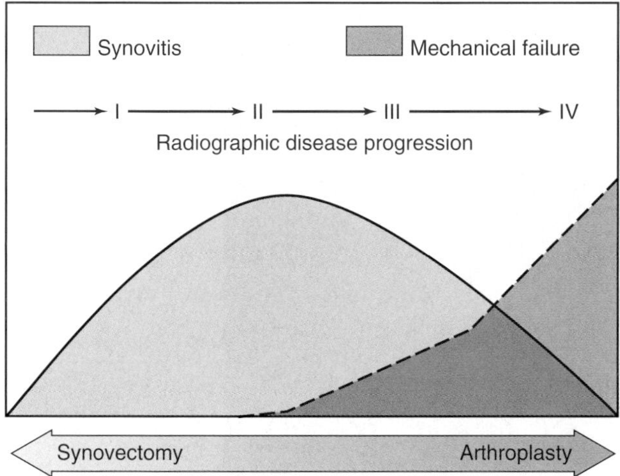

Figure 62-1 Inflammatory arthritis disease progression.

a lateral exposure using the Kocher interval between anconeus and extensor carpi ulnaris. Radial head excision is performed to improve forearm rotation and to increase joint exposure, thereby facilitating synovectomy.

The outcomes from this procedure are satisfactory, with patients reporting diminished pain and improved range of motion. Ferlic et al.[5] reported that 77% of patients described symptom relief following synovectomy and radial head excision. A subgroup of patients treated with silicone radial head arthroplasty was indistinguishable from the patients treated with synovectomy and excision alone. The best results were observed in patients with early disease. In a survivorship analysis, Gendi et al.[6] identified factors associated with a poor outcome following open elbow synovectomy including advanced disease, long duration of symptoms, a significant reduction in the elbow flexion/extension arc, and poor general health. Using severe pain or the need for revision surgery as the end point, 80% of patients had a satisfactory response during the first year following the intervention, but additional failures accumulated at a rate of 2.6% per year.

Another survivorship analysis reported by Mäenpää et al.[7] found that 77% of elbow synovectomies did not require additional surgery at a mean of 5 years following the primary synovectomy. Patients undergoing synovectomy for late-stage arthritis were most likely to be revised to an elbow arthroplasty. Elbow pain and patient satisfaction both improved following synovectomy, but range of motion was unchanged.

Selected reports describing the outcome of open synovectomy are summarized in Table 61-2. Outcomes are difficult to interpret because of methodologic shortcomings including a lack of comparator groups, the use of nonstandardized outcome measures, and deficient statistical measurements. The best indications for elbow synovectomy, based on the papers cited, include pain, early radiographic changes (I and II), and restricted elbow motion. Although early results are rewarding, the durability of the results remains questionable.

Arthroscopic Synovectomy. Arthroscopic elbow synovectomy offers several advantages over open synovectomy. The improved joint visualization achieved with arthroscopy allows for a more thorough synovectomy without sacrificing

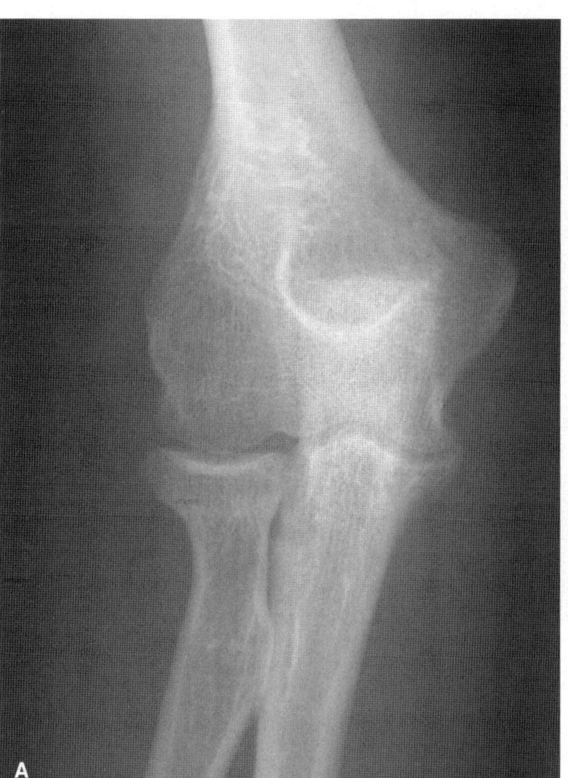

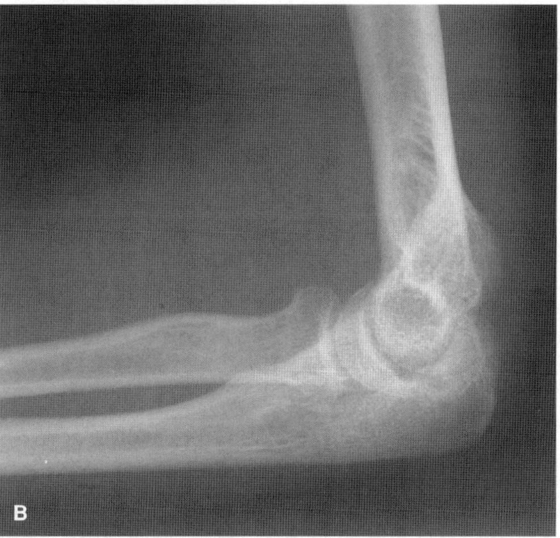

Figure 62-2 A: Stage I rheumatoid arthritis. B: Stage I rheumatoid arthritis.

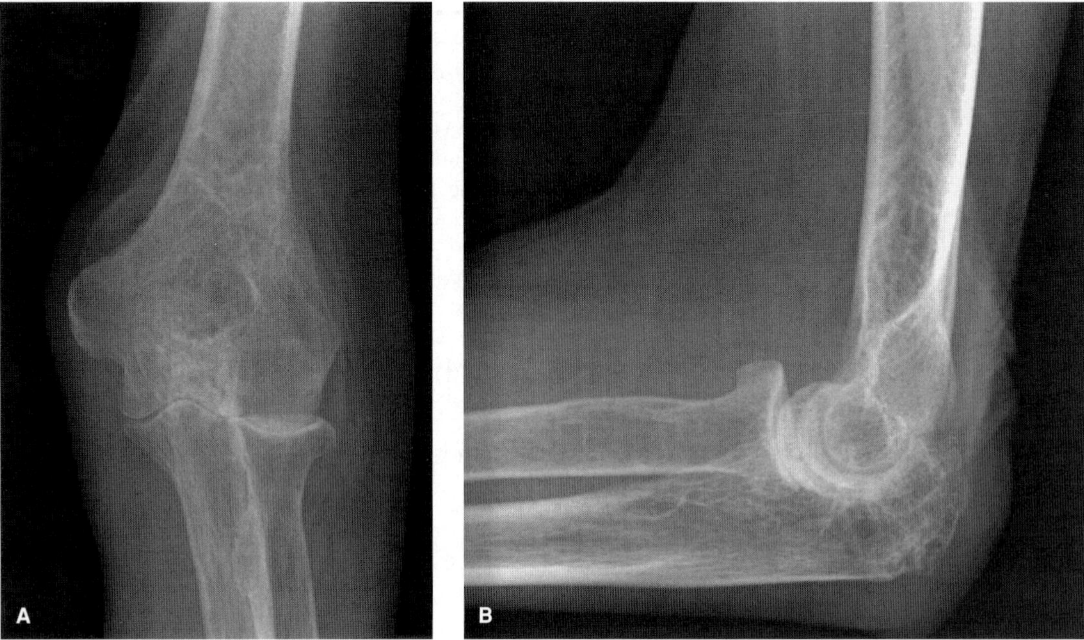

Figure 62-3 A: Stage II rheumatoid arthritis. B: Stage II rheumatoid arthritis.

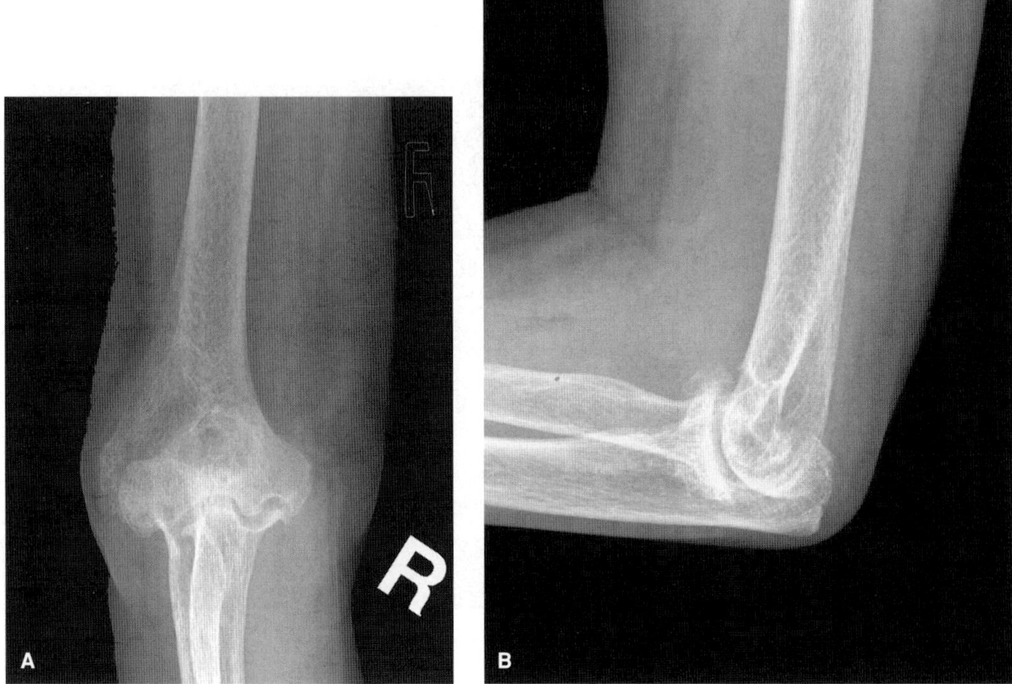

Figure 62-4 A: Stage III rheumatoid arthritis. B: Stage III rheumatoid arthritis.

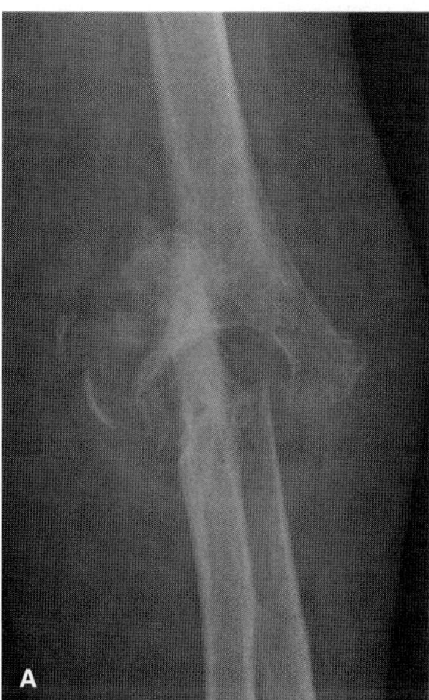

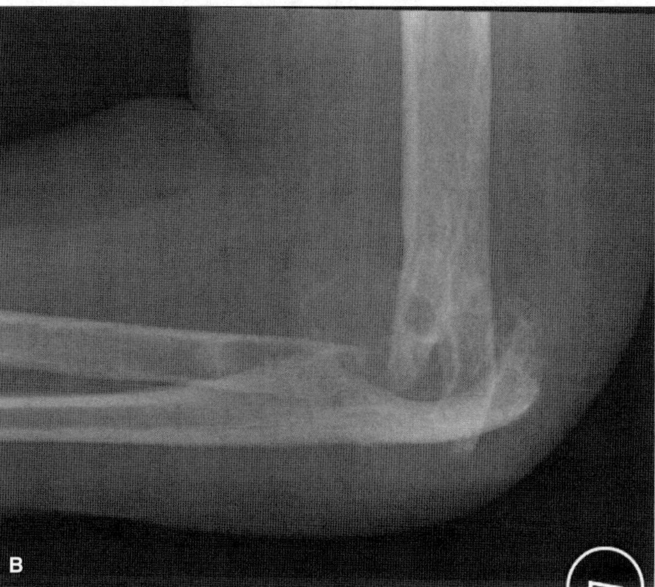

Figure 62-5 A: Stage IV rheumatoid arthritis. B: Stage IV rheumatoid arthritis.

the radial head. The radiocapitellar articulation normally transmits 40% of the forearm axial load across the elbow joint. Radial head excision may result in accelerated wear of the ulnohumeral joint as a consequence of altered joint reaction forces. Radial head excision can still be performed if required using standard arthroscopic techniques. The morbidity of synovectomy is reduced using portals that minimize muscle injury and protect ligamentous stabilizers of the joint.

Despite its many advantages, arthroscopic synovectomy is a technically difficult procedure that requires advanced arthroscopy skills. Furthermore, an assistant is required for limb positioning and for intra-articular retraction of nerves and vessels to avoid neurovascular injury. At the present

TABLE 62-2 OUTCOMES REPORTED FOLLOWING ELBOW SYNOVECTOMY

Author	*N*	Procedure	Follow-Up	Outcome Comments
Brattstrom and Al Khudairy,[8] 1975	105	Open synovectomy, radial head excision	45 months	Pain decreased in 80% of cases. Forearm rotation improved in 60%, and flexion-extension improved in 40% of cases.
Ferlic et al.,[5] 1987	57	Open synovectomy, radial head excision with or without silastic radial head arthroplasty (13 patients)	86 months	Long-term pain relief in 77% of cases. Best results were observed in patients with earlier stages of disease.
Gendi et al.,[6] 1997	171	Open synovectomy, radial head excision	Survivorship analysis	Satisfactory results at 1 year in 81% of cases, but results deteriorated quickly. The most durable outcome was observed in cases with significant preop reduction of forearm rotation.
Lee et al.,[9] 1997	14	Arthroscopic synovectomy	42 months	Early improvement in function as measured by the Mayo Elbow Performance Index was not durable with additional follow-up.
Horiuchi et al.,[10] 2002	21	Arthroscopic synovectomy	97 months	Best results were observed in stage I and stage II disease. The results were not durable in more advanced disease.

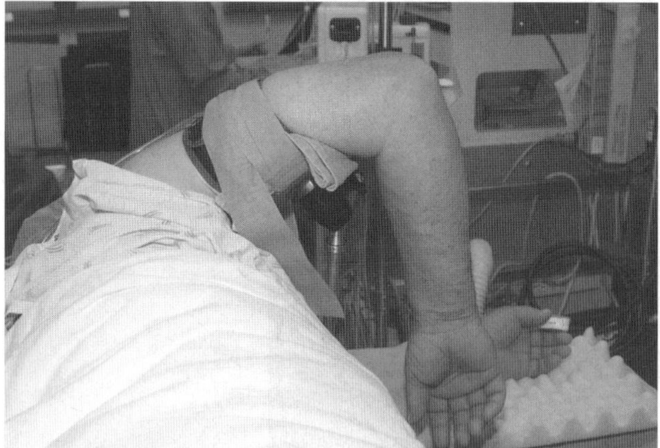

Figure 62-6 Patient positioned for elbow arthroscopy. The elbow is placed high to avoid contact with the arthroscope or other instruments against the patient.

time, the superiority of arthroscopic synovectomy over open synovectomy has not been proven.

Several principles promote the safe performance of an arthroscopic synovectomy. First, the surgeon must possess a thorough knowledge of the three-dimensional anatomic relationships among nerves, vessels, synovium, capsule, and articular structures. This allows for safe portal placement and efficient insertion and removal of surgical instruments. Second, arthroscopic irrigation fluid should not be considered as a means to maintain joint distention but rather as the medium to clear debris from the joint. Ideally, inflow pressure should be minimized to prevent harmful fluid extravasations that obscure surface anatomy landmarks and interfere with the use of arthroscopic instruments. Third, a surgical assistant providing intra-articular retraction helps to maintain joint visualization and to prevent iatrogenic nerve injury. Finally, the procedure must proceed in a sequential manner that minimizes the risk of complication. For example, synovectomy precedes any planned bone resection since the synovium will likely obscure the visualization of osseous structures within the joint. Similarly, bone resection precedes planned capsulectomy since satisfactory

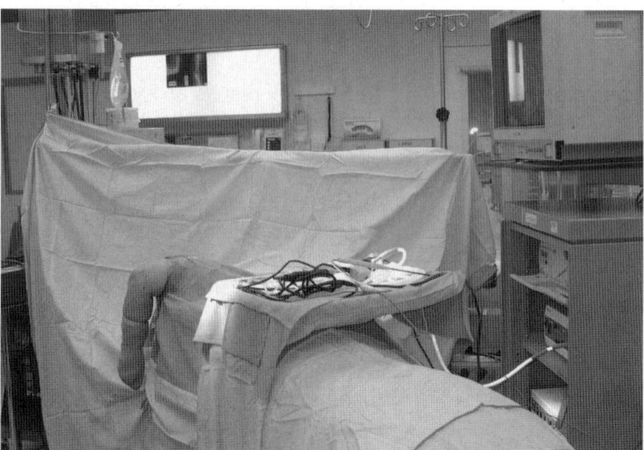

Figure 62-7 View of patient positioned for elbow arthroscopy.

irrigation fluid management is difficult to maintain once the capsule has been removed. By strictly adhering to the above principles and by exercising patience during the procedure, arthroscopic synovectomy can be safely performed.

Lee and Morrey[9] reported the outcome of arthroscopic synovectomy in a series of 11 patients at 42 months following surgery and found that only 6 of the patients continued to report a satisfactory result. Four of the patients required revision surgery and were treated with total elbow arthroplasty. Their recommendation was to cautiously advise patients regarding arthroscopic synovectomy since the initial early satisfactory response did not seem durable.

More recently, Horiuchi et al.[10] described the results of arthroscopic synovectomy in a series of 27 patients. Durable pain relief was observed at a mean follow-up of 97 months. The best results were obtained in patients with early disease whereas the outcome in patients with more advanced disease was unsatisfactory. Their conclusion was that arthroscopic synovectomy could reliably relieve pain in patients with stage I or stage II disease.

Interposition Arthroplasty. Although interposition arthroplasty is a recognized treatment for posttraumatic arthritis, there are several reports of the outcome of interposition arthroplasty for the treatment of RA. A number of interposition materials have been used including autogenous fascia, dermis, and allograft tissue. Distraction with an articulated external fixator is recommended to protect the interposition material during the early postoperative period.

The rationale of interposition arthroplasty is to replace damaged articular surfaces with an interposition material that eventually undergoes transformation into a new fibrocartilage articular surface. This transformation requires biologic robustness that can promote healing and soft tissue integration into the humerus and ulna. In an immunosuppressed host with impaired tissue healing, it is unknown whether the interposed tissue actually undergoes the expected changes.

In general, the results of interposition arthroplasty have not been encouraging. Ljung et al.[11] reported their outcomes following interposition arthroplasty and found that patients reported diminished pain, but that there were no significant improvements in joint motion. Of concern, they observed progressive bone loss in two thirds of humeri and in one third of ulnae. In some instances, the bone loss interfered with their ability to perform revision surgery. Total elbow arthroplasty was favored over interposition arthroplasty based on their comparison of outcomes following both procedures.

OSTEOARTHRITIS OF THE ELBOW

Primary degenerative arthritis of the elbow joint is relatively uncommon.[12,13,14] Primary osteoarthritis of the elbow tends to occur predominantly in manual laborers and those who rely on wheelchairs or crutches for ambulatory assistance.[13,15,16,17] Three main pathologic processes are involved in osteoarthritis of the elbow. Reactive bone and cartilage formation give rise to osteophytes. Loss and fragmentation of cartilage can lead to loose body formation.

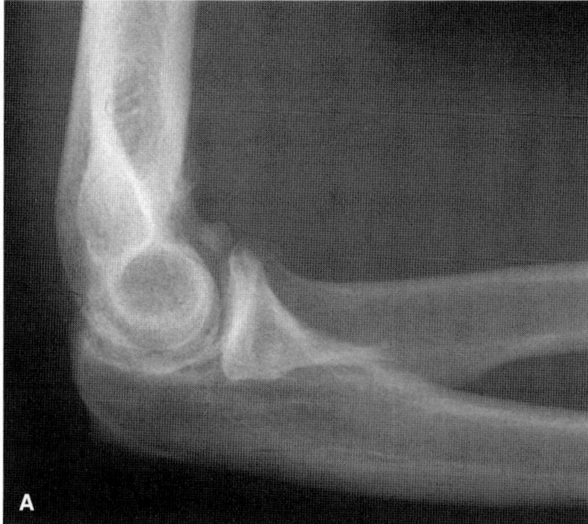

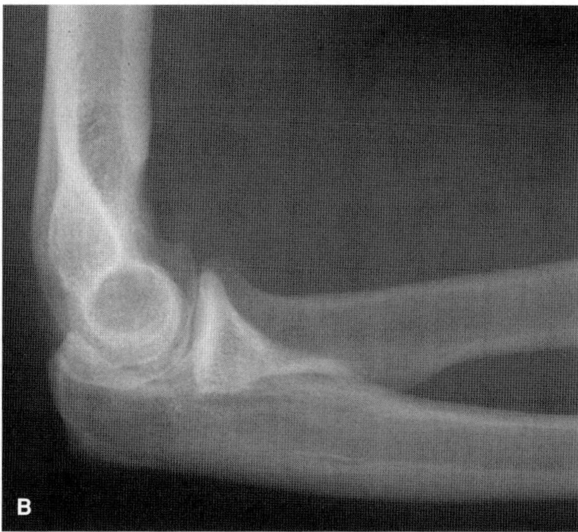

Figure 62-8 A: Preoperative radiograph of a typical patient, a 47-year-old right hand–dominant man with right elbow osteoarthritis, demonstrates osteophyte formation and joint space narrowing. B: Postoperatively, the osteophytes and bony spurs have been removed.

These two processes cause impingement and contribute to the third process of joint contracture.[17,18] Symptoms include pain at the end points of motion, loss of extension, and mechanical symptoms such as catching or locking.[12,15] Other commonly associated conditions include cubital tunnel syndrome with paresthesias and weakness in the ulnar distribution and decreased grip strength.[15,19]

Historical treatments have included nonoperative measures such as anti-inflammatory medications and activity modifications.[13] Total elbow arthroplasty, although it reliably provides pain relief and improved range of motion, may be associated with early aseptic loosening in young active patients and should rarely be done primarily in this group.[20] Elbow arthrodesis is a potential procedure in this population; however, many patients find the restricted motion postoperatively undesirable.[20] Multiple open debridement procedures have been used with good success.[12,15,17,21,22,23,24] Arthroscopic debridement and resection of osteophytes and capsule is a technique that addresses the underlying pathologic processes and provides outcomes similar to open procedures, and is associated with minimal perioperative morbidity.[13,25,26,27,28]

In positioning the patient for elbow arthroscopy, the lateral decubitus position allows for excellent joint access (Figs. 62-6, 62-7). The arm is cradled in a padded arm holder that attaches to the side to the table. A nonsterile tourniquet is then placed high on the arm at the level of the arm holder. The arm should be secured to the arm holder. This is helpful during instrumentation since the arm remains stable, similar to how a knee holder maintains stability during knee arthroscopy. The elbow should be positioned slightly higher than the shoulder. This will allow for 360-degree exposure of the elbow joint, eliminating potential impingement of the arthroscope or shaver against the side of the body.

It is best to mark all potential portal sites before surgery when the elbow is not distended or edematous and palpation of bony landmarks is more precise. Surface landmarks that should be marked with a pen in all patients include the ulnar nerve, the lateral epicondyle, medial epicondyle, the radial head, capitellum, and olecranon.

Distending the elbow with fluid prior to making the starting portal is an important step in contrast to techniques in the shoulder or the knee. The elbow can be injected with 20 to 30 mL of fluid at the location of the anterolateral portal just anterior to the radiocapitellar articulation. With the elbow joint distended, the major neurovascular structures are positioned farther from the starting portal site and entry into the joint is easier.

The choice of starting portal depends on surgeon preference. No starting portal has been shown to be better than another, and ultimately the experience of the surgeon and his or her knowledge of anatomy is the best guide to elbow arthroscopy. Superficial cutaneous sensory nerves are common about the elbow and can be injured during portal placement.

Once the arthroscope has been placed into the joint, visualization can be maintained by pressure distention of the capsule or by mechanical retraction. Retractors for the elbow are simple lever retractors such as a Howarth or a large blunt Steinmann pin. Retractors are placed into the elbow joint via an accessory portal, which is typically 2 to 3 cm proximal to the arthroscopic viewing portal. By holding the capsule and overlying soft tissue away from the bone with retractors, adequate visualization can be achieved with a high-flow, low-pressure system.

Kashiwagi described a procedure, now known as the *Outerbridge-Kashiwagi procedure*, in which a triceps splitting approach is used to access and débride osteophytes and loose bodies from the posterior aspect of the elbow joint. Fenestration of the olecranon fossa allowed access to the anterior aspect of the joint, and loose bodies and osteophyte removal was facilitated by use of an osteotome and irrigation.[22] Others have subsequently described arthroscopic modifications of this procedure and have demonstrated satisfactory clinical outcomes following use for treatment of osteoarthritis.[13,16,28,29] Cohen et al.[28]

compared outcomes following arthroscopic debridement versus open debridement of the elbow for osteoarthritis using the Outerbridge-Kashiwagi procedure and the arthroscopic modification. Both groups demonstrated improved range of elbow flexion, decrease in pain, and a high level of patient satisfaction. Increases in elbow extension, although improved in both groups, were more modest. However, neither procedure included capsular release. Comparison between the open and arthroscopic procedures demonstrated that the open procedure might be more effective in improving flexion whereas the arthroscopic procedure seemed to provide more pain relief. No differences between overall effectiveness of the two procedures were noted.[28] Heterotopic ossification prophylaxis should be considered in these patients, as this complication has been demonstrated to occur in the postoperative period following elbow procedures.[30,31]

Using an arthroscopic approach, all areas in the anterior and posterior aspects of the elbow joint can be visualized and pathology addressed (Fig. 62-8). To obtain a similar view and access using open techniques would require large surgical exposures and incisions with presumably attendant increased morbidity. Despite the many advantages of arthroscopy in addressing elbow pathology, it remains a technically demanding procedure that requires a high level of arthroscopic experience and training to perform safely.

Performing a complete capsular resection provides better range of motion postoperatively and leaves less opportunity for recurrent scar or contracture formation. By removing the capsule, the pliability of the joint and overlying soft tissues is improved, leading to better possible range of motion. The surgeon should exercise caution in performing this procedure owing to the potential for neurovascular injury. In particular, care should be exercised when working about the radial head. The fat pad near the posterior interosseous nerve can be observed and avoided. In addition, the shaver should not be put to suction, which may cause important structures to inadvertently be pulled into the shaver and thus injured. Rather, the outflow of the shaver should be put to gravity only.

All patients after elbow arthroscopic debridement should be placed in immediate postoperative range of motion therapy. The two common forms of treatment are static splinting and continuous passive motion. There are currently no studies that demonstrate that one technique is better than another.

REFERENCES

1. Larsen A. Radiological grading of rheumatoid arthritis. An interobserver study. *Scand J Rheumatol.* 1973;2(3):136–138.
2. Morrey BF, Adams RA. Semiconstrained arthroplasty for the treatment of rheumatoid arthritis of the elbow. *J Bone Joint Surg Am.* 1992;74:479–490.
3. Goldblatt F, Isenberg DA. New therapies for rheumatoid arthritis. *Clin Exp Immunol.* 2005;140(2):195–204.
4. Felson DT, Anderson JJ, Boers M, et al. American College of Rheumatology. Preliminary definition of improvement in rheumatoid arthritis. *Arthritis Rheum.* 1995;38:727–735.
5. Ferlic DC, Patchett CE, Clayton ML, et al. Elbow synovectomy in rheumatoid arthritis. Long-term results. *Clin Orthop Relat Res.* 1987;220:119–125.
6. Gendi NS, Axon JM, Carr AJ, et al. Synovectomy of the elbow and radial head excision in rheumatoid arthritis. Predictive factors and long-term outcome. *J Bone Joint Surg Br.* 1997;79:918–923.
7. Mäenpää HM, Kuusela PP, Kaarela K, et al. Reoperation rate after elbow synovectomy in rheumatoid arthritis. *J Shoulder Elbow Surg.* 2003;12:480–483.
8. Brattstrom H, Al Khudairy H. Synovectomy of the elbow in rheumatoid arthritis. *Acta Orthop Scand.* 1975;46:744–750.
9. Lee BP, Morrey BF. Arthroscopic synovectomy of the elbow for rheumatoid arthritis. A prospective study. *J Bone Joint Surg Br.* 1997;79:770–772.
10. Horiuchi K, Momohara S, Tomatsu T, et al. Arthroscopic synovectomy of the elbow in rheumatoid arthritis. *J Bone Joint Surg Am.* 2002;84-A:342–347.
11. Ljung P, Jonsson K, Larsson K, et al. Interposition arthroplasty of the elbow with rheumatoid arthritis. *J Shoulder Elbow Surg.* 1996;5(pt 1):81–85.
12. Morrey BF. Primary degenerative arthritis of the elbow. Treatment by ulnohumeral arthroplasty. *J Bone Joint Surg Br.* 1992;74:409–413.
13. Stanley D. Prevalence and etiology of symptomatic elbow osteoarthritis. *J Shoulder Elbow Surg.* 1994;3:386–389.
14. Steinmann SP, King GJ, Savoie FH III. Arthroscopic treatment of the arthritic elbow. *J Bone Joint Surg Am.* 2005;87:2114–2121.
15. Antuna SA, Morrey BF, Adams RA, et al. Ulnohumeral arthroplasty for primary degenerative arthritis of the elbow: long-term outcome and complications. *J Bone Joint Surg Am.* 2002;84A:2168–2173.
16. Sarris I, Riano FA, Goebel F, et al. Ulnohumeral arthroplasty: results in primary degenerative arthritis of the elbow. *Clin Orthop.* 2004;420:190–193.
17. Vingerhoeds B, Degreef I, De Smet L. Debridement arthroplasty for osteoarthritis of the elbow (Outerbridge-Kashiwagi procedure). *Acta Orthop Belg.* 2004;70(4):306–310.
18. Tsuge K, Mizuseki T. Debridement arthroplasty for advanced primary osteoarthritis of the elbow. Results of a new technique used for 29 elbows. *J Bone Joint Surg Br.* 1994;76:641–646.
19. Oka Y, Ohta K, Saitoh I. Debridement arthroplasty for osteoarthritis of the elbow. *Clin Orthop.* 1998;351:127–134.
20. McAuliffe JA. Surgical alternatives for elbow arthritis in the young adult. *Hand Clin.* 2002;18(1):99–111.
21. Allen DM, Devries JP, Nunley JA. Ulnohumeral arthroplasty. *Iowa Orthop J.* 2004;4:49–52.
22. Kashiwagi D. Osteoarthritis of the elbow joint. In: Kashiwagi D, ed. *Elbow Joint.* Amsterdam: Elsevier Science; 1986:177–188.
23. Savoie FH 3rd, Nunley PD, Field LD. Arthroscopic management of the arthritic elbow: indications, technique, and results. *J Shoulder Elbow Surg.* 1999;8:214–219.
24. Phillips NJ, Ali A, Stanley D. Treatment of primary degenerative arthritis of the elbow by ulnohumeral arthroplasty. A long-term follow-up. *J Bone Joint Surg Br.* 2003;85:347–350.
25. O'Driscoll SW. Arthroscopic treatment for osteoarthritis of the elbow. *Orthop Clin North Am.* 1995;26:691–706.
26. O'Driscoll SW. Operative treatment of elbow arthritis. *Curr Opin Rheumatol.* 1995;7(2):103–106.
27. Ogilvie-Harris DJ, Gordon R, MacKay M. Arthroscopic treatment for posterior impingement in degenerative arthritis of the elbow. *Arthroscopy.* 1995;11(4):437–443.
28. Cohen AP, Redden JF, Stanley D. Treatment of osteoarthritis of the elbow: a comparison of open and arthroscopic debridement. *Arthroscopy.* 2000;16701–16706.
29. Redden JF, Stanley D. Arthroscopic fenestration of the olecranon fossa in the treatment of osteoarthritis of the elbow. *Arthroscopy.* 1993;9(1):14–16.
29. Suvarna SK, Stanley D. The histologic changes of the olecranon fossa membrane in primary osteoarthritis of the elbow. *J Shoulder Elbow Surg.* 2004;13:555–557.
30. Gofton WT, King GJ. Heterotopic ossification following elbow arthroscopy. *Arthroscopy.* 2001;17(1):E2.
31. Summerfield SL, DiGiovanni C, Weiss AP. Heterotopic ossification of the elbow. *J Shoulder Elbow Surg.* 1997;6:321–332.

INDEX

Note: Page numbers followed by f denote figures and t denotes tabular material.

F

G

H

P

Q

R

S